MEDICAL RADIOLOGY
Radiation Oncology

Editors:
L. W. Brady, Philadelphia
H.-P. Heilmann, Hamburg
M. Molls, Munich

AF065552

Springer-Verlag Berlin Heidelberg GmbH

C. Nieder · L. Milas · K. K. Ang (Eds.)

Modification of Radiation Response

Cytokines, Growth Factors, and Other Biological Targets

With Contributions by

N. Andratschke · K. K. Ang · M. Baumann · E. J. Bernhard · S. Bodis · J. M. Bonner
J. W. Denham · J. F. De Los Santos · W. Dörr · J. Dunst · Z. Fan · A. W. Fyles · S. Goddard
A. K. Gupta · S. M. Hahn · M. Hauer-Jensen · T. Herrmann · C. Herskind · A. Husain
B. Jeremic · C-Y. Li · Z. Liao · T. Licht · F. Lohr · J. Lohr · K. A. Mason · W. G. McKenna
R. E. Meyn · L. Milas · M. Milas · A. Munshi · R. J. Muschel · C. Nieder · M. Pruschy
U. Raju · O. Riesterer · H.-P. Rodemann · J. Schlegel · G. Stüben · M. Stuschke · K.-R. Trott
J. Wang · F. Wenz · F. B. Zimmermann · D. Zips

Foreword by

L. W. Brady · H.-P. Heilmann · M. Molls

With 78 Figures in 106 Separate Illustrations, 14 in Color and 22 Tables

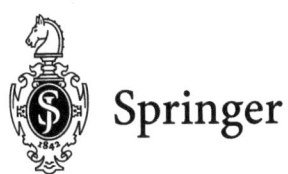

CARSTEN NIEDER, MD
Klinik und Poliklinik für Strahlentherapie und Radiologische Onkologie
Klinikum rechts der Isar der Technischen Universität München
Ismaninger Straße 22
81675 München
Germany

LUKA MILAS, MD, PhD
Department of Experimental Radiation Oncology
UT MD Anderson Cancer Center
1515 Holcombe Blvd.
P.O. Box 66
Houston, TX 77030
USA

K. KIAN ANG, MD, PhD
Department of Radiation Oncology
UT MD Anderson Cancer Center
1515 Holcombe Blvd.
P.O. Box 66
Houston, TX 77030
USA

MEDICAL RADIOLOGY · Diagnostic Imaging and Radiation Oncology
Series Editors: A. L. Baert · L. W. Brady · H.-P. Heilmann · M. Molls · K. Sartor

Continuation of Handbuch der medizinischen Radiologie
Encyclopedia of Medical Radiology

ISBN 978-3-642-62670-8

Library of Congress Cataloging-in-Publication Data
Modification of radiation response : cytocines, growth factors, and other biological
targets / C. Nieder, L. Milas, K. K. Ang, eds. ; with contributions by K. K. Ang ... [et al.] ;
foreword by L. W. Brady, H.-P. Heilmann, and M. Molls.
  p. ; cm. -- (Medical radiology)
  Includes bibliographical references and index.
    ISBN 978-3-642-62670-8   ISBN 978-3-642-55613-5 (eBook)
    DOI 10.1007/978-3-642-55613-5
    1. Cancer--Radiotherapy. 2. Cancer--Adjuvant treatment. 3. Radiation--Physiological
effect. I. Nieder, C. (Carsten), 1964- II. Milas, Luka. III: Ang, K. K. (K. Kian) IV.
Series.
RC271.R3 M5937 2003
616.99'40642--dc21   2002030666

This work is subject to copyright. All rights are reserved, whether the whole or part of the material is concerned, specifically the rights of translation, reprinting, reuse of illustrations, recitations, broadcasting, reproduction on microfilm or in any other way, and storage in data banks. Duplication of this publication or parts thereof is permitted only under the provisions of the German Copyright Law of September 9, 1965, in its current version, and permission for use must always be obtained from Springer-Verlag. Violations are liable for prosecution under the German Copyright Law.

http//www. springer.de
© Springer-Verlag Berlin Heidelberg 2003
Originally published by Springer-Verlag Berlin Heidelberg New York in 2003
Softcover reprint of the hardcover 1st edition 2003

The use of general descriptive names, trademarks, etc. in this publication does not imply, even in the absence of a specific statement, that such names are exempt from the relevant protective laws and regulations and therefore free for general use.

Product liability: The publishers cannot guarantee the accuracy of any information about dosage and application contained in this book. In every case the user must check such information by consulting the relevant literature.

Cover-Design and Typesetting: Verlagsservice Teichmann, 69256 Mauer

21/3150 – 5 4 3 2 1 0 – Printed on acid-free paper

Foreword

Developments in the treatment of cancer have proceeded from periods of major breakthroughs through periods of gradual evolutionary improvement to subsequent dramatic advances predicated on past accomplishments. Clearly the first of the major breakthroughs was the proposal by Halsted for radical mastectomy in the management of patients with cancer of the breast. Following that came gradual evolutionary changes directed toward more precise definition of both the surgical technique and, more importantly, the patients that could be considered for surgical management.

The dramatic breakthrough with the identification of X-rays in 1895 led to the rapid recognition that X-rays had significant biologic characteristics that would allow them to be used in the treatment of cancer. Indeed, patients were treated as early as mid-January of 1896 by these new rays.

In 1922, Coutard and Hautant presented evidence that advanced laryngeal cancer could be cured without disastrous treatment-induced sequelae by using fractioned protracted schemes of treatment, a basic concept for current radiation therapy put forth by Coutard in 1934. The year 1936 saw the advent of publication of the results of treatment not only using external beam radiation therapy but also brachytherapy with radium needles and radium tubes.

Since that point in time, there has been constant development in our understanding of the biologic effects of radiation and of the physics and characteristics of radiation both from radionuclides and from external beam sources, accompanied by the development of new radionuclides for treatment.

The development in chemotherapy was marked by a very slow beginning based on the empirical utilization of nitrogen mustard, triethylenemelanine and then, in 1955, the availability of cytoxan and 5-fluorouracil, followed by a vast array of chemotherapeutic agents from adriamycin to cis-platinum to actinomycin D, methotrexate, etc.

Advances in computer and electronic technology fostered the development of more sophisticated treatment planning and delivery techniques, leading to the development and eventually broad implementation of three-dimensional reconstructed treatment planning and treatment delivery and ultimately the dramatic new advance of intensity-modulated radiation therapy.

It rapidly became apparent that the combination of surgery, radiation therapy and chemotherapy would, at many tumor sites, give rise to greater potential for cure in many patients. This greater interaction among cancer surgeons, radiation oncologists, medical oncologists, pathologists, and diagnostic radiologists further strengthens the need for combined integrated multimodal programs of cancer management.

The present volume by Nieder et al. represents a statement of new biologic factors that will allow for better insights into the molecular processes governing the response of cells and tissues to radiation as well as to chemotherapy. These concepts will lead to better definition of tumor classification and will identify important new initiatives in terms of cancer management. Molecular markers for tumor behavior and response to treatment are now available and are yielding promising results not only in diagnosis but also in follow-up management of patients.

New therapeutic approaches targeting specific molecules for signaling pathways to selectively enhance the response of tumors with distinctive molecular makeup or to protect normal tissues are beginning to emerge.

This volume derives its great significance from this evolving concept and emerging experimental translational research data. These presentations will serve to further stimulate research into cancer management and ultimately will lead to major and dramatic change in the practice of cancer treatment.

Philadelphia	LUTHER W. BRADY
Hamburg	HANS-PETER HEILMANN
Munich	MICHAEL MOLLS

Preface

Though a relatively young medical specialty, radiation oncology has played an increasing role in the treatment of a variety of neoplasms. Its value in the multidisciplinary organ-function-preserving therapy of cancer has recently been firmly established through a number of well-designed randomized clinical trials. The specialty is also experiencing a significant and exciting growth brought about by technological progress and by advances in the insight into tumor biology and the molecular processes governing cellular and tissue responses to ionizing radiation.

Innovations in equipment design and computer technology have dramatically increased the flexibility in dynamic shaping of the radiation portal and in the variation of beam intensity across the field, commonly referred to as intensity-modulated radiation therapy (IMRT). This capacity along with improvements in the accuracy of tumor delineation through progress in diagnostic imaging methodology has introduced an unprecedented era of high-precision radiation therapy. This relatively new technology improves physical targeting of tumors, i.e., delivery of high radiation doses to three-dimensional volumes that conform to the shapes of tumors and involved nodes, thereby reducing the dose administered to normal tissues. IMRT using linear accelerator-generated x-rays (IMXT) is being refined and undergoing clinical testing in many centers. Efforts are also being made to develop IMRT with particle irradiations such as electrons (IMET) and protons (IMPT). Progress in the sensitivity and accuracy of tumor imaging will complement further development of precision radiation therapy.

Parallel with the technical developments, recent advances in the understanding of tumor biology along with improving insights into the molecular processes governing the response of cells and tissues to radiation are leading to new concepts of tumor classification and research initiatives. The search for molecular markers of tumor behavior and response to therapy, for example, is beginning to yield promising results. Appealing therapeutic approaches targeting specific molecules or signaling pathways to selectively enhance the response of tumors with distinct molecular make-up or protect normal tissues from radiation-induced injury are emerging. This volume was put together to give an introductory overview of the evolving concepts and emerging experimental and translational research data, which are expected to stimulate further research and gradually change the practice of radiation oncology. The first part of the book summarizes developing views and data on the pathogenesis and modulation of radiation-induced normal tissue injury. The second part presents some emerging models of tumor biology and targeted therapies.

Munich	CARSTEN NIEDER
Houston	LUKA MILAS
Houston	K. KIAN ANG

Contents

Part I: Normal Tissues 1

1 The Potentional Role of Signaling Proteins in the Acceleration
  of Repopulating Normal and Malignant Tissues
  KLAUS-RÜDIGER TROTT 3

2 Role of Radiation-Induced Signaling Proteins in the Response of Vascular
  and Connective Tissues
  HANS-PETER RODEMANN 15

3 Pathogenetic Mechanisms of Lung Fibrosis
  WOLFGANG DÖRR and THOMAS HERRMANN 29

4 Strategies for Modification of the Radiation Response of the Lung
  C. NIEDER 37

5 Mechanisms and Modification of the Radiation Response
  of Gastrointestinal Organs
  MARTIN HAUER-JENSEN, JUNRU WANG, and JAMES W. DENHAM 49

6 Mechanisms and Modification of the Radiation Response
  of the Central Nervous System
  CARSTEN NIEDER, NICOLAUS ANDRATSCHKE, and K. KIAN ANG 73

7 Hematopoietic Tissue I: Response Modification by Erythropoietin
  JÜRGEN DUNST 89

8 Hematopoietic Tissue II: Role of Colony-Stimulating Factors
  CARSTEN NIEDER, BRANISLAV JEREMIC, THOMAS LICHT, and
  FRANK B. ZIMMERMANN 103

9 Oral Mucosa: Response Modification by Keratinocyte Growth Factor
  WOLFGANG DÖRR 113

Part II: Malignancies 123

10 Role of Growth Factors in Tumor Growth and Progression
   of Gynecological Tumors
   JENNIFER F. DE LOS SANTOS, JAMES M. BONNER, SHANNON GODDARD, and
   ANTHONY W. FYLES 125

11 Growth Factor Expression in Central Nervous System Tumours
   CARSTEN NIEDER, NICOLAUS ANDRATSCHKE, and JUERGEN SCHLEGEL 139

12 Role of Growth Factors and Biological Response Modifiers in Lung, Head
   and Neck and Gastrointestinal Tumors
   G. Stüben and Martin Stuschke 147

13 Role of Signaling Pathway Modification
   Oliver Riesterer, Martin Pruschy, and Stephan Bodis 157

14 Anti-VEGF Strategies in Combination with Radiotherapy
   Daniel Zips and Michael Baumann 179

15 Role of Epidermal Growth Factor Receptor and Its Inhibition in Radiotherapy
   Luka Milas, Z. Fan, Kathy A. Mason, and K. Kian Ang 189

16 Enhancement of the Radiation Response with Interleukins and Interferons
   Frank Lohr, Carsten Herskind, Jens Lohr, Frederik Wenz, and
   Chuan-Yuan Li 205

17 Enhancement of Radiation Response with TNF/TRAIL
   Anupama Munshi and Raymond E. Meyn 227

18 Role of Cyclooxygenase-2 (COX-2) and its Inhibition in Tumor Biology
   and Radiotherapy
   Luka Milas, Kathy Mason, Zhongxing Liao, Uma Raju, Mira Milas,
   Amir Husain, and K. Kian Ang 241

19 Ras Signaling and Its Inhibition with Farnesyltransferase Inhibitors:
   Effects on Radiation Resistance and the Tumor Microenvironment
   Eric J. Bernhard, Anjali K. Gupta, Stephen M. Hahn, Ruth J. Muschel,
   and W. Gillies McKenna 259

Subject Index 275

List of Contributors 279

Part I: Normal Tissues

1 The Potential Role of Signaling Proteins in the Acceleration of Repopulation in Normal and Malignant Tissues

K.-R. Trott

CONTENTS

1.1 The Phenomenon of Accelerated Repopulation 3
1.2 The Nature of the Trigger for Acceleration of Repopulation in Normal and Malignant Squamous Epithelia and Possibilities for Its Modulation 6
1.3 The Mechanism of Accelerated Repopulation and Its Relationship with Cell Proliferation and Cell Differentiation 7
1.4 The Trigger for Acceleration of Repopulation as a Regulated Process 9
1.5 Experimental Strategies for the Study of the Role of Signalling Proteins in the Regulation of Accelerated Repopulation 10
References 12

1.1 The Phenomenon of Accelerated Repopulation

Repopulation is defined as a net increase in stem cell number during cancer treatment, in particular during a course of radiotherapy. Davis and Tannock (2000) recently discussed the importance of repopulation between cycles of chemotherapy, a topic which will not be reviewed here. Since stem cells cannot be identified morphologically, or by molecular methods, they cannot be counted directly. Therefore, they have to be measured by the influence the quantitative destruction of stem cells by radiation has on clinical radiation damage. For the same severity of radiation injury, the tolerated radiation dose or the mean curative radiation dose TCD50 (corrected for fractionation effects using the linear quadratic equation, e.g., by calculating the biologically effective dose (BED) (Shirazi et al. 1995) increases in proportion to the logarithm of the increase in the number of stem cells produced during irradiation.

Accelerated repopulation is the hypothetical mechanism to explain the clinical observation that in some types of tissues and cancers, radioresistance increases dramatically as overall treatment time is increased (Maciejewski et al. 1983). It is measured by the determination of the extra radiation dose, corrected for dose per fraction using the linear quadratic equation needed to compensate the additional duration of treatment (Trott and Kummermehr 1993). Repopulation is thus measured in the unit gray per day. Except for very few special experimental systems in which stem cell regeneration can be measured directly (Hermens and Barendsen 1969; Coggle 1980; Blott and Trott 1989), there is no other way to measure accelerated repopulation. Any study which uses a different criterion has to demonstrate that the results are also obtained when using this criterion.

By making a few assumptions on the underlying mechanism, the measured repopulation rate in gray per day may be converted into a derived, secondary measure: effective doubling time (Maciejewski et al. 1983; Dörr et al. 1994; Denham and Kron 2001). Whereas gray per day is a hard criterion as it is measured directly, the effective doubling time is a soft criterion in that it is based as much on hypothetical cellular parameters as on the measured repopulation rate.

The term "acceleration of repopulation" describes the observation that the repopulation rate is significantly faster, in some tumours by a factor of 10 or more, than would be expected by the pretreatment stem cell production rate (Maciejewski et al. 1983; Fowler 1991). In normal tissues in which tissue structure is maintained by a steady state of cell production and terminal differentiation, repopulation does not exist at all in normal conditions. Yet, any regeneration after injury requires an increase in net stem cell production rate and thus acceleration of repopulation.

The first evidence that tissue regeneration accelerates during a course of daily fractionated radiotherapy was published by Fletcher et al. in 1962. By

K.-R. Trott, MD
Professor, St. Bartholomew's Medical College QMW, Charterhouse Square, London, EC1M 6BQ, UK

carefully recording the development of oral mucositis in patients treated with different schedules of radiotherapy at frequent intervals throughout treatment, they observed that oral mucositis started with erythema by the end of the 1st treatment week and progressed to spotted mucositis in the 3rd treatment week. Yet despite continuing irradiation, mucositis did not get worse but remained at that level of severity for the rest of the treatment period in most patients, and in some patients it even improved towards the end of treatment. These findings suggested that in the human oral mucosa, a regenerative process is stimulated in the 2nd or 3rd week of radiotherapy, which is able to compensate at least 9–10 Gy per week.

The first experimental data on accelerated regeneration were published by DENEKAMP in 1973. She determined the accumulation of radiation damage in mouse epidermis during daily fractionated irradiation using a top-up design and observed that there was little regeneration in the 1st week but pronounced acceleration of regeneration in the 2nd week. Experiments by SHIRAZI et al. (1995) confirmed and extended these early experimental data on accelerated repopulation in mouse skin.

Whereas there was widespread agreement that during fractionated irradiation some normal tissues would mount a regenerative response, this was not expected to occur in cancers. MACIEJEWSKI et al. (1983) were the first to prove that in squamous cell carcinomas of the head and neck the mean curative radiation dose TCD50 would increase dramatically if the overall treatment time was prolonged beyond 5 weeks, by as much as 3.5 Gy per week on average. This was interpreted as being due to an increase in tumour stem cell production rate from the typical pretreatment doubling time of more than 40 days on average to an effective doubling time of 4 days. OVERGAARD et al. (1988) observed a similar increase in TCD50 in those patients who were treated with split-course radiotherapy. Numerous subsequent publications confirmed that, in squamous cell carcinomas, repopulation is accelerated during radiotherapy to an average repopulation rate of 0.5–0.7 Gy per day (WITHERS et al. 1988; FOWLER 1991). In bladder cancer, despite smaller numbers of cases available for analysis and some differences in the time frame observed, similar findings were reported (MACIEJEWSKI and MAJEWSKI 1991). Circumstantial evidence such as the greater damaging effect of a treatment interruption in the last 2 weeks of a normal course of radiotherapy of head and neck cancer compared to weeks 3 and 4 (SKLADOWSKI et al. 1994; HERRMANN et al. 1994) suggested that repopulation accelerated only in the second half of a normal treatment course. Recent analysis of the Gliwice data on head and neck cancer indicated that repopulation was faster during a treatment gap (0.75 Gy/day) than on treatment days (0.2 Gy/day) and that acceleration of repopulation started after 2 weeks of daily irradiation (TARNAWSKI et al. 2002). Yet there is no way to determine the kinetics of repopulation in human tumours directly. This would require a dedicated experimental protocol based on daily irradiation, with fixed doses comparable to those given in clinical radiotherapy. The accumulated effect of fractionated irradiation would then be measured by a top-up dose (given under clamp ischemia to avoid artefacts which might be introduced by variable oxygenation of the tumours). This is clearly not possible in human tumours, yet in transplanted isogeneic mouse tumours (KUMMERMEHR 1992) and in human tumour xenografts (BAUMANN et al. 2002) such a design has been developed and successfully applied. In murine and in human squamous cell carcinomas transplanted into appropriate mice, repopulation accelerated significantly after a delay of 1 week or longer.

These clinical and experimental data demonstrate that in some tissues, repopulation starts at a low rate in the 1st week or weeks of radiotherapy to increase greatly and very suddenly, demonstrating a delayed onset of rapid repopulation acceleration.

Delayed acceleration of repopulation does not occur in all tissues. So far we have good evidence only for acceleration of repopulation during fractionated radiotherapy in normal squamous epithelia (Figs. 11–1.3), in particular in oral mucosa of mice (DÖRR and KUMMERMEHR 1990) and human patients (FLETCHER et al. 1962), in the epidermis of mice (DENEKAMP 1973; SHIRAZI et al. 1995) and in squamous cell carcinomas, in particular in well-differentiated squamous cell carcinomas of mice (KUMMERMEHR 1992) and humans (HANSEN et al. 1997). So far we have no consistent indication that accelerated repopulation occurs in other tissues and in other tumour types. In particular, there is no evidence for accelerated repopulation in mucous membranes or in adenocarcinomas. Delayed acceleration of repopulation appears to occur specifically in normal and malignant squamous epithelia as a tissue-specific response to radiation damage (TROTT 1999).

Fig. 1.1. Squamous cell epithelium from unirradiated human buccal mucosa: regular structure including parakeratosis at the surface, basal cell layer and lamina propria (HE, ×250, reproduced from SEIFERT 2000, with permission)

Fig. 1.2. Squamous cell epithelium from unirradiated floor of the mouth: regular structure including polar basal cell layer and stratum spinosum with keratinocytes (toluidine blue, ×600, reproduced from SEIFERT 2000, with permission)

Fig. 1.3a, b. MIB-1 antibody-detected proliferation-associated antigens in dysplastic squamous cell epithelia and carcinoma. a On the *left side* regular epithelium with slight hyperplasia. Stained cells in basal and parabasal region. On the *right side* epithelium with irregular cell layers and marked dysplasia (carcinoma in situ). Stained cells throughout the epithelium. b Squamous cell carcinoma with staining of the majority of cell nuclei (reproduced from MEYER-BREITING and BURKHARDT 1999, with permission)

1.2
The Nature of the Trigger for Acceleration of Repopulation in Normal and Malignant Squamous Epithelia and Possibilities for Its Modulation

Since the pattern of accelerated repopulation appears to be similar in normal and in malignant squamous epithelia, the hypothesis has been put forward that the mechanism is specific to squamous epithelia and occurs, although it is probably less well regulated, also in tumours which are derived from keratinocytes as long as they have a tendency to maintain the normal differentiation pattern and remember the characteristic response patterns of the tissue of origin. In poorly differentiated squamous cell carcinomas, however, another mechanism based on radiation-induced changes in the microenvironment of the surviving stem cells, in particular reoxygenation, may also play a role (BAUMANN et al. 2002; PETERSEN et al. 2001).

In mouse oral mucosa, acceleration of repopulation is very closely regulated to meet demand (DÖRR and KUMMERMEHR 1990). Examples of histological slides are shown in Fig. 1.4. During fractionated irradiation with different doses per fraction ranging from 2.5 Gy to 4 Gy, there was a linear decrease of mucosal cellularity in the 1st week which was followed by a plateau during the next weeks. Although the maximum rate of repopulation obviously was 20 Gy per week, lower treatment intensities induced only a submaximal repopulation response that was just sufficient to keep mucosal cellularity at the level it had reached at the end of the 1st week. Obviously, the repopulation response of the irradiated tissue involves a mechanism that senses the radiation-induced tissue damage. This sensor is triggered by a certain level of tissue damage to send out signals that alter the proliferation pattern of the tissue for as long as the damage continues to increase the supply of stem cells. The intensity of the signals depends on the intensity of the triggering damage.

Experimental studies in irradiated normal squamous epithelia of mice (POTTEN et al. 2002) and, to a lesser extent, in rodent tumours have provided some information about the nature of the triggering tissue damage to which the sensor responds by accelerating repopulation. While some indication on the nature of the trigger could be derived from a temporal relationship such as the coincidence of acceleration of repopulation in human squamous cell carcinoma xenografts with reoxygenation (BAUMANN et al. 2002) or in oral mucosa and epidermis with the beginning of the inflammatory response (TROTT 1999), evidence for possible causal relationships must be based on interventional studies. Yet such kinetic studies can still rule out hypothetical mechanisms. As an example, TROTT (1999) suggested that radiation-induced alterations in the barrier function of the irradiated epidermis might be related to the triggering event. A massive increase in water permeability of the mouse epidermis irradiated with 3 Gy per day was indeed measured; however, these functional changes occurred only 1 week after the

Fig. 1.4a–c. Histomorphology of the mucosa of the lower surface of mouse tongue. **a** Unirradiated control; **b** after 15×3 Gy/ 3 weeks; **c** at day 10 after a single dose of 17 Gy. Compared to control mucosa, cell numbers are significantly reduced to about 70% after fractionated irradiation with a total dose of 45 Gy, but the stratified tissue architecture is clearly maintained. The corresponding cell numbers are described in DÖRR and KUMMERMEHR (1990). In contrast, after single-dose irradiation with sufficient doses (**c**), complete cell loss is seen, with the erosion covered by a pseudomembrane comprised mainly of cell detritus and fibrinous exudate. In the *right-hand part* of **c**, the remaining epithelium at the margin of the radiation field is seen start of accelerated repopulation and thus could be ruled out as the triggering event. The increase in water permeability is rather a consequence of the defective differentiation that accompanies accelerated repopulation in mouse epidermis (see Sect. 1.3, "The Mechanism of Accelerated Repopulation and Its Relationship with Cell Proliferation and Cell Differentiation").

Several interventional studies designed to modulate the kinetics of acceleration of repopulation have been conducted. In skin as well as in oral mucosa, the timing of acceleration appears to be closely related to the appearance of erythema, i.e., of the inflammatory response of the dermis and submucosa. In mouse skin, the relationship of accelerated repopulation with the dermal inflammatory response has been investigated in some detail, leading to the conclusion that the inflammatory response of the dermis has no significant influence on the acceleration response. For example, treatment with nonsteroidal anti-inflammatory drugs throughout a course of daily irradiation did not delay or decrease accelerated repopulation (TROTT et al. 1999).

Pretreatment of the mouse epidermis with UV-B, on the other hand, caused a significant increase in radioresistance to single radiation doses and, in particular, to 1 week of daily fractionated irradiation (SHIRAZI et al. 1996). These findings were interpreted as being due to two mechanisms, both of which increase radioresistance: a delayed hyperplastic response related to the UVB-induced inflammation (which causes the increased resistance to single radiation doses) and in addition, an earlier trigger to acceleration of repopulation which, in some schedules showed already maximal repopulation rates in the 1st week of daily fractionated irradiation. The delay between UVB and increased repopulation rates suggest that, as in the studies with anti-inflammatory treatment, the inflammatory response itself is not the trigger but alterations in the biological status of the tissue which develops gradually after UV damage.

The only experiments that succeeded in stimulating acceleration of repopulation already during the lag phase of the normal delayed repopulation response were those in which the epithelial surface was damaged, either by tape stripping of the epidermis (TROTT et al. 1999) or by coagulation of the uppermost oral mucosal cell layers using silver nitrate (DÖRR and KUMMERMEHR 1992). Three daily treatments with very diluted silver nitrate solution were also successful in significantly reducing the severity of oral mucositis in patients who received an accelerated course of radiotherapy for head and neck cancer (MACIEJEWSKI et al. 1991). This conditioning treatment was, however, ineffective if it was combined with radiotherapy with a conventional daily treatment (DÖRR et al. 1995). This was probably because in the first case, due to the higher dose intensity used, radiation-induced stimulation already started during the transient repopulation response after local conditioning, which was upheld throughout the treatment course at maximal level, whereas in the second case, the repopulation response induced by the much lower treatment intensity started only after the transient repopulation response after conditioningh add isappeared.

No experiments have been published demonstrating a successful modulation of the kinetics of accelerated repopulation in squamous cell carcinomas.

It may be concluded that the triggering of tissue damage sensed by the tissue leading to a regulated repopulation response is not directly and causally related to the inflammatory tissue response, which often occurs in close temporal relation to the acceleration of repopulation, nor is it related to reduction of the specific tissue function such as the barrier function of the epidermis. This may indicate that the triggered tissue damage is related to reduced cellularity. However, it remains to be shown which subpopulation of cells is critical for the initiation of the accelerated repopulation response.

1.3
The Mechanism of Accelerated Repopulation and Its Relationship with Cell Proliferation and Cell Differentiation

Cellular mechanisms of accelerated repopulation have been investigated in normal squamous epithelia. Since accelerated repopulation is defined as an increased net stem cell production rate, it is obvious that cell proliferation must be involved in the process. However, it is equally clear that in normal tissues under normal steady state, an increased rate of cell proliferation alone would not lead to any net increase in stem cell numbers. More important than the cell turnover rate is the partitioning rate of the daughters of stem cell divisions into stem cells on the one hand and into transit cells destined to enter the differentiation pathway, on the other hand.

Under normal steady state, the stem cell number in a normal tissue remains constant. This is because, on average, 50% of the daughters of stem cell divisions remain stem cells whereas the other 50% progress into transit cell divisions and differentiation. This process of stem cell partitioning appears to be a well-regulated process in which cytokines and growth factors are involved, acting at the level of the stem cell daughters (APPLETON et al. 2002). If any tissue damage occurs that demands stem cell regeneration, proportionally more stem cells are produced than under normal steady-state conditions. This process has been most closely investigated in bone marrow stem cells (CFU) (COGGLE 1980). As soon as damage is recognized, the partitioning factor of stem cell daughters is changed from the normal value of 0.5-1, i.e., all daughters of stem cell divisions remain stem cells and the number of stem cells increases with the same doubling time as the generation time of the stem cells. This process is called the transition from the normal asymmetrical stem cell divisions to symmetrical stem cell divisions (loss of asymmetry). As the defective stem cell pool is gradually replenished, the partitioning factor gradually returns to the normal value of 0.5. In addition to this regulated change of stem cell partitioning, the stem cell proliferation rate increases as well. However, the main factor responsible for the rapid net increase in stem cell numbers is the change in stem cell partitioning into more stem cells at the cost of differentiation. Several growth factors and cytokines have been identified that are involved in the regulation of this regenerative response; however, the exact role of each of this remains to be elucidated.

The processes associated with the increased repopulation rate of squamous epithelia during fractionated irradiation are very similar to those described in the bone marrow. SHIRAZI et al. (1995) demonstrated that the repopulation rate in the irradiated mouse epidermis, 3 weeks after the start of irradiation, increased to 0.6 per day while the cell proliferation rate increased only to 0.15 per day. Also, DÖRR et al. (1994) demonstrated in mouse oral mucosa that the repopulation rate was four times higher than proliferation rate 2-3 weeks after the start of daily irradiation. This demonstrates that the key process leading to acceleration of repopulation is not related to increased cell proliferation but to decreased cell differentiation.

The consequences of this decreased cell differentiation associated with the loss of asymmetry in the process of accelerated repopulation was clearly demonstrated in mouse epidermis by LIU et al. (1996). The expression pattern of biological markers of keratinocyte differentiation such as keratins and involucrin changed dramatically at the time of maximal repopulation rates after a few weeks of daily irradiation, resembling that in hyperproliferative skin disorders such as psoriasis. The defective differentiation has also been associated with decreased barrier function of the irradiated repopulating epidermis. First evidence for impaired differentiation appears only some time after repopulation accelerates, which suggests that the impaired differentiation is not a primary effect of radiation itself and not a trigger for repopulation, but the consequence of the mechanism that increases the rate of production of immature keratinocyte stem cells at the cost of differentiating keratinocytes. Based on these observations, LIU et al. (1996) suggested the following explanation of the processes responsible for accelerated repopulation. In normal epidermis, after asymmetric stem cell divisions the transit cells are programmed by differentiation signals to undergo a defined number of expansion divisions (three in mouse epidermis) before producing terminally differentiated keratinocytes. The key process in the acceleration of repopulation is the disappearance or reduced concentration of the differentiation-inducing signal or its ability to respond to it by impaired receptor concentration or function. As a consequence, most progeny of stem cell divisions remain stem cells and symmetrical stem cell divisions increase. However, most of these stem cells from symmetrical divisions are sterilized by subsequent irradiation, consequently losing their "stemness," and behave like transit cells by performing only a limited number of abortive divisions. But the difference between a sterilized stem cell and a transit cell (both of which have only a limited proliferative potential) is that the sterilized stem cell did not receive or respond to the normal differentiation signals. This, together with an increased proliferation rate, results is a new steady state of epidermal cellularity with constant cell numbers, the majority of which, however, are progeny of abortive divisions of differentiation-impaired radiation-sterilized stem cells, which are functionally defective.

DÖRR (1997) summarized his own observations on the proliferation and repopulation pattern in mouse oral mucosa and the findings of LIU et al. (1996) on the differentiation pattern in repopulating mouse epidermis in a cellular model of the mechanism of accelerated repopulation in oral mucosa based on the normal steady state of stem cell divisions, transit cell proliferation and terminal differentiation. The most important feature of this model is that acceleration of repopulation occurs primarily as a result of a shift in the differentiation pattern of the daughters of stem cell divisions. Under normal steady state, on average one of the two daughters proceeds into transit divisions and finally terminal differentiation whereas, in response to tissue injury from all sorts of causes, regeneration is effected by preventing stem cell daughters from entering the transit to differentiation and remain stem cells. There is no indication that this process is specific to radiation; it is not directly induced by radiation but occurs at a well-defined time point, which appears to be related to a certain level of tissue injury. The effect of the shift from asymmetry to symmetry of stem cell divisions is enhanced by a moderately increased cell production rate (by shortening the cell cycle time) and by the increased use of progeny from abortive divisions of sterilized stem cells (the three As).

Acceleration of repopulation in differentiated squamous cell carcinomas thus is primarily the consequence of changes in stem cell daughter differentiation. This is independent of cell proliferation. In oral mucosa (DÖRR et al. 1994), but less so in epidermis (SHIRAZI et al. 1996), some increase in proliferation rate is measured when acceleration of repopulation starts. Yet, in squamous cell carcinomas the increase in the repopulation rate is associated with a pronounced decrease in the tumour cell proliferation rate (BEGG et al. 1991). Quite obviously, an increase or decrease in proliferation rates has little or no impact on repopulation. This was demonstrated most impressively by the dissociation of the effect of the inhibitor of the epidermal growth factor (EGF)-receptor BIBX1382BS on regrowth delay, on the one hand, and on tumour cure, on the other hand, in xenografts of human squamous cell carcinomas irradiated with daily doses for 6 weeks at University Hospital Dresden. Whereas the radiation effect on regrowth delay was significantly increased no change was observed in the tumour cure assay (KRAUSE and BAUMANN, unpublished data). This may be interpreted as indication that EGF receptor inhibition decreased proliferation rates in surviving tumour cells but had no influence on their repopulationra tes.

1.4
The Trigger for Acceleration of Repopulation as a Regulated Process

Accelerated repopulation in mouse oral mucosa is very well regulated to meet demand and it is switched off when demand is met. Experimental studies in mice (DÖRR 1997) and also various clinical studies (VAN DER SCHUEREN et al. 1990; DENHAM et al. 1996; MACIEJEWSKI et al. 1996) have demonstrated that the repopulation response depends on treatment intensity. In normal squamous epithelia in mice, the triggering event is related to a relatively minor degree of tissue hypoplasia, which does not lead to any measurable changes in tissue function. Functional changes may occur, however, as a consequence of tissue inflammation or of altered tissue differentiation in the epidermis. Although in oral mucosa and in epidermis, the time of acceleration is close to the time of tissue inflammation, suppression of the inflammatory response did not lead to any significant reduction in the repopulation response. Both are related in time but are clearly independent tissue responses to radiation injury.

If changes in tissue function are not the triggering event, it may be the reduction in cellularity, i.e., hypoplasia. In epidermis and oral mucosa, repopulation is triggered when cellularity is decreased to approximately 50%–60% of the normal value (DÖRR et al. 2002). Thus, there must be some mechanism in the tissue that counts the number of specific cells. In mouse oral mucosa, the counted cells are also the target cells for the accelerated repopulation response. This means that the number of stem cells in the tissue at the moment of acceleration is likely to be the critical trigger for acceleration of repopulation. These numbers are remarkably small: in the oral mucosa, the triggering stem cell density would be approximately 1% of the normal value (DÖRR and KUMMERMEHR 1990); in the epidermis it has been estimated to be less than 1% (SHIRAZI et al. 1995) and in murine squamous cell carcinomas, the triggering stem cell density would also be approximately 1% of the normal value, i.e., 1 in 10,000 tumour cells (KUMMERMEHR and TROTT 1997). In human squamous cell carcinomas, acceleration may be delayed until week 4 or 5 of conventional fractionated radiotherapy. This would mean that acceleration of repopulation would start only when there are only about 1000 tumour stem cells left surviving in the slowly disintegrating volume of billions of tumour cells (KUMMERMEHR and TROTT 1997).

Which sort of mechanism could count such small numbers of specific but otherwise not particularly conspicuous cells spread randomly in a hundred to a thousand times greater mass of inactivated stem cells or transit cells of all kinds? It is inconceivable that any signal arising from the disintegrating, dying cells would be the trigger since the difference between acceleration of repopulation or no acceleration of repopulation would be equivalent to a difference in signal intensity from 99.9 or 99.99% in tumours, and a little larger difference in normal tissues. The search for the mechanism that counts the number of surviving stem cells will be the most difficult problem in future experimental research on accelerated repopulation.

1.5
Experimental Strategies for the Study of the Role of Signalling Proteins in the Regulation of Accelerated Repopulation

Accelerated repopulation is a major cause of treatment failure in squamous cell carcinomas and an important factor in increasing radiation tolerance of normal squamous epithelia in radiotherapy. There is good clinical evidence to suggest that by selective manipulation of the acceleration process, clinical results of radiotherapy of some of the most common cancers could be substantially increased. This would, however, require detailed knowledge of the biological and molecular processes involved in the accelerated repopulation response.

The following biological characteristics of accelerated repopulation have been determined in the past and have been described above:
- Accelerated repopulation is a specific response of normal and malignant squamous epithelia to damage inflicted by fractionated irradiation.
- Acceleration of repopulation occurs with a delay of 1 week or longer after start of irradiation. It is not triggered directly by the radiation effect on the repopulating stem cells but is secondary to tissue damage, which develops gradually.
- The trigger to accelerated repopulation is not related to impaired tissue function or to inflammation but to hypoplasia of specific tissue cells, probably stem cells.
- Accelerated repopulation is a well-regulated process to meet demand.
- Accelerated repopulation involves changes in stem cell differentiation regulation.
- Acceleration of repopulation is not due to an increased proliferation rate.
- Accelerated repopulation is a tissue response, not a response of cells in isolation to irradiation.

The primary aims of research into the mechanisms of accelerated repopulation are to identify:
- The nature of the radiation-induced alteration in the irradiated tissue and how is it sensed by the organ or organism or the tumour tissue in order to trigger the acceleration response.
- The signals that are emitted by the sensing system to process this information and regulate the probability of self-maintenance of epithelial stem cells.

As indicated in Sect. 1.2, "The Nature of the Trigger for Acceleration of Repopulation in Normal and Malignant Squamous Epithelia and Possibilities for Its Modulation," the reduced cellularity of stem cells in the irradiated tissue is likely to be the critical factor that is sensed by a tissue-specific mechanism in order to trigger the changes in stem cell differentiation patterns outlined in this chapter. Little information has been published that may be related to this process. LIU et al. (1997) showed that enhanced expression of connexin43, a protein involved in intercellular communication is one of the earliest changes in the irradiated epidermis that occurs shortly before acceleration of repopulation can be measured. They suggested that this increase might be directly related to reduced stem cell density, yet further data in this direction are lacking. Also, a role of the local immune-competent cells such as Langerhans cells in initiation of the acceleration response of the mouse epidermis has been postulated (LIU and TROTT 1996).

From the biological characteristics listed above, it is highly probable that cytokines and their receptors are intimately involved in this process. One would have expected that extensive research has been devoted to this field, yet so far, no experiments specifically designed to explore the role of cytokines in the molecular and cellular processes of accelerated repopulation have been reported.

Experiments to investigate the molecular and cellular processes of accelerated repopulation require dedicated experimental protocols such as those used in the studies listed in Sect. 1.3, "The Mechanism of Accelerated Repopulation and Its Relationship with Cell Proliferation and Cell Differentiation", which explored the biological characteristics of the accelerated repopulation response in mouse oral mucosa (DÖRR 1997), mouse epidermis (SHIRAZI et al. 1995), and mouse squamous cell carcinomas (KUMMERMEHR 1992). The closest any study on the modulation of radiation effects by cytokines has come to this dedicated experimental design is that of DÖRR et al. on the role of keratinocyte growth factor (KGF) in fractionated irradiation of the mouse oral mucosa described in Chap. 9, "Oral Mucosa: Response Modification by Keratinocyte Growth Factor" of this volume and that of KRAUSE and BAUMANN on the role of EGFR in the FaDu squamous cell carcinoma xenograft. Yet these studies do not permit the analysis of specific cytokine effects on the regulation of the repopulation response.

Numerous studies have investigated the regulation of bone marrow stem cell regeneration after irradiation by cytokines (see Chap. 8 "Hematopoietic Tissue II: Role of Colony-Stimulating Factors"), yet, although it is related to the accelerated repopulation response to different clinical processes, the effects of cytokines on bone marrow stem cell proliferation and differentiation/partitioning and other related features might also be important in the accelerated repopulation response in squamous epithelia.

This book describes a plethora of experimental and clinical data on the possibilities of modulating radiosensitivity in vitro and in vivo, yet none of the studies provides any stringent indication for a specific role of any of the investigated cytokines in the accelerated repopulation response of normal and malignant squamous epithelia.

Since acceleration of repopulation is a tissue response to impending radiation injury, only in vivo experiments have any chance of directly yielding relevant results. In vitro experiments are of very limited value and sooner or later need to be backed up with carefully designed and properly conducted experiments in animal tissues or animal tumours. KUMMERMEHR (private communication, 2002) compared the acceleration of repopulation response to daily fractionated irradiation in the same differentiated murine squamous cell carcinoma growing either in vivo after transplantation into isogeneic mice or in vitro in the megacolony system. Although in vivo repopulation accelerated dramatically in the 2nd week of treatment, in vivo little or no acceleration was observed using identical criteria of regrowth delay and tumour control. It remains to be seen whether this absence of a significant repopulation response in a tumour in vitro, which in vivo shows a characteristic repopulation response, is due to the absence of specific stromal, endothelial or immune cells interacting with the surviving tumour stem cells or is due to the need for the complex tissue structure and integrated physiology of a differentiated squamous cell carcinoma in vivo.

Whichever cell or molecule counts the number of surviving stem cells and sets the process of acceleration of repopulation in motion, there must be a profound multiplication of signalling molecules and interaction between many cells. The most surprising event takes place in tumours: all of the few surviving tumour stem cells respond simultaneously although they are randomly spread throughout a disintegrating tumour mass that is about to lose its structural organization. This means that the trigger molecule has to be generally available throughout the tumour volume.

Microarray studies for gene expression might offer fascinating insight into the regulation of repopulation acceleration. Yet, the experiments would need to be very carefully designed to correlate gene expression with acceleration of repopulation. Since the kinetics of acceleration of repopulation cannot be measured precisely in human tumours (and also not well in human normal squamous epithelia), studies using microarrays on accelerated repopulation in human tissues are not possible for the foreseeable future. The only indication for microarray studies on accelerated repopulation is in irradiated mouse squamous cell carcinomas comparing gene expression patterns in the irradiated mouse tumour a few days before acceleration, on the presumed day of acceleration and a few days after acceleration. This requires precise knowledge of the timing of acceleration. Only the experimental protocols used and described by KUMMERMEHR (1992) in mouse tumours and by DÖRR and KUMMERMEHR (1990) and SHIRAZI et al. (1995) in normal squamous epithelia permit the identification of that critical time point with a resolution of approximately 2 days. Yet there are other problems making microarray studies a poor option for future research in accelerated repopulation: many other biological processes change at the same time as repopulation. Thus it will be very difficult to separate out those genes involved in the acceleration of repopulation from those involved in increased transit cell proliferation, in the development of inflammation response and in managing the removal of dying cells. It would be sheer luck to find the key gene(s) – if indeed changes in gene expression by parenchymal or endothelial or immunologically competent cells are important.

Intervention studies, however, i.e., the manipulation of the accelerated repopulation response by physical, chemical or molecular means, including cytokines and receptor blocking molecules, are an alternative, more promising approach. A few examples were reported in the literature and at a recent symposium in Dresden in September 2002. It is, however, essential that dedicated experimental protocols precisely measuring the kinetics of acceleration of repopulationa reu sed.

The results with KGF in mouse oral mucosa (DÖRR and KUMMERMEHR 2002; POTTEN et al. 2002) look promising. The suggested association of the EGF receptor with the acceleration of repopulation has been refuted by the unpublished studies of KRAUSE and BAUMANN, first reported in 2002. The only indication that the EGF receptor might play any role in the accelerated repopulation response are preliminary data from the DAHANCA study (OVERGAARD, personal communication 2002) which showed an association of the expression of the EGF receptor before radiotherapy with a therapeutic gain of accelerated radiotherapy, yet these data are complicated by the association of the EGF receptor with differentiation levels of the squamous cell carcinomas. If these data can be confirmed in a future comprehensive analysis they would be the first and only indication of a possibly successful direction an interventional study could take.

Proper experimental design is the key to successful experimentation and this is of particular importance in the investigation of the mechanisms of accelerated repopulation and the role cytokines and cytokine receptors undoubtedly play in it.

References

Appleton DR, Thomson PJ, Donaghey CE et al (2002) Simulation of cell proliferation in mouse oral epithelium, and the action of epidermal growth factor: evidence for a high degree of synchronization of the stem cells. Cell Prolif 35 [Suppl 1]:68–77

Baumann M, Petersen C, Eicheler W et al (2002) Mechanisms of repopulation in experimental squamous cell carcinomas. In: Kogelnik HD, Lukas P, Sedelmayer E (eds) Progress of radio-oncology VII. Monduzzi, Bologna, pp 417–422

Begg AC, Hofland I, Kummermehr J (1991) Tumour cell repopulation during fractionated radiotherapy: correlation between flow cytometric ADN radiobiological data in three mouse tumours. Eur J Cancer 27:537–543

Blott P, Trott KR (1989) The effect of actinomycin D on split dose recovery and repopulation in jejunal crypt cells in vivo. Radiother Oncol 15:73–78

Coggle JE (1980) Absence of late radiation effects on bone marrow stem cells. Int J Radiat Biol 38:589–595

Davis AJ, Tannock JF (2000) Repopulation of tumour cells between cycles of chemotherapy: a neglected factor. Lancet Oncol 1:86–93

Denekamp J (1973) Changes in the rate of repopulation during multifraction irradiation in mouse skin. Br J Radiol 46:381–387

Denham JW, Kron T (2001) Extinction of the weakest. Int J Radiat Oncol Biol Phys 51:807–819

Denham JW, Walker QJ, Lamb DS et al (1996) Mucosal regeneration during radiotherapy. Radiother Oncol 41:109–118

Dörr W (1997) Three A's of normal tissue repopulation: a review of mechanisms. Int J Radiat Biol 72:635–644

Dörr W, Kummermehr J (1990) Accelerated repopulation of mouse tongue epithelium during fractionated irradiations or following single doses. Radiother Oncol 17:249–259

Dörr W, Kummermehr J (1992) Increased radiation tolerance of mouse tongue epithelium after local conditioning. Int J Radiat Biol 61:369–379

Dörr W, Emmendörfer H, Haide E et al (1994) Proliferation equivalent of accelerated repopulation in mouse oral mucosa. Int J Radiat Biol 66:157–168

Dörr W, Jacubek A, Kummermehr J et al (1995) Effects of stimulated repopulation on oral mucositis during conventional radiotherapy. Radiother Oncol 37:100–107

Dörr W, Hamilton CS, Boyd T et al (2002) Radiation-induced changes in cellularity and proliferation in human oral mucosa. Int J Radiat Oncol Biol Phys 52:911–917

Fletcher GH, MacComb WS, Shalek RJ (1962) Radiation therapy in the management of cancer of the oral cavity and oropharynx. Thomas, Springfield

Fowler JF (1991) The phantom of tumour treatment – continually rapid proliferation unmasked. Radiother Oncol 22:156–167

Hansen O, Overgaard J, Hansen HS et al (1997) Importance of overall treatment time for the outcome of radiotherapy of advanced head and neck carcinoma: dependence on tumour differentiation. Radiother Oncol 4:47–51

Hermens AF, Barendsen GW (1969) Changes of cell proliferation characteristics in a rat rhabdomyosarcoma before and after X-irradiation. Eur J Cancer 5:173–189

Herrmann T, Jacubek A, Trott KR (1994) Importance of the timing of a gap in radiotherapy of squamous cell carcinomas of the head and neck. Strahlenther Onkol 170:545–549

Kummermehr J (1992) Time factors in experimental tumors. In: Fowler JF, Kinsella T (eds) Prediction of response in radiation therapy. American Institute of Physics, Woodbury, NY, pp 217–231

Kummermehr J, Trott KR (1997) Tumour stem cells. In: Potten C (ed) Stem cells. Academic, London, pp 636–699

Liu K, Trott KR (1996) Changes in dendritic epidermal T cells, CD4+ and CD8+ cells in mouse skin during fractionated X-irradiation. Radiat Oncol Invest 4:261–267

Liu K, Kasper M, Trott KR (1996) Changes in keratinocyte differentiation during accelerated repopulation in the irradiated mouse epidermis. Int J Radiat Biol 69:763–769

Liu K, Kasper M, Bierhaus A et al (1997) Connexin 43 expression in normal and irradiated mouse skin. Radiat Res 147:437–441

Maciejewski B, Majewski S (1991) Dose fractionation and tumour repopulation in radiotherapy for bladder cancer. Radiother Oncol 21:163–170

Maciejewski B, Preuss-Bayer G, Trott KR (1983) The influence of the number of fractions and of overall treatment time on local control and late complication rate in squamous cell carcinoma of the larynx. Int J Radiat Oncol Biol Phys 9:321–328

Maciejewski B, Zajusz A, Pilecki B et al (1991) Acute mucositis in the stimulated oral mucosa of patients during radiotherapy for head and neck cancer. Radiother Oncol 22:7–11

Maciejewski B, Skladowski K, Pilecki B et al (1996) Randomized clinical trial on accelerated 7 days per week fractionation in radiotherapy for head and neck cancer. Preliminary report on acute toxicity. Radiother Oncol 40:137–145

Meyer-Breiting E, Burkhardt A (1999) Histologische Begutachtung und spezielle Untersuchungsmethoden. In: Seifert G (ed) HNO-Pathologie. Springer, Berlin Heidelberg New York, pp 573–619

Overgaard J, Hjelm-Hansen M, Johansen LV et al (1988) Comparison of conventional and split-course radiotherapy as primary treatment in carcinoma of the larynx. Acta Oncol 27:147–152

Petersen C, Zips D, Krause M et al (2001) Repopulation of FaDu human squamous cell carcinoma during fractionated radiotherapy correlates with reoxygenation. Int J Radiat Oncol Biol Phys 51:483–493

Potten CS, Booth D, Cragg NJ et al (2002) Cell cinetic studies in the murine ventral tongue epithelium: mucositis induced by radiation and its protection by pretreatment with keratinocyte growth factor (KGF). Cell Prolif 35:32–40

Seifert G (2000) Normale Struktur und Alterswandlungen der Mundschleimhaut. In: Siefert G (ed) Oralpathologie III. Mundhöhle, angrenzendes Weichteil- und Knochengewebe (German). Springer Berlin, Heidelberg, New York, pp 12–20

Shirazi A, Liu K, Trott KR (1995) Epidermal morphology, cell proliferation and repopulation in mouse skin during daily fractionated irradiation. Int J Radiat Biol 68:215–221

Shirazi A, Liu K, Trott KR (1996) Exposure of ultraviolet B radiation increases the tolerance of mouse skin to daily X-irradiation. Radiat Res 145:768–775

Skladowski K, Law MG, Maciejewski B et al (1994) Planned and unplanned gaps in radiotherapy: the importance of gap position and gap duration. Radiother Oncol 30:109–120

Tarnawski R, Fowler J, Skladowski K et al (2002) How fast is repopulation of tumor cells during the treatment gap. Int J Radiat Oncol Biol Phys 54:229–236

Trott KR (1999) The mechanisms of acceleration of repopulation in squamous epithelia during daily irradiation. Acta Oncol 38:153–157

Trott KR, Kummermehr J (1993) The time factor and repopulation in tumors and normal tissues. Semin Radiat Oncol 3:115–125

Trott KR, Shirazi A, Heasman F (1999) Modulation of accelerated repopulation in mouse skin during daily irradiation. Radiother Oncol 50:261–266

Van der Schueren E, van den Bogaert W, Vanuytsel L (1990) Radiotherapy by multiple fractions per day (MFD) in head and neck cancer: acute reactions of skin and mucosa. Int J Radiat Oncol Biol Phys 19:301–311

Withers HR, Taylor JMG, Maciejewski B (1988) The hazard of accelerated tumor clonogen repopulation during radiotherapy. Acta Oncol 27:131–146

2 Role of Radiation-Induced Signaling Proteins in the Response of Vascular and Connective Tissues

H. P. Rodemann

CONTENTS

2.1 Introduction 15
2.2 Radiation Response of the Vascular Tissue and Proteins Involved 16
2.2.1 Cellular and Molecular Responses of Endothelium to Radiation Exposure 16
2.2.2 Pathways and Proteins of Endothelial Cell Death 17
2.2.2.1 DNA-Damage-Independent Ceramide-Mediated Radiation-Induced Apoptosis 17
2.2.2.2 Protection from Radiation-Induced Apoptosis of Endothelial Cells by Fibroblast Growth Factor 19
2.2.2.3 DNA-Damage-Mediated Apoptosis 19
2.3 Radiation Response of the Connective Tissue and Proteins Involved 20
2.3.1 Fibrotic Tissue Alterations as a Result of Radiation-Activated Fibroblasts 20
2.3.2 Molecular Aspects of Radiation-Induced Connective Tissue Remodeling 21
2.3.2.1 TGF-β1 – A Regulator of Cell Growth, Differentiation, and Collagen Synthesis 21
2.3.2.2 TGF-β1 – A Regulator of Cellular Radiation Sensitivity and Radiation-Induced Tissue Remodeling 23
2.3.2.3 TGF-β1 – A Potential Target for Antifibrotic Strategies? 24
References 25

2.1 Introduction

Over the years considerable effort has been made not only to quantify the tolerance of normal tissue to radiation, but also to provide a baseline for radio-

H. P. Rodemann, PhD
Professor, Section of Radiobiology and Molecular Environmental Research, Department of Radiation Oncology, Eberhard-Karls University, Tübingen, Röntgenweg 11, 72076 Tübingen, Germany

therapy at maximum biological effective doses. Normal tissue complications induced by ionizing radiation differ depending on the target organ and cell types. Acute or early reactions are primarily characterized by rapidly occurring changes within hours, such as increased endothelial cell swelling, vascular permeability and edema as well as lymphocyte adhesion and infiltration. Apoptosis of endothelial cells is probably the most important feature in the concert of these radiation-induced acute alterations in the vascular system of irradiated organs. Thus, acute reactions are primarily reflected by the rates of radiation-induced cell death and regeneration by surviving stem cells.

Late reactions occurring months or years after radiation exposure are primarily the result of radiation-dependent depletion of the tissue stem cell or progenitor compartment leading to tissue fibrosis, organ dysfunction and necrosis. Although the early inducing molecular steps, i.e. induction of specific molecular pathways of inter- and intracellular signal transduction, leading to the manifestation of late reactions, may certainly occur shortly after radiation exposure, the cellular events and tissue remodeling processes triggered by these mechanisms present slow time kinetics. This may indicate that acute processes such as radiation-induced cell death and apoptosis are not the major or critical events underlying late tissue reactions. At least for the development of radiation-induced fibrosis, accelerated terminal differentiation of fibroblast progenitor cells is the major driving cellular event. However, independent of whether acute or late reactions of tissues to radiation therapy occur, these tissue remodeling processes are regulated by a number of inter- and intracellular signal transduction proteins. This chapter will thus be focused on the cellular events of acute and late reactions and the specific proteins regulating the molecular pathways primarily involved in triggering these events.

2.2
Radiation Response of the Vascular Tissue and Proteins Involved

The radiation response of the vascular tissue actually occurs in two waves. The acute vascular changes within 24 h are dominated by the radiation-induced apoptotic cell death of endothelial cells (PENA et al. 2000). Late vascular effects occur within months after irradiation and include capillary collapse, thickening of basement membrane, scarring of the surrounding tissue as well as telangiectasia, and a loss of clonogenic capacity (PENA et al. 2000). Based on this radiation-induced late vascular damage, it has been argued that radiation injury of the microvascular system may contribute to the late radiation response of normal tissues (REINHOLD et al. 1974).

Capillaries are the most radiosensitive component of the vasculature; thus, capillary vascular injury may be at the crux of tissue radiosensitivity (FAJARDO and BERTHRONG 1988). For example, renal capillary endothelium responds to radiation by leukocyte attachment, endothelial cell swelling, and increased capillary permeability (JAENKE et al. 1993). Characteristic changes in capillary histology after irradiation include detachment of endothelial cells from the basal lamina, cell pyknosis, thrombosis, and loss of entire capillary segments, resulting in tissue ischemia or regrowth of lost vessels in some organs (FAJARDO 1989). In response to ionizing radiation, capillaries show considerably more morphological changes than larger vessels (DIMITRIEVICH et al. 1984). Radiation also produces a marked shift in the size distribution of the microvasculature to larger diameters, apparently from capillary obliteration with dilation of the remaining vessels (DIMITRIEVICH et al. 1984).

Endothelial cells have generally been regarded as the most radiosensitive cells of the vessel wall (MORRIS et al. 1996), and most research concerning the arterial response to radiation has focused on the endothelium. Endothelium from different tissues shows differential temporal and morphological responses to radiation (REINHOLD and BUISMAN 1973). In mice, ultrastructural changes are noticeable in the lung capillary endothelium after irradiation, but only minimal changes in the ultrastructure of the capillary wall of cerebral cortical vessels were noted at similar doses in rats (MAISIN et al. 1977). Within hours of irradiation, mice lung endothelium shows intracellular changes followed days later by separation from the basement membrane and subsequent platelet aggregation and luminal obstruction (MAISIN et al. 1977).

Endothelial cells can exhibit significant repair capacity and recovery potential after radiation insult (HOPEWELL et al. 1986). After endothelial cell loss from irradiation, remaining viable endothelial cells proliferate abnormally, which may result in luminal occlusion and loss of capillary bed size (HOPEWELL et al. 1986). Proliferative subintimal cell aggregation has been seen to occur along the interstitial side of endothelium in irradiated areas (YANG et al. 1977) and has been associated with swelling at sites of intimal repair (DIMITRIEVICH et al. 1977).

2.2.1
Cellular and Molecular Responses of Endothelium to Radiation Exposure

The cellular and molecular responses of endothelial cells to ionizing radiation have been well characterized by in vitro studies (O'CONNOR and MAYBERG 2000). Within hours of irradiation, specific endothelial-cell structural proteins can be detected, which affect the physiological appearance of these cells as well. Among these structural changes, alterations in the distribution of endothelial cell F-actin (WATERS et al. 1996), cell retraction (FRIEDMAN et al. 1986) and a dose-dependent increase in transendothelial flux of low molecular weight solutes (WATERS et al. 1996; FRIEDMAN et al. 1986) are prominent. Irradiated endothelial cells furthermore exhibit alterations in the synthesis and secretion of a variety of biomolecules, predominantly proteins, including increased synthesis and secretion of growth factors (WITTE et al. 1989) and chemo-attractants (MATZNER et al. 1988). Irradiated endothelial cells secret specific injury markers such as thrombomodulin, von Willebrand factor, heparinase and endothelial cell adhesion factor-1 (ECAM-1) (MATTUCI-CERINIC et al. 1992; NICOLSON et al. 1991; LIN et al. 1992). Surviving irradiated endothelial cells display compensatory cytoplasmic hypertrophy (RUBIN et al. 1989; T'SAO and WARD 1985) and cell formation, which maintain monolayer confluence (FISCHER-DZOGA et al. 1984). Formation of giant endothelial cells following radiation exposure reflects a permanent arrest in the G1 phase or the G0 phase, likely due to a radiation-induced terminal differentiation process of the cell type as has been described for other cell types as well (RODEMANN et al. 1996). Furthermore, irradiated cultures of endothelial cells exhibit increased cellular adhesiveness for neutrophils and promote intracellular platelet deposition.

With respect to cell growth, ionizing radiation induces a dose-dependent induction of proliferation in growing endothelial cell cultures and cell loss in non-growing cultures. On the other hand, endothelial cell migration is unimpaired by irradiation and sufficient to repair occurring cell loss (KLEIN-SOYER et al. 1990). Decreased endothelial cell survival after ionizing radiation most likely reflects both an early apoptotic mechanism and a later clonogenic or reproductive cell death mechanism. Early morphological abnormalities in irradiated endothelial cells are consistent with apoptotic changes beginning at 6–10 h in microvascular endothelium and at 12–16 h in aortic endothelium. Oligonucleosomal DNA analysis during these intervals shows time- and dose-responsive DNA fragmentation consistent with radiation-induced apoptosis. Expression of proteins regulating cell cycle progression, induction of repair processes and apoptosis, such as p53, GADD45, p21 and BAX proteins increase in a time- and dose-dependent manner after radiation exposure, indicating radiation-induced stabilization of the p53 protein and gene transcription of its target genes *GADD45*, *p21* and *BAX*. Likewise intracellular caspases, which are the effector proteins of the apoptosis, show enhanced activity up to 15 h after irradiation. This time course of caspase activation coincides with other indices of endothelial cell apoptosis such as oligonucleosomal DNA degradation and specific morphological changes. Since apoptotic cell death of endothelium is most likely the major cause of radiation-induced vascular damage, the molecular components and pathways of endothelial cell apoptosis need to be addressed in more detail.

2.2.2
Pathways and Proteins of Endothelial Cell Death

Since radiation-induced cell death of endothelial cells seems to be the major cause of the high radiation sensitivity of the vascular system, studies have focused on the specific pathways of this cell death processes. Special attention was drawn to the role of DNA damage and/or membrane damage on the induction of apoptotic processes. DNA-damage-dependent apoptotic processes mainly involve the p53 protein. DNA-damage-independent processes are mediated through radiation-induced membrane damage via the activation of sphingomyelinases and the generation of ceramide. To what precise extent these processes contribute to radiation-induced death of endothelial cells can not clearly be answered at present. The rapid pace of apoptosis research will doubtless ensure that answers to these issues are soon provided. Whether DNA-damage-independent but ceramide-mediated apoptosis or DNA-damage-dependent apoptosis involving functional p53 is the major pathway of radiation-induced endothelial cell death shall not be the topic of this chapter. However, many data indicate that both pathways exist in endothelial cells; therefore, with respect to the most current literature, pathways of ceramide-mediated endothelial cell apoptosis and aspects of interference are primarily discussed.

2.2.2.1
DNA-Damage-Independent Ceramide-Mediated Radiation-Induced Apoptosis

The sphingomyelin (SM) pathway is a ubiquitous, evolutionary highly conserved signaling system, analogous to conventional systems such as the cAMP and phosphoinositol pathways. Ceramide is generated from SM by the action of a neutral or acid sphingomyelinase (SMase), or by de novo synthesis coordinated through the enzyme ceramide synthase. Once generated, ceramide may serve as a second messenger molecule in signaling responses to physiological or environmental stimuli, or it may be converted to a variety of structural or effector molecules.

For endothelial cells, radiation-induced elevation of intracellular levels of ceramide have been attributed to a direct or indirect activation of SMase by membrane damage (LIN et al. 2000). As outlined in Fig. 2.1, in this context ceramide released from membrane-bound sphingosine either by activation of SMase, binding of death receptor ligands, or by radiation damage to the membrane feeds into three major cascades: the mitogen-activated protein kinase-8 (MAPK8) pathway, the mitochondrial pathway and the death receptor pathway.

Released ceramide specifically targets and activates the ceramide-activated protein kinase (CAPK) and the ceramide-activated phosphatase (CAPP) (DRESSLER et al. 1992; REYES et al. 1996). CAPK can directly activate RAC1, a component of the stress pathway, and can also activate RAF1, a component of the PKC/RAF1/MAPK cytoprotective pathway (ZHANG et al. 1997). CAPP, through its phosphates function, can directly inactivate protein kinase C (PKC) an enzyme involved in anti-apoptotic signaling (MULLER et al. 1995). For maintaining ceramide's key role in triggering apoptosis, inactivation of the anti-apoptotic PKC seems essential since this kinase can block the hydrolysis of sphingomyelin and thus the release of ceramide from cellular membranes (HAIMOVITZ-FRIEDMAN et al. 1994a,b). With respect

Fig. 2.1. DNA-damage-independent and DNA-damage-dependent pathways of apoptosis

to apoptosis, however, the most important target of ceramide is the RAC1/MEKK1 pathway, which directly leads to activation of MAPK8. This protein kinase has been implicated in apoptosis induced by tumor necrosis factor (TNF) the cytokine activating the TNF receptor and other environmental stresses (VERHEIJ et al. 1996). Activation of the MAPK8 pathway results in apoptosis through the activation of effector caspases, namely caspases 1, 3 and 6, as well as the autocrine stimulation of the death receptor pathway.

Ceramide may also initiate pro-apoptosis proteins in the mitochondria that facilitate apoptosis through an alternative activation pathway of caspases, mainly via caspase 9. This pathway is initiated by ceramide-dependent activation of CAPK and promotes apoptosis through processes involving the pro-apoptotic proteins BAX and BAD (BASU et al. 1998). BAD exerts its function by binding to the anti-apoptotic proteins BCL2 and BCL2L1 and preventing them from inhibiting cell death mediated by BAX (ZHA et al. 1996). The anti-apoptotic action of BCL2 and BCL2L1 is based on their ability to maintain mitochondrial function, i.e. stabilizing mitochondrial membrane integrity and preventing release of cytochrome C into the cytoplasm (YANG et al. 1997; BELKA and BUDACH 2002). Release of cytochrome C would result in the activation of the so-called apoptosome complex composed of APA1, cytochrome C and dATP, which activates caspase 9. This enzyme will then cleave and activate downstream effector caspases, such as caspase 3. Activated caspase 3 degrades a variety of cell death substrates, such as poly(adenosyine-5'-diphosphate-ribose)polymerase (PARP), the retinoblastoma protein (RB), or the DNA fragmentation factors A (DFFA) or B (DFFB) and thereby initiate apoptosis (STROH and SCHULZE-OSTHOFF 1998).

Ceramide released through the action of death or TNF receptor may mediate a direct pathway to apoptosis through various adapter protein complexes such as FADD (Fas-associated death domain) and TRADD (TNFaR-associated death domain). These complexes initiate the activation of cytoplasmic promoters of apoptosis, notably the pro-caspase 8. This enzyme in turn activates caspases 1, 3 and 6. As outlined above, activated caspases 1, 3 and 6 initiate apoptosis through degradation of cell death substrates.

That ionizing radiation acts on cellular membranes of endothelial cells to generate ceramide and initiate apoptosis was firstly described by HAIMOVITZ-FRIEDMAN et al. in 1994. This study provided conclusive evidence that apoptotic signals can be generated as a result of radiation-induced membrane damage and release of ceramide and suggested thus an alternative to the hypothesis that direct DNA damage mediates radiation-induced cell kill.

Interestingly, a second source of ceramide resulting from ceramide synthase activation may be directly related to DNA damage induced by ionizing radiation. Recent data published by LIAO et al. (1999) indicate that radiation-induced DNA double-strand breaks may also trigger the activation of ceramide synthase and thus production of ceramide, which will then induce apoptotic cell death. However, since this ceramide synthase pathway requires de novo protein synthesis, this pro-apoptotic mechanism exerts slower kinetics and may thus be responsible for more sustained effects as compared to those resulting from immediate release of ceramide after SMase activation.

2.2.2.2
Protection from Radiation-Induced Apoptosis of Endothelial Cells by Fibroblast Growth Factor

Several mechanisms and strategies have been proposed to protect endothelial cells from radiation effects. As in any other cell, anoxic conditions increase radioresistance in endothelial cells by diminishing the free radical formation. Furthermore, the tripeptide protease inhibitor z-Val-Ala-Asp blocks proteolytic cleavage of poly(adenosyine-5'-diphosphate-ribose)polymerase, i.e. PARP, which functions as a death substrate (Fig. 2.1) and the cleavage of which is needed to execute the apoptotic process. As a result, DNA fragmentation and all other morphological features of apoptotic cells can be prevented (GAJDUSEK et al. 2001). Finally the basic fibroblast growth factor (bFGF) protects endothelial cells in vitro and in vivo from radiation-induced apoptosis (FUKS et al. 1994; PENA et al. 2000; PARIS et al. 2001).

The radioprotective effect of bFGF on endothelial cells seems to be directly related to the inhibition of ceramide-mediated apoptosis (FUKS et al. 1994; HAIMOVITZ-FRIEDMAN et al. 1994a,b; LANGLEY et al. 1997). It could be demonstrated that mutations which inactivate SMase activity or treatment with bFGF can abrogate ceramide generation and apoptosis induced by irradiation. Although the precise mechanism involved in the bFGF-mediated radioprotective and anti-apoptotic effect needs to be clarified, evidence exists that protein kinase C serves as the effector system mediating bFGF radioprotection. This has been postulated by studies indicating that PKC blocks the hydrolysis of sphingomyelin and thus the release of ceramide from cellular membranes (HAIMOVITZ-FRIEDMAN et al. 1994a,b). In addition to the already discussed complex processes leading to ceramide-induced cell death, ZUNDEL and GIACCIA (1998) have shown that stress-induced apoptosis is associated with ceramide-mediated down-regulation of phosphatidyl-inositol-3'-kinase (PI3K) and subsequent inhibition of the kinase Akt. The inhibition of this pathway resulted in decreased phosphorylation of the BAD protein, which is essential for the mitochondrial pathway of apoptosis. Hence, radiation-induced apoptotic signaling through ceramide appears to involve multiple, coordinated pathways, and the apoptotic outcome in vitro as well as in vivo depends on the balance between the activities of pro- and anti-apoptotic signaling systems (PENA et al. 2000).

The specific sensitivity of microvascular versus large vessel endothelium to ionizing radiation may be associated with the distribution of bFGF with the vascular basement membranes. BFGF is highly expressed and present in basement membranes of large and intermediate-sized blood vessels. However, microvascular basement membranes have only minimal or absent bFGF deposits (PARIS et al. 2001). Yet it is not surprising that, as indicated by ultrastructural studies, capillaries represent the most radiation-sensitive sections of the vascular system (REINHOLD et al. 1990). Since basement membrane-bound bFGF protects endothelial cells against radiation-induced apoptosis in vitro, the lack of bFGF expression in microvascular basement membranes may render this section of the vascular system highly sensitive to radiation apoptosis mediated through SMase activity and ceramide. These data suggest that depending upon the tumor type and tumor sensitivity to bFGF, this growth factor may provide a strategy to protect the vascular system from radiation damage and especially apoptosis of endothelial cells in the microvasculature of the normal tissues in patients undergoing radiotherapy.

2.2.2.3
DNA-damage-Mediated Apoptosis

As has long been demonstrated by many investigators, radiation-induced DNA damage can lead to apoptosis through p53-dependent processes. As is outlined in Fig. 2.1 and Table 2.1, DNA damage, mainly DNA double-strand breaks, are able to activate the protein kinases ATM and DNA-PK, both located in the nucleus. ATM and DNA-PK will then phosphorylate p53 in specific serine residues, which results in the stabilization and activation of the p53 protein. Then activated p53 will exert different functions with respect to regulation of the cell cycle progression and transactivation of genes involved in pro- and anti-apoptotic cascades. The direct regulation of BAX and BCL2 proteins leads to the activation or blockage of the mitochondrial pathway which will

Table 2.1. p53-dependent components of apoptosis

Components of DNA-damage-dependent and p53-mediated apoptosis
p53 directly regulates pro- and anti-apoptotic members of the BCL-2 family, e.g. BAX, BCL-2, BCL-2X$_L$
p53-dependent up-regulation of death receptor-ligand system

result in the activation of the apoptosome and induction of effector caspases, as addressed above, through the release of cytochrome C from mitochondria (MIYASHITA et al. 1994; MIYASHITA and REED 1995; ZHAN et al. 1994; JOHNSTONE et al. 2002).

In addition to this classical p53-dependent apoptosis program, evidence has accumulated over the recent years that p53, when activated, is also able to up-regulate the death receptor–ligand system and thereby stimulate apoptosis as described above and outlined in Fig. 2.1 (KASTAN 1997; HERR and DEBATIN 2001; RYAN et al. 2001).

2.3
Radiation Response of the Connective Tissue and Proteins Involved

A serious complication of radiotherapy in the treatment of cancer patients is the late onset of fibrosis in normal tissues that can lead to marked morbidity and even death. Radiation-induced fibrotic lesions can occur in parenchymal and connective tissues of lung, kidney, liver and skin. Since blood vessels in irradiated normal tissue often undergo adverse changes, as discussed in Sect. 2.2, and since these changes often precede the development of fibrosis, it has been hypothesized that vascular radiation damage could be an important first step in the pathogenesis of late radiation fibrosis. Clear evidence to this hypothesis is still lacking, however.

Based on current knowledge from in vitro and in vivo analyses, the fibrotic process is thought to involve the stimulatory response of connective tissue fibroblasts, resulting in an increased proliferation as well as differentiation and especially collagen synthesis, secretion and extracellular deposition (REMY et al. 1991). Although fibroblasts represent the cell type biochemically responsible for fibrotic tissue remodeling, other cell types of the irradiated tissue are involved in the primary events, leading to induction of fibrosis as well. It has been shown that in tissues composed of a variety of individual cell types, multicellular interactions occur through the release of cell communication mediators such as eicosanoid metabolites, destructive proteolytic enzymes, and inflammatory growth and differentiation factors (GAULDIE et al. 1993). These factors act directly on resident tissue cells to modify their behavior and alter matrix gene expression. During the onset of manifestation and progression of fibrotic connective tissue remodeling, it is now clear that specific cytokines and growth factors, including transforming growth factor b1 (TGF-β1) and platelet-derived growth factor (PDGF) play an important part in the overall tissue distortion, fibroblast proliferation and differentiation, and the alterations of tissue structure (RODEMANN 1989; RUBIN et al. 1992; RODEMANN and BAMBERG 1995; RODEMANN et al. 1996; MARTIN et al. 2000). The cellular and especially the molecular aspects of the processes leading to radiation-induced alterations in connective tissue will be discussed in the following paragraphs.

2.3.1
Fibrotic Tissue Alterations as a Result of Radiation-activated Fibroblasts

Like any other fibrotic tissue response, radiation-induced connective tissue remodeling is a multicellular process driven by intercellular communication via cytokines and growth factors, which are induced during the radiation response of each participating cell type (Fig. 2.2) (RODEMANN and BAMBERG 1995). The fibrosis-specific biochemical changes such as accumulation of collagen and other extracellular matrix proteins are predominantly based on the reactivity of the fibroblast cell system (RODEMANN and BAYREUTHER 1984; RUBIN et al. 1992; RODEMANN and BAMBERG 1995). It has been demonstrated that ionizing radiation induces premature terminal differentiation of potentially mitotic progenitor fibroblasts to irreversible postmitotic fibrocytes (RODEMANN et al. 1992, 1996; BUMAN et al. 1995; LARA et al. 1996; BURGER et al. 1998; HERSKIND et al. 1998; HAKENJOS et al. 2000; FOURNIER et al. 2001). Terminally differentiated fibrocytes are the biochemically functioning and active cells of the fibroblast system responsible for the production of tissue specific collagen and matrix molecules as well as growth factors and cytokines (BAYREUTHER et al. 1988a,b; RODEMANN et al. 1989, 1992, 1996; BAYREUTHER et al. 1992; HERSKIND et al. 2000; ALALUF et al. 2000; FOURNIER et al. 2001). Based on these functional properties of the different cell types of the fibroblast/fibrocyte cell system, it can be concluded that the radiation-induced accumulation of postmitotic fibrocytes results in the pronounced elevation of synthesis and extracellular deposition of collagen characteristic for fibrotic tissue alteration.

Fig. 2.2. Cytokine-mediated multicellular interactions in connective tissue remodeling

2.3.2
Molecular Aspects of Radiation-Induced Connective Tissue Remodeling

In light of the recent developments in cell and molecular biology, the concept of a single target cell which can explain the dynamic sequence of events occurring after radiation exposure is supplanted by that of multiple cell systems interacting. Thus, as already addressed (Fig. 2.2), radiation-induced fibrotic remodeling of connective tissues represents a multicellular process initiating and sustaining the fibrogenic process through an intercommunication between different cell types, leading to the activation of fibroblasts as the biochemically responsible executer cell type. As described by various authors for different cell systems in vivo and in vitro, an immediate and transient expression of a number of proto-oncogenes, e.g. *c-fos* and *c-jun* (HALLAHAN et al. 1991; SHERMAN et al. 1990; WOLOSCHAK and CHANG-LIU 1990), *c-myc* (ANDERSON and WOLOSCHAK 1992) as well as growth factors such as PDGF, interleukin-1 (IL-1), TNF-α (HALLAHAN et al. 1991), and especially TGF-β1 (LANGBERG et al. 1994; RANDALL and COGGLE 1996; SEONG et al. 2000) occurs within hours of irradiation. This early modulation of gene expression has profound effects on the pathophysiology of the late radiation effect. Altered expression of growth factors and cytokines may thus result in a modulation of the cellular interactions of cell types involved, e.g. in fibrotic reaction.

For example, TGF-β1 has been shown to influence the proliferation pattern of early progenitor fibroblasts and myofibroblasts, which may be one initial step in the onset of fibrosis (MARTIN et al. 1993; RODEMANN et al. 1995). On the other hand, it has been shown that radiation exposure of fibroblasts accelerates the terminal differentiation process of progenitor fibroblasts into postmitotic functioning fibrocytes producing and depositing collagen at elevated levels (RODEMANN et al. 1996). Furthermore, radiation-exposed fibroblasts significantly increase the production and secretion of TGF-β1. Although the complete molecular mechanisms of TGF-β1 in the process of radiation-induced fibroblast differentiation/activation and connective tissue remodeling is not completely understood at present, it can be stated that this factor plays an important role in radiation-induced tissue reactions.

2.3.2.1
TGF-β1 – A Regulator of Cell Growth, Differentiation, and Collagen Synthesis

As observed in a variety of cell systems, TGF-β is a prominent regulator of cellular growth and differentiation during embryonic development and tissue regeneration (ROBERTS and SPORN 1990, 1996; SHULL et al. 1992). It has been described to inhibit growth of epithelial cells (PONCELET et al. 1999; MARTIN et al. 2000; LAWRENCE 1996), to promote proliferation of progenitor fibroblasts and myofibroblasts (MARTIN et al. 2000; RODEMANN et al. 1995) and to induce terminal differentiation of normal human skin and lung fibroblasts (RODEMANN et al. 1996; BURGER et al. 1998; HAKENJOS et al. 2000; HERSKIND et al. 2000). Furthermore, TGF-β1 exerts strong modulatory effects on cells of the immune system as well as apoptosis of specific cell types (WAHL 1994; SITNICKA et al. 1996; MARTIN et al. 2000).

TGF-β is synthesized by several cell types, including platelets, macrophages, lymphocytes, epithelial and endothelial cells as well as fibroblasts (MARTIN et al. 2000). Three isoforms of TGF-β exist, TGF-β1, 2 and 3, with specific as well as overlapping activities in various cellular processes (ROBERTS and SPORN 1990, 1996; MARTIN et al. 2000). TGF-β1, a 25-kDa protein, is the most prominent isoform of TGF-β1. It is synthesized as an inactive, latent form which associates to the latency-associated peptide (LAP) before secretion into the extracellular space (Fig. 2.3) (DERYNCK et al. 1986; EHRHART et al. 1997; LEITLEIN et al. 2001). Through disulphide bonds, LAP can bind to the latent TGF-β-binding protein (LTBP) which is linked to the extracellular matrix (EHRHART et al. 1997). Latent and inactive TGF-β can be activated by the function of specific extracellular proteases (BARCELLOS-HOFF 1998; EHRHART et al. 1997; LEITLEIN et al. 2001). Activation of extracellular matrix-bound latent TGF-β1 can also be a consequence of radiation exposure, i.e. ionizing radiation, as was shown in the stroma of mammary glands (BARCELLOS-HOFF 1998; BARCELLOS-HOFF et al. 1994). This mechanism involves the activation of specific proteolytic enzymes from inactive pro-enzymes and is most likely dependent on the presence of reactive oxygen species.

Once activated, TGF-β1 can bind to specific TGF-β1 receptors, the TGF-β1 receptor types I and II, which are located on the cell membrane (Fig. 2.3). Both receptors exhibit serine/threonine kinase activities. The TGF-β1 receptor II first binds active TGF-β1 and presents it to the receptor type I to form a heteroterameric receptor complex, which is the active form of the TGF-β1 receptor. Activation of the receptor kinase activity generates the first step of the TGF-β1 signaling pathway, which is the phosphorylation of specific Smad proteins, namely Smad2 and/or Smad3. Upon phosphorylation activation these two proteins can form a complex with another Smad-protein, Smad4. This protein complex is able to translocate from the cytoplasm to the nucleus. Within the nucleus the activated Smad-complex acts together with other transcription factors as transactivator complex for specific target genes to be activated in response to the TGF-β1 stimulus (KRETSCHMAR and MASSAGUE 1998).

Depending upon the cell type, TGF-β1 promotes and regulates a number of rapid responses in cells, including alterations in proliferation, differentiation and apoptosis. The most pronounced effect of TGF-β1, which is observable in epithelial, endothelial, and hematopoietic cells as well as fibroblasts, is the inhibition of cell growth by inducing a reversible and/or irreversible G1-cell cycle arrest. In this context, TGF-β1 induces through TGF-β1 receptor- and Smad signaling the transactivation of inhibitor proteins of the cyclin-dependent kinases such as p15, p21, and p27 (DATTO et al. 1995; HANNON and BEACH 1994).

Although the main effect of TGF-β1 with respect to cell cycle control is inhibition of cell proliferation, TGF-β1 can at least to a certain degree also promote proliferation of mesenchymal cells such as early progenitor fibroblasts and osteoblasts. This growth stimulatory effect of TGF-β1 has been shown in highly proliferative populations of human embryonic progenitor

Fig. 2.3. TGF-β1-receptor-dependent signal transduction

fibroblasts and mouse fibroblasts, which present an infinite growth in vitro (RAYNAL and LAWRENCE 1995; RAVITZ et al. 1996). In these cells, TGF-β1 down-regulates the cyclin-dependent kinase inhibitors p21 and p27. Thus, concerning cell proliferation, TGF-β1 can be a bifunctional cytokine at least for certain cell types. Apart from regulating cell growth, TGF-β1 can also induce apoptosis, especially in hepatocytes, endometrial cells and keratinocytes (MARTIN et al. 2000). The mechanisms of TGF-β1-mediated apoptosis are, however, poorly understood, but they may involve generation of reactive oxygen species.

In addition to the strong modulatory effect of TGF-β1 on cells of the immune system (WAHL 1994; SITNICKA et al. 1996) with respect to the aspect of tissue remodeling, the most important function of TGF-β1 is to control homeostasis of the extracellular matrix (MARTIN et al. 2000). Remodeling of the extracellular matrix is caused through TGF-β1 ability to simultaneously stimulate the synthesis of most matrix proteins, decrease the production of matrix degrading enzymes, increase the production of inhibitors of these enzymes and by modulating the expression of integrins. Thus, through these multiple functions, TGF-β1 has a central role in development and normal wound healing and was proposed to be involved in the development of fibrotic tissue alterations.

2.3.2.2
TGF-β1 – A Regulator of Cellular Radiation Sensitivity and Radiation-induced Tissue Remodeling

The function of TGF-β1 in the regulation of cell growth and differentiation as well as homeostasis of extracellular matrix proteins has instigated investigations into the role of this growth factor during the induction, progression and manifestation of radiation-induced late tissue complications such as fibrosis. In a variety of tissues and in vitro cell systems, the immediate and maintained gene expression, synthesis and secretion of TGF-β1 in response to radiation exposure has been described (RUBIN et al. 1992; RODEMANN et al. 1996; KRÜSE et al. 1999; HAKENJOS et al. 2000; MARTIN et al. 2000; VON PFEIL et al. 2002). Especially in the skin, elevated TGF-β1 expression is observable and can be related to the progressing connective tissue remodeling. Likewise up to 40 weeks after irradiation, pathological changes of late radiation damage in non-tumor-bearing tissues of patients who had received pre-operative radiotherapy have been reported (CANNEY and DEAN 1990).

Since the fibroblast cell system is the relevant cell system in connective tissues able to produce the biochemical features of fibrosis, this cell system has been investigated in detail to clarify whether TGF-β1 exerts a modulatory role with respect to radiation sensitivity and collagen synthesis. To approach these questions, fibroblast cultures established from mice of different TGF-β1 genotypes, i.e. TGF-β1 wild-type cells (TGF-β1$^{+/+}$), heterozygous TGF-β1 knockout cells (TGF-β1$^{+/-}$), and homozygous TGF-β1 knockout cells (TGF-β1$^{-/-}$) were analyzed. It was shown that TGF-β1 not only regulates the clonogenic potential of fibroblasts by inducing terminal differentiation into postmitotic fibrocytes, but also is especially a potent determinant of the intrinsic radiation sensitivity of fibroblasts (VON PFEIL et al. 2002). Radiation sensitivity as tested by clonogenic cell survival was significantly reduced in homozygous TGF-β1$^{-/-}$ knockout fibroblasts as compared to wild type fibroblasts (TGF-β1$^{+/+}$). Most interestingly, heterozygous TGF-β1 knockout fibroblasts (TGF-β1$^{+/-}$) presented essentially the same radioresistance as homozygous TGF-β1$^{-/-}$ knockout fibroblasts. In accordance with earlier data of radiation-induced TGF-β1-production in normal skin and lung fibroblasts (RODEMANN et al. 1996; HAKENJOS et al. 2000), TGF-β1-production was stimulated in TGF-β1 wild type fibroblasts upon radiation exposure but not in heterozygous TGF-β1$^{+/-}$ knockout fibroblasts. As expected due to the knockout condition TGF-β1$^{-/-}$ fibroblasts did not produce any TGF-β1. Application of active TGF-β1 to radioresistant homozygous TGF-β1$^{-/-}$ knockout fibroblasts restored the normal radiation sensitivity of TGF-β1-wild type cells. Analyses of the differentiation pattern and collagen synthesis of normal fibroblasts revealed that TGF-β1 and radiation exposure not only induces the accumulation of postmitotic biochemically active fibrocytes but also up-regulates collagen production and deposition through the process of induced terminal differentiation (RODEMANN et al. 1996; BURGER et al. 1994; HAKENJOS et al. 2000). Inhibition of TGF-β1 both in treated and irradiated fibroblasts by the application of TGF-β1-neutralizing antibodies abolishes the effect of TGF-β1 on fibroblast differentiation and collagen production. Based on these results, in can be concluded that TGF-β1 is a major regulator of radiation sensitivity and differentiation of fibroblasts and is the key cytokine that induces the cellular events responsible for late connective tissue remodeling processes in response to radiation such as fibrosis.

The presented experimental data are supported by clinical studies indicating the importance of alterations in TGF-β1 levels following radiation. ANSCHER et al. (1997) demonstrated that radiation-induced pneumonitis is associated with an increase in plasma TGF-β1 at the end of radiation therapy. Furthermore, clinical evidence for the role of TGF-β1 in the development of radiogenic lung fibrosis has been reported by BENTZEN et al. (1996). Breast cancer patients undergoing radiation therapy and treated with the anti-estrogen, Tamoxifen, presented a higher risk for radiation fibrosis than patients who did not receive the drug. BENTZEN et al. (1996) suggested that this result may be due to the known induction of TGF-β1 expression by Tamoxifen.

Consequently, on the basis of the experimental and clinical data sets, the following scenario for the cellular and molecular processes underlying the late fibrotic connective tissue remodeling process in patients after radiation therapy can be established. In response to the radiation insult, cells of the connective tissue present a stimulated production and secretion of TGF-β1. With respect to the fibroblast cell system, in a paracrine and autocrine manner this cytokine is then responsible for a short wave of proliferation of early progenitor fibroblasts, which primarily undergo differentiation divisions into postmitotic fibrocytes. The main function of TGF-β1, however, is the immediate transition of already existing late progenitor fibroblasts into terminally differentiated fibrocytes (RODEMANN and BAMBERG 1995; RODEMANN et al. 1996; FOURNIER et al. 2001). Thus, these proliferation and differentiation events result in the accumulation of postmitotic biochemically activated fibrocytes producing and secreting collagens and other extracellular matrix proteins at a high level. Consequently, the radiation-induced and TGF-β1-mediated alterations in cellular homeostasis of the fibroblast system are the basis for the biochemical changes of connective tissue remodeling, i.e. enhanced production and extracellular deposition of interstitial collagen molecules by activated terminally differentiated fibrocytes.

2.3.2.3
TGF-β1 – A Potential Target for Antifibrotic Strategies?

Understanding that TGF-β1 is a key factor in fibrogenesis offered a new possible target for therapeutic agents with potential antifibrotic effects. Until very recently, fibrotic tissue was considered as irreversible tissue that could not be cured. Drugs of several categories have been tried in the management of fibrosis, including anti-inflammatory agents (steroids, colchicine, D-penicillamine), drugs acting on blood flow (heparin, pentoxifylline), and interferons. Corticosteroids are still the first-line therapeutics, even though they essentially reduce symptoms associated with inflammatory reactions. Several drugs were effective in preventing the occurrence of fibrosis in experimental models, whereas only very few were able to reduce an established fibrotic tissue (PETER et al. 1999; CUTRONEO et al. 1981; BENYAHA et al. 1996; LEFAIX et al. 1996; DELANIAN et al. 1999). Among the latter, several, such as interferons, produced significant clinical improvement in various fibrotic disorders, but were associated with toxicity and side effects.

Recent data challenged the postulate of the irreversibility of established radiation fibrosis. Liposomal Cu/Zn superoxide dismutase (SOD) was shown to be the first agent effective in reducing long-standing fibrosis in patients treated by radiotherapy (DELANIAN et al. 1994). Although this so far successful treatment approach could be reproduced in a pig fibrosis model, further clinical proof needs to be established before this treatment can be recommended for routine clinical use.

The importance of TGF-β1 as a target for antifibrotic strategies has been found in fibrotic disorders of various origins, including those in kidney, skin, lung, joint, and arterial wall (BORDER et al. 1990; SHAH et al. 1992; WOLF et al. 1994; GIRI et al. 1993; CHOI et al. 1996; BOTTINGER et al. 1996). Various approaches have been tested to down-regulate TGF-β. Thus, administration of TGF-β neutralizing antibodies significantly reduced glomerulonephritis in rats (BORDER et al. 1990), cutaneous scarring of rat wounds (SHAH et al. 1992), intimal hyperplasia in a rat model of carotid artery injury (WOLF et al. 1994), and lung fibrosis induced by bleomycin in mice (GIRI et al. 1993). Similarly, the application of TGF-β1-antisense mRNA on dermal wounds resulted in markedly reduced scarring and fibrosis and was associated with decreased TGF-β1 expression (CHOI et al. 1996). Furthermore, recombinant LAP, the latency-associated peptide of TGF-β1, was shown to be a potent inhibitor of bioactive TGF-β, both in vitro and in vivo, in transgenic mice with elevated TGF-β1 in liver (BOTTINGER et al. 1996). These examples indicate that with respect to the function and role of TGF-β1 in fibrotic tissue remodeling based on mechanistic data, clinical strategies can be developed and optimized to establish target-specific interventional therapies.

References

Alaluf S, Muir-Howie H, Hu HL, Evans A, Green MR (2000) Atmospheric oxygen accelerates the induction of a postmitotic phenotype in human dermal fibroblasts: the key protective role of glutathione. Differentiation 66:147–155

Anderson A, Woloschak GE (1992) Cellular proto-oncogene expression following exposure of mice to g-rays. Radiat Res 130:340–344

Anscher MS, Kong FM, Marks LB, Bentel GC, Jirtle RI (1997) Changes in plasma transforming growth factor b during radiotherapy and the risk of symptomatic radiation-induced pneumonitis. Int J Radiat Oncol Biol Phys 37:253–258

Barcellos-Hoff MH (1998) How do tissues respond to damage at the cellular level? The role of cytokines in irradiated tissues. Radiat Res 150:109–120

Barcellos-Hoff MH, Derynck R, Tsang ML (1994) Transforming growth factor-β activation in irradiated murine mammary gland. J Clin Invest 93:892–899

Basu S, Bayoumy S, Zhang Y, Lozano J, Kolesnick R (1998) BAD enables ceramide to signal apoptosis via Ras and Raf-1. J Biol Chem 273:30419–30426

Bayreuther K, Rodemann HP, Francz PI, Maier K (1988a) Differentiation of fibroblast stem cells. J Cell Sci [Suppl] 10:115–130

Bayreuther K, Rodemann HP, Hommel R, Dittmann K, Albiez M, Francz PI (1988b) Human skin fibroblasts in vitro differentiate along a terminal cell lineage. Proc Natl Acad Sci U S A 85:5112–5116

Bayreuther K, Francz PI, Rodemann HP (1992) Fibroblasts in normal and pathological terminal differentiation, ageing, apoptosis and transformation. Arch Gerontol Geriatr [Suppl] 3:47–74

Belka C, Budach W (2002) Anti-apoptotic Bcl-2 proteins: structure, function and relevance for radiation biology. Int J Radiat Biol 78:643–658

Bentzen SM, Skoczylas JZ, Overgaard M, Overgaard J (1996) Radiotherapy-related lung fibrosis enhanced by tamoxifen. J Natl Cancer Inst 88:918–922

Benyaha B, Campana F, Perdereau B (1996) Effects of superoxide dismutase topical treatment on human skin radiofibrosis: a pathological study. Breast 5:75–81

Border WA, Okuda S, Languino LR (1990) Suppression of experimental glomerulonephritis by antiserum against transforming growth factor-beta1. Nature 346:371–374

Bottinger EP, Factor VM, Tsang ML (1996) The recombinant proregion of TGF-β1 (latency-associated peptide) inhibits active TGF-β1 in transgenic mice. Proc Natl Acad Sci U S A 93:5877–5882

Bumann J, Santo-Hoeltje L, Löffler H, Bamberg M, Rodemann HP (1995) Radiation-induced alterations of the proliferation dynamics of human skin fibroblasts after repeated irradiation in the subtherapeutic dose range. Strahlenther Onkol 1:35–41

Burger A, Güven N, Hämmerle H, Bamberg M, Rodemann HP (1994) Co-culture systems of alveolar type II pneumocytes and lung fibroblasts as a model for radiation-induced lung fibrosis. Eur J Cell Biol 63:113–114

Burger A, Löffler H, Bamberg M, Rodemann HP (1998) Molecular and cellular basis of radiation fibrosis. Int J Radiat Biol 73:401–408

Canney PA, Dean S (1990) Transforming growth factor b. A promoter of late connective tissue injury following radiotherapy? Br J Radiol 63:620–623

Choi BM, Kwak HJ, Jun CD (1996) Control of scarring in adults' wounds using antisense TGF-β1 oligodeoxynucleotides. Immunol Cell Biol 74:144–150

Cutroneo KR, Rokowski R, Counts DF (1981) Glucocorticoids and collagen synthesis: comparison of in vivo and cell culture studies. Coll Rel Res 1:557–568

Datto MB, Li Y, Panus JF (1995) TGF-β induces the cyclin-dependent kinase inhibitor p21 through a p53-independent mechanism. Proc Natl Acad Sci U S A 92:5545–5549

Delanian S, Baillet F, Huart J (1994) Successful treatment of radiation-induced fibrosis using liposomal Cu/Zn superoxide dismutase: clinical trial. Radiother Oncol 32:12–20

Delanian S, Balla-Mekias S, Lefaix JL (1999) Striking regression of chronic radiotherapy damage in a clinical trial of combined pentoxifylline and a tocopherol. J Clin Oncol 17:3283–3290

Derynck R, Jarrett JA, Chen EY, Goeddel DV (1986) The murine transforming growth factor-β precursor. J Biol Chem 261:4377–4379

Dimitrievich GS, Hausladen SL, Kuchnir FT, Griem ML, Yang VV, Stearner SP (1977) Radiation damage and subendothelial repair to rabbit ear chamber microvasculature: an in vivo and histologic study. Radiat Res 69:276–292

Dimitrievich GS, Fischer-Dzoga K, Griem ML (1984) Radiosensitivity of vascular tissue I. Differential radiosensitivity of capillaries: a quantitative in vivo study. Radiat Res 99:511–535

Dressler KA, Mathias S, Kolesnick RN (1992) TNF-a activates the sphingomyelin pathway in a cell free system. Science 255:1715–1718

Ehrhart EJ, Carroll A, Segarini P (1997) Latent transforming growth factor b1 activation in situ: quantitative and functional evidence after low-dose γ-irradiation. Fed Am Soc Exp Biol 11:991–1002

Fajardo LF (1989) Morphological patterns of radiation injury. Front Radiat Ther Oncol 23:75–84

Fajardo LF, Berthrong M (1988) Vascular lesions following radiation. Pathol Annu 1:297–330

Fischer-Dzoga K, Dimitrievich GS, Griem ML (1984) Radiosensitivity of vascular tissue II. Differential radiosensitivity of aortic cells in vitro. Radiat Res 99:536–546

Fournier C, Scholz M, Kraft-Weyrather W, Kraft G, Rodemann HP (2001) Changes of fibrosis-related parameters after high and low LET irradiation of fibroblasts. Int J Radiat Biol 77:713–722

Friedman M, Ryan US, Davenport WC, Chaney EL, Strickland DL, Kwock L (1986) Reversible alterations in cultured pulmonary artery endothelial cell monolayer morphology and albumin permeability induced by ionizing radiation. J Cell Physiol 129:237–249

Fuks Z, Persaud RS, Alfieri A, McLoughlin M, Ehleiter D, Schwartz JL, Seddon AP, Cordon-Cardo C, Haimovitz-Friedman A (1994) Basic fibroblast growth factor protects endothelial cells against radiation-induced programmed cell death in vitro and in vivo. Cancer Res 54:2582–2590

Gajdusek C, Onoda K, London S, Johnson M, Morrison R, Mayberg M (2001) Early molecular changes in irradiated aortic endothelium. J Cell Physiol 188:8–23

Gauldie J, Jordana M, Cox G (1993) Cytokines and pulmonary fibrosis. Thorax 48:931–935

Giri SN, Hyde DM, Hollinger MA (1993) Effect of antibody to

TGF-β on bleomycin-induced accumulation of lung collagen in mice. Thorax 48:959-966

Haimovitz-Friedman A, Kan CC, Ehleiter D, Persaud RS, McLoughlin M, Fuks Z, Kolesnick RN (1994a) Ionizing radiation acts on cellular membranes to generate ceramide and initiate apoptosis. J Exp Med 180:525-535

Haimovitz-Friedman A, Balaban N, McLoughlin M, Ehleiter D, Michaeli J, Vlodavsky I, Fuks Z (1994b) Protein kinase C mediates basic fibroblast growth factor protection of endothelial cells against radiation-induced apoptosis. Cancer Res 54:2591-2597

Hakenjos L, Bamberg M, Rodemann HP (2000) TGF-β1-mediated alterations of rat lung fibroblast differentiation resulting in the radiation-induced fibrotic response. Int J Radiat Biol 76:503-509

Hallahan DE, Sukhatme VP, Sherman ML, Virudachalam S, Kufe D, Weichselbaum RR (1991) Protein kinase C mediates x-ray inducibility of nuclear signal transducers EGR1 and JUN. Proc Natl Acad Sci U S A 88:2156-2160

Hannon GJ, Beach D (1994) p15INK4B is a potential effector of TGF-β-induced cell cycle arrest. Nature 371:257-261

Herr I, Debatin KM (2001) Cellular stress response and apoptosis in cancer therapy. Blood 98:2603-2614

Herskind C, Bentzen SM, Overgaard J, Overgaard M, Bamberg M, Rodemann HP (1998) Differentiation state of skin fibroblast cultures versus risk of subcutaneous fibrosis after radiotherapy. Radiother Oncol 47:263-269

Herskind C, Johansen J, Bentzen SM, Overgaard M, Overgaard J, Bamberg M, Rodemann HP (2000) Fibroblast differentiation in subcutaneous fibrosis after postmastectomy radiotherapy. Acta Oncol 39:383-388

Hopewell JW, Campling D, Calvo W, Reinhold HS, Wilkinson JH, Yeung TK (1986) Vascular irradiation damage: its cellular basis and likely consequences. Br J Cancer 53:181-191

Jaenke RS, Robbins ME, Bywaters T, Whitehouse E, Rezvani M, Hopewell JW (1993) Capillary endothelium: target site of renal radiation injury. Lab Invest 68:396-405

Johnstone RW, Ruefi AA, Lowe SW (2002) Apoptosis: a link between cancer genetics and chemotherapy. Cell 108:153-164

Kastan M (1997) On the TRAIL from p53 to apoptosis? Nat Genet 17:130-131

Klein-Soyer C, Beretz A, Cazenave JP, Driot F, Maffrand JP (1990) Behavior of confluent endothelial cells after irradiation: modulation of wound repair by heparin and acidic fibroblast growth factor. Biol Cell 68:231-238

Kretschmar M, Massague J (1998) Smads: mediators and regulators of TGF-β signaling. Curr Opin Genet Dev 8:102-111

Krüse JJ, Bart CI, Visser A, Wondergem J (1999) Changes in transforming growth factor-β (TGF-β1), procollagen types I and II mRNA in the rat heart after irradiation. Int J Radiat Biol 75:1429-1436

Langberg CW, Hauer-Jensen M, Sung S-S, Kane C (1994) Expression of fibrogenic cytokines in rat small intestine after fractionated irradiation. Radiother Oncol 32:29-36

Langley RE, Bump EA, Quartuccio SG, Medeiros D, Braunhut SJ (1997) Radiation-induced apoptosis in microvascular endothelial cells. Br J Cancer 75:666-672

Lara PC, Russell NS, Smolders IJ, Bartelink H, Begg AC, Cocomartin JM (1996) Radiation-induced differentiation of human skin fibroblasts: relationship with cell survival and collagen production. Int J Radiat Biol 70:683-692

Lawrence A (1996) Transforming growth factor-β: a general review. Eur Cytokine Net 7:363-374

Lefaix JL, Delanian S, Leplat JJ (1996) Successful treatment of radiation-induced fibrosis using Cu/Zn-SOD and Mn-SOD: an experimental study. Int J Radiat Oncol Biol Phys 35:305-312

Leitlein J, Aulwurm S, Waltereit R, Naumann U, Wagenknecht B, Garten W, Weller M, Platten M (2001) Processing of immunosuppressive pro-TGF-β12 by human glioblastoma cells involves cytoplasmic and secreted furin-like proteases. J Immunol 166:7238-7243

Liao WC, Haimovitz-Friedman A, Persaud RS, McLoughlin M, Ehleiter D, Zhang N, Gatei M, Lavin M, Kolesnick R, Fuks ZJ (1999) Ataxia telangiectasia-mutated gene product inhibits DNA damage-induced apoptosis via ceramide synthase. J Biol Chem 274:17908-17917

Lin PS, Ho KC, Sung SJ, Gladding J (1992) Effect of tumour necrosis factor, heat, and radiation on the viability and microfilament organization in cultured endothelial cells. Int J Hyperthermia 8:667-677

Lin T, Genestier L, Pinkoski MJ, Castro A, Nicholas S, Mogil R, Paris F, Fuks Z, Schuchman EH, Kolesnick RN, Green DR (2000) Role of acidic sphingomyelinase in Fas/CD95-mediated cell death. J Biol Chem 275:8657-8663

Maisin JR, Reyners H, de Reyners EG (1977) Changes in the ultrastructure and the permeability of the capillaries after irradiation. Bibl Anat 15:311-314

Martin M, Lefaix J-L, Pinton P, Crechet F, Daburon F (1993) Temporal modulation of TGF-β1 and b-actin gene expression in pig skin and muscular fibrosis after ionizing radiation. Radiat Res 134:63-70

Martin M, Lefaix J-L, Delanian S (2000) TGF-β1 and radiation fibrosis: a master switch and a specific therapeutic target? Int J Radiat Oncol Biol Phys 47:277-290

Matucci-Cerinic M, Jaffa A, Kahaleh B (1992) Angiotensin converting enzyme: an in vivo and in vitro marker of endothelial injury. J Lab Clin Med 120:428-433

Matzner Y, Cohn M, Hyam E, Razin E, Fuks Z, Buchanan MR, Haas TA, Vlodavsky I, Eldor A (1988) Generation of lipid neutrophil chemoattractant by irradiated bovine aortic endothelial cells. J Immunol 140:2681-2685

Miyashita T, Reed JC (1995) Tumor suppressor p53 is a direct transcriptional activator of the human bax gene. Cell 80:293-299

Miyashita T, Krajewski S, Krajewska M, Wang HG, Lin HK, Liebermann DA, Hoffman B, Reed JC (1994) Tumor suppressor p53 is a regulator of bcl-2 and bax gene expression in vitro and in vivo. Oncogene 9:1799-1805

Morris GM, Coderre JA, Bywaters A, Whitehouse E, Hopewell JW (1996) Boron neutron capture irradiation of the rat spinal cord: histopathological evidence of a vascular-mediated pathogenesis. Radiat Res 146:313-320

Muller G, Ayoub M, Storz P, Rennecke J, Fabbro D, Pfizenmaier K (1995) PKC zeta is a molecular switch in signal transduction of TNF-a, bifunctionally regulated by ceramide and arachidonic acid. EMBO J 14:1961-1969

Nicolson GL, Custead SE, Dulski KM, Milas L (1991) Effects of g-irradiation on cultured rat and mouse microvessel endothelial cells: metastatic tumor cell adhesion, subendothelial matrix degradation, and secretion of tumor cell growth factors. Clin Exp Metastasis 9:457-468

O'Connor MM, Mayberg MR (2000) Effects of radiation on cerebral vasculature: a review. Neurosurgery 46:138–145

Oursler MJ, Riggs BL, Spelsberg TC (1993) Glucocorticoid-induced activation of latent TGF-β by normal human osteoblast-like cells. Endocrinology 133:2187–2196

Paris F, Fuks Z, Kang A, Capodieci P, Juan G, Ehleiter D, Haimovitz-Friedman A, Cordon-Cardo C, Kolesnick R (2001) Endothelial apoptosis as the primary lesion initiating intestinal radiation damage in mice. Science 293:293–297

Pena LA, Fuks Z, Kolesnick RN (2000) Radiation-induced apoptosis of endothelial cells in the murine central nervous system: protection by fibroblast growth factor and sphingomyelinase deficiency. Cancer Res 60:321–327

Peter RU, Gottlöber P, Nadeshina GK (1999) Interferon g in survivors of the Tchernobyl power plant accident: new therapeutic option for radiation-induced fibrosis. Int J Radiat Oncol Biol Phys 45:147–152

Poncelet A-C, de Caestecker MP, Schnaper HW (1999) The transforming growth factor-β/SMAD signaling pathway is present and functional in human mesangial cells. Kidney Int 56:1354–1365

Randall K, Coggle JE (1995) Expression of transforming growth factor b1 in mouse skin during the acute phase of radiation damage. Int J Radiat Biol 68:301–309

Randall K, Coggle JE (1996) Long-term expression of transforming growth factor TGF-β1 in mouse skin after localized b-irradiation. Int J Radiat Biol 70:351–360

Ravitz MJ, Yan S, Dolce C (1996) Differential regulation of p27 and cyclin D1 by TGF-β and EGF in C3H10T1/2 mouse fibroblasts. J Cell Physiol 168:510–520

Raynal S, Lawrence DA (1995) Differential effects of TGF-β1 on protein levels of p21WAF and cdk2-kinase activity in human RD and CCL64 mink lung cells. Int J Oncol 7:337–341

Reinhold HS, Buisman GH (1973) Radiosensitivity of capillary endothelium. Br J Radiol 46:54–57

Reinhold HS, Keyeux A, Dunjic A, Jovanovic D, Maisin JR (1974) The influence of radiation on blood vessels and circulation XII. Discussion and conclusions. Curr Top Radiat Res Q 10:185–198

Reinhold HS, Calvo W, Hopewell JW, van der Berg AP (1990) Development of blood vessel-related radiation damage in the fimbria of the central nervous system. Int J Radiat Oncol Biol Phys 18:37–42

Remy J, Wegrowski J, Crechet F, Martin M, Daburon F (1991) Long-term overproduction of collagen in radiation-induced fibrosis. Radiat Res 125:14–19

Reyes JG, Robayna IG, Delgado PS, Gonzalez IH, Aguiar JQ, Rosas FE, Fanjul LF, Galaretta CMR (1996) c-Jun is a downstream target for ceramide-activated protein phosphatase in A431 cells. J Biol Chem 271:21375–21380

Roberts AB, Sporn MB (1990) The transforming growth factor-βetas In: Sporn MB, Roberts AB (eds) Peptide growth factors and their receptors. Springer, Berlin Heidelberg New York, pp 419–472

Roberts AB, Sporn MB (1996) Transforming growth factor b. In: Clark RAF (ed) The molecular and cellular biology of wound repair. Plenum, New York, pp 275–308

Rodemann HP (1989) Differential degradation of intracellular proteins in human skin fibroblasts of mitotic and mitomycin C(MMC)-induced postmitotic differentiation states. Differentiation 42:37–43

Rodemann HP, Bamberg M (1995) Cellular basis of radiation-induced fibrosis. Radiother Oncol 35:83–90

Rodemann HP, Bayreuther K (1984) Abnormal collagen metabolism in cultured skin fibroblasts from patients with Duchenne muscular dystrophy. Proc Natl Acad Sci U S A 81:5130–5134

Rodemann HP, Bayreuther K, Francz PI, Dittmann K, Albiez M (1989) Selective enrichment and biochemical characterisation of seven fibroblast cell types of human skin fibroblast populations in vitro. Exp Cell Res 180:84–93

Rodemann HP, Peterson H-P, Schwenke K, von Wangenheim K-H (1992) Terminal differentiation of human fibroblasts is induced by radiation. Scan Micr 5:1135–1143

Rodemann HP, Binder A, Bamberg M (1995) Radiation-induced fibrosis: experimental studies. In: Dunst J, Sauer R (eds) Medical radiology. Springer, Berlin Heidelberg New York, pp 93–99

Rodemann HP, Binder A, Burger A, Güven N, Löffler H, Bamberg M (1996) The underlying cellular mechanism of fibrosis. Kidney Int 49:32–36

Rubin DB, Drab EA, Bauer KD (1989) Endothelial cell subpopulations in vitro: cell volume, cell cycle, and radiosensitivity. J Appl Physiol 67:1585–1590

Rubin P, Finkelstein J, Schapiro D (1992) Molecular biology mechanisms in the radiation induction of pulmonary injury syndromes: interrelationship between the alveolar macrophage and the septal fibroblast. Int J Radiat Oncol Biol Phys 24:93–101

Ryan KM, Phillips AC, Vousden KH (2001) Regulation and function of the p53 tumor suppressor protein. Curr Opin Cell Biol 13:332–337

Seong J, Kim SH, Chung EJ, Lee WJ, Suh CO (2000) Early alteration in TGF-β mRNA expression in irradiated rat liver. Int J Radiat Oncol Biol Phys 46:639–643

Shah M, Forman DM, Ferguson MW (1992) Control of scarring in adult wounds by neutralizing antibody to TGF-β. Lancet 339:213–214

Sherman ML, Datta R, Hallahan DE, Weichselbaum RR, Kufe DW (1990) Ionizing radiation regulates expression of the c-jun protooncogene. Proc Natl Acad Sci U S A 87:5663–5666

Shull MM, Ormsby I, Kier AB, Pawlowski S, Diebold FJ, Yin M, Allen R, Sidman C, Proetzel G, Calvin D, Annunziata N, Doetschmann T (1992) Targeted disruption of the mouse transforming growth factor-β1 gene results in multifocal inflammatory disease. Nature 359:693–699

Sitnicka E, Ruscetti FW, Priestley GV (1996) Transforming growth factor b1 directly and reversibly inhibits the initial cell divisions of long-term repopulating hematopoietic stem cells. Blood 88:82–88

Stroh C, Schulze-Osthoff K (1998) Death by a thousand cuts: an ever increasing list of caspase substrates. Cell Death Differ 5:997–1000

Ts'ao C, Ward WF (1985) Acute radiation effects on the content and release of plasminogen activator activity in cultured aortic endothelial cells. Radiat Res 101:394–401

Verheij M, Bose R, Lin XH, Yao B, Jarvis WD, Grant S, Birrer MJ, Szabo E, Zon LI, Kolesnick RN (1996) Requirement for ceramide-initiated SAPK/JNK signaling in stress-induced apoptosis. Nature 380:75–79

Von Pfeil A, Hakenjos L, Herskind C, Dittmann K, Weller M, Rodemann HP (2002) Irradiated homozygous TGF-β1 knockout fibroblasts show enhanced clonogenic survival as compared with TGF-βeta1 wild-type fibroblasts. Int J Radiat Biol 78:331–339

Wahl SM (1994) Transforming growth factor β: the good, the bad and the ugly. J Exp Med 180:1587–1590

Waters CM, Taylor JM, Molteni A, Ward WF (1996) Dose-response effects of radiation on the permeability of endothelial cells in culture. Radiat Res 146:321–328

Witte L, Fuks Z, Haimovitz-Friedman A, Vlodavsky I, Goodman DS, Eldor A (1989) Effects of irradiation on the release of growth factors from cultured bovine, porcine, and human endothelial cells. Cancer Res 49:5066–5072

Wolf YG, Rasmussen LM, Ruoslahti E (1994) Antibodies against TGF-β1 suppress intimal hyperplasia in a rat model. J Clin Invest 93:1172–1178

Woloschak GE, Chang-Liu CM (1990) Differential modulation of specific gene expression following high- and low-LET radiations. Radiat Res 124:183–187

Yang VV, Stearner SP, Dimitrievich GS, Griem ML (1977) Radiation damage to the microvasculature in the rabbit ear chamber: an electron microscope study. Radiat Res 70:107–117

Yang J, Liu X, Bhalla K, Kim CN, Ibrado AM, Cai J, Peng TI, Jones DP, Wang X (1997) Prevention of apoptosis by Bcl-2: release of cytochrome c from mitochondria blocked. Science 275:1129–1132

Zha J, Harada H, Yang E, Jockel J, Korsmeyer SJ (1996) Serine phosphorylation of death agonist BAD in response to survival factor results in binding to 14-3-3 not Bcl-x_L. Cell 87:619–628

Zhan Q, Fan S, Bae I, Guillouf C, Liebermann DA, O'Connor PM, Fornace AJ (1994) Induction of bax by genotoxic stress in human cells correlates with normal p53 status and apoptosis. Oncogene 9:3743–3751

Zhang Y, Yao B, Delikat S, Bayoumy S, Lin XH, Basu S, McGinley M, Chan-Hui PY, Lichenstein H, Kolesnick R (1997) Kinase suppressor of Ras is ceramide-activated protein kinase. Cell 89:63–72

Zhou Q, Zhao Y, Li P, Bai X, Ruan C (1992) Thrombomodulin as a marker of radiation-induced endothelial cell injury. Radiat Res 131:285–289

Zundel W, Giaccia A (1998) Inhibition of the anti-apoptotic PI(3)K/Akt/Bad pathway by stress. Genes Dev 12:1941–1946

3 Pathogenetic Mechanisms of Lung Fibrosis

W. Dörr and T. Herrmann

CONTENTS

3.1 Introduction 29
3.2 Gross Lung Reactions to Irradiation 30
3.3 Radiation Effects on Pneumocytes 30
3.4 Radiation Effects in Fibroblasts 31
3.5 Radiation Effects on
     Endothelial Cells and Capillaries 31
3.6 Radiation Response of Macrophages,
     Lymphocytes, Eosinophils and Neutrophils 32
3.7 Mediators in the
     Radiation Response of the Lung 32
3.7.1 Growth Factors 32
3.7.2 Cytokines 32
3.7.3 Chemokines 33
3.7.4 Adhesion Molecules 33
3.8 The Role of Superoxide 33
3.9 Conclusion 33
     References 34

3.1 Introduction

The lung is one of the most important dose-limiting organs in radiotherapy. Substantial research efforts have been undertaken over the past decades to understand the radiobiology and radiopathology of lung tissue, to define mechanisms of radiation responses in the lung, and to transfer experimental results into clinical trials and practice.

A variety of animal models, including mice, rats, pigs and dogs, have been used in radiobiological studies in the lung. The lung structure of some of these models is very close to humans, while others – including all rodents – differ in several important aspects

W. Dörr, DVM, PhD
Professor, Medical Faculty Carl Gustav Carus, Technical University of Dresden, Fetscherstrasse 74, PF 58, 01307 Dresden, Germany
T. Herrmann, MD
Medical Faculty Carl Gustav Carus, Technical University of Dresden, Fetscherstrasse 74, PF 58, 01307 Dresden, Germany

from the clinical situation (Hopewell et al. 2000). Thus, while many basic questions can be addressed using small laboratory animals, other problems probably are better studied in large animals or, if appropriate, in clinical investigations (Dörr et al. 2000).

Target structures for radiation injury in the lung are the alveolar sacculi, i.e. the alveolar membranes. Radiation exposure of lung tissue with relevant doses results in a specific sequence of gross reactions, which include pneumonitis and eventually result in fibrotic remodelling within the irradiated volume. The radiation response is associated with characteristic radiological changes. The functional consequences of these reactions, however, are predominantly dependent on the volume irradiated, i.e. the residual functional capacity of the organ after the clinical manifestation of radiation injury. As a rule of thumb, if lung function is not severely impaired by other factors, 30% of the lung volume can be irradiated with a dose of 20 Gy, and 20% with a dose of 30 Gy without exceeding clinical lung tolerance.

Radiation-induced lung injury represents the manifestation of highly complex processes, which involve interactions between a variety of cell populations present in the lung, which amount to approximately 40 (Gross 1977; Movsas et al. 1997). These include pneumocytes II and I, which represent the parenchymal component, fibroblasts, and endothelial cells. Moreover, macrophages and other cells are involved in the inflammatory element of the tissue response. Also, interactions between the various phases of the lung response, with consequences of pneumonitis on the development of fibrosis, play a major role.

Morphological changes in the irradiated lung and the reactions of the individual cell populations will be summarized before their interactions and external factors influencing their response to tissue injury are reviewed. Fibrosis development starts with interstitial oedema and inflammatory cell infiltration, which then lead to proliferation of fibroblasts and increased collagen deposition. This sequence of events is similar for all interstitial lung diseases, independent of the aetiology (Kuwano et al. 2001; Fajardo et al. 2001).

3.2
Gross Lung Reactions to Irradiation

The radiation response of the lung is a continuous process with early changes progressing to acute radiation pneumonitis at 8–16 weeks after onset of radiotherapy, and to pulmonary fibrosis after months to years. Typical changes, which may not result in clinical consequences, can be detected best by diagnostic X-radiographs or CT scans. At very early time points, congestion, perivascular and intra-alveolar oedema and early transmigration of macrophages into the alveolar lumen (Fajardo et al. 2001; Spencer 1968; Ts'ao et al. 1983a, b) can be observed.

The *acute radiation pneumonitis* is similar to the response to any other alveolar injury. The lung presents firm and uniformly dense, with septal oedema. The alveolar lumen is filled with hyaline membranes, i.e. fibrin-like material (Fajardo et al. 2001). In the development of radiation fibrosis, the hyaline membranes are fragmented and decreased or, less frequently and mainly associated with infections, becomes organized into connective tissue. The collagen content of the lung increases. The originally irradiated volume shows a strong tendency for shrinkage.

The radiation response proper must be differentiated from the *lymphocytic alveolitis*, which can occur outside the radiation volume, and hence represents an abscopal radiation effect (Bennett et al. 1969). The induction of this response by radiation is, in most instances, hard to prove, because concomitant infections, which are promoted by the breakdown of the alveolar epithelial barrier (see Section 3.3.) can yield a similar response. One plausible mechanism, however, is that the acute pneumonitis is associated with accumulation of T lymphocytes (CD4+/CD8+/ICAM-1+), which can be demonstrated in the broncho-alveolar lavage, and which may result in alveolitic reactions out of field.

3.3
Radiation Effects on Pneumocytes

The alveolar epithelium represents a tissue with a hierarchical proliferative structure, with type II pneumocytes representing the stem cell compartment, which gives rise to the functional, differentiated epithelial cells, i.e. pneumocytes I. Hence, the target cells for radiation effects in the pneumocyte system are type II pneumocytes. Their proliferative impairment, in face of ongoing cell loss from the pneumocyte I compartment, results in progressive cell depletion and loss of function of the alveolar epithelium. The turnover time of the system is in the range of 20–35 days in mice (Gross 1977) and hence the clinical symptoms become manifest slightly after this time period (Dörr und Herrmann 2002). The main function of the alveolar epithelium is the protection against external factors from inhaled air, which is based on the mechanical barrier by the presence of epithelium, but also on the phagocytotic activity of the pneumocytes I. Radiation-induced epithelial hypo- or aplasia results in a reduced barrier function.

Moreover, the alveolar epithelium also represents a barrier between the interstitium and the alveoli. Therefore, cell depletion results in exudation of tissue fluids (mainly fibrin) into the alveolar space (Fig. 3.1), but also in increased transmigration of various cells, predominantly macrophages. These processes can be demonstrated and diagnosed by broncho-alveolar lavages (Herrmann and Knorr 1995). Thickening of the alveolocapillary membrane, due to interstitial oedema, results in an additional impairment of the gas exchange. The transmigration of fibroblasts can result in intra-alveolar fibrosis (Fukuda et al. 1987; Basset et al. 1986).

The second major function of pneumocytes type II is the synthesis of surfactant factor, stored in lamellar bodies. Release of this factor into the alveolar space maintains the low surface tension of the alveolar sac and hence is the basis for the compliance of the lung.

Fig. 3.1. Electron-microscopic appearance of the alveolocapillary membrane after irradiation. The alveolar lumen is filled with fluid (*F*). The interstitial oedema results in thickening of the alveolocapillary membrane. *E*, erythrocyte

Radiation damage of the pneumocytes II results in an initial release of surfactant, with a decrease in cellular content and an increase in alveolar concentration, which in rodent models lasts for about 1 week (McDonald et al. 1995). This is followed by increased cellular levels, with increased numbers of lamellar bodies (Fig. 3.2) and normal alveolar concentrations. These changes can also be shown in bronchoalveolar lavages (Herrmann and Knorr 1995).

3.4
Radiation Effects in Fibroblasts

Radiation effects on fibroblasts have been extensively studied both in vitro and in vivo (see Chap. 2, "Role of Radiation-Induced Signaling Proteins in the Response of Vascular and Connective Tissues"). Their main response is stimulated proliferation (Kuwano et al. 2001), which results in an early transition into postmitotic fibrocytes. These deposit collagen at a significantly increased rate, which eventually results in fibrotic tissue remodelling. TGF-β1 is a key modulator of these post-irradiation cellular events (Burger et al. 1998; Hakenjos et al. 2000; Martin et al. 2000).

3.5
Radiation Effects on Endothelial Cells and Capillaries

Capillaries in the lung are end segments of the pulmonary artery tree. They form a dense network and can – in the adult – contain up to 50% of all endothelial cells of the body, which illustrates the particular relevance of radiation damage to these cells in the lung. The vascular network in the lung, in contrast to most organs, has a dual function: supply of lung tissue with nutrients and gas exchange.

Radiation exposure of capillaries results in initial swelling of endothelial cells and their detachment from the basement membrane, which in experimental animals occurs as early as 5 days after single-dose exposure (Adamson and Bowden 1983; Adamson et al. 1970; Philips 1966), which progresses into interruption of the continuity of the capillaries. Recanalization at later time points (6 months) is possible. However, in most cases progressive perivascular fibrosis, which in the lung represents septal fibrosis, develops, which is associated with impaired blood flow.

Fig. 3.2. Pneumocyte type II (*N*, nucleus) with an increased number of lamellar bodies (examples labelled by *arrows*) after irradiation. The pneumocyte is slightly protruding into the alveolar lumen (*L*)

Capillary radiation effects are also associated with increased permeability. This response occurs – as shown in experimental models (Evans et al. 1986) – in two waves, with a first peak at 24 h and a second peak at 19 days after single-dose irradiation. The vascular leakage significantly contributes to exudation of protein-rich fluids into the alveolar lumen (see Section 3.2).

Functional changes in endothelial cells result in a decreased synthesis of plasminogen-activating factor (Ts'ao et al. 1983b) and angiotensin-converting enzyme (Ward et al. 1983). A consequence of the reduction in plasminogen-activating factor is a diminished fibrinolytic activity, which contributes to the formation of hyaline membranes (see Section 3.2). The varying radiosensitivity of the plasminogen-activator system may be one of the reasons for strain and species differences in the fibrotic response (Fajardo et al. 2001). Moreover, changes in prostaglandin I2 levels, with an initial decrease and a subsequent, continuous increase to supernormal levels are seen, which is inversely correlated with arterial perfusion (Ts'ao et al. 1983a).

Capillary radiation effects are associated with significant changes in perfusion. In rats, arterial perfusion to the irradiated right lung increased during the first 2 weeks after irradiation, then decreased to approximately 40% of the control blood flow in the left lung by 150 days.

These changes result in nutritional impairment of downstream lung structures, which represents a continuing trauma. Also, the decrease in capillary density causes an impairment of the exchange of oxygen and carbon monoxide through the alveolar wall, i.e. a reduction in functional capacity of the respective lung volume.

3.6
Radiation Response of Macrophages, Lymphocytes, Eosinophils and Neutrophils

In irradiated *macrophages*, increased levels of arachidonic acid are observed, with consequences for the prostaglandin and leukotriene metabolism. Also, reactive oxygen species are produced during the so-called respiratory burst. Moreover, a number of chemo- and cytokines (e.g. TGF-β, PDGF) are released.

Lymphocytes respond to radiation exposure with interstitial infiltration and production of a number of factors, such as IL-4 or IFN-gamma. The relevance of the lymphocyte response in the lung is illustrated by the observation that depletion of CD4+CD8+ lymphocytes attenuated the fibrotic response in rodent models (PIGUET et al. 1989).

Similarly to other cell types, *eosinophils* release a number of cytokines, e.g. TGF-β. Reactions of neutrophils are mainly seen after total body irradiation, where these cells represent the earliest infiltration. *Neutrophils*, like macrophages, produce prostaglandins and leukotrienes, reactive oxygen species and cytokines (G-CSF, IL-8).

3.7
Mediators in the Radiation Response of the Lung

The mediators involved in the late fibrotic response of lung tissue to injury have extensively been studied in idiopathic pulmonary fibrosis. However, as the pathways eventually resulting in pulmonary fibrosis are grossly independent of the aetiology, similar processes are involved in the development of radiation fibrosis. Changes in growth factors, cytokines, chemokines and adhesion molecules in fibrotic lung disease have comprehensively been reviewed by KUWANO et al. (2001).

3.7.1
Growth Factors

Transforming growth factor-β (TGF-β), particularly the isoform TGF-β1, is a key cytokine in radiation fibrosis (RODEMANN and BAMBERG 1995; BURGER et al. 1998; HAKENJOS et al. 2000; MARTIN et al. 2000), which promotes differentiation of fibroblasts and deposition of collagen and fibronectin. Moreover, TGF-β1 has an anti-proliferative effect on epithelial cells, is chemotactic for monocytes and macrophages and stimulates their production of PDGF, IL-1β, bFGF, TNF-α and TGF-β itself, and suppresses production of nitric oxide (TOOMEY et al. 2001). TGF-β1 is produced by epithelial cells and macrophages in bleomycin-induced fibrosis (RAGHOW et al. 1989). In a recent report (RUBIN et al. 1995) found altered gene expression from day 1 after irradiation, in parallel to altered fibroblast gene expression of collagens 1, 3, 4 and fibronectin. The effect of TGF-β seems to be controlled by cyclin-kinase inhibitors p21, p27, p15 and p16. In vitro, neutralizing antibodies to TGF-β1 inhibit this differentiation process after irradiation (HAKENJOS et al. 2000). Following thoracic radiotherapy, the manifestation of pulmonary injury corresponds to permanently elevated plasma levels of TGF-β after the end of therapy (ANSCHER et al. 1998).

Proliferation of fibroblasts, endothelial and epithelial cells is stimulated by *TGF-α* from alveolar macrophages and epithelial cells in bleomycin-induced fibrosis (MADTES et al. 1994).

Platelet-derived growth factor (PDGF), produced by macrophages, epithelial cells type II and mesenchymal cells, induces fibroblast proliferation and synthesis of extracellular matrix (TOOMEY et al. 2001). *Insulin-like growth factor-1* (IGF-1) from alveolar macrophages acts synergistically with PDGF (ROM et al. 1988).

Basic fibroblast growth factor (bFGF) stimulates proliferation of fibroblasts and endothelial cells. This bFGF is produced by a variety of cells, predominantly macrophages (HENKE et al. 1993), but also endothelial cells, fibroblasts and mast cells (TOOMEY et al. 2001).

Vascular endothelial growth factor (VEGF) in normal lung is expressed by type II epithelial cells, smooth muscle cells and myofibroblasts (FEHRENBACH et al. 1999). VEGF attracts mast cells into radiation-induced fibrotic tissue (THRALL and SCALISE 1995). Their number correlates with the degree of fibrosis (PESCI et al. 1993).

3.7.2
Cytokines

Tumour necrosis factor-alpha (TNF-α) is predominantly synthesized by type II epithelial cells of the thickened alveolar septa, as well as by macrophages in fibrotic tissue (PIGUET et al. 1993b). TNF-α activates leukocytes and endothelial cells and stimulates the expression of adhesion molecules. Moreover, stimulation of fibroblasts results in proliferation and synthesis of PDGF, prostaglandin E2, collagenase, GM-CSF, IL-β1 and IL-6. Soluble TNF-receptor protects mice against bleomycin-induced fibrosis (PIGUET et al. 1993a; PIGUET and VESIN 1994).

Interleukin-1 (IL-1) induces fibroblast proliferation and affects collagen synthesis (RAINES et al. 1989). In parallel, fibroblast proliferation is counteracted by synthesis of prostaglandin E2 (PGE2). Decreased levels of IL-1 are found in interstitial fibrosis. *IL-1 receptor antagonist* (IL-1ra), in contrast, is significantly increased in type II pneumocytes, macrophages and fibroblasts (SMITH et al. 1995). This imbalance may significantly contribute to the progressive nature of lung fibrosis.

Cytokines of T-helper cells type 1 (Th1) are *interferon-gamma* (IFN-γ) and IL-12, while *IL-4, IL-5 and IL-10* are found in type 2 helper cells (Th2). IL-4 stimulates fibroblast proliferation and collagen deposition. In fibrotic tissue, Th2 cytokines dominate, while IFN-γ, which normally inhibits collagen deposition, is decreased (WALLACE et al. 1995).

Interleukin-6 is – among others – produced by endothelial cells and fibroblasts, and stimulates fibroblast proliferation and collagen deposition (FRIES et al. 1994).

3.7.3
Chemokines

Macrophage inflammatory protein-1alpha (MIP-1α) and *monocyte chemotactic protein-1* (MCP-1) are produced by macrophages, pneumocytes and endothelial cells in response to stimulation by IL-1, IL-6 or TNF-α. Increased levels are found in the bronchoalveolar lavage from fibrosis patients (ANTIONIADES et al. 1990; IYONAGA et al. 1994). The effect is recruitment and activation of lymphocytes, eosinophils and macrophages. MIP-1α also modifies ICAM-1 expression, while MCP-1 stimulates the expression of CD11b and CD11c by monocytes (JIANG et al. 1992; STANDIFORD et al. 1995). Neutralizing antibodies against MIP-1α reduce bleomycin-induced fibrosis (SMITH et al. 1994).

Interleukin-8 (IL-8), increased prior to development of fibrosis (DONELLY et al. 1993), is mainly produced by macrophages, attracts and activates neutrophils, and hence indirectly results in production of proteases and leukotriene B4.

RANTES is produced by macrophages, eosinophils and epithelial cells in response to TNF-α and IL-1β, attracts monocytes and T lymphocytes and activates eosinophils. Increased levels were found in lavages from patients with idiopathic fibrosis (KODAMA et al. 1998).

3.7.4
Adhesion Molecules

Leukocyte and endothelial cell adhesion molecules are up-regulated by inflammatory mediators in areas of active inflammation within the fibrotic tissue. *Intercellular adhesion molecule-1* (ICAM-1), expressed on endothelial cells, is essential for the adherence of CD11a/CD18-positive inflammatory cells. Anti-CD11 antibodies inhibit the manifestation of bleomycin-induced fibrosis (PIGUET et al. 1993). Recently, it could be shown that irradiated ICAM-1 knock-out mice, in comparison to ICAM-1 wild type mice, had significantly lower leukocyte numbers in the lung and also developed less pulmonary fibrosis (HALLAHAN et al. 2002).

Integrins regulate, via interaction between parenchymal cells and extracellular matrix (ECM), cellular proliferation, migration and ECM production. They are expressed on all major cell types involved in fibrosis development. Definition of the precise role of integrins in radiation-induced lung fibrosis requires further research (TOOMEY et al. 2001).

3.8
The Role of Superoxide

Recently, it was demonstrated that gene therapy with plasmid/liposome or adenovirus delivery of *manganese superoxide dismutase* (MnSOD) transgene to the lungs of mice resulted in protection from early cytokine changes and development of fibrosis at 150 days after irradiation (EPPERLY et al. 1998, 1999; ZWACKA et al. 1998). This suggests a role of the reactive oxygen species, produced by a variety of cell types in response to stimulation, in the development of acute and late radiation effects in the lung. MnSOD gene therapy modulates the expression of IL-1 as well as of TGF-β (EPPERLY et al. 1999).

3.9
Conclusion

In conclusion, biological research during the recent years has resulted in a substantial increase in our knowledge of the processing and the structural manifestation of radiation effects in the lung. The response of this organ to radiation exposure represents a complex scenario in which a variety of cell types are involved, which interact via a large variety of mediators in an extremely complex network (Fig. 3.3). At present, there is no closed pathogenetic circuit detectable, which would allow for effective therapeutic intervention into the processes underlying the clinical manifestation of lung reactions to radiotherapy. Interruption of one of the potentially involved cascades of events, e.g. TGF-β signalling, might probably result in modification of the response, but not necessarily in amelioration or even prevention.

Detailed knowledge of the individual pathogenetic steps requires further experimental studies, in vitro and in relevant animal models, which must comprise modern molecular biological techniques. This knowledge will then result in novel treatment approaches, in addition to those, which are currently tested experimentally or clinically, like MnSOD gene therapy, anti-ICAM-1 antibodies, etc. However, it must be demonstrated carefully, in appropriate models including experimental animal tumours, that these new protocols for the prevention of treatment of lung injury are selective for normal tissue.

References

Adamson IYR, Bowden DH (1983) Endothelial injury and repair in radiation-induced pulmonary fibrosis. Am J Pathol 112:224–230

Adamson IYR, Bowden DH, Wyatt JP (1970) A pathway to pulmonary fibrosis: an ultrastructural study of mouse and rat following radiation to the whole body and hemithorax. Am J Pathol 58:481–487

Anscher MS, Kong FM, Andrews K, Clough R, Marks LB, Bentel G, Jirtle RL (1998) Plasma transforming growth factor beta1 as a predictor of radiation pneumonitis. Int J Radiat Oncol Biol Phys 41:1029–1035

Antoniades HN, Bravo MA, Avila RE, Galanopoulos T, Neville-Golden J, Maxwell M, Selman M (1990) Platelet-derived growth factor in idiopathic pulmonary fibrosis. J Clin Invest 86:1055–1064

Basset F, Ferrans VJ, Soler P, Takemura T, Fukuda Y, Crystal RG (1986) Intraluminal fibrosis in interstitial lung disorders. Am J Pathol 122:443–461

Bennett DE, Million RR, Ackerman IV (1969) Bilateral radiation pneumonitis. A complication of the radiotherapy of bronchogenic carcinoma. Cancer 23:1001–1018

Burger A, Loffler H, Bamberg M, Rodemann HP (1998) Molecular and cellular basis of radiation fibrosis. Int J Radiat Biol 73:401–408

Dörr W, Herrmann T (2002) Akute Strahlenveränderungen der Gewebe. In: Bamberg M, Molls M, Sack H (eds) Radio-Onkologie, 5th edn. Zuckschwerdt, Munich

Dörr W, Baumann M, Herrmann T (2000) Radiation-induced lung damage: a challenge for radiation biology, experimental and clinical radiotherapy. Int J Radiat Biol 76:443–446

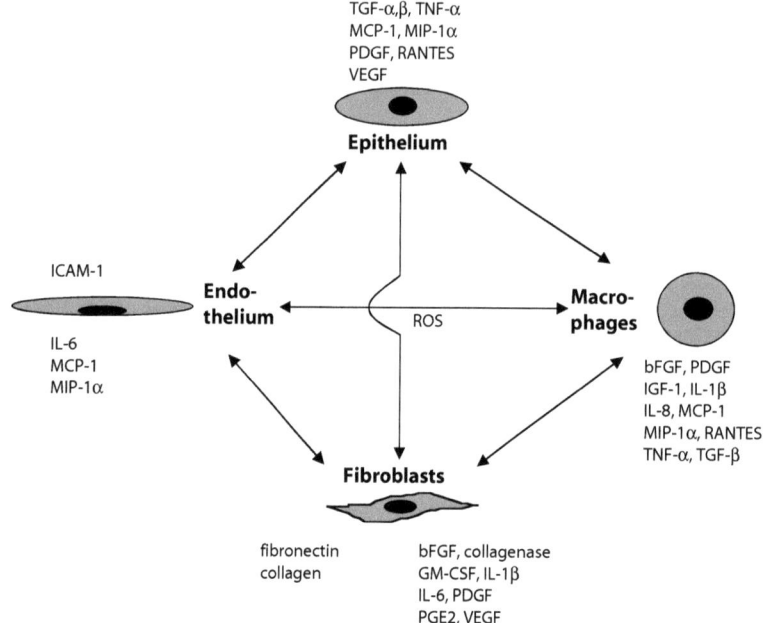

Fig. 3.3. Cell populations dominating the radiation response in lung tissue, i.e. epithelial cells, fibroblasts, endothelial cells and macrophages, and their most important mediators. For abbreviations see text. Reactive oxygen species (ROS) are produced by a large variety of cells. Intense interaction between the various cell types establishes a complex network

Donnelly SC, Strieter RM, Kunkel SL, Walz A, Robertson CR, Carter DC, Grant IS, Pollok AJ, Haslett C (1993) Interleukin-8 and development of adult respiratory distress syndrome in at-risk patient groups. Lancet 341:643-647

Epperly MW, Bray JA, Krager S, Berry LM, Gooding W, Engelhardt JF, Zwacka R, Travis EL, Greenberger JS (1998) Intratracheal injection of adenovirus containing the human MnSOD transgene protects athymic nude mice from irradiation-induced organizing alveolitis. Int J Radiat Oncol Biol Phys 1999 43:169-181

Epperly MW, Travis EL, Sikora C, Greenberger JS (1999) Manganese (correction of Magnesium) superoxide dismutase (MnSOD) plasmid/liposome pulmonary radioprotective gene therapy: modulation of irradiation-induced mRNA for IL-I, TNF-alpha, and TGF-beta correlates with delay of organizing alveolitis/fibrosis. Biol Blood Marrow Transpl 5:204-214

Evans ML, Graham MM, Mahler PA, Rasey JS (1986) Changes in vascular permeability following thorax irradiation in the rat. Radiat Res 107:262-271

Fajardo LFL-G, Berthrong M, Andrson RE (2001) Radiation pathology. Oxford University Press, Oxford, pp 198-208

Fehrenbach H, Kasper M, Haase M, Schuh D, Müller M (1999) Differential immunolocalization of VEGF in rat and human adult lung, and in experimental rat lung fibrosis: light, fluorescence, and electron microscopy. Anat Rec 254:61-73

Fries KM, Felch ME, Phipps RP (1994) Interleukin-6 is an autocrine growth factor for murine lung fibroblast subsets. Am J Respir Cell Mol Biol 11:552-560

Fukuda Y, Ishizaki M, Masuda Y, Kimura G, Kawanami O, Masugi Y (1987) The role of intraalveolar fibrosis in the process of pulmonary structural remodeling in patients with diffuse alveolar damage. Am J Pathol 126:171-182

Gross NJ (1977) Pulmonary effects of radiation therapy. Ann Intern Med 129:81-92

Hakenjos L, Bamberg M, Rodemann HP (2000) TGF-beta1-mediated alterations of rat lung fibroblast differentiation resulting in the radiation-induced fibrotic phenotype. Int J Radiat Biol 76:503-509

Hallahan DE, Geng L, Shyr Y (2002) Effects of intercellular adhesion molecule 1 (ICAM-1) null mutation on radiation-induced pulmonary fibrosis and respiratory insufficiency in mice. J Natl Cancer Inst 94:733-741

Henke C, Marineili W, Jessurun J, Fox J, Harms D, Peterson M, Chiang L, Doran P (1993) Macrophage production of basic fibroblast growth factor in the fibroproliferative disorder of alveolar fibrosis after lung injury. Am J Pathol 143:1189-1199

Herrmann T, Knorr A (1995) Radiogenic lung reactions. Pathogenesis-prevention-therapy. Strahlenther Onkol 171:490-498

Hopewell JW, Rezvani M, Moustafa HF (2000) The pig as a model for the study of radiation effects on the lung. Int J Radiat Biol 76:447-452

Jiang Y, Beller DI, Frendl G, Graves DT (1992) Monocyte chemoattractant protein-1 regulates adhesion molecule expression and cytokine production in human monocytes. J Immunol 148:2423-2428

Iyonaga K, Takeya M, Saita N, Sakamoto O, Yoshimura T, Ando M, Takahashi K (1994) Monocyte chemoattractant protein-1 in idiopathic pulmonary fibrosis and other interstitial lung diseases. Hum Pathol 25:455-463

Kodama N, Yamaguchi E, Hizawa N, Furuya K, Kojima J, Oguri M, Takahashi T, Kawakami Y (1998) Expression of RANTES by bronchoalveolar lavage cells in nonsmoking patients with interstitial lung diseases. Am J Respir Cell Mol Biol 18:526-531

Kuwano K, Hagimoto N, Hara N (2001) Molecular mechanisms of pulmonary fibrosis and current treatment. Curr Mol Med 1:551-573

Madtes DK, Busby HK, Strandjord TP, Clark JG (1994) Expression of transforming growth factor-alpha and epidermal growth factor receptor is increased following bleomycin-induced lung injury in rats. Am J Respir Cell Mol Biol 11:540-551

Martin M, Lefaix J-L, Delanian S (2000) TGF-β1 and radiation fibrosis: a master switch and a specific therapeutic target? Int J Radiat Oncol Biol Phys 47:277-290

McDonald S, Rubin P, Phillips TL, Marks LB (1995) Injury to the lung from cancer therapy: clinical syndromes, measurable endpoints and potential scoring systems. Int J Radiat Oncol Biol Phys 31:1187-1203

Movsas B, Raffin TA, Epstein AH, Link CJ Jr (1997) Molecular mechanisms of pulmonary fibrosis and current treatment. Chest 111:1061-1076

Pesci A, Bertorelli G, Gabrielli M, Olivieri D (1993) Mast cells in fibrotic lung disorders. Chest 103:989-996

Philips TL (1966) An ultrastructural study of the development of radiation injury in the lung. Radiol 87:49-54

Piguet PF, Vesin C (1994) Treatment by human recombinant soluble TNF receptor of pulmonary fibrosis induced by bleomycin or silica in mice. Eur Respir J 7:515-518

Piguet PF, Collart MA, Grau GE, Kapanci Y, Vassalli PJ (1989) Tumor necrosis factor/cachectin plays a key role in bleomycin-induced pneumopathy and fibrosis. J Exp Med 170:655-663

Piguet PF, Rosen H, Vesin C, Grau GE (1993a) Effective treatment of the pulmonary fibrosis elicited in mice by bleomycin or silica with anti-CD-11 antibodies. Am Rev Respir Dis 147:435-441

Piguet PF, Ribaux C, Karpuz V, Grau GE, Kapanci Y (1993b) Expression and localization of tumor necrosis factor-alpha and its mRNA in idiopathic pulmonary fibrosis. Am J Pathol 143:651 655

Raghow R, Irish P, Kang AH (1989) Coordinate regulation of transforming growth factor beta gene expression and cell proliferation in hamster lungs undergoing bleomycin-induced pulmonary fibrosis. J Clin Invest 84:1836-1842

Raines EW, Dower SK, Ross R (1989) Interleukin-1 mitogenic activity for fibroblasts and smooth muscle cells is due to PDGF-AA. Science 243:393-396

Rodemann HP, Bamberg M (1995) Cellular basis of radiation-induced fibrosis. Radiother Oncol 35:83-90

Rom WN, Basset P, Fells GA, Nukiwa T, Trapnell BC, Crysal RG (1988) Alveolar macrophages release an insulin-like growth factor I-type molecule. J Clin Invest 82:1685-1693

Rubin P, Johnston CJ, Williams JP, McDonald S, Finkelstein JN (1995) A perpetual cascade of cytokines postirradiation leads to pulmonary fibrosis. Int J Radiat Oncol Biol Phys 33:99-109

Smith DR, Kunkel SL, Standiford TJ, Rolfe MW, Lynch JP III, Arenberg DA, Wilke CA, Burdick MD, Martinez FJ, Hampton JN, Whyte RI, Orringer MB, Strieter RM (1995) Increased interleukin-1 receptor antagonist in idiopathic pulmonary fibrosis. A compartmental analysis. Am J Respir Crit Care Med 151:1965-1973

Smith RE, Strieter RM, Phan SH, Lukacs NW, Huffnagle GB, Wilke CA, Burdick MD, Lincoln P, Evanoff H, Kunkel SL (1994) Production and function of murine macrophage inflammatory protein-1 alpha in bleomycin-induced lung injury. J Immunol 153:4704–4712

Spencer H (1968) Pathology of the lung, 2nd edn. Pergamon, Oxford, pp 472–478

Standiford TJ, Kunkel SL, Lukacs NW, Greenberger MJ, Danforth JM, Kunkel RG, Strieter RM (1995) Macrophage inflammatory protein-1 alpha mediates lung leukocyte recruitment, lung capillary leak, and early mortality in murine endotoxemia. J Immunol 155:1515–1524

Thrall RS, Scalise PJ (1995) Bleomycin. In: Phan SH, Thrall RS (eds) Pulmonary fibrosis. Dekker, New York

Toomey D, Condron C, Wu QD, Kay E, Harmey J, Broe P, Kelly C, Bouchier-Hayes D (2001) TFG-beta1 is elevated in breast cancer tissue and regulates nitric oxide production from a number of cellular sources during hypoxia re-oxygenation injury. Br J Biomed Sci 58:177–183

Ts'ao CH, Ward WF, Port CD (1983a) Radiation injury in the rat lung. I. Prostacyclin (PGI2) production, arterial perfusion and ultrastructure. Radiat Res 96:284–293

Ts'ao CH, Ward WF, Port CD (1983b) Radiation injury in the rat lung. III. Plasminogen activator and fibrinolytic inhibitor activities. Radiat Res 96:301–308

Wallace WA, Ramage EA, Lamb D, Howie SE (1995) A type 2 (Th2-like) pattern of immune response predominates in the pulmonary interstitium of patients with cryptogenic fibrosing alveolitis (CFA). Clin Exp Immunol 101:436–441

Ward WF, Solliday NH, Molteni A, Port CD (1983) Radiation injury in the rat lung. II. Angiotensin converting enzyme activity. Radiat Res 96:294–300

Zwacka RM, Dudus L, Epperly MW, Greenberger JS, Engelhardt JF (1998) Redox gene therapy protects human IB-3 lung epithelial cells against ionizing radiation-induced apoptosis. Hum Gene Ther 9:1381–1386

4 Strategies for Modification of the Radiation Response of the Lung

C. NIEDER

CONTENTS

4.1 Introduction 37
4.2 Risk Factors for Radiation-Induced Lung Changes, Dysfunction and Morbidity 38
4.2.1 Treatment of Lung Cancer 38
4.2.2 Treatment of Breast Cancer 40
4.3 Technical Aspects of Modern Treatment Planning for Thoracic Radiotherapy 40
4.4 Strategies for Response Modification 42
4.4.1 Angiotensin-Converting Enzyme Inhibitors and Other Antihypertensive Drugs 42
4.4.2 Pentoxifylline 43
4.4.3 Amifostine 43
4.4.4 Other Response-Modulating Agents 44
References 46

4.1
Introduction

Successful clinical application of radiation therapy to malignant tumors of the thoracic region represents a major challenge. On the one hand, many of the common tumors arise in this location, for example breast cancer, lung cancer, esophageal cancer and various types of lymphomas. Radiation therapy is an effective treatment modality for these diseases and dose-response curves have been characterized over the last decades. However, evidence from a large number of clinical trials led to paradigm changes that resulted in implementation of combination treatment protocols. These may include neoadjuvant, definitive and adjuvant radiochemotherapy with a variety of active compounds as well as hormonal treatment in breast cancer. On the other hand, organ systems with restricted radiation tolerance such as the cardiovascular system, spinal cord and lungs must be taken into consideration when planning thoracic radiation

C. NIEDER, MD
Department of Radiation Oncology, Klinikum rechts der Isar, Technical University Munich, Ismaninger Strasse 22, 81675 Munich, Germany

therapy. It has long been recognized that the lung is among the most radiosensitive organs in the human body, especially if a larger volume has to be included in the treatment fields.

Clinical radiation pneumonitis is a common acute side effect, occurring in 5%–20% of patients treated for lung cancer (HERRMANN and KNORR 1995; VUJASKOVIC et al. 2000). Both acute and delayed toxicity might add significantly to the overall morbidity of cancer treatment, with potentially severe consequences on daily activities and quality of life. This is particularly true for elderly or unfit patients with medically inoperable lung cancer. Under several clinical circumstances, lung toxicity might even result in mortality. This point has played a major role in the recent discussion on the usefulness of postoperative radiation treatment for non-small cell lung cancer (NSCLC) which has been discussed in more detail by SAWYER and BONNER (2000). The mortality rate of NSCLC patients with severe radiation pneumonitis is high, and survival is much shorter in patients with out-of-field radiation pneumonitis (WANG et al. 2002).

Integration of newly available additional agents into current multimodality treatment might have a profound influence on irreversible side effects and this must be taken into account when designing early clinical trials. The same holds true for radiation-dose escalation trials with established cytotoxic drugs. Basic research on radiation-induced lung reactions significantly improved our understanding of the molecular and cellular mechanisms underlying acute radiation pneumonitis and the tissue remodeling leading to lung fibrosis. The emerging role of mediators such as various adhesion molecules, cytokines and growth factors in the pathophysiological cascades is the subject of ongoing laboratory studies. Current radiobiological models are reviewed in depth in Chap. 2 and 3 of this book. The search for predictive factors of normal tissue radiosensitivity has been hampered by, for example, the clinical feasibility of such tests and the prolongation of time to treatment. For example, DILETO and TRAVIS (1996) did not find a correlation between in vitro radiosensitivity of lung fibroblasts as assayed by survival at 2 Gy with the development of lung fibrosis in their mouse model. Serum marker evaluations are currently under investigation. The following paragraphs deal with translational research data, clinical strategies of response modification and response prediction.

4.2 Risk Factors for Radiation-Induced Lung Changes, Dysfunction and Morbidity

4.2.1 Treatment of Lung Cancer

Risk factors may roughly be divided into patient-associated (age, etc.), comorbidity-associated (emphysema, chronic obstructive pulmonary disease, etc.) and treatment-associated (Table 4). After curative radiation therapy for lung cancer, 40% of patients in a large series of 935 patients from different European Organisation for the Research and Treatment of Cancer (EORTC) studies were free from complications after 4 years. Mean time to late toxicity was 13 months. Age was not a significant risk factor (Pignon et al. 1998). The incidence of clinical radiation pneumonitis was increased for patients with low performance status, comorbid lung disease, smoking history, low pulmonary function tests, and

Table 4.1. Risk factors and predictive factors for radiation-induced lung damage derived from clinical trials

Treatment-associated factors	Other factors
Mean lung dose	Reduced performance status
V20 or V30	Comorbid lung disease
Contralateral lung dose (?)	Low pulmonary function tests
Dose per fraction	Smoking history (except in breast cancer)
Fractions per day	Genetic determinants
NTCP model indices	High IL-1, IL-6 or maybe TGF-beta
Chemotherapy (especially high-dose or certain drugs such as paclitaxel)	Age (?, perhaps only in breast cancer)
Tamoxifen	Inflammatory disease (?) Diabetes mellitus (?)

V20: lung volume receiving +20 Gy
NTCP normal tissue complication probability; *IL* interleukin TGF-beta: transforming growth factor-beta; *?* influence not proven

for those patients who were treated with primary rather than adjuvant radiotherapy (Monson et al. 1998).

Geara et al. (1998) examined a group of 25 patients with small cell lung cancer (SCLC) who had serial computerized tomography (CT) examinations of the chest after combined chemoradiotherapy. The severity of lung fibrosis was recorded for each patient from the CT images using an arbitrary scale at 1 year after treatment. Radiographic fibrosis scores were recorded on one to three CT slices in three different dose areas (20–30 Gy, 30–40 Gy; and >40 Gy) that were defined using the corresponding CT slices from the patient's CT treatment plan. Of these patients, 23 (92%) had at least two slices scored; 11 patients had all three slices scored. Among the clinical and treatment parameters investigated (including type of chemotherapy), only total dose and fractionation schedule were identified as significant and independent determinants of lung fibrosis. Radiographic fibrosis scores were higher in high-dose areas and among patients treated with an accelerated radiation therapy schedule. Using a fit of the proportional odds (PO) model based on the total dose and fractionation schedule, fibrosis score residuals were calculated for each patient. The residual for each score was defined as the difference between the observed and expected score based on the dose and treatment schedule received. Average residuals varied significantly among patients. Using a modified version of the PO model, the coefficient of variation in patient heterogeneity was estimated to be 10.1% (95% confidence interval, 6.2%–14.9%). Inclusion of the heterogeneity factor, in addition to total dose and fractionation schedule, improved the fit of the PO model to an extremely high level of significance. These data indicate that the risk and severity of lung fibrosis analyzed radiographically on CT images increases with total dose and with the use of an accelerated radiation schedule, for patients treated with chemoradiation for SCLC. There was also demonstrable patient-to-patient heterogeneity, suggesting that the risk of lung fibrosis is strongly affected by inherent factors that vary among individuals. Experimental data on radiosensitivity of mouse lungs of two inbred strains of mice, shown to differ markedly in their susceptibility to radiation-induced lung fibrosis, also indicate genetic determinants of variability in normal tissue reactions (Dileto and Travis 1996).

It is common practice to evaluate treatment-associated risk factors on the basis of dose–volume histograms (DVH), which, however, are generated with considerable interinstitutional differences with regard to contouring and planning algorithms. Differences in imaging protocols and breathing instructions might also contribute to heterogeneity. A large study of three-dimensional (3D) conformal radiation therapy in 201 patients (19% developed pneumonitis) by HERNANDO et al. (2001) concluded that dosimetric factors were the best predictors of pneumonitis. Clinical parameters did not substantially improve accuracy of mean lunge dose (Table 4.2), V30 (volume exposed to 30 Gy) and normal tissue complication probability (NTCP) models (Lyman and Kutcher models). Data from Memorial Sloan Kettering Cancer Center on 49 patients with NSCLC were reported by YORKE et al. (2002a). 3D conformal radiation therapy to doses ranging from 57.6 to 81 Gy was administered. Acute lung toxicity data were correlated with various parameters. Yet only nine patients had Radiation Therapy Oncology Group (RTOG) grade 3 or higher pneumonitis. For the whole lung, grade 3 or higher toxicity was significantly correlated with mean dose and Lyman and parallel NTCP model indices. It was significantly correlated with these indices and with V20 for the ipsilateral lung and with mean dose and effective dose for the inferior half of the lungs. The same parameters were also analyzed for the superior half of the lungs and the contralateral lung, yet no significant influence was seen.

CHEN et al. (2002) measured plasma cytokine levels before, during and after thoracic radiotherapy by enzyme-linked immunosorbent assays (ELISA) in 24 patients. Thirteen had symptomatic radiation pneumonitis grade 2 according to common toxicity criteria (CTC). They found significant elevations of interleukin (IL)-1alpha and IL-6 compared to the patients without such side effects. Other cytokines, including basic fibroblast growth factor (bFGF) and transforming growth factor (TGF)-beta1 did not correlate with pneumonitis. A dose-escalation study by ANSCHER et al. (2001) used TGF-beta for monitoring of toxicity risk. Patients with locally advanced or medically inoperable NSCLC received 3D conformal radiation therapy to the primary tumor and radiographically involved nodes to a dose of 73.6 Gy (1.6 Gy twice daily). If the plasma TGF-beta level was normal after 73.6 Gy, additional twice daily radiation therapy was delivered at successively higher total doses. Thirty-eight patients were enrolled. Twenty-four patients were not eligible for radiation dose escalation beyond 73.6 Gy because of persistently abnormal TGF-beta levels. Fourteen patients whose TGF-beta levels were normal after 73.6 Gy were escalated to 80 Gy ($n=8$) and 86.4 Gy ($n=6$). At the highest dose level, two patients developed grade 3 late toxicity. This strategy was based on their finding that patients whose TGF-beta-1 level was higher at the end of radiation therapy than at the beginning were at higher risk of toxicity than other patients (FU et al. 2001). The same group investigated loss of heterozygosity (LOH) at the mannose 6-phosphate/insulin-like growth factor-2 receptor (*M6P/IGF2R*) gene locus (KONG et al. 2001). Twelve of 13 patients with LOH had increased pre-treatment plasma TGF-beta-1 levels vs 3 of 12 patients without LOH ($p<0.01$). A decrease or loss of M6P/IGF2R protein in the malignant cell accompanied by increased latent TGF-beta-1 protein in extracellular matrix and tumor stroma was found in tumors with LOH, suggesting that this mutation resulted in loss of function of the receptor (Fig. 4.1). Seven of 13 (54%) LOH patients developed symptomatic radiation-induced lung injury (CTC) vs 1 of 12 (8%) of patients without LOH ($p=0.05$). In another report, 19 of 86 patients who received thoracic radiation treatment to 30–76 Gy developed symptomatic pneumonitis according to CTC (SASAKI et al. 2001). The authors found that monitoring serum surfactant protein D by ELISA might facilitate early diagnosis of pneumonitis.

Table 4.2. Rate of lung toxicity at different levels of mean lung dose (MLD) for patients from 4 studies (patients from different institutions included in the study by KWA et al.)

Author	Number of patients	Rate of lung toxicity in %			
		MLD 5-10 Gy	MLD 11-20 Gy	MLD 21-30 Gy	MLD >30 Gy
KWA et al. 1998	400 (paired organ analysis)*	8%	16%	35%	40%
OETZEL et al. 1995	66 (separate organ analysis)	0%	13%	30%	43%
GRAHAM et al. 1999	99 (paired organ analysis)	0%	9%	24%	25%
HERNANDO et al. 2001	201 (paired organ analysis)	10%	16%	27%	44%

* both lungs regarded as a single organ

Non LOH　　　　　　　　　LOH

Fig. 4.1. Immunofluorescence staining for latent (LAP) TGF-beta-1. Immunofluorescence staining for LAP-TGFbeta-1 in patients without loss of heterozygosity (LOH) and with LOH is shown. LAP-TGF-beta-1 staining (*green*) was located predominantly in the tumor cell (*T*) in patients without LOH and predominantly in the stromal cells (*S*) in the LOH patients. Tissues were counterstained with propidium iodide, X500. Reproduced with permission from Kong et al. (2001)

4.2.2
Treatment of Breast Cancer

High-dose chemotherapy with stem cell rescue largely failed to improve the outcome in breast cancer. Notably, the incidence of pneumonitis appears to be higher in patients who receive radiation therapy after such intense pretreatment. Lind et al. described serial lung function tests (forced expiratory volume at one second, diffusing capacity of carbon monoxide) in 68 patients. Complications grade 2 or higher (World Health Organization [WHO] classification) occurred in 46% and were correlated with several potential predictive factors. Preradiotherapy function test values did not predict subsequent development of pneumonitis. However, if no recovery from nadir value of diffusing capacity of carbon monoxide after carmustine-based high-dose therapy was seen, complications occurred more frequently. The same holds true for shorter intervals between chemotherapy and radiation therapy.

Besides high-dose chemotherapy, concurrent treatment with radiation therapy and certain cytotoxic agents might increase the risk of pulmonary toxicity. For example, there was a rate of 20% radiation pneumonitis in a small study of paclitaxel during radiation treatment following doxorubicin-containing combinations (Hanna et al. 2002). Sequential chemotherapy as well as concurrent tamoxifen did not significantly influence the risk of lung toxicity in the study by Wennberg et al. (2002). They evaluated the course of 121 patients and performed CT scans before and 4 months after radiation therapy. Changes in mean lung density in the anterior third of the central CT slice correlated with clinical pneumonitis. Changes in the apical part of the lung had no appreciable influence. Furthermore, age but not smoking habits significantly influenced density changes. Radiation doses of 16–30 Gy were associated with CT abnormality.

Different results were obtained by Huang et al. (2000). They analyzed 109 patients treated after modified radical mastectomy. The patients received single-portal electron-beam treatment to the chest wall and lymphatics to 46–50.4 Gy plus or minus chemotherapy (CMF or CEF). Follow-up included regular chest X-rays. According to the RTOG/EORTC score, 29% of patients developed grade 1 pulmonary fibrosis. More severe lung changes were not found. Risk factors were evaluated in uni- and multivariate tests. However, risk factors could be determined only for the group treated without chest wall bolus because bolus use significantly reduced the incidence of fibrosis. Significant factors included lower body mass index and use of tamoxifen, but not age, diabetes, hypertension or chemotherapy. A potential contribution of tamoxifen to the development of lung fibrosis has already been discussed by Bentzen et al. (1996). Interestingly, smoking apparently depresses the frequency of radiation-induced pneumonitis in breast and esophageal cancer patients (Bjermer et al. 1990; Johansson et al. 1998).

4.3
Technical Aspects of Modern Treatment Planning for Thoracic Radiotherapy

Despite all the advances in imaging technology, definition of the appropriate gross tumor volume (GTV) and microscopic tumor extension remains the basic prerequisite of successful radiation treatment planning. What needs to be included in the clinical target volume (CTV) in an individual patient is not always perfectly clear. In addition, organ and patient movement represents a major obstacle in creating small planning target volumes (PTV) for thoracic radiation therapy. The first steps in treatment planning should be based on rational concepts, which should be derived from a careful and comprehensive pattern of failure and organ movement studies. SENAN et al. (2002) recently published an analysis of recurrences in 50 patients with stage III NSCLC treated with sequential chemotherapy and conventionally fractionated 3D conformal radiotherapy to 70 Gy. The GTV consisted of the prechemotherapy tumor volume and lymph nodes with a short-axis diameter of 1 cm or more. This strategy was considered involved-field radiotherapy by the authors. While in-field recurrence was common and distant metastases were detected during follow-up in 18% of patients, no elective nodal failure was observed. In the larger series by ROSENZWEIG et al. (2001), 171 patients with NSCLC had been treated with 3D conformal radiotherapy. Only lymph node regions initially involved with tumor either by biopsy (55%) or radiographic criteria (node +15 mm in the short axis on CT) were included in the CTV. Elective nodal failure was defined as a recurrence in an initially uninvolved lymph node in the absence of local failure. Only 11 patients (6.4%) with elective nodal failure were identified. With a median follow-up of 21 months in survivors, the 2-year actuarial rates of elective nodal control and primary tumor control were 91% and 38%, respectively. Thus, omitting elective mediastinal irradiation did result in very low rates of isolated nodal failure, yet facilitates dose-escalation studies by reducing lung exposure. These facts contributed to the increasing acceptance of omitting elective nodal treatment.

PTVs derived using slow CT scans consistently produce superior target coverage than those using conventional scans (VAN SORNSEN DE KOSTE et al. 2001). In their study, a conventional planning CT scan and two limited scans of the tumor region were performed in seven patients with peripheral tumors. Three slow scans (slice thickness 4 mm, index 3 mm, revolution time 4 s/slice) were then performed, followed by 3D image registration. Methods to improve target coverage also include real-time tumor tracking by means of insertion of a gold marker using bronchofiberscopy (HARADA et al. 2002). Treatment planning might be improved further by taking advantage of physiological information complementing the information obtainable from CT scans, such as lung perfusion. The latter method was found to correlate with reduction in pulmonary function tests (FAN et al. 2001; THEUWS et al. 2000). A recent study of a virtual phantom and five patients with NSCLC at the Netherlands Cancer Institute used perfusion-weighted dose–volume histograms after a planning procedure where the weight of the beams that were directed through the hypoperfused lung regions was increased in order to optimize lung exposure (SEPPENWOOLDE et al. 2002). It was possible to create clinically well applicable treatment plans causing less toxicity to functioning lung for patients with large perfusion defects.

Functional imaging by positron emission tomography, for example with the tracer fluorodeoxyglucose, has also been shown to alter the target volume definition in lung cancer in a high proportion of patients (VANUYTSEL et al. 2000; ERDI et al. 2002).

Dose escalation might be accomplished by several different strategies. Among these, there is the deep inspiration breath-hold technique which, compared to free-breathing CT planning showed decreased target coverage, but higher radiation doses without violating normal tissue constraints (YORKE et al. 2002b). In this Monte Carlo dose calculation example of five NSCLC patients, where margins were not reduced despite more degradation of target coverage, higher total doses to GTV and greater than 99% PTV could be administered. The advantage of the deep inspiration breath-hold technique has also been described by ROSENZWEIG et al. (2000). Another method is the use of hypofractionated stereotactic radiotherapy for relatively small targets. Initial results suggest encouraging local control without intolerable toxicity for carefully selected patients (WULF et al. 2001; NAGATA et al. 2002). The use of intensity-modulated radiation therapy (IMRT) might not necessarily result in improved lung sparing, as shown in a planning example for esophageal cancer (NUTTING et al. 2001). With IMRT, the planning results are highly dependent on technique.

In adjuvant radiotherapy after breast-conserving surgery, CT-based 3D treatment planning for conformal tangential irradiation is increasingly being used. When less than 2–2.5 cm of the lung are included inside the treatment fields, the risk for pulmonary morbidity is expected to be very low, i.e. less than 1% (MUREN et al. 2002). Nevertheless, several institutions have started to investigate the use of IMRT in such patients, a more complex and often time-consuming technique. In the study by HURKMANS et al. (2002) of 17 left-sided breast cancer patients, the NTCP for radiation pneumonitis ranged from 0.3%–0.5% with IMRT vs non-IMRT 3D planning. However, the probability of cardiac toxicity was significantlyr educed.

4.4
Strategies for Response Modification

In clinical routine, strategies are based on avoiding morbidity by means of advanced treatment planning and on treating symptomatic pneumonitis in those patients where it occurs with a course of corticosteroid treatment with or without antibiotics. Lung fibrosis is a chronic state of damage and established methods for amelioration are not yet available. In 1990, GRAHAM et al. studied the prospects of rather nonspecific pharmacological alteration of lung reactions after radiation therapy. Lungs of rats exposed to single-dose hemithorax irradiation were evaluated. Thirteen different drugs were studied. Dexamethasone, indomethacin, cromolyn, cyproheptadine, Vitamin D3, theophylline, and diethylcarbamazine were all effective at reducing vascular-mediated lung damage on the irradiated side. Further data on some of these agents are discussed in Sect. 4.4.4. Besides pharmacological intervention, hyperfractionation might increase the therapeutic ratio (PENNEY et al. 1994; ROACH et al. 1995; ITOH et al. 1999). Bearing the progress in cellular and molecular research on radiation reactions in mind, a very important question is how many crucial early events that need to be targeted eventually cause lung toxicity and how specific any type of prevention or intervention must be.

4.4.1
Angiotensin-Converting Enzyme Inhibitors and Other Antihypertensive Drugs

In experimental settings mRNA production of TGF-b1 in the lungs of C57Bl6 mice after low-dose whole-body irradiation was determined (OLEJAR et al. 2000). Control (irradiated) and irradiated angiotensin-converting enzyme (ACE) inhibitor-treated animals were simultaneously examined. The ACE inhibitor group received butylaminiperindopril for 9 days after irradiation (7 Gy) at a daily dose of 0.1 mg/kg per rectum. On day 9 all mice were killed and the production of mRNA TGF-beta-1 in lung tissue was determined semiquantitatively. In butylaminiperindopril-treated mice, a decrease in transcript of TGF-beta-1 (to 59% in comparison with controls) was observed. Another group of researchers exposed rats to a single dose of either 20 or 30 Gy to a hemithorax port (MOLTENI et al. 2000). Perfusion scans and autopsies were performed at intervals up to 12 months after radiation. Three different ACE inhibitors and penicillamine were given as radiation protectors and their activity compared. All drugs were administered in the rats' drinking water. In the irradiated rats, pulmonary damage progressed to severe arteritis and interstitial collagen deposition at 3 months, and then on to severe pneumonitis and extensive pulmonary fibrosis at 6 months. A marked increase in hydroxyproline was also found in the lungs at 6 months. These morphological changes were associated with a significant decrease in ACE and plasminogen activator activity (PLA) and a marked increase of prostaglandins (PGI2) and thromboxane (TXA2), substances considered as indicators of endothelial pulmonary damage. ACE inhibitors prevented the markers of endothelial dysfunction. Penicillamine, a sulfhydryl-containing compound with weak ACE inhibitory activity was also a strong antifibrotic agent but showed only modest anti-inflammatory activity.

A study where patients taking ACE inhibitors while receiving radiation therapy for lung cancer with curative intent at Duke University Medical Center was reported by WANG et al. (2000). Of the 213 patients, 26 (12.2%) were on ACE inhibitors (usually for the management of hypertension) during radiotherapy. Patients were irradiated with total doses of 50–80 Gy. After treatment, patients were generally followed every 3 months for 2 years, then every 6 months thereafter. Symptomatic radiation pneumonitis was scored according to modified CTC (i.e., radiographic changes alone were not sufficient for the diagnosis of pneumonitis). There was no difference in the incidence of pneumonitis between the two groups. Fifteen percent of the patients on ACE inhibitors developed symptomatic radiation-induced lung injury compared to 12% of the patients not receiving these drugs. Comparable findings were published by FLECKENSTEIN et al. (2000) who retrospectively evaluated the NSCLC patients included in a randomized trial of two different radiation treatment schedules. In conclusion, within the dose range prescribed for treating hypertension, ACE inhibitors do not appear to either decrease the incidence or delay the onset of symptomatic radiation pneumonitis among lung cancer patients. However, this evidence is based on retrospective data only and several different drugs were included.

Carvedilol, an antihypertensive drug with activity on adrenoceptors as well as on calcium channel activity, has also been investigated with irradiation in vitro as well as in vivo (JONSSON et al. 1999). A daily injection of carvedilol in clinically relevant concentrations (3 mg/kg subcutaneously), 4 days before and 3 days after a single radiation dose of 20 Gy significantly decreased the inflammatory reaction in the rat lung, evaluated as the number of inflammatory cells in the perivascular area. The density of mast cells was also slightly reduced. In vitro studies revealed that carvedilol caused different radioprotective effects, dependent on dose (1–7 Gy) used and cell line studied. The effects were especially pronounced in a malignant mesothelioma cell line, and somewhat less evident in a prostatic carcinoma cell line. No significant effect was seen in a highly radiosensitive small cell lung cancer cell line. Thus, it remains questionable from these data whether carvedilol truly could improve the therapeutic ratio.

4.4.2
Pentoxifylline

Pentoxifylline down-regulates the production of proinflammatory cytokines, particularly tumor necrosis factor (TNF)-alpha, in response to noxious stimuli and may therefore provide protection against radiation-induced, cytokine-mediated cellular damage. RUBE et al. (2002) investigated the temporal and spatial release of TNF-alpha in the lung tissue of C57BL/6J mice after thoracic irradiation with a single fraction of 12 Gy. In addition, they evaluated the ability of the drug to reduce the radiation-induced TNF-alpha release in this animal model. The TNF-alpha mRNA expression in the lung tissue was quantified by real-time quantitative reverse transcriptase polymerase chain reaction (RT-PCR). Immunohistochemical detection methods and automated image analysis were used for objective quantification of TNF-alpha protein expression. Following thoracic irradiation with a single dose of 12 Gy, radiation-induced TNF-alpha mRNA release in the lung tissue was significantly increased during the acute phase of pneumonitis. The elevated levels of TNF-alpha mRNA during the pneumonic phase correlated with a significant increase in positive inflammatory cells, predominantly macrophages, in the lung parenchyma. In contrast to the radiation-only group, the lung tissue of the pentoxifylline-treated mice showed only a minor radiation-mediated TNF-alpha response on mRNA and protein level. Therefore, the results indicate that pentoxifylline down-regulates the TNF-alpha mRNA and protein production in the lung tissue in response to radiation.

In 1992, WARD et al. performed experiments in rats which were exposed to single doses of radiation to one hemithorax. Half of each dose group consumed only a regular diet, and half consumed feed containing pentoxifylline (50 mg/kg/day). Two months after irradiation the animals were killed and pulmonary endothelial function was monitored by the activity of lung ACE and PLA, and by production of PGI2 and TXA2. The amount of hydroxyproline in the lung served as an index of pulmonary fibrosis. Radiation produced a dose-dependent decrease in ACE and PLA activity in the treated lung and an increase in the production of PGI2 and TXA2. This endothelial dysfunction was accompanied by an increase in wet weight and in protein and hydroxyproline content in the irradiated lung. Pentoxifylline spared only the increase in lung wet weight and protein content, and actually elevated the radiation-induced hyperproduction of PGI2 and TXA2. Thus, contradictory preclinical data have been published.

In a clinical phase III trial, 64 patients with stage I–III NSCLC were randomly divided into a pentoxifylline plus radiotherapy group and a radiotherapy alone group (KWON et al. 2000). However, only 47 patients who had measurable tumors on chest X-ray views were included in the analysis. A total dose of 65–70 Gy was delivered as conventional fractionated radiation schedule. Pentoxifylline was given to the patients 3×400 mg/day, with a daily dose of 1200 mg during treatment for the purpose of sensitizing tumor cells. The median time to relapse in the drug plus radiation therapy group was 11 months, which was 2 months longer than for the radiation therapy alone group ($p>0.05$). All the patients in both groups showed lower than or equal to grade 2 dysphagia, odynophagia, pulmonary fibrosis, and pneumonitis. The median survival was 18 months in the pentoxifylline group and 7 months in the radiation therapy alone group. Survival differences were not statistically significant. This study suggests that pentoxifylline could be a modestly effective radiation sensitizer for the treatment of NSCLC. Protection against toxicity needs to be addressed in further trials.

4.4.3
Amifostine

Currently, both experimental and clinical data suggest a possible role of amifostine (WR-2721) for radioprotection of the lung. In a rat model of fractionated lung irradiation (five daily fractions of 7 Gy), amifostine was administered intraperitoneally at a dose of 150 mg/kg (Vujaskovic et al. 2002a). Follow-up was 6 months. Compared to radiation alone, radiation plus amifostine resulted in a significant delay in increased breathing frequency and a significantly lower peak. Hydroxyproline content was also significantly lower. The plasma TGF-beta levels after irradiation were significantly lower in the group that received the drug. Further data from this group suggest that amifostine also reduces the accumulation of macrophages after irradiation (Vujaskovic et al. 2002b). In addition, mammary adenocarcinoma-bearing animals were treated in these experiments. Tumor growth delay and regrowth rate after radiation therapy were not significantly different. These data suggest both efficacy of amifostine in reducing functional and histological lung injury and the usefulness of TGF-beta for monitoring intervention strategies. In contrast, inhaled aerosol of amifostine failed to influence the development of radiation-induced lung damage at 14–16 weeks as assessed by a rise in the breathing rate in the mouse by Lockhart (1990).

Amifostine has been studied clinically in phase I/II studies of radiochemotherapy (Koukourakis et al. 2002), where it was administered subcutaneously at 500 mg. However, the nature of such studies is less conclusive than randomized trials such as those reported by Antonadou (2002). The first one included 146 patients with NSCLC treated with conventional radiation therapy to a maximum dose of 60 Gy and randomized to either 340 mg/m^2 amifostine or no radioprotection. Grade 2 or higher pneumonitis occurred in 9% vs 43%. Significant reduction was also seen for fibrosis rate at 6 months, whereas tumor response was unchanged. Comparable results were obtained in a smaller randomized trial of 45 patients who received the same radiotherapy schedule after platinum-based induction chemotherapy. The randomized study by Komaki et al. (2002) was different with respect to radiation therapy (two daily fractions of 1.2 Gy up to a total dose of 69.6 Gy), chemotherapy (concurrent) and administration of amifostine (500 mg IV twice weekly). Nonetheless, in this trial of 60 NSCLC patients, acute pneumonitis was also significantly reduced. In conclusion, important open questions (also related to cost) regarding the dose and schedule of application for lung protection remain to be resolved in further randomized studies. One of these is the ongoing phase III trial RTOG 98-01. As recently reviewed, the selectivity of amifostine for normal tissue is still a matter of debate (Lindegaard and Grau 2000). This is one more reason to continue with prospective clinical trials before recommending a widespread use. Another aspect when a costly prevention strategy is being considered is the upfront ability to perform risk estimates that could help to avoid unnecessary treatment in low-risk groups.

4.4.4
Other Response-Modulating Agents

Ward et al. (1993) used a model of bilateral radiation-induced lung disease in the rat to study the effects of corticosteroids. This model is characterized by interstitial edema at 2 weeks after treatment followed by florid alveolitis with an alveolar protein leak, which peaks at 4 weeks. Mast cell density peaks at 7 weeks, and there is a progressive increase in lung collagen (fibrosis) from 5–20 weeks. Intraperitoneal corticosteroids or saline were given at the time of irradiation or sham irradiation (protocol 1) every second day during weeks 3 and 4 (protocol 2), or three times weekly during weeks 3–8 (protocol 3). In protocol 1, steroids protected the lung from interstitial edema at 2 weeks, delayed the alveolitis without reducing its intensity, and significantly reduced the alveolar protein leak. However, radiation fibrosis was not reduced at 20 weeks. Longer steroid administration (protocol 2) suppressed the alveolar protein leak and delayed and significantly reduced the severity of the inflammatory cell response. Although the tissue mast cell and fibrotic responses were suppressed during and for at least 3 weeks after steroids, the ultimate fibrotic reaction was the same in both irradiated groups. In protocol 3, steroids suppressed the alveolitis and delayed the rise in tissue mast cell density, but did not affect the fibrotic response at 20 weeks. These studies suggest that steroids can suppress the alveolitis provided they are used throughout the period of alveolitis. Although they also delay the tissue mast cell response to radiation, the ultimate fibrosis is not altered. This is in concordance with observations from the management of radiation-induced lung disease in humans.

Protective effects of indomethacin, a prostaglandin-inhibiting agent, against early and late sequelae of radiation injury in mice were investigated by Milas et al. (1992). Radiation was delivered as a single dose. Indomethacin led to significant protection against radiation-induced pneumonitis (protection factor of 1.2). This protection was smaller than that observed with amifostine. However, indomethacin combined with amifostine produced a radioprotective effect greater than the radioprotection achieved by individual treatments. Compared to the use of cytotoxic treatment for tumor control, where combination strategies have shown their potential, combination treatment targeting several pathways for normal tissue protection has rarely been studied so far.

Besides the clinically investigated agents reviewed in Sect. 4.4, experimental strategies continue to evolve. Using a mouse model of radiation-induced lung toxicity, a monoclonal anti-CD40L antibody (MR1) that disrupts CD40–CD40L interactions was tested for the ability to reduce lung injury (ADAWI et al. 1998). C57BL/6 mice were pretreated with either nothing, MR1, or hamster immunoglobulin G (IgG) 24 h prior to a single dose of 15 Gy to the thorax. During the following 26 weeks, mice continued to receive MR1 or hamster IgG twice a week. MR1 protected against death from radiation pneumonitis and fibrosis and dramatically reduced lung pathology as evidenced by a limited influx of inflammatory cells, minimal collagen deposition, and septal thickening. MR1 also prevented radiation-induced pulmonary mastocytosis and blunted expression of cyclooxygenase-2, a proinflammatory enzyme responsible for prostaglandin synthesis.

An animal model of radiation-induced lung injury in the hamster and the effects of pretreatment with recombinant human CuZn superoxide dismutase (SOD) on the development of the lesion were evaluated by BREUER et al. (1992). Hamsters exposed to a single irradiation dose of 20 Gy delivered to the thorax were treated with 150 mg/kg body weight of SOD or saline intraperitoneally 75 min and subcutaneously 5 min before receiving irradiation. At 4, 8, and 16 weeks following irradiation, pulmonary injury was evaluated by the grading of morphological changes semiquantitatively, measurement of lung hydroxyproline content, and analysis of bronchoalveolar lavage fluid for total and differential cell counts and total protein concentration. Radiation-induced lung injury in saline-pretreated animals was documented at 16 weeks by histological morphology and increased protein in bronchoalveolar lavage fluid. SOD protected against radiation-induced pulmonary injury as indicated by the absence of severe histopathological changes and prevention of elevation in bronchoalveolar lavage protein levels.

EPPERLY et al. (2002) administered manganese superoxide dismutase-plasmid/liposome intratracheally 24 h before single-dose irradiation to both lungs in a mouse model and found a reduction in lung fibrosis. This treatment delayed the expression of vascular cell adhesion molecule-1 and intracellular adhesion molecule-1 (ICAM-1) which were first detectable in endothelial cells several months after irradiation, suggesting that the pulmonary vascular endothelium can be considered as a target for interventional strategies. Further arguments for studying agents that block ICAM-1 function or expression can be derived from the experiments in mice bearing a null mutation of ICAM-1, which had less pulmonary fibrosis than ICAM-1 (+/+) mice (HALLAHAN et al. 2002).

In the light of such data, it remains to be shown that Ukrain, an alkaloid thiophosphoric acid derivative of *Chelidonium majus* L., which has shown radioprotection of lung fibroblasts in early in vitro studies (CORDES et al. 2002), can lead to comparable findings. There is also a lack of confirmatory data on the effectiveness of vitamin A to reduce radiation-induced pneumonitis. This strategy was discussed by REDLICH et al. (1998), who performed dietary supplement studies in rats treated with 15 Gy whole-thorax irradiation. The same authors compared the survival of IL-11 and vehicle-treated control mice after 25 Gy of thoracic irradiation, and initiated studies to elucidate the mechanism of the observed protection. This dose of radiation killed 50% of the control mice during the first 2 weeks after irradiation. In contrast, the subcutaneous administration of rIL-11 resulted in significant radioprotection, with 89% of the IL-11-treated animals surviving the study interval. It was described that IL-11 inhibits both radiation-induced TNF mRNA expression in vivo and macrophage TNF protein production and mRNA accumulation in vitro (REDLICH et al. 1996).

Intravenous application of bFGF was initially reported to confer significant protection against death from radiation pneumonitis in C3H/HeJ mice (FUKS et al. 1995). Although the mechanism of this protection remained unclear, one hypothesis, based on in vitro data, was that bFGF protects against radiation-induced apoptosis in pulmonary endothelial cells. TEE and TRAVIS (1995) repeated the experiments in two strains of mice with differing sensitivities to radiation pneumonitis. One mouse strain, C3Hf/Kam, originated from the same C3H/He strain as the C3H/HeJ mouse used by FUKS et al. in their study. The other strain, the NCR/Sed-nu/+ strain, is a white mouse heterozygous for the nude trait. The LD50 for radiation pneumonitis between 12 and 28 weeks after irradiation, the standard assay time for this phase of radiation-induced lung damage, was

12.5 Gy in the C3Hf/Kam and 8.5 Gy in the NCR/Sed-nu/+ strain. Contrary to the previous results, it was found that bFGF did not protect against radiation pneumonitis in either C3Hf/Kam or NCR/Sed-nu/+ mice. Quantitation of apoptosis after both doses to the lungs of the two strains showed that the incidence of apoptosis was less than 1% in C3Hf/Kam mice and 0.5% in NCR/Sed-nu/+ mice.

References

Adawi A, Zhang Y, Baggs R et al (1998) Blockade of CD40–CD40 ligand interactions protects against radiation-induced pulmonary inflammation and fibrosis. Clin Immunol Immunopathol 89:222–230

Anscher MS, Marks LB, Shafman TD et al (2001) Using plasma transforming growth factor beta-1 during radiotherapy to select patients for dose escalation. J Clin Oncol 19:3758–3765

Antonadou D (2002) Radiotherapy or chemotherapy followed by radiotherapy with or without amifostine in locally advanced lung cancer. Semin Radiat Oncol 12 [Suppl 1]:50–58

Bentzen SM, Skoczylas JZ, Overgaard M et al (1996) Radiotherapy-related lung fibrosis enhanced by tamoxifen. J Natl Cancer Inst 88:918–922

Bjermer L, Franzen L, Littbrand B et al (1990) Effects of smoking and irradiated volume on inflammatory response in the lung of irradiated breast cancer patients evaluated with bronchoalveolar lavage. Cancer Res 50:2027–2030

Breuer R, Tochner Z, Conner MW et al (1992) Superoxide dismutase inhibits radiation-induced lung injury in hamsters. Lung 170:19–29

Chen Y, Williams J, Ding I et al (2002) Radiation pneumonitis and early circulatory cytokine markers. Semin Radiat Oncol 12 [Suppl 1]:26–33

Cordes N, Plasswilm L, Bamberg M et al (2002) Ukrain, an alkaloid thiophosphoric acid derivative of Chelidonium majus L. protects human fibroblasts but not human tumour cells in vitro against ionising radiation. Int J Radiat Biol 78:17–27

Dileto CL, Travis EL (1996) Fibroblast radiosensitivity in vitro and lung fibrosis in vivo: comparison between a fibrosis-prone and fibrosis-resistant mouse strain. Radiat Res 146:61–67

Epperly MW, Sikora CA, DeFilippi SJ et al (2002) Pulmonary irradiation-induced expression of VCAM-1 and ICAM-1 is decreased by manganese superoxide dismutase-plasmid/liposome (MnSOD-PL) gene therapy. Biol Blood Marrow Transplant 8:175–187

Erdi YE, Rosenzweig K, Erdi AK et al (2002) Radiotherapy treatment planning for patients with non-small cell lung cancer using positron emission tomography (PET). Radiother Oncol 62:51–60

Fan M, Marks LB, Lind P et al (2001) Relating radiation-induced regional lung injury to changes in pulmonary function tests. Int J Radiat Oncol Biol Phys 51:311–317

Fleckenstein J, Nestle U, Walter K et al (2000) Influence of ACE-inhibitors on the risk of radiation-induced lung injury in patients with lung cancer (abstract). Radiother Oncol 56 [Suppl 1]:S130

Fu XL, Huang H, Bentel G et al (2001) Predicting the risk of symptomatic radiation-induced lung injury using both the physical and biologic parameters V(30) and transforming growth factor beta. Int J Radiat Oncol Biol Phys 50:899–908

Fuks Z, Alfieri A, Haimovitz-Friedman A (1995) Intravenous bFGF protects the lung but not mediastinal organs against radiation-induced apoptosis in vivo. Cancer J Sci Am 1:62–72

Geara FB, Komaki R, Tucker SL et al (1998) Factors influencing the development of lung fibrosis after chemoradiation for small cell carcinoma of the lung: evidence for inherent interindividual variation. Int J Radiat Oncol Biol Phys 41:279–286

Graham MM, Evans ML, Dahlen DD et al (1990) Pharmacological alteration of the lung vascular response to radiation. Int J Radiat Oncol Biol Phys 19:329–339

Graham MV, Purdy JA, Emami B et al (1999) Clinical dose-volume histogram analysis for pneumonitis after 3D treatment for non-small cell lung cancer (NSCLC). Int J Radiat Oncol Biol Phys 45:323–329

Hallahan DE, Geng L, Shyr Y (2002) Effects of intercellular adhesion molecule 1 (ICAM-1) null mutation on radiation-induced pulmonary fibrosis and respiratory insufficiency in mice. J Natl Cancer Inst 94:733–741

Hanna YM, Baglan KL, Stromberg JS et al (2002) Acute and subacute toxicity associated with concurrent adjuvant radiation therapy and paclitaxel in primary breast cancer therapy. Breast J 8:149–153

Harada T, Shirato H, Ogura S et al (2002) Real-time tumor-tracking radiation therapy for lung carcinoma by the aid of insertion of a gold marker using bronchofiberscopy. Cancer 95:1720–1727

Hernando ML, Marks LB, Bentel GC et al (2001) Radiation-induced pulmonary toxicity: a dose-volume histogram analysis in 201 patients with lung cancer. Int J Radiat Oncol Biol Phys 51:650–659

Herrmann T, Knorr A (1995) Radiogenic lung reactions. Pathogenesis – prevention – therapy (German). Strahlenther Onkol 171:490–498

Huang EY, Wang CJ, Chen HC et al (2000) Multivariate analysis of pulmonary fibrosis after electron beam irradiation for postmastectomy chest wall and regional lymphatics: evidence for non-dosimetric factors. Radiother Oncol 57:91–96

Hurkmans CW, Cho BC, Damen E et al (2002) Reduction of cardiac and lung complication probabilities after breast irradiation using conformal radiotherapy with or without intensity modulation. Radiother Oncol 62:163–171

Itoh S, Inomata T, Ogawa Y et al (1999) Serial histopathological changes in irradiated guinea pig lung receiving conventional fractionated and hyperfractionated irradiation. Radiat Med 17:227–233

Johansson S, Bjermer L, Franzen L et al (1998) Effects of ongoing smoking on the development of radiation-induced pneumonitis in breast cancer and oesophagus cancer patients. Radiother Oncol 49:41–47

Jonsson OE, Bjermer L, Denekamp J et al (1999) Perivascular cell protection in vivo and increased cell survival in vitro by the antihypertensive agent carvedilol following radiation. Eur J Cancer 35:1268–1273

Komaki R, Lee JS, Kaplan B et al (2002) Randomized phase III study of chemoradiation with or without amifostine for patients with favorable performance status inoperable stage II–III non-small cell lung cancer: preliminary results. Semin Radiat Oncol 12 [Suppl 1]:46–49

Kong FM, Anscher MS, Sporn TA et al (2001) Loss of heterozygosity at the mannose 6-phosphate insulin-like growth factor 2 receptor (M6P/IGF2R) locus predisposes patients to radiation-induced lung injury. Int J Radiat Oncol Biol Phys 49:35–41

Koukourakis MI, Romanidis K, Froudarakis M et al (2002) Concurrent administration of Docetaxel and Stealth liposomal doxorubicin with radiotherapy in non-small cell lung cancer: excellent tolerance using subcutaneous amifostine for cytoprotection. Br J Cancer 87:385–392

Kwon HC, Kim SK, Chung WK et al (2000) Effect of pentoxifylline on radiation response of non-small cell lung cancer: a phase III randomized multicenter trial. Radiother Oncol 56:175–179

Lind PA, Marks LB, Jamieson TA et al (2002) Predictors for pneumonitis during locoregional radiotherapy in high-risk patients with breast carcinoma treated with high-dose chemotherapy and stem-cell rescue. Cancer 94:2821–2829

Lindegaard JC, Grau C (2000) Has the outlook improved for amifostine as a clinical radioprotector? Radiother Oncol 57:113–118

Lockhart SP (1990) Inhaled thiol and phosphorothiol radioprotectors fail to protect the mouse lung. Radiother Oncol 19:187–191

Milas L, Nishiguchi I, Hunter N et al (1992) Radiation protection against early and late effects of ionizing irradiation by the prostaglandin inhibitor indomethacin. Adv Space Res 12:265–271

Molteni A, Moulder JE, Cohen EF et al (2000) Control of radiation-induced pneumopathy and lung fibrosis by angiotensin-converting enzyme inhibitors and an angiotensin II type 1 receptor blocker. Int J Radiat Biol 76: 523–532

Monson JM, Stark P, Reilly JJ et al (1998) Clinical radiation pneumonitis and radiographic changes after thoracic radiation therapy for lung carcinoma. Cancer 82:842–850

Muren LP, Maurstad G, Hafslund R et al (2002) Cardiac and pulmonary doses and complication probabilities in standard and conformal tangential irradiation in conservative management of breast cancer. Radiother Oncol 62: 173–183

Nagata Y, Negoro Y, Aoki T et al (2002) Clinical outcomes of 3D conformal hypofractionated single high-dose radiotherapy for one or two lung tumors using a stereotactic body frame. Int J Radiat Oncol Biol Phys 52:1041–1046

Nutting CM, Bedford JL, Cosgrove VP et al (2001) A comparison of conformal and intensity-modulated techniques for oesophageal radiotherapy. Radiother Oncol 61: 157–163

Oetzel D, Schraube P, Hensley F et al (1995) Estimation of pneumonitis risk in three-dimensional treatment planning using dose-volume histogram analysis. Int J Radiat Oncol Biol Phys 33:455–460

Olejar T, Pouckova P, Zadinova M (2000) Butylaminiperindopril decreases transforming growth factor-beta 1 messenger RNA production in lungs of C57Bl6 mice after low-dose whole-body irradiation. Drugs Exp Clin Res 26:113–117

Penney DP, Siemann DW, Rubin P et al (1994) Morphological correlates of fractionated radiation of the mouse lung: early and late effects. Int J Radiat Oncol Biol Phys 29:789–804

Pignon T, Gregor A, Schaake Koning C et al (1998) Age has no impact on acute and late toxicity in curative thoracic radiotherapy. Radiother Oncol 46: 239–248

Redlich CA, Gao X, Rockwell S et al (1996) IL-11 enhances survival and decreases TNF production after radiation-induced thoracic injury. J Immunol 157:1705–1710

Redlich CA, Rockwell S, Chung JS et al (1998) Vitamin A inhibits radiation-induced pneumonitis in rats. J Nutr 128: 1661–1664

Roach M 3rd, Gandara DR, Yuo HS (1995) Radiation pneumonitis following combined modality therapy for lung cancer: analysis of prognostic factors. J Clin Oncol 13: 2606–2612

Rosenzweig KE, Hanley J, Mah D et al (2000) The deep inspiration breath-hold technique in the treatment of inoperable non-small-cell lung cancer. Int J Radiat Oncol Biol Phys 48:81–87

Rosenzweig KE, Sim SE, Mychalczak B et al (2001) Elective nodal irradiation in the treatment of non-small-cell lung cancer with three-dimensional conformal radiation therapy. Int J Radiat Oncol Biol Phys 50:681–685

Rube CE, Wilfert F, Uthe D et al (2002) Modulation of radiation-induced tumour necrosis factor alpha (TNF-alpha) expression in the lung tissue by pentoxifylline. Radiother Oncol 64:177–187

Sasaki R, Soejima T, Matsumoto A et al (2001) Clinical significance of serum pulmonary surfactant proteins A and D for the early detection of radiation pneumonitis. Int J Radiat Oncol Biol Phys 50:301–307

Sawyer TE, Bonner JA (2000) Postoperative irradiation in non-small cell lung cancer. Semin Radiat Oncol 10:280–288

<Senan S, Burgers S, Samson MJ et al (2002) Can elective nodal irradiation be omitted in stage III non-small-cell lung cancer? Analysis of recurrences in a phase II study of induction chemotherapy and involved-field radiotherapy. Int J Radiat Oncol Biol Phys 54:999–1006

Seppenwoolde Y, Engelsman M, De Jaeger K et al (2002) Optimizing radiation treatment plans for lung cancer using lung perfusion information. Radiother Oncol 63:165–177

Tee PG, Travis EL (1995) Basic fibroblast growth factor does not protect against classical radiation pneumonitis in two strains of mice. Cancer Res 55:298–302

Theuws JC, Seppenwoolde Y, Kwa SL et al (2000) Changes in local pulmonary injury up to 48 months after irradiation for lymphoma and breast cancer. Int J Radiat Oncol Biol Phys 47:1201–1208

Van Sornsen de Koste JR, Lagerwaard FJ, Schuchhard-Schipper RH et al (2001) Dosimetric consequences of tumor mobility in radiotherapy of stage I non-small cell lung cancer – an analysis of data generated using 'slow' CT scans. Radiother Oncol 61:93–99

Vanuytsel LJ, Vansteenkiste JF, Stroobants SG et al (2000) The impact of (18)F-fluoro-2-deoxy-D-glucose positron emission tomography (FDG-PET) lymph node staging on the radiation treatment volumes in patients with non-small cell lung cancer. Radiother Oncol 55:317–324

Vujaskovic Z, Marks LB, Anscher MS (2000) The physical parameters and molecular events associated with radiation-induced lung toxicity. Semin Radiat Oncol 10: 296–307

Vujaskovic Z, Feng QF, Rabbani ZN et al (2002a) Assessment

of the protective effect of amifostine on radiation-induced pulmonary toxicity. Exp Lung Res 28:577–590

Vujaskovic Z, Feng QF, Rabbani ZN et al (2002b) Radioprotection of lungs by amifostine is associated with reduction in profibrogenic cytokine activity. Radiat Res 157:656–660

Wang LW, Fu XL, Clough R et al (2000) Can angiotensin-converting enzyme inhibitors protect against symptomatic radiation pneumonitis? Radiat Res 153:405–410

Wang JY, Chen KY, Wang JT et al (2002) Outcome and prognostic factors for patients with non-small-cell lung cancer and severe radiation pneumonitis. Int J Radiat Oncol Biol Phys 54:735–741

Ward WF, Kim YT, Molteni A et al (1992) Pentoxifylline does not spare acute radiation reactions in rat lung and skin. Radiat Res 129:107–111

Ward HE, Kemsley L, Davies L et al (1993) The effect of steroids on radiation-induced lung disease in the rat. Radiat Res 136:22–28

Wennberg B, Gagliardi G, Sundbom L et al (2002) Early response of lung in breast cancer irradiation: radiologic density changes measured by CT and symptomatic radiation pneumonitis. Int J Radiat Oncol Biol Phys 52: 1196–1206

Wulf J, Hadinger U, Oppitz U et al (2001) Stereotactic radiotherapy of targets in the lung and liver. Strahlenther Onkol 177:645–655

Yorke ED, Jackson A, Rosenzweig KE et al (2002a) Dose-volume factors contributing to the incidence of radiation pneumonitis in non-small-cell lung cancer patients treated with three-dimensional conformal radiation therapy. Int J Radiat Oncol Biol Phys 54:329–339

Yorke ED, Wang L, Rosenzweig KE et al (2002b) Evaluation of deep inspiration breath-hold lung treatment plans with Monte Carlo dose calculation. Int J Radiat Oncol Biol Phys 53:1058–1070

5 Mechanisms and Modification of the Radiation Response of Gastrointestinal Organs

M. Hauer-Jensen, J. Wang, and J. W. Denham

CONTENTS

5.1 Introduction 49
5.2 Radiation Enteropathy as a Clinical Problem 49
5.2.1 Incidence 50
5.2.2 Prevalence 50
5.3 Pathology and Pathophysiology of Radiation Enteropathy 51
5.4 Mechanisms of Radiation Enteropathy 52
5.4.1 Clonogenic Cell Death and Apoptosis 53
5.4.2 Inflammation 53
5.4.3 Cytokines and Growth Factors 53
5.4.4 Endothelial Dysfunction 54
5.4.5 Mast Cells 56
5.4.6 Neuroimmune Interactions 57
5.5 Modification of Gastrointestinal Radiation Responses 58
5.5.1 Antioxidants, Free Radical Scavengers, and Cytoprotective Agents 59
5.5.2 Modulation of the Effects of Cytokines, Growth Factors, and Chemokines 60
5.5.3 Enterotrophic Strategies 62
5.5.4 Anti-inflammatory Strategies 62
5.5.5 Modulation of Intraluminal Contents 63
5.5.6 Topical Agents 63
5.5.7 Amelioration of Endothelial Dysfunction 64
5.5.8 Neuroimmune Modulation 64
5.6 Future Directions and Priorities 64
5.6.1 Models and Endpoints 64
5.6.2 Physiological Versus Pathological Responses 65
5.6.3 Predictive Assays 65
5.6.4 Low-molecular-weight Compounds 65
5.6.5 Translation to the Clinic 65
References 66

M. Hauer-Jensen, MD, PhD
Arkansas Cancer Research Center, 4301 West Markham, Slot 725, Little Rock, AR 72205, USA
J. Wang, MD, PhD
Department of Surgery, University of Arkansas for Medical Sciences, Little Rock, AR 72205, USA
J. W. Denham, MD
Department of Radiation Oncology, Newcastle University, Newcastle, NSW, Australia

5.1 Introduction

The alimentary canal extends from the mouth to the anus. It comprises the upper aerodigestive tract (oral cavity and pharynx), the esophagus, and the gastrointestinal (GI) tract proper (stomach, duodenum, jejunum, ileum, colon, rectum, and anus). In radiation therapy, toxicities of the small intestine, colon, and rectum are more important in terms of quantitative and clinical significance than toxicities of the proximal GI tract. Therefore, this review will largely address the radiation response of the small bowel, colon, and rectum. Although the mechanisms and pathophysiology of radiation injury in these segments of the GI tract are similar in many respects, there are also anatomical and physiological differences that result in unique features of radiation toxicity and strategies for modulation in each segment.

Excellent textbooks on the subjects of normal tissue radiation injury in general (Fajardo 1982b; Fajardo et al. 2001b), radiation injury of the intestine (Galland and Spencer 1990; Potten and Hendry 1995), and important cellular aspects of radiation injury, such as endothelial injury (Rubin 1998), are already available. Rather than duplicating existing literature, this review will focus on issues that deserve additional consideration such as strategies with potential for clinical translation, aspects of the intestinal radiation response that have not been sufficiently addressed in the past; as well as recent contributions to our understanding of the mechanisms of the intestinal radiation response.

5.2 Radiation Enteropathy as a Clinical Problem

The intestine is highly radiosensitive. Because it is almost invariably exposed during abdominal radiation therapy, the small or large bowel is often dose-limiting during treatment of patients with tumors in the abdomen or pelvis. Depending on the time between radiation therapy and clinical presentation of symptoms of intestinal toxicity, it is customary to classify radiation enteropathy as early (acute) or delayed (chronic).

Transient symptoms of acute intestinal toxicity are very common in patients who undergo treatment for intra-abdominal or pelvic neoplasms. While severe chronic injury is less common, it is clinically highly important because it is associated with high morbidity and mortality. Symptoms of delayed radiation enteropathy appear after a latency period of variable length, usually 6 months to 3 years, although, in the occasional patient, chronic symptoms may occur as a direct continuation of the acute symptoms. Delayed radiation enteropathy is characterized by intestinal dysfunction (i.e., malabsorption and dysmotility) and often leads to complications that require surgical intervention, mainly intestinal obstruction, fistula formation, and perforation.

The prognosis of patients with radiation enteropathy is poor. Corrective surgery is associated with high postoperative morbidity and mortality. In the long term, the majority of patients have persistent or recurrent symptoms, and about 10% of patients with radiation enteropathy die as a direct result of the disease (GALLAND and SPENCER 1985; HARLING and BALSLEV 1988; SILVAIN et al. 1992; FISCHER et al. 1989; KIMOSE et al. 1989; REGIMBEAU et al. 2001).

Improvements in radiation therapy equipment and treatment planning over the years have helped limit the exposure of intestine during treatment and may reduce the frequency of radiation enteropathy. Nevertheless, radiation therapy of tumors will always be dose-limited by the tolerance of adjacent normal tissues. Therefore, radiation enteropathy will remain an important obstacle to the radiocurability of abdominal or pelvic tumors and continue to adversely impact the quality of life of long-term cancer survivors.

5.2.1
Incidence

The risk of intestinal complications depends on radiation dose, volume of bowel irradiated, fractionation schedule, and use of concomitant chemotherapy. Exposure of limited amounts of intestine to less than 40 Gy using conventionally fractionated radiation without pertinent comorbidity or concomitant chemotherapy rarely causes severe chronic injury. Above this threshold, however, there is a clear relationship between total dose delivered and intestinal complications. Postoperative treatment of rectal cancer is associated with a 5-year actuarial incidence of chronic diarrhea of 30%–40%, and late small-bowel obstruction requiring surgery of 9%–30% (LETSCHERT et al. 1994; MAK et al. 1994). The incidence of severe intestinal toxicity among women treated for cervical cancer is about 9% at 5 years and 14% at 20 years (EIFEL et al. 1995).

It is important to recognize that the number of patients who seek medical attention for chronic symptoms of radiation enteropathy represents the tip of an iceberg. Systematic studies of patients who have undergone abdominal or pelvic radiation therapy reveal that 60%–90% have chronic symptoms and/or signs of GI dysfunction, including bile acid and vitamin B_{12} malabsorption (YEOH et al. 1993, 1996; FRANSSON and WIDMARK 1999). In other words, as pointed out by YEOH, intestinal dysfunction is an almost inevitable consequence of abdominal radiation therapy.

5.2.2
Prevalence

Clinical trials and cohort studies have provided estimates of the incidence of acute and chronic toxicities in different organs after specific radiation regimens. However, the prevalence of injury, rather than its incidence, reflects the burden of radiation enteropathy on patients and their families, the health care system, and society. Surprisingly, there is very limited information about the prevalence of chronic radiation toxicities among the steadily increasing number of patients who are cancer survivors. The prevalence of chronic complications depends on a number of factors in addition to individual and organ radiosensitivity, including (1) the relative incidence of specific tumors (i.e., common cancers will contribute more to the overall prevalence of late effects in the population than rare cancers), (2) long-term survival rate (i.e., cancers that have favorable long-term survival rates will contribute more to the overall prevalence of late effects than cancers with notoriously poor prognosis), and (3) patient age (i.e., tumors that occur predominantly in younger patients will contribute more to the overall prevalence [greater number of patient-years at risk] than tumors that occur predominantly in older patients).

The prevalence of delayed radiation toxicity in GI organs likely exceeds that of other organ systems. Abdominal and pelvic tumors are relatively common malignancies and have better prognosis than many other malignancies. These features, coupled with the high incidence of intestinal dysfunction after radiation therapy, make delayed intestinal toxicity a major determinant of quality of life in a large cohort of cancer survivors. Data from the Surveillance, Epidemiology, and End Results (SEER) Program of the National Cancer Institute show that of approximately 8 million cancer survivors in the United States, more than 50% are survivors of abdominal or pelvic cancers. Assuming that about one-half of these patients have undergone radiation therapy, a conservative estimate of the number of patients with postradiation intestinal dysfunction living in the United States clearly exceeds 1 million and likely approaches 2 million. How many of these suffer from socially, functionally, medically significant complications as a result is unknown, however. There is a definite need for clinical-epidemiological and outcomes studies in well-defined cohorts of cancer survivors to define the overall and organ-specific prevalence of radiation late effects, as well as the medical, quality of life-related, social, and financial consequences of radiation late effects. Such studies are critical in determining priorities for prophylactic and interventional clinical trials, as well as for selecting focus areas and optimal strategies for future preclinical and basic research.

tionated radiation therapy in the clinic. In fact, there is significant restitution of the intestinal mucosa during ongoing fractionated radiation therapy. Hence, despite increasing symptoms of bowel toxicity and continued daily irradiation, intestinal permeability and histological injury (Fig. 5.1) are maximal in the middle of the radiation course, but may regress significantly toward the end (CARRATU et al. 1998; HOVDENAK et al. 2000). These observations not only demonstrate the powerful compensatory responses of epithelial proliferation and mucosal adaptation but also show that mechanisms other than obvious changes in mucosal structure and function must be responsible for symptoms in patients who undergo pelvic or abdominal radiation therapy.

The pathogenesis of chronic radiation enteropathy is more complex than that of the acute response. Mechanisms of injury involve vascular and connective tissue damage, and structural alterations occur in most compartments of the intestinal wall, as depicted in Fig. 5.2.

On gross examination, affected intestine exhibits gray, roughened peritoneal surfaces, fibrinous deposits, and fibrous adhesions. Bowel wall and mesentery are indurated and thickened. Ulceration and stenosis of the intestinal lumen are common. Histopathologi-

5.3
Pathology and Pathophysiology of Radiation Enteropathy

The pathology and pathophysiology of radiation enteropathy will be discussed only briefly. For more in-depth reviews, the reader is referred to the many excellent review articles, two radiation pathology textbooks by FAJARDO (FAJARDO 1982a,b; FAJARDO et al. 2001a), and an exceptionally thorough review of the morphology of intestinal radiation injury by CARR (2001).

Acute radiation enteropathy occurs as a result of mitotic and apoptotic cell death in the crypt epithelium, resulting in insufficient replacement of the surface epithelium. Breakdown of the mucosal barrier facilitates penetration of antigens, bacterial products, and digestive enzymes from the intestinal lumen into the intestinal wall, thus initiating an intense inflammatory response. Changes in motility, which may precede the development of histopathology, appear to play an important role in the symptomatology of acute radiation enteropathy (ERICKSON et al. 1994).

Important compensatory physiological and proliferative responses occur during a course of frac-

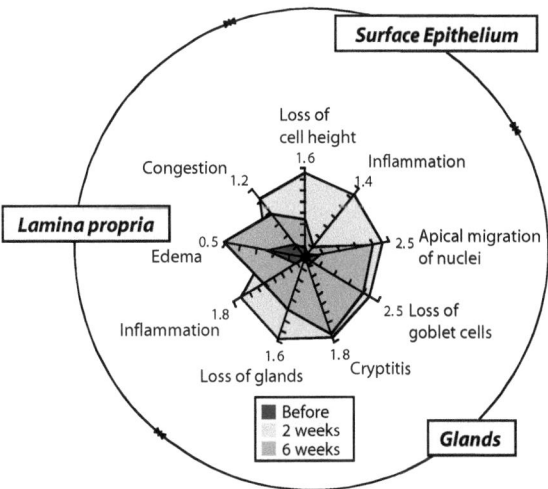

Fig. 5.1. Sequential histological changes in the rectal mucosa during pelvic radiation therapy. The spider chart shows the average score for nine alterations, each scored from 0 to 4 according to severity. The changes are grouped according to compartment (surface epithelium; glands; lamina propria) and time of biopsy (before irradiation [*black*]; 2 weeks after initiation of radiation therapy [*light gray*]; and 6 weeks after initiation of radiation therapy [*dark gray*]). There is highly significant improvement of structural changes from 2 to 6 weeks, despite ongoing radiation therapy and worsening clinical symptoms. (From HOVDENAK et al. 2000, with permission)

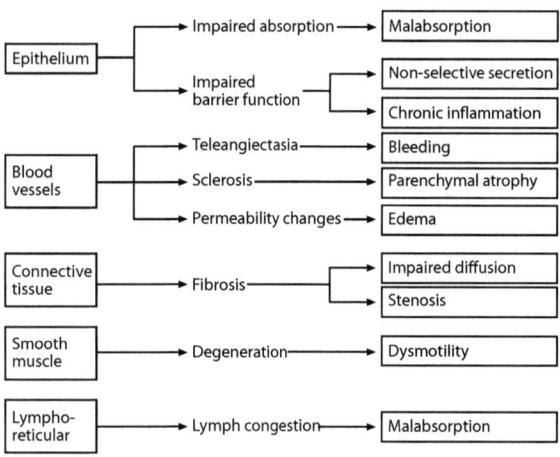

Fig. 5.2. Simplified diagram of important aspects of the pathology and pathophysiology of delayed radiation enteropathy

cal features also include mucosal atrophy, atypical hyperplastic or cystic glands, intestinal wall fibrosis, vascular sclerosis (most prominent in small arteries and arterioles), and lymphatic dilation. Intestinal dysmotility causing proximal bacterial overgrowth may contribute to diarrhea and malabsorption (HUSEBYE et al. 1994, 1995). Low-power photomicrographs of normal small intestine and a resection specimen of chronic radiation enteropathy are shown in Fig. 5.3.

5.4
Mechanisms of Radiation Enteropathy

Radiation responses in normal tissues represent a combination of three different injury processes: (1) direct cytocidal effects (clonogenic cell death, apoptotic cell death), (2) direct functional (noncytocidal) effects, and (3) indirect (reactive) effects. Reactive oxygen species play critical roles in the mechanisms of injury, as each fraction of ionizing radiation generates a burst of free radicals in the irradiated tissue. This does not directly rearrange or destroy the integrity of tissue components, but substantial damage occurs in cellular DNA, as well as in proteins, lipids, carbohydrates, and other complex molecules. While the actual amount of energy deposited is small, each exposure thus inflicts considerable injury. Another important characteristic of normal tissue toxicity associated with radiation therapy is that a series of insults is delivered over a period of several weeks to tissues that undergo a dynamic spectrum of cellular injury, repair, inflammation, and other pathophysiological responses. Therefore, during a course of fractionated radiation therapy, many cellular and molecular responses will be substantially exacerbated, suppressed, or altered in comparison with the situation after a single exposure of unperturbed tissue.

Fig. 5.3. Structural changes in delayed radiation enteropathy. Normal small intestine (*left*) and small-bowel resection specimen from patient with chronic radiation enteropathy. Original magnification of both images 20×. Note severe mucosal atrophy and massive submucosal and subserosal fibrosis in irradiated intestine

In terms of the tissue specificity of the response, the mechanisms of injury and repair in the intestine differ in several important ways from those in other organs. For example, the intestinal wall beneath the mucosa contains relatively few fibroblasts, and collagen is produced largely by smooth muscle cells and, after the initial phase of injury, by myofibroblasts. Another organ-specific feature pertinent to intestinal remodeling after radiation injury is the presence of pluripotent fibroblasts with the capacity to undergo transformation into smooth muscle cells, histiocyte-like cells, or vasoformative cells.

5.4.1
Clonogenic Cell Death and Apoptosis

The intestinal mucosa undergoes continuous, rapid turnover, with epithelial cells proliferating in the crypts, migrating along the villi, and eventually being shed into the intestinal lumen. The crypt epithelium is considered the main target-cell compartment responsible for the acute effects of radiation. Classically, cytocidal effects relate to the well-known phenomenon characterized by the target-cell model. Hence, the time between irradiation and manifestation of injury depends on target-cell characteristics (radiation sensitivity, repair capacity, proliferation rate, etc.) and tissue organization. In rapidly renewing tissues, such as the intestinal epithelium, injury manifests itself clinically within days of the first radiation exposure when cells in the so-called differentiated cellular compartment are no longer replaced by cells from the progenitor compartment.

The relative significance of clonogenic death and apoptosis in the intestine and their relation to the intestinal radiation response in the clinical situation are unclear. The issue is further complicated by the fact that many preclinical studies have been performed in models utilizing single lethal doses of total-body or abdominal radiation, a situation that differs significantly from the clinical treatment situation. Temporal shifts in the relative significance of clonogenic cell death, apoptosis, compensatory proliferation, and cell migration during courses of fractionated irradiation are factors that further complicate the extrapolation of such animal experiments to the clinical situation.

5.4.2
Inflammation

Mucosal epithelia are the primary sites for antigen entry. Although intestinal epithelium consists of only a single layer of cells, it controls the access of potential antigens and pathogens and at the same time plays a critical role in the absorption of nutrients. Not surprisingly, the intestine is by far the largest immunological organ in the body: 50%–80% of immunoglobulin-producing cells are found in the gut, and 40% of T cells reside in intraepithelial lymphoid tissue. Furthermore, because of the constant bombardment by antigens, some degree of intestinal inflammation is always present in the normal situation. In situations where the epithelial barrier is compromised, such as by radiation injury, inflammatory cell recruitment and transmigration increase by several orders of magnitude (RICHTER et al. 1997a).

Whether inflammatory processes play direct roles in the mechanisms of radiation enteropathy is not clear, however. On the one hand, radiation enteropathy is definitely not primarily an infectious or inflammatory process. This is clearly evident by the inability of anti-inflammatory strategies to effectively ameliorate radiation enteropathy. Furthermore, while there is substantial mucosal inflammation during the early phase of injury, inflammation is much less prominent during the later stages and mainly present in areas of chronic mucosal ulcerations. On the other hand, there is strong correlation between the severity of acute mucosal inflammation and subsequent delayed radiation enteropathy (consequential injury) (RICHTER et al. 2001). Hence, while inflammation is an integral part of the acute intestinal radiation response and certainly develops secondary to epithelial barrier breakdown, other aspects of the acute injury, rather than inflammation itself, are likely responsible for the pathology that develops in the irradiated tissue.

5.4.3
Cytokines and Growth Factors

Irradiation of normal tissues elicits prominent cellular responses, as well as changes in endogenous cytokines, growth factors, and chemokines (small cytokines with chemotactic activity). Some changes are epiphenomena secondary to tissue injury and inflammation, others are counteractive responses to injury, while yet others relate mechanistically to specific pathophysiologic processes.

Cytokines regulate a vast array of biological processes, including inflammation, cell proliferation, tissue remodeling, coagulation, and angiogenesis. They are critically involved in key aspects of early and delayed radiation injury. Rather than an orderly cascade leading to distinct cellular responses, however, the network of biological activities of cytokines is complex and depends on cell–cell interactions within and among tissue compartments and on the local microenvironment. Cytokines have been the subject of intense study in radiation injury in many organ systems, including the GI tract. Studies in transgenic animal models and in models involving modulation of cytokine levels or cytokine activities support a role for many cytokines in the mechanisms of intestinal radiation injury and also demonstrate the feasibility of modulating cytokine levels or activity to influence the radiation response in vivo. In the acute setting, focus has been mainly on anti-inflammatory and enterotrophic cytokine manipulations, while fibrogenic cytokines, especially transforming growth factor β (TGF-β), have been the target in strategies aimed at reducing intestinal radiation fibrosis.

TGF-β1 is one of the best documented paradigms of a cytokine playing an important role in radiation fibrosis in many organs, including intestine. TGF-β1 stimulates mesenchymal cell proliferation and collagen production, inhibits epithelial cell proliferation, and is the strongest chemotactic factor known for granulocytes and mast cells (Gruber et al. 1994; Parekh et al. 1994). TGF-β1 also acts as a potent immunosuppressor by inhibiting the proliferation and/or function of T cells, B cells, and natural killer (NK) cells (Kehrl et al. 1986a,b; Rook et al. 1986) and by inhibiting the expression of monocyte chemoattractant protein-1 (MCP-1) and tumor necrosis factor-α (TNF-α) receptors by endothelial cells (Weiss et al. 1999).

A possible sequence of events that may explain the role of TGF-β1 in radiation enteropathy is depicted in Fig. 5.4.

A direct role for TGF-β1 in radiation enteropathy is supported by several lines of evidence: (1) TGF-β1 expression in irradiated intestine is consistently increased and independently associated with levels of fibrosis (Richter et al. 1997b); (2) pharmacological induction of TGF-β1 exacerbates intestinal radiation fibrosis (Hauer-Jensen et al. 2000); and (3) scavenging active TGF-β1 after intestinal irradiation ameliorates radiation fibrosis (Zheng et al. 2000b).

While TGF-β1 is a potent immunosuppressive cytokine, it is also the most potent chemotactic factor known for mast cells and granulocytes. Chronic inflammation with continued release of TGF-β1 from inflammatory cells, increased TGF-β1 half-life in the extracellular matrix as a result of mast cell mediator release, and TGF-β1 auto-induction may thus sustain the increased levels of TGF-β1 and provide a continued stimulus of fibroblast proliferation and extracellular matrix accumulation. Unlike many other ulcerative conditions, radiation injury is associated with prominent vascular sclerosis. Once vascular sclerosis has developed, chronic low tissue pH due to local ischemia may stimulate additional TGF-β1 production and conversion of latent to active TGF-β1, thus sustaining both epithelial cell depletion and fibrosis.

5.4.4
Endothelial Dysfunction

An important unanswered question with regard to normal tissue radiation toxicity is why the injury does not resolve over time as do most other injury-repair processes. There is evidence to suggest that endothelial dysfunction may be the motor that drives the vicious cycle of progressive radiation fibrosis.

Vascular sclerosis was recognized as a prominent feature of radiation fibrosis only 4 years after the discovery of the X-ray (Gassmann 1899). The high radiation sensitivity of vasculature is mainly linked

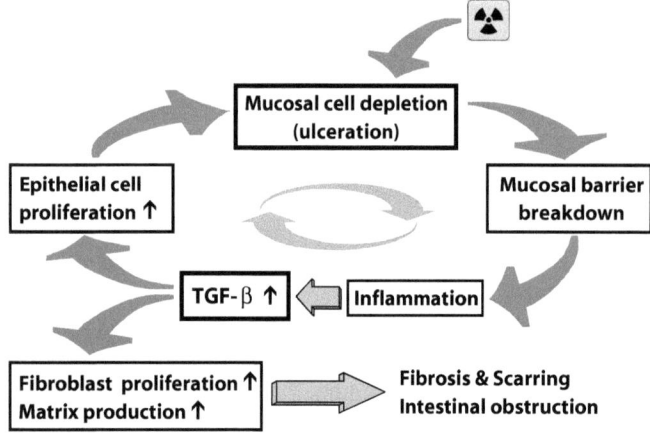

Fig. 5.4. Proposed role of TGF-β in radiation enteropathy. Model showing the putative role of TGF-β1 in the vicious cycle leading to progressive intestinal radiation fibrosis. Radiation causes breakdown of the mucosal barrier, inflammation, and increased TGF-β1 production. TGF-β1 inhibits epithelial restitution and increases extracellular matrix deposition, leading to intestinal fibrosis and obstruction

to endothelial cells, a critical target cell for radiation injury (FAJARDO 1989; PARIS et al. 2001). However, direct molecular links between endothelial injury and radiation-induced tissue fibrosis have not yet been established in vivo.

There is ample evidence that radiation causes a state of local microvascular hypercoagulability. Radiation induces a plethora of microvascular alterations, including endothelial cell swelling, increased permeability, interstitial fibrin deposition, and development of platelet-fibrin thrombi. At the cellular level, radiation causes apoptosis (LANGLEY et al. 1997; PARIS et al. 2001), increased permeability (LAW 1985), inflammatory cell adhesion and emigration (DUNN et al. 1986; HALLAHAN et al. 1995), and decreased fibrinolysis (SVANBERG et al. 1976). Radiation also greatly enhances endothelial prothrombotic properties by increasing the expression of tissue factor (VERHEIJ et al. 1995) and von Willebrand factor (JAHROUDI et al. 1996) and decreasing the expression of prostacyclin (RUBIN et al. 1985) and thrombomodulin (ZHOU et al. 1992).

Prothrombotic (hypercoagulable) states are associated with increased generation of thrombin, a serine protease that plays a central role in coagulation. Thrombin removes fibrinopeptides A and B from fibrinogen (to generate fibrin) and also activates platelets, thus forming the fibrin-platelet clot. However, thrombin is not only a coagulation factor but also an important regulator of cell proliferation, inflammation, and tissue remodeling. For example, thrombin mediates lipopolysaccharide-induced tissue injury (MOULIN et al. 1996) and regulates endothelial permeability (DEMICHELE and MINNEAR 1992), chemotaxis of neutrophils (BIZIOS et al. 1986) and monocytes (BAR-SHAVIT et al. 1983), and TGF-β1 production (YAMABE et al. 1997) by mechanisms that are independent of coagulation. Thrombin also increases production of platelet-activating factor (PAF), PAF-mediated neutrophil adhesion to endothelial cells, and smooth muscle cell migration and proliferation. Hence, specific inhibitors of thrombin decrease smooth muscle cell proliferation, migration, and collagen production both in vitro (NODA-HEINY and SOBEL 1995) and in vivo (RAGOSTA et al. 1996).

Most noncoagulant thrombin effects are mediated through activation of receptors that belong to the recently discovered family of protease-activated receptors (PAR), of which PAR-1 is the best studied and likely the most relevant biologically (DERY et al. 1998).

Knowledge about thrombin's effects on smooth muscle cells comes mainly from studies of vascular smooth muscle. However, strikingly analogous processes and interactions occur in the smooth muscle of the GI tract. As mentioned, intestine is unique in that collagen is produced largely by smooth muscle cells rather than fibroblasts (GRAHAM et al. 1987). Collagen production by intestinal smooth muscle is increased during inflammation and augmented by TGF-β1 (GRAHAM et al. 1990). In our own laboratory, smooth muscle cells in irradiated intestine were observed to exhibit increases in (1) proliferation rate (ZHENG et al. 2000a), (2) procollagen mRNA (WANG et al. 2001a), (3) TGF-β1 mRNA (WANG et al. 1998), and (4) PAR-1 protein and transcript levels (WANG et al. 2002b). This sets the stage for a positive feedback loop, because up-regulation of PAR-1 by TGF-β1 may increase the effects of thrombin at sites of injury (SCHINI-KERTH et al. 1997), while PAR-1 activation serves to further up-regulate TGF-β1 (BACHHUBER et al. 1997).

Additional data from our laboratory suggest that an important reason for increased thrombin effects in irradiated intestine is a deficiency of endothelial cell thrombomodulin (TM), a potent natural anticoagulant. TM is a transmembrane protein that is abundant on the luminal surface of endothelial cells. It binds and changes the substrate specificity of thrombin so that thrombin no longer converts fibrinogen to fibrin but instead activates protein C with protein S as a cofactor (Fig. 5.5).

The protein C anticoagulant pathway is critical for maintaining coagulation-anticoagulation homeostasis in normal blood vessels. Deficient TM levels are therefore associated with decreased protein C activation, increased clotting, and enhanced mitogenic, proinflammatory, and fibrogenic effects of thrombin (ESMON et al. 1991). A shift toward a procoagulant state may also contribute to local release of TGF-β1 from aggregating platelets (ASSOIAN et al. 1983).

Several aspects of TM gene regulation and function supports its role in radiation enteropathy: (1) endothelial cell TM is directly down-regulated by radiation (ZHOU et al. 1992), as well as by interleukin-1 (IL-1), TNF-α, TGF-β1, and endotoxin (NAWROTH et al. 1986; OHJI et al. 1995; MOORE et al. 1987); (2) TM is inactivated and/or released from endothelial cells by the concerted action of reactive oxygen species and granulocyte products (GLASER et al. 1992; BOEHME et al. 1996, 1997); (3) TM down-regulation is a premorbid alteration (i.e., it occurs before evidence of structural injury); and (4) TM is up-regulated by IL-4 (KAPIOTIS et al. 1991) and compounds that increase intracellular cAMP, including pentoxifylline (SEIGNEUR et al. 1995).

It is important to recognize, however, that although the procoagulant endothelium is the initial trigger, the mitogenic, proinflammatory, and fibrogenic effects of thrombin are likely more important in the pathogen-

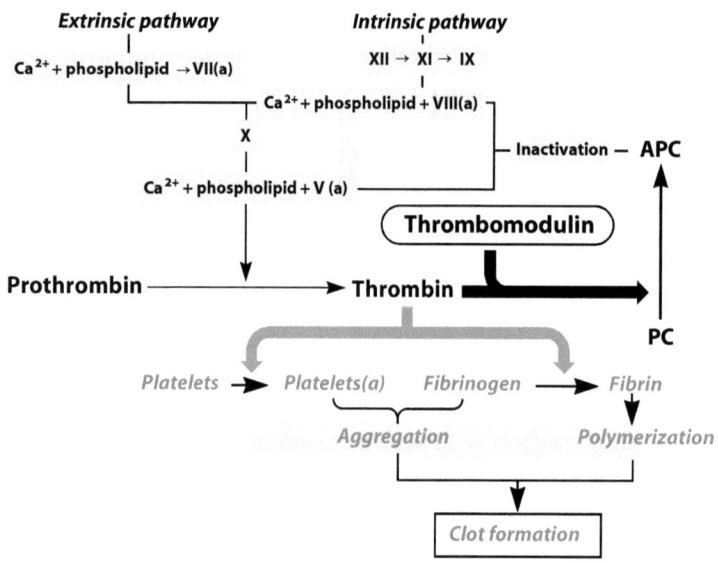

Fig. 5.5. The coagulation cascade. Simplified diagram of the coagulation cascade with the intrinsic, extrinsic, and common pathways. Note how thrombomodulin, located on the luminal surface of endothelial cells, forms a complex with thrombin, which is converted from a pro-coagulant to an anticoagulant. See text for further details

esis of delayed intestinal fibrosis than changes in the thrombohemorrhagic balance (Wang et al. 2002b). A model for how endothelial dysfunction may be involved in the mechanisms of chronicity of radiation injury is depicted in Fig. 5.6.

5.4.5
Mast Cells

Recent evidence suggests that mast cells play critical roles in the intestinal radiation response both in the acute (inflammatory) phase and in the chronic (fibroproliferative) phase. Mast cells are part of the innate immune system that provides the first line of defense against tissue damage. In addition to their critical role in immunoglobulin E (IgE)-dependent, histamine-mediated hypersensitivity, mast cells release and modulate cytokines, growth factors, chemokines, and other mediators, which in turn regulate a vast array of important biological processes.

Mast cells in the mucosa of the digestive canal differ from mast cells in the skin, lung, and peritoneal cavity in terms of proteoglycan and proteinase content, response to secretagogues and mitogens, monoamine storage capacity, turnover rate, and radiosensitivity (Fukuzumi et al. 1990). The two types of mast cells are commonly referred to as mucosal mast cells (MMCs) and connective tissue mast cells (CTMCs).

Injury to the intestinal mucosa is associated with MMC activation and degranulation. Mast cell degranulation contributes to mucosal inflammation in inflammatory bowel disease models and after intestinal irradiation (Stein et al. 1998; Sedgwick and Ferguson 1994). However, studies in mast cell-

Fig. 5.6. Proposed role of endothelial dysfunction in radiation enteropathy. Model showing how radiation-induced endothelial dysfunction may be linked to subsequent vascular sclerosis and intestinal radiation fibrosis. Radiation causes TM deficiency in endothelial cells, leading to insufficient scavenging of locally formed thrombin, which exerts its pro-coagulant, pro-inflammatory, mitogenic, and pro-fibrogenic effects on smooth muscle cells, fibroblasts, myofibroblasts, and other cell types in the irradiated tissue. Feed-back by cytokines sustains the endothelial TM deficiency and thus contributes to the chronicity of radiation injury. (From Wang et al. 2002b, with permission) deficient mice and rats have demonstrated that resident MMCs also play a critical physiological role in host defense (ECHTENACHER et al. 1996; MALAVIYA et al. 1996) and that their absence exacerbates acute radiation injury in the intestinal mucosa (ZHENG et al. 2000a).

In contrast to MMCs, CTMCs appear to play an important role in fibrogenesis (Fig. 5.7). CTMC hyperplasia is a prominent feature of many fibrotic disorders, including radiation fibrosis of the lung and intestine. A role for CTMCs in intestinal radiation fibrosis is unequivocally demonstrated in experiments in mast cell-deficient rats, which develop minimal intestinal wall fibrosis (ZHENG et al. 2000a).

Preclinical studies suggest that the fibrogenic effects of TGF-β1 and mast cells are, at least to some extent, interdependent; that is, mast cells exert their full fibrogenic effect only in the presence of TGF-β1, and vice versa. In vitro studies of interactions between mast cells and TGF-β1 provide likely explanations for these observations: TGF-β1 is the strongest known chemotactic agent for mast cells (GRUBER et al. 1994). TGF-β1 increases the production of stem cell factor by fibroblasts, thereby affecting both mast cell proliferation and function through interactions with c-Kit, the receptor for stem cell factor on mast cells.

Other mast cell-dependent effects of TGF-β1 include up-regulation and release of chymase (MILLER et al. 1999) and down-regulation of matrix metalloproteinase-9 (FANG et al. 1999). Conversely, mast cells stabilize and enhance the activation of TGF-β1 by (1) producing tissue plasminogen activator and activating urokinase plasminogen activator to increase plasmin activity, thereby activating TGF-β; (2) releasing heparin, which stabilizes activated TGF-β1; and (3) secreting chymase, the peptidase that releases TGF-β1 from the extracellular matrix. Furthermore, chymase contributes to generating angiotensin II (URATA et al. 1990; TAKAI et al. 1999), thus indirectly amplifying the effects of TGF-β through up-regulation of its type II receptor (WOLF et al. 1999).

Mast cell tryptase is a main activator of PAR-2, a receptor expressed in normal intestine that mediates many inflammatory, mitogenic, and fibroproliferative responses to injury (MACFARLANE et al. 2001). The activation of PAR-2 appears to be important in several other aspects of GI pathophysiology, including the regulation of intestinal ion secretion and absorption (MALL et al. 2002; CUFFE et al. 2002), nociception (COELHO et al. 2002), motility (LINDEN et al. 2001), and inflammation (FIORUCCI et al. 2001; MIIKE et al. 2001). Recent preclinical evidence from our laboratory suggests that PAR-2 activation may also contribute to the fibroproliferative responses in irradiated intestine (WANG et al. 2001b).

5.4.6
Neuroimmune Interactions

The nervous system of the intestine is the second largest in the body, with more neurons than the spinal cord. Of the various components of the enteric nervous system, sensory (afferent) nerves may be particularly important in the context of radiation toxicity. Sensory nerves were traditionally thought of as recipients of various stimuli and conveyors of these stimuli from the periphery to the central nervous system or some peripheral neural circuitry; that is, they were assumed to act in a purely unidirectional manner. However, research during the past 2 decades has clearly documented that sensory nerves also have important local effector functions, that they are involved in maintaining the integrity of the intestinal mucosa, and that there are important

Fig. 5.7. Various mechanisms by which mast cells may promote fibroblast proliferation and collagen production interactions between sensory nerves and various cell types, including mast cells.

Mast cells exhibit particularly close (almost synaptic) anatomical and functional associations with sensory nerve endings (SKOFITSCH et al. 1985), and bidirectional interactions between mast cells and afferent nerves are critical for maintaining mucosal homeostasis and ensuring an appropriate response to injury. Hence, sensory nerves regulate the activation threshold of mast cells. Conversely, signaling from mast cells to enteric nerves by histamine and/or nerve growth factor is critical for afferent nerve function and for the intestinal defense against injury (FRIELING et al. 1994; LEON et al. 1994; NILSSON et al. 1997).

The physiological significance of sensory nerves can be studied experimentally by ablating afferent neurons with capsaicin, the pungent ingredient of hot peppers. Capsaicin administration in rats causes complete functional and morphological ablation of thin sensory nerve fibers lasting several months (HOLZER 1991). Capsaicin pretreatment augments most types of acute GI injury, including experimental inflammatory bowel disease and acute intestinal toxicity after whole-body (PICARD et al. 1999) or localized irradiation (WANG et al. 2002c). Interestingly, while capsaicin pretreatment exacerbates acute mucosal injury, it ameliorates chronic radiation fibrosis (WANG et al. 2002c).

The mechanisms by which capsaicin pretreatment dissociates the intestinal radiation response in this way are unclear. In the acute setting, capsaicin destabilizes and reduces the number of enteroprotective MMCs in jejunum (ELIAKIM et al. 1995; GOTTWALD et al. 1997; WANG et al. 2002c), thus disrupting the physiological crosstalk between afferent nerves and mast cells.

While afferent nerves are required for normal mucosal homeostasis, inappropriate stimulation of these nerves causes neurogenic inflammation and structural injury. Among the mediators released by afferent nerves, substance P, an undecapeptide of the tachykinin peptide family, appears to be particularly important. Several lines of evidence support a role for substance P in GI inflammation and fibrosis. Substance P exacerbates GI inflammation by increasing mast cell production of TNF-α and impairing the hyperemic response to injury (COCCHIARA et al. 1999; MATSUDA et al. 1989; KARMELI et al. 1991). Substance P receptor antagonists and mast cell stabilizers ameliorate these changes (RYDNING et al. 1999; DI SEBASTIANO et al. 1999; KARMELI et al. 1991). Substance P may also promote fibrosis by increasing the production of TGF-β1 by mast cells (KATAYAMA and NISHIOKA 1997).

Substance P exerts its effects by binding to its receptor, the neurokinin-1 (NK-1) receptor. The NK-1 receptor, a G-protein-coupled receptor, is expressed on a wide variety of cells, including epithelial cells, fibroblasts, inflammatory cells, and mast cells. NK-1-receptor knockout mice are protected against intestinal inflammation (CASTAGLIUOLO et al. 1998; CAO et al. 1999). Conversely, mice deficient in neutral endopeptidase (the enzyme that degrades substance P to terminate inflammation) sustain increased injury, which is ameliorated by administration of either recombinant neutral endopeptidase or an NK-1 receptor blocker (STURIALE et al. 1999). Mast cell mediators released during mast cell degranulation directly stimulate sensory nerve endings (NOZDRACHEV et al. 1999). Mast cells may enhance delayed radiation injury by stimulating postradiation sprouting of substance P-containing axons (CROWE et al. 1996). These data support the notion that substance P is a central mediator in the crosstalk between mast cells and enteric nerves during development of radiation enteropathy and may be a target for prophylactic and/or therapeutic strategies.

5.5 Modification of Gastrointestinal Radiation Responses

The goal of strategies aimed at ameliorating intestinal radiation injury is to increase the therapeutic ratio (tumor control/normal tissue toxicity) of abdominal or pelvic radiation therapy. An equally important objective, but one that has received less attention, is to increase the number of uncomplicated cancer cures. While these objectives are closely related and to some extent inseparable, they pertain to different aspects of the cancer situation. Hence, while the therapeutic ratio relates to the incidence and severity of toxicity for specific sites and treatments, the uncomplicated cure concept reflects the prevalence of chronic side effects in the cancer survivor population. Whichever way the problem is looked at, it is axiomatic that prevention is a better strategy than treatment of established enteropathy. As pointed out above, the medical and surgical management of established enteropathy is fraught with difficulty. Hyperbaric oxygen therapy, while possibly helpful in the management of severe radiation proctopathy (ZIMMERMANN and FELD-

MANN 1998) and fistulae (FELDMEIER et al. 1996), rarely restores normal bowel function and has not yet been adequately tested in prospective, randomized trials.

An obvious way to reduce the incidence and severity of intestinal radiation injury is to minimize the radiation dose to the intestine and/or the volume of intestine irradiated. This can be achieved by the use of more sophisticated radiation equipment and treatment-planning techniques, optimized patient positioning and other physical methods to displace intestine out of the radiation field, or by partial or complete exclusion of intestine from the radiation field by a variety of surgical abdominopelvic partitioning procedures. The details and pros and cons of these methods will not be discussed in this review.

Pharmacological–dietary interventions aimed at modulating radiation injury in the intestine and other normal tissues can be categorized into two conceptually different approaches. The first includes strategies aimed at interfering with more or less radiation-specific mechanisms of injury, such as the administration of antioxidants, free radical scavengers, or other cytoprotective agents. The second, fundamentally different approach is to apply modifiers that are intended to ameliorate specific processes that are considered to be important in normal tissue radiation responses. The latter category includes strategies aimed at increasing normal tissue tolerance; ameliorating normal tissue injury at the pathophysiological, cellular, or molecular level; or even treating established complications.

In the forthcoming sections, a number of highly diverse, but promising approaches are briefly described. Most of these approaches are in early stages of evaluation, and many have not even been subject to phase 1 clinical trials. Proven preventive strategies, shown to be of benefit in large-scale controlled clinical trials, have not yet been established, and none of the approaches described in the following sections of this chapter can presently be considered standard of care.

5.5.1
Antioxidants, Free Radical Scavengers, and Cytoprotective Agents

It is a generally accepted notion that tissue injury in response to low linear-energy-transfer radiation is largely mediated by the action of reactive oxygen species. Therefore, antioxidants, free radical scavengers, and even methods to render normal tissues temporarily ischemic during radiation therapy (LOTE 1981; FORSBERG and JUNG 1978; FORSBERG et al. 1978) have been investigated as potential protective strategies.

Superoxide dismutase (SOD), the class of enzymes that converts superoxide to hydrogen peroxide, has been the subject of active investigation for many years. SOD exists in three main forms: mitochondrial manganese SOD (MnSOD), cytoplasmic copper-zinc SOD (Cu/ZnSOD), and extracellular SOD (EC-SOD). Gene therapy with MnSOD in lung and esophagus effectively ameliorates several aspects of radiation toxicity in these organs (EPPERLY et al. 1999; STICKLE et al. 1999). Interestingly, SOD administration has also been suggested as a postradiation antifibrotic strategy in skin (LEFAIX et al. 1996; DELANIAN et al. 1994). There is little information about the efficacy of SOD as a radioprotector in the intestine. However, a small pilot study using a low-molecular-weight SOD mimic, administered after localized intestinal irradiation, was unsuccessful in reversing fibrosis in the intestine (unpublished data).

The most thoroughly studied radioprotective agent is the aminothiol amifostine (WR2721, Ethyol) a free radical scavenger, developed after the Second World War to prevent injury to troops on the nuclear battlefield. Parenterally administered amifostine reduces the severity of early and delayed radiotherapeutic injuries at several anatomical sites. However, the many trials that have been undertaken have been limited in size due to the cost of amifostine, the practicalities of administering the drug 30 min prior to each radiation exposure, and side effects such as hypotension. In addition, tumor protection has not been adequately ruled out in the limited randomized studies performed to date (LINDEGAARD and GRAU 2000). Nevertheless, a clinical role in the protection of bowel injury may yet eventuate. Preclinical studies have shown that parenteral amifostine protects both small and large intestine (ITO et al. 1986; CAROLL et al. 1995) and that topical application of the compound also protects the gut (DELANEY et al. 1994b). Emphasizing the potential importance of the latter finding, a recent clinical phase I trial by BEN-JOSEF et al. (2002) found that intrarectal installation of an aqueous solution of amifostine 30 min prior to irradiation of the prostate caused no toxicity at any of the dose levels tested, and that patients receiving the higher doses of amifostine experienced less proctitis. Larger-scale randomized trials using this approach during prostatic irradiation are clearly warranted.

In addition to amifostine, a number of antioxidants, free radical scavengers, and cytoprotective compounds have undergone testing to assess their efficacy as modifiers of intestinal radiation responses. For example, the L-cysteine prodrug, ribose-cysteine, which stimulates glutathione biosynthesis, affords protection against small- and large-bowel injury in rats and pigs (CAROLL et al. 1995; ROWE et al. 1993).

Tirilazad, a lazaroid or 21-aminosteroid, is a steroid-like compound that, while lacking corticosteroid and mineralocorticoid effects, localizes within cell membranes and inhibits lipid peroxidation. Tirilazad, applied topically in the intestine, is highly protective against radiation toxicity, but the drug does not confer protection when administered systemically (FELEMOVICIUS et al. 1998). Similarly, topical application of other inhibitors of lipid peroxidation also protects against experimental intestinal radiation toxicity (DELANEY et al. 1992), and vitamin E (alpha-tocopherol) is protective whether given as oral pretreatment or as a brief topical application (EMPEY et al. 1992; BEYZADEOGLU et al. 1997; CAROLL et al. 1995; FELEMOVICIUS et al. 1995). Probucol, another antioxidant that inhibits the formation of peroxides, confers intestinal protection in rats when given either intraluminally or systemically (BONSACK et al. 1999).

The phosphodiesterase inhibitor pentoxifylline has a variety of biochemical and antioxidant properties. While the initial impetus for investigating this compound was its presumed rheological properties, other effects are more likely to be responsible for its efficacy in models of injury. Pentoxifylline appears to reduce gut injury in ischemia-reperfusion and sepsis models, but it does not ameliorate intestinal radiation toxicity (TAMOU and TROTT 1994). Pentoxifylline in combination with vitamin E has been reported to promote reversal of fibrosis in chronic radiation skin damage (DELANIAN et al. 1999), but, to our knowledge, this concept has not yet been tested in intestinal radiation fibrosis.

Many studies have assessed modification of cyclooxygenase activity or components of the arachidonic acid cascade in the context of radiation responses in normal tissues, including intestine. The best documented protective agents are prostaglandin E (PGE) and its synthetic analogues, although the exact mechanisms by which these compounds confer cytoprotection are still not known. In animal studies, PGE2 is radioprotective in the intestine (HANSON and THOMAS 1983; TOMAS-DE LA VEGA et al. 1984). Oral administration of enprostil (a PGE2 analogue) or luminal application of misoprostol (a PGE1 analogue) protects against intestinal radiation toxicity (KEELAN et al. 1992; DELANEY et al. 1994a). A recent small, but provocative clinical study showed misoprostol suppositories to be highly effective in reducing symptoms of radiation proctitis in patients with prostate cancer (KHAN et al. 2000).

5.5.2
Modulation of the Effects of Cytokines, Growth Factors, and Chemokines

Cytokines are soluble signaling proteins produced by a variety of cell types. They act on a wide spectrum of target cells to modulate their activity under normal and pathological conditions. Cytokines resemble hormones in that they mediate actions between cells, regulate processes in the extracellular environment, and often produce their effects as circulating mediators. They regulate a vast array of cellular functions including growth, differentiation, chemotaxis, mediator release, and gene expression. Not surprisingly, cytokines have been extensively studied as potential radiation-response modifiers in tumors and normal tissues.

Interleukin-1 (IL-1) has a wide range of biological activities. The two distinct forms of IL-1 (IL-1α and IL-1β) are derived from different genes; the amino acid sequences are only 20% homologous, but both IL-1s bind to the same receptor and have similar biological properties. Both also have modest and highly schedule-dependent radioprotective effects in mouse intestine (WU and MIYAMOTO 1990; HANCOCK et al. 1991).

IL-7, which plays critical roles in the development of B and T cells, also influences the function of mature NK cells and monocytes/macrophages. In the intestine, IL-7 protects intraepithelial lymphocytes (IELs) from undergoing apoptosis (YADA et al. 2001). It may also protect the intestinal stem cell compartment from radiation, as demonstrated indirectly by the increased crypt-cell sensitivity of IL-7-receptor knockout mice to whole-body irradiation (WELNIAK et al. 2001).

The multifunctional cytokine, interleukin-11 (IL-11), in addition to its hematopoietic and immunomodulating activities, also serves to protect and restore the GI mucosa. Administration of IL-11 protects mice against the intestinal effects of total-body irradiation (POTTEN 1995, 1996; ORAZI et al. 1996). It is possible that at least part of the protective effect is simply the result of induction of transient cell cycle arrest (PETERSON et al. 1996), somewhat similar to TGF-β, which is assumed to protect intestinal crypt cells by inhibiting their progression through G1 (POTTEN et al. 1997). At any rate, despite the encouraging preclinical results, severe side effects, including significant fluid retention and multisystem organ failure, appear to be a limiting factor in the clinical implementation of IL-11 as a radioprotective strategy.

IL-15 is widely expressed in epithelial cells, stromal cells, and immune cells. Because IL-15 shares some biological properties with IL-2 (which causes, rather than ameliorates, mucositis), it is not known whether inhibition or stimulation of IL-15 activities is beneficial in the context of radiation. However, IL-15 promotes IEL survival, inhibits epithelial expression of IL-8 and monocyte MCP-1 (LAI et al. 1999; LUGERING et al. 1999), and stimulates proliferation of intestinal epithelial cells (REINECKER et al. 1996). While IL-15 has not been systematically studied in radiation enteropathy, it confers an impressive degree of protection against the intestinal toxicity of irinotecan (CPT-11), a chemotherapeutic agent that is notorious for GI toxicity, mainly due to dose-limiting diarrhea (CAO et al. 1998).

The angiogenic growth factors, acidic fibroblast growth factor (aFGF; FGF-1), basic fibroblast growth factor (bFGF; FGF-2), and vascular endothelial growth factor, have all been shown to be radioprotective in the small intestine of mice exposed to total-body irradiation (OKUNIEFF et al. 1998; PARIS et al. 2001). The mechanisms of protection are unclear. The many documented effects of bFGF include protection of endothelial cells from apoptosis, enhanced repair of DNA damage, and increased proliferation and enhanced restitution of intestinal epithelium. It remains to be determined whether the enteroprotective effect of bFGF is primarily a direct effect on epithelial cells, as suggested by HOUCHEN et al. (1999), secondary to reduced endothelial cell apoptosis, as suggested by PARIS et al. (2001), or a combination of the two. The potent pro-angiogenic effects of bFGF would make the use of this growth factor in cancer patients highly problematic.

The keratinocyte growth factors, KGF-1 (FGF-7) and KGF-2 (FGF-10), are two other members of the FGF superfamily in which there is significant interest. In contrast to aFGF and bFGF, which activate several FGF receptors, KGF only activates the receptor FGFR2IIIb in epithelial cells and thus has much greater target cell specificity. Recombinant human KGF-1, administered either subcutaneously or intravenously to mice before single-dose, total-body or fractionated abdominal irradiation, increased crypt survival and LD50 (FARRELL et al. 1998; KHAN et al. 1997). KGF-2 is under investigation as a radioprotective agent in head and neck and lung. While KGF-2 has not yet been studied in irradiated intestine, it has shown efficacy in indomethacin-induced ulceration and dextran sulfate-induced colitis (HAN et al. 2000; MICELI et al. 1999).

Of the three mammalian TGF-β isoforms, TGF-β1 is assumed to be the biologically most relevant in the fibrotic response to injury. Approaches to reducing TGF-β1 action in order to counteract fibrosis include, for example, administration of neutralizing TGF-β antibodies (BORDER et al. 1990; GIRI et al. 1993; SHAH et al. 1992), decorin as a TGF-β sequestering agent (BORDER et al. 1992), mannose-6-phosphate to block TGF-β activation (FERGUSON 1994), antisense TGF-β oligonucleotides (FERGUSON 1994), and vector-mediated expression of a dominant-negative type II receptor (TβR-II) (QI et al. 1999). A particularly promising strategy involves the use of a soluble cytokine receptor peptide. Hence, administration of a recombinant TβR-II fusion protein, consisting of the extracellular portion of mouse TβR-II fused to the Fc portion of mouse IgG, in a mouse model of radiation enteropathy greatly reduced structural radiation injury and intestinal wall fibrosis.

Stem cell factor (SCF, mast cell growth factor, c-Kit ligand) functions to promote stem/progenitor cell survival, proliferation and differentiation, adhesion, activation, and migration/chemoattraction. SCF is a less effective radioprotectant in the gut than most of the other cytokines discussed in this section but appears to confer some protection in the proximal intestine in the mouse model (LEIGH et al. 1995; KHAN et al. 1997).

The growth hormone (GH)/insulin-like growth factor-1 (IGF-1) axis plays a critical role in the growth, development, and restitution of many different organ systems, including intestine. Both GH and IGF-1 are generally considered growth-promoting. Rats fed a high-protein diet and receiving daily subcutaneous administration of recombinant human GH beginning 3 days before irradiation showed increased mucosal height and crypt-cell proliferation and reduced mortality and epithelial apoptosis 2–7 days after an LD50 (12 Gy) of abdominal radiation (VAZQUEZ et al. 1999). GH has also been shown to enhance anastomotic healing in irradiated bowel (SILVER et al. 1999). Analogously, IGF-1, administered by mini-osmotic pumps, was enteroprotective after abdominal irradiation in rats (HOWARTH et al. 1997).

Chemokines, technically considered members of the cytokine superfamily, have unique and very distinct effects. The name originates from the combination of "chemotaxis" and "cytokine." The central concept of chemokines is their ability to induce directed migration of cells, such as inflammatory cells, to sites of tissue injury. Depending on the situation, this can have both beneficial and detrimental effects. Studies of the role of various chemokines in the context of GI radiation toxicity are still in their early stages.

Chemokines are often remarkably specific for certain cell types. For example, IL-8 is mainly chemotactic for granulocytes, but not for monocytes, and is thus important mainly during the acute inflammatory phase. In contrast, MCP-1 is chemotactic primarily to mononuclear leukocytes, but not granulocytes, and appears to play a more important role in chronic inflammatory processes. MCP-1, eotaxin, and RANTES are chemokines that are of particular interest in chronic radiation responses, because of their chemotactic effects on mast cells.

Macrophage inflammatory protein-1α (MIP-1α) is a chemokine with a wide range of biological activities. MIP-1α plays potential roles in monocyte chemotaxis in tissue responses to injury, including radiation injury. BB-10010, a MIP-1α analogue, administered 3 h before total-body irradiation of mice, conferred a statistically significant (albeit unimpressive in magnitude) protection in terms of increased crypt survival (ARANGO et al. 2001).

Several other cytokines have growth-promoting effects on the intestinal mucosa, but concerns about tumor protection or tumor growth promotion would likely preclude their use in cancer patients. These cytokines include, for example, epidermal growth factor/TGF-α and hepatocyte growth factor. Nevertheless, these cytokines could be useful in other situations, such as accidental radiation exposure, and therefore investigation into these scenarios may be indicated.

5.5.3
Enterotrophic Strategies

The goal of enterotrophic (growth-promoting) strategies in intestinal radiation protection is to increase the resistance of the mucosa to radiation injury and/or to enhance its capacity for recovery. Enterotrophic strategies fall into one of the following three categories: nutrients, GI peptides, and cytokines.

The category of enterotrophic nutrients includes a variety of substances and compounds, such as fiber, short-chain fatty acids, and certain amino acids, for example, glutamine and arginine. Glutamine is perhaps the best-studied enterotrophic nutrient but remains controversial both in terms of efficacy and differential protection (concerns about tumor protection). In general, glutamine supports mucosal structure and recovery. It ameliorates intestinal radiation toxicity after abdominal irradiation in some studies (KLIMBERG et al. 1990; CAMPOS et al. 1996), although other authors have been unable to confirm a significant protective effect in similar models (MCARDLE 1994). Due to the nature of glutamine as a so-called fuel for epithelial cells, it is not surprising that intravenous glutamine is not protective (SCOTT and MOELLMAN 1992). Similar to glutamine, oral arginine supplementation also enhances mucosal recovery and bacterial clearance after abdominal irradiation (GURBUZ et al. 1998).

Many GI peptide hormones have potent enterotrophic activities. In addition to GH, this category includes neurotensin, cholecystokinin, bombesin, peptide YY, and glucagon-like peptide-2. While these peptides have protective effects in various types of intestinal injury, they have not yet been subjected to systematic testing in radiation enteropathy.

A common concern with enterotrophic strategies is that they may also enhance the growth or metastatic potential of tumors, especially those of epithelial origin. This is an issue that is difficult to resolve. There are few clinically relevant animal studies, as well as a lack of clinical studies, that, while assessing radioprotection as the main endpoint, are of sufficient duration and have sufficient statistical power to be able to detect a clinically significant degree of tumor protection.

5.5.4
Anti-inflammatory Strategies

The use of traditional anti-inflammatory drugs to ameliorate acute or chronic radiation enteropathy has been generally disappointing. Acetylsalicylic acid (aspirin) may ameliorate intestinal radiation toxicity to some extent (MENNIE et al. 1975), while other nonsteroidal anti-inflammatory drugs do not appear to be effective at all (STRYKER et al. 1979). Sulfasalazine may also be of some benefit in the reduction of acute radiation-induced intestinal side effects (KILIC et al. 2000). In contrast, salicylic acid derivatives, developed specifically for therapy of inflammatory bowel disease, while having potent anti-inflammatory effects, are ineffective and possibly even harmful in radiation enteropathy (FREUND et al. 1987; BAUGHAN et al. 1993; MARTENSON et al. 1996; RESBEUT et al. 1997). These compounds given topically as enemas also have no effect on chronic radiation proctitis (BAUM et al. 1989). It is possible that future agents, targeted to specific aspects of the inflammatory process, may prove more effective in modifying the intestinal radiation response.

5.5.5
Modulation of Intraluminal Contents

Breakdown of the mucosal barrier during the acute phase of radiation enteropathy exposes subepithelial tissues to the detrimental actions of the contents of the intestinal lumen. The significance of the intestinal contents in acute radiation-induced mucosal damage has been recognized for almost a century. Not surprisingly, modifications of the various intraluminal factors have been explored as strategies to ameliorate intestinal radiation injury.

A possible role for intestinal bacteria in the development of the acute intestinal radiation response was already proposed in 1906 (KRAUSE and ZIEGLER 1906). Subsequently, the role of the bacterial flora has been extensively studied in germ-free animal models (BEALMEAR et al. 1984; WILSON et al. 1968; MASTROMARINO and WILSON 1976b), as well as in models involving more or less selective decontamination with different antimicrobial agents (MASTROMARINO and WILSON 1976a; SPRATT et al. 1961; TOOROP-BOUMA and VAN DER WAAIJ 1985; GERACI et al. 1985). These studies suggest that protection is likely conferred by two different mechanisms. In germ-free animals, the epithelial cell proliferation rate is lower than in normal animals, survival after abdominal irradiation is directly related to cellular transit time (WILSON et al. 1968), and enteral infusion of bile acids restores both proliferation rate and radiosensitivity to control levels (MASTROMARINO and WILSON 1976b). In other words, the relative radioresistance of germ-free animals seems to be the result of a lack of bile salt-deconjugating bacteria. On the other hand, treatment of conventional animals with antibiotics before irradiation increases survival without significant changes in epithelial cell transit time or excretion of deconjugated bile salts (MASTROMARINO and WILSON 1976a). In the clinical situation, it is likely that the proper balance in the bacterial flora is optimal in terms of minimizing radiation toxicity. Hence, probiotic therapy also has a beneficial effect on acute intestinal radiation toxicity (SALMINEN et al. 1988).

Of the various intraluminal factors, pancreatic enzymes exert the most pronounced influence on intestinal radiation toxicity (MORGENSTERN and HIATT 1967). Reducing pancreatic enzyme secretion by surgical or dietary methods attenuates acute mucosal injury after abdominal irradiation (SOKOL et al. 1967; MORGENSTERN et al. 1970; RACHOOTIN et al. 1972), and pancreatic duct occlusion in rats confers protection against both early mucositis and delayed fibrosis (HAUER-JENSEN et al. 1985). Furthermore, the reduced levels of intestinal injury seen in dogs fed an elemental diet before and during pelvic irradiation is at least partly due to feedback inhibition of the exocrine pancreas (MCARDLE et al. 1985).

The most promising method of reducing intraluminal pancreatic secretions in patients may be by administration of a synthetic somatostatin receptor analogue. These drugs act as so-called universal gastrointestinal inhibitors and are essentially capable of producing a pharmacological, reversible exocrine pancreatectomy. Short-term administration of the somatostatin analogue, octreotide, markedly ameliorates both acute mucosal radiation injury in the small bowel, as well as the subsequent development of chronic structural alterations (WANG et al. 1999, 2001a). While octreotide is a highly effective compound, it is exceptionally well tolerated clinically, with almost no side effects and, for all practical purposes, no maximal tolerated dose. Moreover, not only are there no concerns about possible tumor protection, but octreotide actually has intrinsic antitumor and antiangiogenic effects (WECKBECKER et al. 1992a,b, 1994; PATEL et al. 1994), which make it particularly suitable as a protector against normal-tissue injury during cancer therapy. The only obvious drawback of octreotide as a modulator of normal tissue injury is that its protective effect is likely to be confined to the small intestine.

5.5.6
Topical Agents

As can be expected, agents that have to be applied topically have shown the most promise in the prevention or treatment of radiation toxicity in the rectum.

Butyric acid has interesting anti-inflammatory properties, including potent inhibition of nuclear factor (NF)-κB activation and a shift in the Th1/Th2 cytokine balance toward a type 2 cytokine profile. A small but interesting randomized study showed that butyrate enemas were highly effective in reducing symptoms and endoscopic signs of radiation proctitis (VERNIA et al. 2000).

The aluminum hydroxide complex of sulfated sucrose, sucralfate, is effective in the treatment of peptic ulcer disease. Its postulated mechanism of action is to provide a protective film by forming a complex with proteins in injured mucosa. Initial studies reported a protective effect of oral sucralfate in patients undergoing pelvic radiation therapy (Henriksson et al. 1992). Only one study has been able to reproduce a modest benefit for this regimen (Valls et al. 1999), while other published studies have found no effect (Kneebone et al. 2001; Denham et al. 1996; Martenson et al. 2000). Topical application of sucralfate is also ineffective in preventing acute radiation proctitis (O'Brien et al. 1997).

In contrast to the lack of effect of sucralfate in acute radiation enteropathy, sucralfate is highly effective in chronic radiation proctitis when applied topically as mini-enemas (Kochhar et al. 1991). It is particularly effective in the hemorrhagic form of proctitis, where it is currently the first-line therapy of choice.

5.5.7
Amelioration of Endothelial Dysfunction

As discussed above, radiation induces a plethora of changes in the microvascular endothelium. Some of these changes are transient but may be involved in aspects of acute intestinal radiation toxicity. Other changes are more sustained and may play direct roles in radiation fibrosis and in the mechanisms of chronicity of injury. The postradiation shift in the thrombohemorrhagic balance toward procoagulation and the accompanying cellular effects of thrombin discussed above are particularly promising targets for modulation.

Administration of so-called traditional antithrombotics, such as heparin, warfarin, or acetylsalicylic acid, may confer some, albeit inconsistent, protection against radiation injury in some organs, including intestine. Recent studies have also shown that inhibition of ADP-induced platelet aggregation with clopidogrel, as well as direct thrombin inhibition with hirudin, markedly reduced acute and chronic intestinal radiation injury in a rat model (Wang et al. 2002a; Albertson et al. 2000). When these agents are administered in effective doses, however, their use is also associated with a significant risk of bleeding complications, and thus the potential for clinical use may be limited. Restoring endothelial cell TM or blocking PAR-1, on the other hand, would be more attractive and presumably safer approaches to modulate radiation-induced endothelial dysfunction or its downstream detrimental effects. Investigations of these strategies are, however, still at the very early preclinical stage.

5.5.8
Neuroimmune Modulation

Evidence is accumulating that interactions between the enteric nervous system and various cell types in the intestinal wall are critically important in the intestinal response to injury, including radiation injury. As a result, modulation of these interactions is emerging as a strategy for ameliorating acute radiation toxicity, and perhaps chronic radiation fibrosis in the gut.

Atropine, for example, ameliorates the effects of radiation on mouse villus morphology and reduces crypt depletion, supporting a role for neurogenic mechanisms and suggesting the involvement of parasympathetic effector sites (Carr et al. 1991). However, it is the previously discussed interactions between sensory (afferent) nerves and various types of immune cells, notably mast cells, that have been the most studied and appear to hold the most promise.

The extent to which substance P and/or calcitonin gene-related peptide (CGRP), the other major tachykinin released by enteric sensory nerves, play direct roles in radiation enteropathy remains to be determined. Correlative clinical and animal studies implicate substance P in the intestinal radiation response (Christensen and Haley 1968; Esposito et al. 1996; Hockerfelt et al. 2000; Forsgren et al. 2000). Furthermore, NK-1 receptor antagonists reduce substance P-induced production of TNF-α and TGF-β by mast cells and ameliorate some aspects of acute GI toxicity after whole-body irradiation (Esposito et al. 1998; Alfieri and Gardner 1998). An NK-1 receptor antagonist (GR203040) has been shown to ameliorate radiation- and cisplatin-induced intestinal injury in a ferret model (Alfieri and Gardner 1998). CGRP has thus far been less well studied than substance P. However, indirect evidence suggests that CGRP may be as important and possibly even more important in the intestinal radiation response than substance P.

5.6
Future Directions and Priorities

5.6.1
Models and Endpoints

In the past, many studies have been performed with lethal doses of total-body or abdominal irradiation, with crypt-cell survival as an endpoint. To the extent that the phenomenon of interest is acute epithelial cell death, such studies have provided the desired information, that is, whether or not a specific modifier has an effect. On the other hand, as discussed above, some modifiers that confer striking protection do not protect the epithelium. In some cases, there is even a dissociation in the radiation response, with the early response being clearly exacerbated, while the delayed response is significantly blunted (ZHENG et al. 2000a, 2002; WANG et al. 2002c). To study these types of processes, interactions, and pathophysiological phenomena, it is preferable to use localized radiation, so that animals can be observed over the long term without the confounding of systemic morbidity. For preclinical proof of principle of differential protection, orthotopic tumor models in immunocompetent animals are preferable to xenograft models. New structural, molecular, and functional endpoints using imaging and other emerging technologies will likely enhance our ability to develop effective response modifiers in preclinical models and translate them to the clinic.

5.6.2
Physiological Versus Pathological Responses

Many early postradiation cellular and molecular phenomena are part of the physiological response to injury. These changes are only harmful if they progress beyond a certain level or fail to regress to normal levels at the appropriate time. Hence, it is likely that the detrimental effects of cytokine overexpression occur when cellular and molecular responses are exaggerated and/or prolonged beyond the early phase. Ideally, postradiation interventions should not perturb physiological (beneficial) processes, but rather target the mechanisms responsible for exaggerating or sustaining them.

Mechanistic and interventional studies are needed to elucidate differences between physiological and pathological responses, as well as optimal interventional strategies. Specific issues relating to cytokine modulation include (1) optimal dosing of the modulator, (2) timing of modulation relative to irradiation, (3) duration of administration, (4) mode of administration, and (5) influence of time-dose-fractionation parameters. While such experiments may seem quite tedious and unexciting, the are nevertheless essential in the drug development process.

5.6.3
Predictive Assays

The so-called ideal protector of normal tissues is one that has high efficacy, low toxicity, low cost, and no concerns about the possibility of tumor protection. In the case of this ideal protector, it would be justified to treat all patients who receive radiation therapy, because it is currently not possible to reliably predict whether a specific patient will or will not develop long-term side effects. However, because most available strategies for reducing intestinal radiation toxicity fail to fulfill one or more of the above criteria, it is reasonable to attempt to narrow the target group to high-risk patients. Hence, an important area of investigation is the development of methods (predictive assays) by which patients at high risk of radiation toxicity can be identified with reasonable precision before or during radiation therapy so that protective measures can be instituted.

5.6.4
Low-molecular-weight Compounds

Many response modifiers, especially those used for cytokine modification, are large peptides. These compounds are often associated with significant pharmacological and immunological problems. While these hurdles can be overcome, major improvements in modifying inflammatory and fibrotic processes are likely to be associated with the development of synthetic low-molecular-weight compounds. Such compounds can be designed to optimize biodistribution and half-life, and produced at a fraction of the cost of most peptides.

5.6.5
Translation to the Clinic

While many radiation response modifiers have shown promise in preclinical studies, few have been tested clinically. One reason for this is the logistical difficulties arising from the lack of informative clinical surrogate endpoints (i.e., current endpoints are nonspecific and not very sensitive). Moreover, in the absence of reliable surrogate endpoints, the studies would require inordinately lengthy follow-up. To facilitate translation of promising preclinical data to the clinic, it is essential to have access to specific and sensitive surrogate markers that predict the development of chronic radiation-induced intestinal dysfunction. This is best done through close collaboration with other medical disciplines with expertise in the specific organ system of interest, as in the case of radiation enteropathy, gastroenterologists and GI physiologists.

Another reason for the relative lack of clinical trials is the indifference of the pharmaceutical and biotechnology industry. To a large extent, this lack of interest is largely based on misconceptions about the size of the market. Hence, industry frequently views the potential market as the occasional patient who develops serious toxicity. With some effort from the clinical scientific community to quantify the burden of radiation induced gastrointestinal problems among cancer survivors, this is a misunderstanding that can be corrected. To strengthen collaborative research with the pharmaceutical and biotechnology industry, it is essential to emphasize that, for compounds that potentially fulfill the criteria for an ideal intestinal protector, the market is the entire cohort of patients who undergo pelvic or abdominal radiation therapy, estimated at more than 200,000 patients per year in the United States alone.

References

Albertson CM, Wang J, Zheng H et al (2000) Recombinant hirudin, a direct thrombin inhibitor, ameliorates radiation enteropathy (abstract). Am J Clin Pathol 114:300

Alfieri AB, Gardner CJ (1998) Effects of GR203040, an NK1 antagonist, on radiation- and cisplatin-induced tissue damage in the ferret. Gen Pharmacol 31:741–746

Arango V, Ettarh RR, Holden G et al (2001) BB-10010, an analog of macrophage inflammatory protein-1a, protects murine small intestine against radiation. Dig Dis Sci 46:2608–2614

Assoian RK, Komoriya A, Meyers CA et al (1983) Transforming growth factor-beta in human platelets. J Biol Chem 258:7155–7160

Bachhuber BG, Sarembock IJ, Gimple LW et al (1997) a-thrombin induces transforming growth factor-b1 mRNA and protein in cultured vascular smooth muscle cells via a proteolytically activated receptor. J Vasc Res 34:41–48

Bar-Shavit R, Kahn A, Fenton JW et al (1983) Chemotactic response of monocytes to thrombin. J Cell Biol 96:282–285

Baughan CA, Canney PA, Buchanan RB et al (1993) A randomized trial to assess the efficacy of 5-aminosalicylic acid for the prevention of radiation enteritis. Clin Oncol 5:19–24

Baum CA, Biddle WL, Miner PB (1989) Failure of 5-aminosalicylic acid enemas to improve chronic radiation proctitis. Dig Dis Sci 34:758–760

Bealmear PM, Holtermann OA, Mirand EA (1984) Radiation pathology and treatment. In: Coates ME, Gustafsson BE (eds) The germ-free animal in biomedical research. Laboratory Animals, London, pp 413–434

Ben-Joseph E, Han S, Tobi M et al (2002) Intrarectal application of amifostine for the prevention of radiation-induced rectal injury. Semin Radiat Oncol 12:81–85

Beyzadeoglu M, Balkan M, Demiriz M et al (1997) Protective effect of vitamin A on acute radiation injury in the small intestine. Radiat Med 15:1–5

Bizios R, Lai L, Fenton JW et al (1986) Thrombin-induced chemotaxis and aggregation of neutrophils. J Cell Physiol 128:485–490

Boehme MWJ, Deng Y, Raeth U et al (1996) Release of thrombomodulin from endothelial cells by concerted action of TNF-α and neutrophils: in vivo and in vitro studies. Immunology 87:134–140

Boehme MWJ, Autschbach F, Zuna I et al (1997) Elevated serum levels and reduced immunohistochemical expression of thrombomodulin in active ulcerative colitis. Gastroenterology 113:107–117

Bonsack ME, Felemovicius I, Baptista ML et al (1999) Radioprotection of the intestinal mucosa of rats by probucol. Radiat Res 151:69–73

Border WA, Okuda S, Languino LR et al (1990) Suppression of experimental glomerulonephritis by antiserum against transforming growth factor b1. Nature 346:371–374

Border WA, Noble NA, Yamamoto T et al (1992) Natural inhibitor of transforming growth factor b protects against scarring in experimental kidney disease. Nature 360:361–364

Campos FG, Waitzberg DL, Mucerino DR et al (1996) Protective effects of glutamine-enriched diets on acute actinic enteritis. Nutricion Hospitalaria 11:167–177

Cao S, Black JD, Troutt AB et al (1998) Interleukin 15 offers selective protection from irinotecan-induced intestinal toxicity in a preclinical animal model. Cancer Res 58:3270–3274

Cao T, Gerard NP, Brain SD (1999) Use of NK1 knockout mice to analyze substance P-induced edema formation. Am J Physiol 277:R476–R481

Caroll MP, Zera RT, Roberts JC et al (1995) Efficacy of radioprotective agents in preventing small and large bowel radiation injury. Dis Colon Rectum 38:716–722

Carr KE (2001) Effects of radiation damage on intestinal morphology. Int Rev Cytol 208:1–119

Carr KE, Bullock C, Ryan SS et al (1991) Radioprotectant effects of atropine on small intestinal villus shape. J Submicrosc Cytol Pathol 23:569–577

Carratu R, Secondulfo M, de Magistris L et al (1998) Assessment of small intestinal damage in patients treated with pelvic radiotherapy. Oncol Rep 5:635–639

Castagliuolo I, Riegler M, Pasha A et al (1998) Neurokinin-1 (NK-1) receptor is required in clostridium difficile-induced enteritis. J Clin Invest 101:1547–1550

Christensen HD, Haley TJ (1968) Distribution of substance P in the central nervous system and small intestine of the rat after X-irradiation. Radiat Res 33:588–595

Cocchiara R, Lampiasi N, Albeggiani G et al (1999) Mast cell production of TNF-α induced by substance P: evidence for a modulatory role of substance P-antagonists. J Neuroimmunol 101:128–136

Coelho AM, Vergnolle N, Guiard B et al (2002) Proteinases and proteinase-activated receptor 2: a possible role to promote visceral hyperalgesia in rats. Gastroenterology 122:1035–1047

Crowe R, Vale J, Trott KR et al (1996) Radiation-induced changes in neuropeptides in the rat urinary bladder. J Urol 156:2062–2066

Cuffe JE, Bertog M, Velazquez-Rocha S et al (2002) Basolateral PAR-2 receptors mediate KCl secretion and inhibition of Na$^+$ absorption in the mouse distal colon. J Physiol (Lond) 539:209–222

Delaney JP, Bonsack M, Hall P (1992) Intestinal radioprotection by two new agents applied topically. Ann Surg 216: 417–422

Delaney JP, Bonsack ME, Felemovicius I (1994a) Misoprostol in the intestinal lumen protects against radiation injury of the mucosa of the small bowel. Radiat Res 137:405–409

Delaney JP, Bonsack ME, Felemovicius I (1994b) Radioprotection of the rat small intestine with topical WR-2721. Cancer 74:2379–2384

Delanian S, Baillet F, Huart J et al (1994) Successful treatment of radiation-induced fibrosis using liposomal Cu/Zn superoxide dismutase: clinical trial. Radiother Oncol 32:12–20

Delanian S, Balla-Mekias S, Lefaix JL (1999) Striking regression of chronic radiotherapy damage in a clinical trial of combined pentoxifylline and tocopherol. J Clin Oncol 17: 3283–3290

DeMichele MAA, Minnear FL (1992) Modulation of vascular endothelial permeability by thrombin. Semin Thromb Hemost 18:287–295

Denham JW, Walker QJ, Lamb DS et al (1996) Mucosal regeneration during radiotherapy. Radiother Oncol 41:109–118

Dery O, Corvera CU, Steinhoff M et al (1998) Proteinase-activated receptors: novel mechanisms of signaling by serine proteases. Am J Physiol 274:C1429–C1452

Di Sebastiano P, Grossi L, Di Mola FF et al (1999) SR140333, a substance P receptor antagonist, influences morphological and motor changes in rat experimental colitis. Dig Dis Sci 44:439–444

Dunn MM, Drab EA, Rubin DB (1986) Effects of irradiation on endothelial cell-polymorphonuclear leukocyte interactions. J Appl Physiol 60:1932–1937

Echtenacher B, Mannel DN, Hultner L (1996) Critical protective role of mast cells in a model of acute septic peritonitis. Nature 381:75–77

Eifel PJ, Levenback C, Wharton JT et al (1995) Time course and incidence of late complications in patients treated with radiation therapy for FIGO stage IB carcinoma of the uterine cervix. Int J Radiat Oncol Biol Phys 32:1289–1300

Eliakim R, Karmeli F, Okon E et al (1995) Ketotifen ameliorates capsaicin-augmented acetic acid-induced colitis. Dig Dis Sci 40:503–509

Empey LR, Papp JD, Jewell LD et al (1992) Mucosal protective effects of vitamin E and misoprostol during acute radiation-induced enteritis in rats. Dig Dis Sci 37:205–214

Epperly MW, Travis EL, Sikora C et al (1999) Magnesium superoxide dismutase (MnSOD) plasmid/liposome pulmonary radioprotective gene therapy: modulation of irradiation-induced mRNA for IL-I, TNF-α, and TGF-β correlates with delay of organizing alveolitis/fibrosis. Biol Blood Marrow Transplant 5:204–214

Erickson BA, Otterson MF, Moulder JE et al (1994) Altered motility causes the early gastrointestinal toxicity of irradiation. Int J Radiat Oncol Biol Phys 28:905–912

Esmon CT, Taylor FB, Snow TR (1991) Inflammation and coagulation: linked processes potentially regulated through a common pathway mediated by protein C. Thromb Haemost 66:160–165

Esposito V, Linard C, Maubert C et al (1996) Modulation of gut substance P after whole-body irradiation. A new pathological feature. Dig Dis Sci 41:2070–2077

Esposito V, Linard C, Wysocki J et al (1998) A substance P receptor antagonist (FK 888) modifies gut alterations induced by ionizing radiation. Int J Radiat Biol 74:625–632

Fajardo LF (1982a) Alimentary tract. In: Fajardo LF (ed) Pathology of radiation injury. Masson Publishing, New York, pp 47–76

Fajardo LF (1982b) Pathology of radiation injury. Masson Publishing, New York

Fajardo LF (1989) The unique physiology of endothelial cells and its implication in radiobiology. In: Vaeth JM, Meyer JL (eds) Radiation tolerance of normal tissues. Front Ther Oncol. Basel, Karger, pp 96–112

Fajardo LF, Berthrong M, Anderson RE (2001a) Alimentary tract. In: Fajardo LF, Berthrong M, Anderson RE (eds) Radiation pathology. Oxford University Press, New York, pp 209–247

Fajardo LF, Berthrong M, Anderson RE (2001b) Radiation pathology. Oxford University Press, Oxford

Fang KC, Wolters PJ, Steinhoff M et al (1999) Mast cell expression of gelatinase A and B is regulated by kit ligand and TGF-β. J Immunol 162:5528–5535

Farrell CL, Bready JV, Rex KL et al (1998) Keratinocyte growth factor protects mice from chemotherapy and radiation-induced gastrointestinal injury and mortality. Cancer Res 58:933–939

Feldmeier JJ, Heimbach RD, Davolt DA et al (1996) Hyperbaric oxygen an adjunctive treatment for delayed radiation injuries of the abdomen and pelvis. Undersea Hyperb Med 24: 215–216

Felemovicius I, Bonsack ME, Baptista ML et al (1995) Intestinal radioprotection by vitamin E (alpha-tocopherol). Ann Surg 222:504–510

Felemovicius I, Bonsack ME, Griffin RJ et al (1998) Radioprotection of the rat intestinal mucosa by tirilazad. Int J Radiat Biol 73:219–223

Ferguson MW (1994) Skin wound healing: transforming growth factor b antagonists decrease scarring and improve quality. J Interferon Res 14:303–304

Fiorucci S, Mencarelli A, Palazzetti B et al (2001) Proteinase-activated receptor 2 is an anti-inflammatory signal for colonic lamina propria lymphocytes in a mouse model of colitis. Proc Natl Acad Sci U S A 98:13936–13941

Fischer L, Kimose HH, Spjeldnaes N et al (1989) Late radiation injuries of the small intestine – management and outcome. Acta Chir Scand 155:47–51

Forsberg JO, Jung B (1978) Abdominal radiation response modified by hypoxia after intra-arterial injection of starch microspheres. Acta Radiol Oncol 17:353–361

Forsberg JO, Jung B, Larsson B (1978) Mucosal protection during irradiation of exteriorized rat ileum: effect of hypoxia induced by starch microspheres. Acta Radiol Oncol 17:485–496

Forsgren S, Hockerfelt U, Norrgard O et al (2000) Pronounced substance P innervation in irradiation-induced enteropathy – a study on human colon. Regul Pept 88:1–13

Fransson P, Widmark A (1999) Late side effects unchanged 4–8 years after radiotherapy for prostate carcinoma. Cancer 85: 678–688

Freund U, Scholmerich J, Siems H et al (1987) Unwanted side-effects in using mesalazine (5-aminosalicylic acid) during radiotherapy. Strahlenther Onkol 163:678–680

Frieling T, Cooke HJ, Wood JD (1994) Neuroimmune communication in the submucous plexus of guinea pig colon after sensitization to milk antigen. Am J Physiol 267: G1087–G1093

Fukuzumi T, Waki N, Kanakura Y et al (1990) Differences in irradiation susceptibility and turnover between mucosal and connective tissue-type mast cells of mice. Exp Hematol 18:843–847

Galland RB, Spencer J (1985) The natural history of clinically established radiation enteritis. Lancet 1:1257–1258

Galland RB, Spencer J (1990) Radiation enteritis. Arnold, London

Gassmann A (1899) Zur Histologie der Röntgenulcera. Fortschr Geb Roentgenstr 2:199–207

Geraci JP, Jackson KL, Mariano MS (1985) Effect of pseudomonas contamination or antibiotic decontamination of the GI tract on acute radiation lethality after neutron or gamma irradiation. Radiat Res 104:395–405

Giri SN, Hyde DM, Hollinger MA (1993) Effect of antibody to transforming growth factor b on bleomycin-induced accumulation of lung collagen in mice. Thorax 48:959–966

Glaser CB, Morser J, Clarke JH et al (1992) Oxidation of a specific methionine in thrombomodulin by activated neutrophil products blocks cofactor activity. J Clin Invest 90:2565–2573

Gottwald T, Lhotak S, Stead RH (1997) Effect of truncal vagotomy and capsaicin on mast cells and IgA-positive plasma cells in rat jejunal mucosa. Neurogastroenterology 9:25–32

Graham MF, Drucker DEM, Diegelmann RF et al (1987) Collagen synthesis by human intestinal smooth muscle cells in culture. Gastroenterology 92:400–405

Graham MF, Bryson GR, Diegelmann RF (1990) Transforming growth factor b1 selectively augments collagen synthesis by human intestinal smooth muscle cells. Gastroenterology 99:447–453

Gruber BL, Marchese MJ, Kew RR (1994) Transforming growth factor-beta1 mediates mast cell chemotaxis. J Immunol 152:5860–5867

Gurbuz AT, Kunzelman J, Ratzer EE (1998) Supplemental dietary arginine accelerates intestinal mucosal regeneration and enhances bacterial clearance following radiation enteritis in rats. J Surg Res 74:149–154

Hallahan D, Clark ET, Kuchibhotla J et al (1995) E-selectin gene induction by ionizing radiation is independent of cytokine induction. Biochem Biophys Res Commun 217:784–795

Han DS, Li F, Holt L et al (2000) Keratinocyte growth factor-2 (FGF-10) promotes healing of experimental small intestinal ulceration in rats. Am J Physiol 279:G1011–G1022

Hancock SL, Chung RT, Cox RS et al (1991) Interleukin 1 beta initially sensitizes and subsequently protects murine intestinal stem cells exposed to photon radiation. Cancer Res 51:2280–2285

Hanson WR, Thomas C (1983) 16,16-Dimethyl Prostaglandin E2 increases survival of murine intestinal stem cells when given before photon radiation. Radiat Res 96:393–398

Harling H, Balslev I (1988) Long-term prognosis of patients with severe radiation enteritis. Am J Surg 155:517–519

Hauer-Jensen M, Sauer T, Berstad T et al (1985) Influence of pancreatic secretion on late radiation enteropathy in the rat. Acta Radiol Oncol 24:555–560

Hauer-Jensen M, Zheng H, Wang J (2000) Pharmacologic induction of transforming growth factor-β enhances intestinal radiation toxicity (abstract). Radiat Res Soc 47:143

Henriksson R, Franzen L, Littbrand B (1992) Effects of sucralfate on acute and late bowel discomfort following radiotherapy of pelvic cancer. J Clin Oncol 10:969–975

Hockerfelt U, Franzen L, Kjorell U et al (2000) Parallel increase in substance P and VIP in rat duodenum in response to irradiation. Peptides 21:271–281

Holzer P (1991) Capsaicin: cellular targets, mechanisms of action, and selectivity for thin sensory neurons. Pharmacol Rev 43:143–201

Houchen CW, George RJ, Sturmoski MA et al (1999) FGF-2 enhances intestinal stem cell survival and its expression is induced after radiation injury. Am J Physiol 39:G249–G258

Hovdenak N, Fajardo LF, Hauer-Jensen M (2000) Acute radiation proctitis: a sequential clinicopathologic study during pelvic radiotherapy. Int J Radiat Oncol Biol Phys 48:1111–1117

Howarth GS, Fraser R, Frisby CL et al (1997) Effects of insulin-like growth factor-I administration on radiation enteritis in the rat. Scand J Gastroenterol 32:1118–1124

Husebye E, Hauer-Jensen M, Kjorstad K et al (1994) Severe late radiation enteropathy is characterized by impaired motility of proximal small intestine. Dig Dis Sci 39:2341–2349

Husebye E, Skar V, Hoverstad T et al (1995) Abnormal intestinal motor patterns explain enteric colonization with gram-negative bacilli in late radiation enteropathy. Gastroenterology 109:1078–1089

Ito H, Meistrich ML, Barkley T et al (1986) Protection of acute and late radiation damage of the gastrointestinal tract by WR-2721. Int J Radiat Oncol Biol Phys 12:211–219

Jahroudi N, Ardekani AM, Greenberger JS (1996) Ionizing radiation increases transcription of the von Willebrand factor gene in endothelial cells. Blood 88:3801–3814

Kapiotis S, Besemer J, Bevec D et al (1991) Interleukin-4 counteracts pyrogen-induced downregulation of thrombomodulin in cultured human vascular endothelial cells. Blood 78:410–415

Karmeli F, Eliakim R, Okon E et al (1991) Gastric mucosal damage by ethanol is mediated by substance P and prevented by ketotifen, a mast cell stabilizer. Gastroenterology 100:1206–1216

Katayama I, Nishioka K (1997) Substance P augments fibrogenic cytokine-induced fibroblast proliferation: possible involvement of neuropeptide in tissue fibrosis. J Dermatol Sci 15:201–206

Keelan M, Walker K, Cheeseman CI et al (1992) Two weeks of oral synthetic E2 prostaglandin (enprostil) improves the intestinal morphological but not the absorptive response in the rat to abdominal irradiation. Digestion 53:101–107

Kehrl JH, Roberts AB, Wakefield LM et al (1986a) Transforming growth factor b is an important immunomodulatory protein for human B lymphocytes. J Immunol 137:3855–3860

Kehrl JH, Wakefield LM, Roberts AB et al (1986b) Production of transforming growth factor b by human T lymphocytes and its potential role in the regulation of T-cell growth. J Exp Med 163:1037–1050

Khan AM, Birk JW, Anderson JC et al (2000) A prospective randomized placebo-controlled double-βlinded pilot study of misoprostol rectal suppositories in the prevention of acute and chronic radiation proctitis syndrome in prostate cancer patients. Am J Gastroenterol 95:1961–1966

Khan WB, Shui C, Ning S et al (1997) Enhancement of murine intestinal stem cell survival after irradiation by keratinocyte growth factor. Radiat Res 148:248–253

Kilic D, Egehan I, Ozenirler S et al (2000) Double-βlinded, randomized, placebo-controlled study to evaluate the effectiveness of sulphasalazine in preventing acute gas-

trointestinal complications due to radiotherapy. Radiother Oncol 57:125–129
Kimose HH, Fischer L, Spjeldnaes N et al (1989) Late radiation injury of the colon and rectum: surgical management and outcome. Dis Colon Rectum 32:684–689
Klimberg VS, Souba WW, Olson DJ et al (1990) Prophylactic glutamine protects intestinal mucosa from radiation injury. Cancer 66:62–68
Kneebone A, Mameghan H, Bolin T et al (2001) The effect of oral sucralfate on the acute proctitis associated with prostate radiotherapy: a double-βlind, randomized trial. Int J Radiat Oncol Biol Phys 51:628–635
Kochhar R, Patel F, Dhar A et al (1991) Radiation-induced proctosigmoiditis. Prospective, randomized, double-blind controlled trial of oral sulfasalazine plus rectal steroids versus rectal sucralfate. Dig Dis Sci 36:103–107
Krause P, Ziegler K (1906) Experimentelle Untersuchungen über die Einwirkung der Roentgenstrahlen auf tierische Gewebe. A. Übersicht über die in der Litteratur niedergelegten Angaben über die Wirkung der Roentgenstrahlen auf innere Organe. Fortschr Geb Roentgenstr 10:126–182
Lai YG, Gelfanov V, Gelfanova V et al (1999) IL-15 promotes survival but not effector function differentiation of CD8+ TCRalphabeta+ intestinal intraepithelial lymphocytes. J Immunol 163:5843–5850
Langley RE, Bump EA, Quartuccio SG et al (1997) Radiation-induced apoptosis in microvascular endothelial cells. Br J Cancer 75:666–672
Law MP (1985) Vascular permeability and late radiation fibrosis in mouse lung. Radiat Res 103:60–76
Lefaix JL, Delanian S, Leplat JJ et al (1996) Successful treatment of radiation-induced fibrosis using Cu/ZN-SOD and Mn-SOD: an experimental study. Int J Radiat Oncol Biol Phys 35:305–312
Leigh BR, Khan W, Hancock SL et al (1995) Stem cell factor enhances the survival of murine intestinal stem cells after photon irradiation. Radiat Res 142:12–15
Leon A, Buriani A, Dal Taso R et al (1994) Mast cells synthesize, store, and release nerve growth factor. Proc Natl Acad Sci U S A 92:3739–3743
Letschert JGJ, Lebesque JV, Aleman BMP et al (1994) The volume effect in radiation-related late small bowel complications: results of a clinical study of the EORTC Radiotherapy Cooperative Group in patients treated for rectal carcinoma. Radiother Oncol 32:116–123
Lindegaard JC, Grau C (2000) Has the outlook improved for amifostine as a clinical radioprotector? Radiother Oncol 57:113–118
Linden DR, Manning BP, Bunnett NW et al (2001) Agonists of proteinase-activated receptor 2 excite guinea pig ileal myenteric neurons. Eur J Pharmacol 431:311–314
Lote K (1981) Hypoxic radioprotection by temporary intestinal ischemia: degradable starch microsphere embolization in the cat. AJR 137:909–914
Lugering N, Kucharzik T, Maaser C et al (1999) Interleukin-15 strongly inhibits interleukin-8 and monocyte chemoattractant protein-1 production in human colonic epithelial cells. Immunology 98:504–509
MacFarlane SR, Seatter MJ, Kanke T et al (2001) Proteinase-activated receptors. Pharmacol Rev 53:245–282
Mak AC, Rich TA, Schultheiss TE et al (1994) Late complications of postoperative radiation therapy for cancer of the rectum and rectosigmoid. Int J Radiat Oncol Biol Phys 28:597–603
Malaviya R, Ikeda T, Ross E et al (1996) Mast cell modulation of neutrophil influx and bacterial clearance at sites of infection through TNF-α. Nature 381:77–80
Mall M, Gonska T, Thomas J et al (2002) Activation of ion secretion via proteinase-activated receptor-2 in human colon. Am J Physiol 282:G200–G210
Martenson JA, Hyland G, Moertel CG et al (1996) Olsalazine is contraindicated during pelvic radiation therapy: results of a double-blind randomized clinical trial. Int J Radiat Oncol Biol Phys 35:299–303
Martenson JA, Bollinger JW, Sloan JA et al (2000) Sucralfate in the prevention of treatment-induced diarrhea in patients receiving pelvic radiation therapy: a North Central Cancer Treatment Group phase III double-blind placebo-controlled trial. J Clin Oncol 18:1239–1245
Mastromarino AJ, Wilson R (1976a) Antibiotic radioprotection of mice exposed to supralethal whole-body irradiation independent of antibacterial activity. Radiat Res 68:329–338
Mastromarino AJ, Wilson R (1976b) Increased intestinal mucosal turnover and radiosensitivity to supralethal whole-body irradiation resulting from cholic acid-induced alterations of the microecology of germfree CFW mice. Radiat Res 66:393–400
Matsuda H, Kawakita K, Kiso Y et al (1989) Substance P induces granulocyte infiltration through degranulation of mast cells. J Immunol 142:927–931
McArdle AH (1994) Elemental diets in treatment of gastrointestinal injury. Adv Biosci 94:201–206
McArdle AH, Wittnich C, Freeman CR et al (1985) Elemental diet as prophylaxis against radiation injury. Arch Surg 120:1026–1032
Mennie AT, Dalley VM, Dinneen LC et al (1975) Treatment of radiation-induced gastrointestinal distress with acetylsalicylate. Lancet 2:942–943
Miceli R, Hubert M, Santiago G et al (1999) Efficacy of keratinocyte growth factor-2 in dextran sulfate sodium-induced murine colitis. J Pharmacol Exp Ther 290:464–471
Miike S, McWilliam AS, Kita H (2001) Trypsin induces activation and inflammatory mediator release from human eosinophils through proteinase-activated receptor-2. J Immunol 167:6615–6622
Miller HRP, Wright SH, Knight PA et al (1999) A novel function for transforming growth factor-β1: upregulation of the expression and the IgE-independent extracellular release of a mucosal mast cell granule-specific b-chymase, mouse mast cell protease-1. Blood 93:3473–3486
Moore KL, Andreoli SP, Esmon NL et al (1987) Endotoxin enhances tissue factor and suppresses thrombomodulin expression of human vascular endothelium in vitro. J Clin Invest 79:124–130
Morgenstern L, Hiatt N (1967) Injurious effect of pancreatic secretions on postradiation enteropathy. Gastroenterology 53:923–929
Morgenstern L, Patin CS, Krohn HL et al (1970) Prolongation of survival in lethally irradiated dogs. Arch Surg 101:586–589
Moulin F, Pearson JM, Schultze AE et al (1996) Thrombin is a distal mediator of lipopolysaccharide-induced liver injury in the rat. J Surg Res 65:149–158
Nawroth PP, Handley DA, Esmon CT et al (1986) Interleukin

1 induces endothelial cell procoagulant while suppressing cell-surface anticoagulant activity. Proc Natl Acad Sci U S A 83:3460–3464

Nilsson G, Forsberg-Nilsson K, Xiang Z et al (1997) Human mast cells express functional TrkA and are a source of nerve growth factor. Eur J Immunol 27:2295–2301

Noda-Heiny H, Sobel BE (1995) Vascular smooth muscle cell migration mediated by thrombin and urokinase receptor. Am J Physiol 268:C1195–C1201

Nozdrachev AD, Akoev GN, Filippova LV et al (1999) Changes in afferent impulse activity of small intestine mesenteric nerves in response to antigen challenge. Neuroscience 94:1339–1342

O'Brien PC, Franklin CI, Dear KBG et al (1997) A phase III double-blind randomised study of rectal sucralfate suspension in the prevention of acute radiation proctitis. Radiother Oncol 45:117–123

Ohji T, Urano H, Shirahata A et al (1995) Transforming growth factor beta1 and beta2 induce down-modulation of thrombomodulin in human umbilical vein endothelial cells. Thromb Haemost 73:812–818

Okunieff P, Mester M, Wang J et al (1998) In vivo radioprotective effects of angiogenic growth factors on the small bowel of C3H mice. Radiat Res 150:204–211

Orazi A, Du X, Yang Z et al (1996) Interleukin-11 prevents apoptosis and accelerates recovery of small intestinal mucosa in mice treated with combined chemotherapy and radiation. Lab Invest 75:33–42

Parekh T, Saxena B, Reibman J et al (1994) Neutrophil chemotaxis in response to TGF-β isoforms (TGF-β1, TGF-β2, TGF-β3) is mediated by fibronectin. J Immunol 152:2456–2466

Paris F, Fuks Z, Kang A et al (2001) Endothelial apoptosis as the primary lesion initiating intestinal radiation damage in mice. Science 293:293–297

Patel PC, Barrie R, Hill N et al (1994) Postreceptor signal transduction mechanisms involved in octreotide-induced inhibition of angiogenesis. Surgery 116:1148–1152

Peterson RL, Bozza MM, Dorner AJ (1996) Interleukin-11 induces intestinal epithelial cell growth arrest through effects on retinoblastoma protein phosphorylation. Am J Pathol 149:895–902

Picard C, Wysocki J, Griffiths NM et al (1999) Sensory nerve ablation modulates abdominal irradiation effects in the rat (abstract). Int Cong Radiat Res 11:159

Potten CS (1995) Interleukin-11 protects the clonogenic stem cells in murine small-intestinal crypts from impairment of their reproductive capacity by radiation. Int J Cancer 62:356–361

Potten CS (1996) Protection of the small intestinal clonogenic stem cells from radiation-induced damage by pretreatment with interleukin 11 also increases murine survival time. Stem Cells 14:452–459

Potten CS, Hendry JH (1995) Radiation and gut. Elsevier Science, Amsterdam

Potten CS, Booth D, Haley JD (1997) Pretreatment with transforming growth factor b-3 protects small intestinal stem cells against radiation damage in vivo. Br J Cancer 75:1454–1459

Qi Z, Atsuchi N, Ooshima A et al (1999) Blockade of type b transforming growth factor signaling prevents liver fibrosis and dysfunction in the rat. Proc Natl Acad Sci U S A 96:2345–2349

Rachootin S, Shapiro S, Yamakawa T et al (1972) Potent antiprotease from Ascaris lumbricoides: efficacy in amelioration of post-radiation enteropathy (abstract). Gastroenterology 62:796

Ragosta M, Barry WL, Gimple LW et al (1996) Effect of thrombin inhibition with desulfatohirudin on early kinetics of cellular proliferation after balloon angioplasty in atherosclerotic rabbits. Circulation 93:1194–1200

Regimbeau J-M, Panis Y, Gouzi J-L et al (2001) Operative and long term results after surgery for chronic radiation enteritis. Am J Surg 182:237–242

Reinecker HC, MacDermott RP, Mirau S et al (1996) Intestinal epithelial cells both express and respond to interleukin 15. Gastroenterology 111:1706–1713

Resbeut M, Marteau P, Cowen D et al (1997) A randomized double blind placebo controlled multicenter study of mesalazine for the prevention of acute radiation enteritis. Radiother Oncol 44:59–63

Richter KK, Fagerhol MK, Carr JC et al (1997a) Association of granulocyte transmigration with structural and cellular parameters of injury in experimental radiation enteropathy. Radiat Oncol Invest 5:275–282

Richter KK, Langberg CW, Sung C-C et al (1997b) Increased transforming growth factor b (TGF-β) immunoreactivity is independently associated with chronic injury in both consequential and primary radiation enteropathy. Int J Radiat Oncol Biol Phys 39:187–195

Richter KK, Wang J, Fagerhol MK et al (2001) Radiation-induced granulocyte transmigration predicts development of delayed structural changes in rat intestine. Radiother Oncol 59:81–85

Rook AH, Kehrl JH, Wakefield LM et al (1986) Effects of transforming growth factor b on the functions of natural killer cells: depressed cytolytic activity and blunting of interferon responsiveness. J Immunol 136:3916–3920

Rowe JK, Zera RT, Madoff RD et al (1993) Protective effect of RibCys following high-dose irradiation of the rectosigmoid. Dis Colon Rectum 36:681–688

Rubin DB (1998) The radiation biology of the vascular endothelium. CRC Press, Boca Raton

Rubin DB, Drab EA, Ts'ao C et al (1985) Prostacyclin synthesis in irradiated endothelial cells cultured from bovine aorta. J Appl Physiol 58:592–597

Rydning A, Lyng O, Aase S et al (1999) Substance P may attenuate gastric hyperemia by a mast cell-dependent mechanism in the damaged gastric mucosa. Am J Physiol 277:G1064–G1073

Salminen E, Elomaa I, Minkkinen J et al (1988) Preservation of intestinal integrity during radiotherapy using live Lactobacillus acidophilus cultures. Clin Radiol 39:435–437

Schini-Kerth VB, Bassus S, Fissithaler B et al (1997) Aggregating human platelets stimulate the expression of thrombin receptors in cultured vascular smooth muscle cells via the release of transforming growth factor-β1 and platelet-derived growth factor. Circulation 96:3888–3896

Scott TE, Moellman JR (1992) Intravenous glutamine fails to improve gut morphology after radiation injury. JPEN J Parenter Enteral Nutr 16:440–444

Sedgwick DM, Ferguson A (1994) Dose-response studies of depletion and repopulation of rat intestinal mucosal mast cells after irradiation. Int J Radiat Biol 65:483–495

Seigneur M, Dufourcq P, Belloc F et al (1995) Influence of pentoxifylline on membrane thrombomodulin levels in

endothelial cells submitted to hypoxic conditions. J Cardiovasc Pharmacol 25:S85–S87
Shah M, Foreman DM, Ferguson MWJ (1992) Control of scarring in adult wounds by neutralising antibody to transforming growth factor beta. Lancet 339:213–214
Silvain C, Besson I, Ingrand P et al (1992) Long-term outcome of severe radiation enteritis treated by total parenteral nutrition. Dig Dis Sci 37:1065–1071
Silver DF, Simon A, Dubin NH et al (1999) Recombinant growth hormone's effects on the strength and thickness of radiation-injured ileal anastomoses: a rat model. J Surg Res 85:66–70
Skofitsch G, Savitt JM, Jacobowitz DM (1985) Suggestive evidence for a functional unit between mast cells and substance P fibers in the rat diaphragm and mesentery. Histochemistry 82:5–8
Sokol AB, Lipson LW, Morgenstern L et al (1967) Protection against lethal irradiation injury by pancreatic enzyme exclusion. Surg Forum 18:387–389
Spratt JS, Heinbecker P, Saltzstein SL (1961) The influence of succinylsulphathiazole (Sulfasuxidine) upon the response of canine small intestine to irradiation. Cancer 14:862–874
Stein J, Ries J, Barrett KE (1998) Disruption of intestinal barrier function associated with experimental colitis: possible role of mast cells. Am J Physiol 274:G203–G209
Stickle RL, Epperly MW, Klein E et al (1999) Prevention of irradiation-induced esophagitis by plasmid/liposome delivery of the human manganese superoxide dismutase transgene. Radiat Oncol Invest 7:204–217
Stryker JA, Demers LM, Mortel R (1979) Prophylactic ibuprofen administration during pelvic irradiation. Int J Radiat Oncol Biol Phys 5:2049–2052
Sturiale S, Barbara G, Qiu B et al (1999) Neutral endopeptidase (EC 3.4.24.11) terminates colitis by degrading substance P. Proc Natl Acad Sci U S A 96:11653–11658
Svanberg L, Åstedt B, Kullander S (1976) On radiation-decreased fibrinolytic activity of vessel walls. Acta Obstet Gynecol Scand 55:49–51
Takai A, Jin D, Sakaguchi M et al (1999) Chymase-dependent angiotensin II formation in human vascular tissue. Circulation 100:654–658
Tamou S, Trott KR (1994) Modification of late radiation damage in the rectum of rats by deproteinized calf blood serum (ActoHorm) and pentoxifylline (PTX). Strahlenther Onkol 170:415–420
Tomas-de la Vega JE, Banner BF, Hubbard M et al (1984) Cytoprotective effect of prostaglandin E2 in irradiated rat ileum. Surg Gynecol Obstet 158:39–45
Toorop-Bouma AG, Van der Waaij D (1985) The effect of selective decontamination of the GI tract of mice on the survival of intestinal mucosa during X-irradiation. In: Wostmann BS (ed) Germfree research. Liss, New York, pp 271–273
Urata H, Kinoshita A, Misono KS et al (1990) Identification of a highly specific chymase as the major angiotensin II-forming enzyme in the human heart. J Biol Chem 265:22348–22357
Valls A, Pestchen I, Prats C et al (1999) Multicenter double-blind clinical trial comparing sucralfate vs placebo in the prevention of diarrhea secondary to pelvic irradiation. Med Clin 113:681–684
Vazquez I, Gomez-de-Segura IA, Grande AG et al (1999) Protective effect of enriched diet plus growth hormone administration on radiation-induced intestinal injury and on its evolutionary pattern in the rat. Dig Dis Sci 44:2350–2358
Verheij M, Dewit LGH, van Mourik JA (1995) The effect of ionizing radiation on endothelial tissue factor activity and its cellular localization. Thromb Haemost 73:894–895
Vernia P, Fracasso PL, Casale V et al (2000) Topical butyrate for acute radiation proctitis: randomised, crossover trial. Lancet 356:1232–1235
Wang J, Zheng H, Sung C-C et al (1998) Cellular sources of transforming growth factor b (TGF-β) isoforms in early and chronic radiation enteropathy. Am J Pathol 153:1531–1540
Wang J, Zheng H, Sung C-C et al (1999) The synthetic somatostatin analogue, octreotide, ameliorates acute and delayed intestinal radiation injury. Int J Radiat Oncol Biol Phys 45:1289–1296
Wang J, Zheng H, Hauer-Jensen M (2001a) Influence of short-term octreotide administration on chronic tissue injury, transforming growth factor b (TGF-β) overexpression, and collagen accumulation in irradiated rat intestine. J Pharmacol Exp Ther 297:35–42
Wang J, Zheng H, Hollenberg MD et al (2001b) Role of protease activated receptor-2 in intestinal radiation toxicity (abstract). Radiat Res Soc 48:106
Wang J, Albertson CM, Zheng H et al (2002a) Short-term inhibition of ADP-induced platelet aggregation by clopidogrel ameliorates radiation-induced toxicity in rat small intestine. Thromb Haemost 87:122–128
Wang J, Zheng H, Ou X et al (2002b) Deficiency of microvascular thrombomodulin and upregulation of protease-activated receptor 1 in irradiated rat intestine: possible link between endothelial dysfunction and chronic radiation fibrosis. Am J Pathol 160:2063–2072
Wang J, Zheng H, Ou X et al (2002c) Neuroimmune modulation of early and delayed radiation responses in rat small intestine. Radiat Res Soc 49:103
Weckbecker G, Liu R, Tolcsvai L et al (1992a) Antiproliferative effects of the somatostatin analogue octreotide (SMS 201-995) on ZR-75-1 human breast cancer cells in vivo and in vitro. Cancer Res 52:4973–4978
Weckbecker G, Tolcsvai L, Liu R et al (1992b) Preclinical studies on the anticancer activity of the somatostatin analogue octreotide (SMS 201-995). Metab Clin Exp 41 [Suppl 2]:99–103
Weckbecker G, Tolcsvai L, Pollak M et al (1994) Somatostatin analogue octreotide enhances the antineoplastic effects of tamoxifen and ovariectomy on 7,12-dimethylbenz(a)anthracene-induced rat mammary carcinomas. Cancer Res 54:6334–6337
Weiss JM, Cuff CA, Berman JW (1999) TGF-β downmodulates cytokine-induced monocyte chemoattractant protein (MCP)-1 expression in human endothelial cells. A putative role for TGF-β in the modulation of TNF receptor expression. Endothelium 6:291–302
Welniak LA, Khaled AR, Anver MR et al (2001) Gastrointestinal cells of IL-7 receptor null mice exhibit increased sensitivity to irradiation. J Immunol 166:2923–2928
Wilson R, Bealmear P, Matsuzawa T (1968) Acute intestinal radiation death in germfree and conventional mice. In: Sullivan MF (ed) Gastrointestinal radiation injury. Excerpta Medica Foundation, Amsterdam, pp 148–158
Wolf G, Ziyadeh FN, Stahl RAK (1999) Angiotensin II stimulates expression of transforming growth factor b receptor type II in mouse proximal tubular cells. J Mol Med 77:556–564

Wu SG, Miyamoto T (1990) Radioprotection of the intestinal crypts of mice by recombinant human interleukin-1 alpha. Radiat Res 123:112–115

Yada S, Nukina H, Kishihara K et al (2001) IL-7 prevents both capsase-dependent and -independent pathways that lead to the spontaneous apoptosis of i-IEL. Cell Immunol 208:88–95

Yamabe H, Osawa H, Inuma H et al (1997) Thrombin stimulates production of transforming growth factor-beta by cultured human mesangial cells. Nephrol Dial Transplant 12:438–442

Yeoh E, Horowitz M, Russo A et al (1993) Effect of pelvic irradiation on gastrointestinal function: a prospective longitudinal study. Am J Med 95:397–406

Yeoh E, Sun WM, Russo A et al (1996) A retrospective study of the effects of pelvic irradiation for gynecological cancer on anorectal function. Int J Radiat Oncol Biol Phys 35:1003–1010

Zheng H, Wang J, Hauer-Jensen M (2000a) Role of mast cells in early and delayed radiation injury in rat intestine. Radiat Res 153:533–539

Zheng H, Wang J, Koteliansky VE et al (2000b) Recombinant soluble transforming growth factor-β type II receptor ameliorates radiation enteropathy in the mouse. Gastroenterology 119:1286–1296

Zheng H, Wang J, Letterio JJ et al (2002) Dissociation of early and delayed intestinal radiation toxicity in TGF-β1 heterozygous mice. Radiat Res Soc 49:103

Zhou Q, Zhao Y, Li P et al (1992) Thrombomodulin as a marker of radiation-induced endothelial cell injury. Radiat Res 131:285–289

Zimmermann FB, Feldmann HJ (1998) Radiation proctitis. Clinical and pathological manifestations, therapy and prophylaxis of acute and late injurious effects of radiation on the rectal mucosa. Strahlenther Onkol 174:85–89

6 Mechanisms and Modification of the Radiation Response of the Central Nervous System

C. Nieder, N. Andratschke, and K. K. Ang

CONTENTS

6.1 Introduction 73
6.2 Models of Radiation Necrosis 73
6.3 Cytokine Production After
    Central Nervous System Irradiation 74
6.4 Glial Reactions After
    Central Nervous System Irradiation 76
6.5 Vascular Changes After
    Central Nervous System Irradiation 77
6.6 Effects of Growth Factors 78
6.7 From Previous Pharmacological
    Prophylactic Approaches to New Perspectives 80
6.8 Early Results of
    Growth Factor-Based Strategies 82
6.9 Conclusions 83
    References 83

6.1 Introduction

Radiobiological advances and technical developments have contributed significantly to reduce the risk of radiation-induced central nervous system damage. In some instances, utilization of both fractionation parameters and methods to decrease the irradiated volume of normal tissue may even allow for administration of an increased dose to the target volume without exceeding the usually accepted tolerance limits of surrounding critical structures. However, there are some situations where current strategies remain unsatisfactory. If innovative approaches could be developed, many patients would be able to receive more effective treatment. Rational biological prevention strategies, which might represent one possible approach, require a detailed understanding of the complex and dynamic pathophysiological changes, possibly resulting in manifestation of radiation-induced neurotoxicity. Considerable research efforts focused on histological as well as cellular and biochemical alterations have been undertaken over the last decades. Most of these experimental studies evaluated the development of late neurotoxicity, for example radiation necrosis either in the brain or the spinal cord (i.e., radiation myelopathy). Acute reactions, which mainly are the result of increased blood-brain-barrier permeability and edema, are self-limiting, of short duration, and treatable by corticosteroid administration. Early delayed reactions after 2–6 months are caused by transient demyelination, often combined with perturbance of the blood-brain barrier. In patients, they might result in somnolence and headache or Lhermitte's syndrome for a limited time span. Compared to these, the clinical implications of late reactions such as radionecrosis or leukencephalopathy are much more important. In addition to their potentially severe consequences for the patients' quality of life, they represent a major therapeutic challenge. So far, treatment is limited to a few strategies with inconsistent outcome, such as anticoagulation or sometimes surgical removal of necrosis. This chapter contains a review of current pathogenetic models of radiation necrosis as well as a discussion of the perspectives of newly developed preclinical prevention strategies.

6.2 Models of Radiation Necrosis

In 1934, first experimental data suggested a primary vascular pathogenesis (Scholz 1934). Later, numerous histopathological studies described both vascular changes (endothelial alterations, teleangiectasia, hyaline degeneration, edema, perivascular fibrosis and inflammation, fibrinoid necrosis, thrombosis),

C. Nieder, MD; N. Andratschke, MD
Department of Radiation Oncology, Klinikum rechts der Isar, Technical University Munich, Ismaningerstrasse 22, 81675 Munich, Germany
K. K. Ang, MD, PhD
Department of Radiation Oncology, The University of Texas M.D. Anderson Cancer Center, 1515 Holcombe Blvd., Box 97, Houston, TX 77030, USA

which might progress to hemorrhagic necrosis or infarction, and areas of demyelination, white matter necrosis, and glial reactions (activated astro- and microglia). Combinations of different changes are commonly observed (reviewed by Schultheiss et al. 1995). Classically, reproductive (or mitotic or clonogenic) cell death resulting from persistent genetic damage (DNA double-strand breaks, genetic instability from non- or misrepaired DNA lesions) was thought to cause a reduction in clonogenic cell numbers in parenchymal or vascular target cells. The long latent period was explained by long survival times of differentiated functional cells such as oligodendrocytes which turn over very slowly. The growth fraction of glial cells in the adult organism is approximately 0.1%–0.4% (Van der Kogel 1986; Li and Wong 1998). Comparable figures can be found for vascular endothelial cells.

More recently, radiation-induced cell killing by apoptosis or programmed cell death which is characterized by activation of a cascade of biochemical processes has been shown in the central nervous system (Larocca et al. 1997; Pena et al. 2000). In general, several apoptotic pathways could be identified, apparently sharing a common final mechanism that involves the interleukin 1β-converting enzyme (ICE/Ced-3) family of cysteine proteases (Dewey et al. 1995). Besides p53-mediated reactions (Chow et al. 2000), sphingomyelinase-mediated release of ceramide from cell membranes is one of the most important pro-apoptotic stimuli (Billis et al. 1998). The latter process was found after irradiation in endothelial cells of the central nervous system (Pena et al. 2000) as well as in oligodendrocytes (Larocca et al. 1997). Ultimately, a balance between pro- and anti-apoptotic mechanisms determines the magnitude of the apoptotic response. In vitro studies recently provided some evidence that neurons also undergo apoptotic cell death after irradiation (Gobbel et al. 1998). In addition, electrophysiological data derived from animal studies have shown that neurons react to clinically relevant radiation doses (Gangloff and Haley 1960; Pellmar and Lepinski 1993). Well-known clinical effects of central nervous system irradiation, e.g., intellectual deficits, memory loss, and dementia certainly suggest involvement of neurons in the pathogenetic process of late injury as well.

Currently, three different categories of radiation-induced effects that might interact in various ways can be described (Fig. 6.1). Cytocidal effects (killing of so-called target cells), reactive changes such as inflammation and perfusion deficit from vascular damage, and nonlethal functional effects such as activation of gene expression. Based on these categories, radiation necrosis is thought to result from complex dynamic interactions between parenchymal and vascular endothelial cells within the central nervous system (Tofilon and Fike 2000). In addition, impairment of the reproductive capacity of stem cells, for example in the subventricular zone, might contribute to development of late injury (Tada et al. 1999; Belka et al. 2001). The latent time, preceding the clinical manifestation of damage, is viewed as an active phase where cytokines and growth factors play important roles in inter- and intracellular communication. However, the molecular basis of this multicellular model has not been completely identified yet.

6.3
Cytokine Production After Central Nervous System Irradiation

Central nervous system irradiation might induce the production of tumor necrosis factor (TNF)-α and interleukin (IL)-1 by microglia and astrocytes (Chiang and McBride 1991; Merrill 1991). Release of IL-1 leads to further activation and proliferation of these cells via autocrine mechanisms (Merrill 1991; Ganter et al. 1992). As shown in vivo, a consecutive astrogliosis may develop (Otero and Merrill 1994). TNF-α is a cytokine with pro-apoptotic properties, which is produced and released mainly by activated macrophages and monocytes, but also by T and B cells. Besides radia-

Fig. 6.1. Radiation-induced effects in the central nervous system, which contribute to the development of neurotoxicity in a different radiation dose-dependent amount tion exposure, bacterial and viral infection might lead to production of TNF-α. The cytokine binds to its receptors (TNFR1/2). Figure 6.2 shows the signal transduction cascade after binding to the TNF-α-R1.

Already 2 h after single-fraction irradiation (25 Gy) of the midbrain in mice, an increase in mRNA levels of TNF-α and IL-1 was found (peak after 4 h, decrease after 24 h) (Hong et al. 1995). Recently, increased activity of the apoptosis-mediating enzymes caspase-1 (or ICE) and caspase-3 3 h after in vitro irradiation of oligodendrocytes was described (Akassoglou et al. 1998). Other data suggest that radiation-induced apoptosis in rat brain in turn leads to increased numbers of microglial cells with phagocytic properties (Ferrer et al. 1995). Besides its cytotoxic effects on oligodendrocytes (Chiang and McBride 1991; Merrill 1991; Cammer 2000), e.g., via induction of caspase-mediated apoptosis (Akassoglou et al. 1998), TNF-α prevents differentiation of oligodendrocyte progenitor cells towards oligodendrocytes in vitro (Baron et al. 1998). Furthermore, TNF-α might cause damage to endothelial cells, resulting in increased vascular permeability and inhibition of cell proliferation (Slungaard et al. 1990; Chiang and McBride 1991). TNF-α and IL-1 induce the expression of intercellular adhesion molecule-1 (ICAM-1) on oligodendrocytes and microvascular endothelial cells, possibly leading to autoimmune reactions (Satoh et al. 1991; Wong and Dorovini 1992). Increased levels of ICAM-1 mRNA were found after midbrain irradiation with 2 Gy in vivo (Hong et al. 1995). However, simple extrapolation of in vitro data to in vivo conditions might not be justified. It has been recently discussed, for example, that the role of TNF might be more complex than thought initially (Tofilon and Fike 2000), because this factor has now been shown to have a wide variety of biological functions that include mediation of antioxidative defense mechanisms and induction of anti-apoptotic proteins such as Bcl-2 (Tamatani et al. 1999). Interestingly, TNFRp75 knockout mice were more sensitive to radiation-induced brain damage after 25-Gy midbrain irradiation than TNFR p55 knockout mice and intact C57BL/6 animals (Daigle et al. 2001). TNF-α mRNA in irradiated TNFRp75 knockout mouse brain rose to levels that were consistently two to three times higher than the other two strains at 2 h. At later time points up to 6 months, the other two strains showed elevated TNF-α mRNA levels. Damage manifested in TNFR p75 knockout mice as early apoptosis in putative stem cell regions of the brain, followed by decreased proliferative responses in the same regions. After 3 months, seizures and other neurological abnormalities developed and histological examination revealed extensive demyelination. Demyelination was present in both TNFR p55 knockout mice and C57BL/6 mice, but it was far less marked and more focal. None of these strains exhibited marked hemorrhagic necrosis or other vascular damage.

Fig. 6.2. TNF-α-mediated apoptosis results from activation of TNF-α-receptor 1 and various signal transduction proteins (*TRADD*, TNFR-associated protein; *FADD*, Fas-associated protein). This results in activation of a cascade of caspases initiating apoptosis

Irradiation of the rat cerebral cortex was shown to increase the Nfkb-DNA-binding activity in a dose- and time-dependent fashion (Raju et al. 1999, 2000). This increased activity of Nfkb after irradiation (Fig. 6.3) is consistent with the activity of recovery and repair processes. For example, Nfkb can protect against apoptotic death and mediates the neuroprotective effects of insulin-like factor-1 (IGF-1) and nerve growth factor (NGF) (Maggirwar et al. 1998; Heck et al. 1999). Benekou et al. reported decreased IGF-1 gene expression after in utero irradiation of developing rat brain (Benekou et al. 2001). Pregnant animals were sacrificed 4 or 24 h after low-dose irradiation (10–40 cGy) and the fetal brain was examined for IGF-1 gene expression. Despite an increase in knowledge about the radioresponse of the central nervous system, the current data are still not sufficient. We need further research to decipher the pathways of the reactions after irradiation to develop protective strategies. In this context, we have to realize that in vitro systems do not allow simulation of the complex interactions between various cell types in vivo and that they are not suitable to reproduce both the volume effects and the time course of late neurotoxicity.

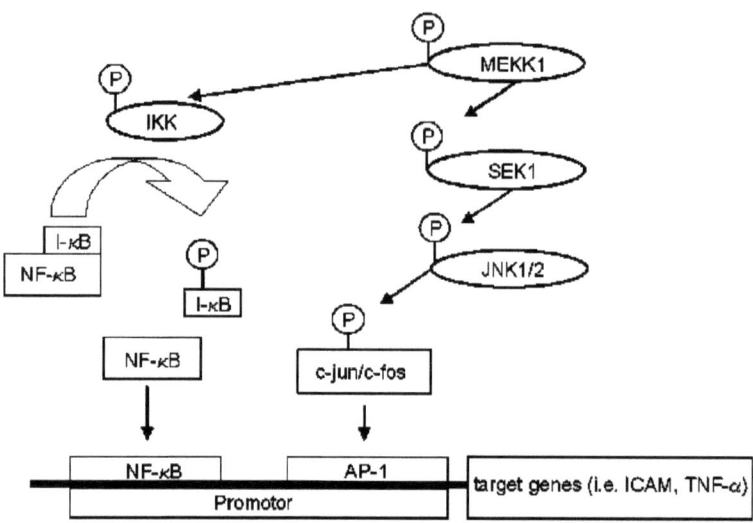

Fig. 6.3. Two basic mechanisms regulate gene expression in response to stress. Activation of *NF-kB* transcription factors is triggered by phosphorylation and degradation of *I-kB*. Degradation of *I-kB* masks the nuclear localization sequence of *NF-kB*, allowing nuclear import. The phosphorylation of *I-kB* is mediated by a kinase complex (*IKK*), which is activated by kinases belonging to stress kinase pathway (*MEKK-1*). In parallel, stress activates the stress kinase pathway, resulting in the activation of the transcription factor *AP-1*. The hallmark of this pathway is the signal transmission via subsequent phosphorylations. The most upstream kinase *MEKK-1* activates *SEK-1* which in turn phosphorylates and activates the jun-N terminal kinases (*JNK1/2*). These kinases phosphorylate the c-jun part of the *AP-1* transcription factor and thereby strongly increase the transcriptional activity (figure reproduced from BELKA et al. 2001, with permission)

6.4
Glial Reactions After Central Nervous System Irradiation

Magnitude and time course of glial reactions are dose-dependent (HORNSEY et al. 1981; CHIANG et al. 1993; SIEGAL and PFEFFER 1995; LI and WONG 1998). Within the first few hours after irradiation, glial cells undergo apoptosis, as has been extensively investigated in rat spinal cord (LI et al. 1996a,b; LI and WONG 1997, 1998), where the maximum (1%) was observed after 8 h (LI and WONG 1997). After 24 h, the baseline level of 0.05% was reached again. Within 24 h a total of approximately 9% of glial cells died via apoptosis. Split-course treatment with two fractions of 8 Gy was more effective than a single fraction of 16 Gy, regardless of the interval (LI and WONG 1997). Apoptosis occurred predominantly in the white matter, especially involving oligodendrocytes (LI et al. 1996a). The density of these cells decreased by 24%. Several studies have shown that oligodendrocyte-type-2-astrocyte (O-2 A) progenitor cells showed reduced clonogenic capacity after irradiation in vitro with doses as low as 5 Gy (VAN DER MAAZEN et al. 1992; VRDOLJAK et al. 1992). These data suggest that doses leading to apoptosis of oligodendrocytes will also decrease the clonogenic capacity of their progenitor cells.

Other studies showed that glial cell proliferation is inhibited for several hours or days (HORNSEY et al. 1981; CHIANG et al. 1993), followed by an early proliferative response without functional consequences. After treatment with 8 Gy, proliferation started after 2 days (maximum after 14 days) (LI and WONG 1998). Following 15 Gy, it started after 14 days (SIEGAL and PFEFFER 1995; SIEGAL et al. 1996), following 20 Gy after 16 days (HORNSEY et al. 1981). When looking at the different cell types, phagocytic cells and microglia were seen after 1–2 weeks, whereas astrocyte numbers increased shortly thereafter (NAKAGAWA et al. 1996). A second proliferative response was found after more than 120 days following treatment with 20 Gy (HORNSEY et al. 1981) or 22 Gy (LI and WONG 1998), i.e., before white matter necrosis and neurological symptoms were recorded (reviewed by STEWART and VAN DER KOGEL 1997). After lower doses, the second wave appeared with some delay, e.g., after 180–240 days following a dose of 15 Gy (SIEGAL and PFEFFER 1995; SIEGAL et al. 1996). As seen earlier, the number of both astrocytes and microglia increased (CHIANG et al. 1993). The latter cells play important roles in antigen presentation and production of cytokines and cytotoxins.

6.5
Vascular Changes After Central Nervous System Irradiation

Microvascular networks, consisting of arterioles, capillaries, and venules, are of critical importance for the supply with oxygen and nutrients. They represent the most radiosensitive part of the vasculature (ROTH et al. 1999). Doses within the usual therapeutic range lead to functional and structural damage such as increased permeability, changes in shape and diameter, and fibrous proliferation, eventually resulting in perfusion deficits. As early as 3 h after irradiation of the thoracolumbar cord with 15 Gy, abrupt increases in prostaglandin E_2, thromboxane, and prostacyclin (PGI_2) synthesis, lasting for 3 days have been described (SIEGAL and PFEFFER 1995). After both 7 and 14 days, synthesis of these molecules decreased significantly. At 28–240 days, continuously increasing abnormal synthesis of thromboxane and simultaneously decreasing production of PGI_2 were observed. The level of serotonin was increased after more than 120 days. Associated with these changes, two phases of increased vascular permeability (at least 70%) were present 24 h and 120–240 days after irradiation (SIEGAL and PFEFFER 1995). Levels of endothelin, a vasoconstrictive molecule, decreased within the first 10 days, followed by a continuous increase thereafter (SIEGAL et al. 1996). These observations suggest that impaired function of microvessels (increased permeability and coagulability, vasoconstriction) can be found in histologically normal spinal cord after irradiation with doses which do not cause structural changes. Comparable results were published for whole-brain irradiation of rats (five fractions of 4 Gy) (MILDENBERGER et al. 1990). There was, however, a localized significant increase in microglial cells, possibly caused by a loss of axons in the striatal white matter after 6 months. The anatomical pattern of changes was suggestive of vascular damage to the few small vessels, exclusively feeding this particular part of the brain.

A decrease of endothelial cell numbers has been observed within 1 week after single-fraction irradiation of the rat plexus choroideus (17.5–25 Gy) (HOPEWELL et al. 1989). The reduction persisted for the observation period of 52 weeks, being dose-dependent from week 26 on and amounting to approximately 40% after 17.5 Gy and 65% after 22.5 or 25 Gy. Recent results provide some evidence that endothelial cells in the central nervous system of mice undergo apoptosis after irradiation in a dose- and time-dependent manner (maximum after 12 h, involving 16%–20% of endothelial cells) (PENA et al. 2000). In addition, a dose-dependent atrophy of smooth muscle cells has been observed, which increased over time (HOPEWELL et al. 1989), possibly explaining why the early functional reduction of the diameter of blood vessels is followed by an increase later on. Teleangiectasia can be commonly observed, e.g., 12 months after single-fraction treatment with 25 Gy (PLOTNIKOVA et al. 1988).

With further increasing doses, latency of vascular damage decreases more and more, as shown after stereotactic irradiation of rat parietal cortex with a 4-mm collimator (doses of 50, 75, or 120 Gy, latency of 12 months to 3 weeks) (KAMIRYO et al. 1996). The extent of damage increased accordingly. RUBIN et al. performed careful magnetic resonance imaging and histological examinations of rat brains 2–24 weeks after high-dose irradiation (single fraction of 60 Gy) (RUBIN et al. 1994). After 2 weeks, the permeability of the blood–brain barrier was significantly increased. After 6 weeks, this increase was even more pronounced. After 8–12 weeks, some recovery occurred. However, at the time of the next examination after 24 weeks, a dramatic impairment was shown. At that time, vessel density was also significantly decreased. Necrosis was observed after more than 24 weeks. Interestingly, this study demonstrated a biphasic time course, comparable to the data for proliferation and activation of glial cells (HORNSEY et al. 1981; SIEGAL and PFEFFER 1995; SIEGAL et al. 1996; LI and WONG 1998).

In general, the biphasic time course might be the result of initial apoptotic processes in a certain proportion of parenchymal and vascular cells as well as a release of cytokines (WITTE et al. 1989; LI et al. 1996a, b; LI and WONG 1997, 1998), both leading to activation of microglia and astrocytes in an attempt to initiate regenerative and proliferative responses. After a period of stabilization and beginning approximately 8 weeks after irradiation, a second wave of cell death (mitotic-linked cell death) initiates progressive vascular dysfunction, again accompanied by complex glial reactions. Following irradiation of the spinal cord in newborn rats, an increase in vascular endothelial growth factor (VEGF) mRNA in astrocytes in areas showing vascular changes later on was shown (BARTHOLDI et al. 1997). In adult rat spinal cord, TSAO et al. (1999) found some evidence that white-matter astrocytes up-regulate VEGF several weeks after single-dose irradiation with 22 Gy and that dysfunction of the blood–spinal cord barrier is associated with this phenomenon. Meanwhile, extension of this study suggests that VEGF up-regulation starting at 16 weeks after irradiation is a result of hypoxia (Li et al. 2001). Unfortunately, these data do not include examinations within 3 months of irradiation. As a result of loss of endothelial cells and blood vessels as well as hyperpermeability, perivascular edema and consecutive ischemia will develop (Hopewell and Van der Kogel 1999). These changes are likely to result in permanent oxidative stress. Due to the particular susceptibility of the myelin membrane for oxidative damage, radiation-induced changes will predominately affect the white matter (Tofilon and Fike 2000). Table 6.1 summarizes the dose-dependent time course of functional and structural changes, cell death, and proliferation in irradiated spinal cord.

The important role of the vasculature is emphasized by results of experimental boron-neutron-capture therapy. By use of pharmacological compounds that do not cross the blood–brain barrier, the vascular wall can be irradiated almost selectively. Morris et al. administered physical doses of approximately 19–35 Gy intravascularly (Morris et al. 1996). The physical dose inside the central nervous system parenchyma was much lower (by a factor of 6), as was the biologically effective dose (by a factor of 2.7). Histologically, spinal cord lesions were indistinguishable from those caused by conventional treatment, which, of course, is not selective to the vasculature. With respect to latency, no difference was observed.

Genetic heterogeneity, age differences between the animals, variations in techniques of anesthesia and radiotherapy, different fractionation schedules, and variations in both irradiated part and volume of the spinal cord might account for some differences in the results from distinct studies.

6.6
Effects of Growth Factors

Both developing and adult central nervous system contains multipotent neuroepithelial stem cells, the source of either neuron- or glia-specific precursor cells which give rise to neurons, astrocytes and oligodendrocytes (Craig et al. 1996; McKay 1997; Brüstle et al. 1999; Rao 1999). Stem cell populations can be expanded by treatment with growth factors, e.g., platelet-derived growth factor (PDGF), basic fibroblast growth factor (FGF-2), IGF-1, and glial growth factor-2 (GGF-2) (Noble et al. 1988; Raff et al. 1988; Craig et al. 1996; Calver et al. 1998; Rao 1999). The same holds true for O-2A progenitor cells (Fig. 6.4) which also have been identified in the adult central nervous system of rodents and humans (Wolswijk and Noble 1989; Levine et al. 1993; Hunter et al. 1997). Astrocytes and microglia represent the most important source of growth factors, which regulate, for example, the function of neurons and the proliferation, differentiation, migration, and survival of oligodendrocytes (Tofilon and Fike 2000). Growth factor receptors

Table 6.1. Time course of pathogenetic processes after central nervous system irradiation in animal models

Time after irradiation	Vascular changes	Consequences	Glial changes
First few hours	Thromboxane, prostacyclin, and prostaglandin production ↑	Vessel dilation and slowing of blood flow	Apoptosis of cells, especially oligodendrocytes
	Endothelin production ↓		
	Apoptosis of endothelial cells		
Within 3 days		Perivascular edema	Inhibition of proliferation
After 1 week	Levels of vasoactive substances decrease again		Activation and proliferation of microglia and astrocytes
After 1 week (and single fraction irradiation >15 Gy)	Continuously increasing loss of endothelial cells and atrophy of smooth muscle cells	Eventually teleangiectasia	
After 2 weeks	Endothelin production ↑	Vasoconstriction starts	Maximum proliferation of glial cells
After 4 weeks	Thromboxane production ↑	Slowing of blood flow and decrease of vascular permeability	Glial proliferation no longer increased
	Prostacyclin production ↓		
After 8 weeks			Continuous reduction of oligodendrocyte number
After 17 weeks	Serotonin production ↑	Permeability increases again (perivascular edema)	2nd phase of glial proliferation
	Vessel density ↓	Ischemia	

```
                    Multipotent Stem Cells
                             ↓
         Type-1 Astrocytes ← ↓ → Neurons
                             ↓
Type-2 Astrocytes ← Oligodendrocyte-Type-2-Astrocyte  Progenitor  Cells
         Proliferation:      ↓         Survivial:
         + NT-3, IGF-1, GGF-2 ↓        +CNTF, IGF-1, PDGF
         ++ FGF-2, PDGF      ↓         Differentiation:
         +++ FGF-2/PDGF Combination ↓  - FGF-2/PDGF Combination
         Migration:          ↓         FGF-2, NT-3
         + PDGF, FGF-2       ↓         +IGF-1, CNTF, LIF, TGF-β
                             ↓
                        Oligodendrocytes
                   (postmigratory, without PDGF-receptors)
                        Survival:
                        FGF-2
                        + IGF-1, CNTF, NT-3, NGF
```

Fig. 6.4. Growth factor effects on oligodendroglial cells. +, stimulation; –, inhibition; NT-3, neurotrophin-3; IGF-1, insulin-like growth factor-1; GGF-2, glial growth factor-2; CNTF, ciliary neurotrophic factor; PDGF, platelet-derived growth factor; FGF-2, basic fibroblast growth factor; LIF, leukemia inhibitory factor; TGF-β, transforming growth factor-β; NGF nerve growth factor

were identified in neurons, astrocytes, microglia, oligodendrocytes and their progenitors (REDWINE et al. 1997). As a general rule, these tyrosine kinase receptors dimerize after binding their respective ligand, followed by autophosphorylation and activation of several possible secondary signal transduction mechanisms (KIRSCH et al. 1997).

IGF-1 is an important survival factor for O-2A progenitor cells and oligodendrocytes in vitro, whereas PDGF stimulates survival of progenitor cells only, because mature cells cease to express PDGF-receptors (RAFF et al. 1993; BUTT et al. 1997; SCOLDING et al. 1998). Signals are being mediated by a pathway that includes the enzyme phosphatidylinositol 3-kinase (PI-3 K) (Fig. 6.5). Inhibition of the enzyme resulted in apoptosis despite the presence of growth factors (VEMURI and MCMORRIS 1996). Regarding the antiapoptotic effect of IGF-1, other possible downstream events include inhibition of caspase-3 activity via activation of Bcl-2, inhibition of Bax, and the mitogen-activated protein kinase (MAPK/ERK) pathway (GROTHEY et al. 1999; PARRIZAS et al. 1997). Conversely, inhibition of stress-activated protein kinase (SAPK/JNK) by IGF-1 has also been described (OKUBO et al. 1998). Increasing the concentration of several factors such as IGF-1 and ciliary neurotrophic factor (CNTF) delayed apoptotic cell death of oligodendrocytes in the postnatal optic nerve of rats in vivo (BARRES et al. 1993). IGF-1 receptors were also found on endothelial cells (BAR et al. 1988). Recent data provide evidence that IGF-1 might regulate the permeability of the blood–brain barrier (PAN and KASTIN 2000).

Fig. 6.5. Activation of protein kinase B/Akt by growth factor receptors via the PI3 kinase pathway

VEGF, initially thought to act exclusively on endothelial cells, regulates embryonic de novo vasculogenesis from angioblasts and later occurring angiogenetic processes (ROSENSTEIN et al. 1998). Endothelial progenitor cells have been identified in adult individuals of several species (ASAHARA et al. 1997). In the adult central nervous system, where virtually no angiogenesis takes place, the choroid plexus, cells in the area postrema, and in the cerebellum physiologically produce low levels of VEGF or VEGF-receptor mRNA. Intracerebral VEGF treatment (0.01 µg for 1 week) caused neoangiogenesis in adult rats as well as reactive astrocytosis. Those perivascular astrocytes expressed VEGFR, suggesting that cells forming a part of the blood–brain barrier might also be involved in mediation of angiogenesis (ROSENSTEIN et al. 1998). Permeability of these new vessels was higher than in controls. Increased permeability caused by VEGF is also thought to cause perifocal tumor edema (HAYASHI et al. 1998; PROESCHOLDT et al. 1999). VEGF showed anti-apoptotic properties, e.g., in endothelial cells exposed to TNF-α (SPYRIDOPOULOS et al. 1997). It prevented apoptosis by activation of MAPK/ERK or inhibition of SAPK/JNK in human microvascular endothelial cells (GUPTA et al. 1999). FGF-2, which also activates MAPK (D'ANGELO et al. 1995), was less effective. In vitro, VEGF increased the proliferation of Schwann cells and the survival of neurons. Retinal astrocytes expressed VEGF in case of hypoxia (STONE et al. 1995). In several animal models, administration of $VEGF_{165}$ led to improved perfusion of ischemic extremities and myocardium as well as to reduced damage after temporary occlusion of the cerebral middle artery (DEWEY et al. 1995). It also protected neuronal cell lines from hypoxia and glucose deprivation (JIN et al. 2000) and showed proliferation- and survival-promoting effects on neural cells in the peripheral nervous system (SONDELL et al. 1999).

Human endothelial cells produce PDGF (KAVANAUGH et al. 1988) and express its receptors, with some variation dependent on vessel size and location (EDELBERG et al. 1998). Capillary endothelial cells proliferated in vitro after stimulation with PDGF (BAR et al. 1989). ZHANG and HUTCHINS (1997) described some of the effects of PDGF in neurons and astrocytes.

FGF receptors were found in capillaries from mouse brain and in vitro studies showed mitogenic responses after FGF-2 treatment (BASTAKI et al. 1997). This effect might depend on vessel size (D'AMORE and SMITH 1993). FGF-2 induced repair of radiation damage in bovine aortic endothelial cells via an extracellular autocrine mechanism (HAIMOVITZ-FRIEDMAN et al. 1991). After irradiation in vitro (2–6 Gy), cells secreted FGF-2, followed by repair of potentially lethal damage and recovery of clonogenicity. The same group showed that human umbilical vein endothelial cells also secreted FGF-2 (WITTE et al. 1989). Additional data suggest that FGF-2 inhibits radiation-induced apoptosis in endothelial cells from large vessels more effectively than in microvascular cells (LANGLEY et al. 1997). FGF-2 activated the 1,2-diacylglycerol (DAG)-PKC system, causing inhibition of sphingomyelinase-mediated apoptosis (HAIMOVITZ-FRIEDMAN 1994).

PENA et al. (2000) demonstrated that three IV injections of FGF-2 5 min before, immediately after, and 1 h after total-body irradiation in mice significantly reduced the apoptotic cell number within the central nervous system, protecting both endothelial and glial cells. The results were not influenced by the dose of FGF-2 (0.45 or 4.5 µg per animal). In vitro, FGF-2 stimulates proliferation of astrocytes (SCHERER and SCHNITZER 1994) as well as microglia, provided that astrocytes are present (GIULIAN and INGLEMAN 1988). FGF-2 has previously been shown to reduce central nervous system damage after ischemia in rats (TANAKA et al. 1995).

6.7
From Previous Pharmacological Prophylactic Approaches to New Perspectives

Considering radiation myelopathy as a consequence of a dynamic and complex cytokine-mediated process, therapeutic intervention in its earliest phase might inhibit progression of these pathological cascades. So far, several pragmatic but nonspecific approaches have been undertaken. Prophylactic treatment with dexamethasone 24 and 1 h before irradiation may reduce expression of TNF-α, IL-1, and ICAM-1 (HONG et al. 1995). In vitro, corticosteroids inhibit the function of microglial cells and their proliferation (TANAKA et al. 1997). Other compounds, e.g., glutathione and cysteine, interact with free radicals. N-acetyl-L-cysteine (NAC) increases intracellular cysteine levels and protected oligodendrocytes against TNF-α-induced death (NOBLE and MAYER-PROESCHEL 1996). WR-2721 (amifostine) was administered intrathecally before single-dose spinal cord irradiation in rats (SPENCE et al. 1986). A dose-modifying factor of 1.3 and a prolongation of median latency to myelopathy by 63% at the

ED$_{50}$ were reported. FIKE et al. (1994) showed that α-difluoromethylornithine (DFMO, a polyamine-synthesis inhibitor given IV 2 days before to 14 days after ^{125}I brachytherapy) reduced the volume of radionecrosis and the contrast-enhancement in dog brain. Compared to controls who received NaCl, DFMO-treated dogs had reduced labeling indices and a delayed increase of phagocytic cells and microglia (NAKAGAWA et al. 1996). KONDZIOLKA et al. (1999) implanted C6 glioma into rat brain and performed a single fraction gamma-knife treatment, with or without IV administration of U-74389G, a 21-aminosteroid that is largely selective to endothelium (50–60 min before radiosurgery). The drug prevented development of perifocal edema and radiation-induced vessel damage in the healthy brain region within the steep dose gradients just outside the target volume. This effect might be caused by antioxidative and membrane-stabilizing properties, leading to reduced secretion of arachidonic acid from damaged cell membranes. Vascular hyperpermeability after radiation was reduced when rh-MnSOD (manganese superoxide dismutase) was given in vivo, emphasizing the possible role of free oxygen radicals for microvessel dysfunction. HOPEWELL et al. (1994) administered unsaturated fatty acids which modulate prostaglandin and thromboxane levels. Oral application for 20 weeks (starting 1 day after 22 Gy) reduced the incidence of radiation myelopathy in pigs and delayed paresis in rats (HOPEWELL et al. 1994; EL-AGAWAMI et al. 1996). The use of gamma linolenic acid in humans with large arteriovenous malformations (AVM) of the brain treated with stereotactic radiosurgery significantly reduced the risk for complications (SIMS and PLOWMAN 2001). However, the therapeutic ratio was not improved due to a reduction in AVM obliteration rate. It has to emphasized that in this particular study, protection of targets in the vasculature might be responsible for both effects. If the primary target of radiotherapy was tumor tissue rather than blood vessels, a therapeutic gain might be obtained. HORNSEY et al. (1990) showed that the vasoactive drug dipyridamole (starting 17 weeks after single dose irradiation) reduced the incidence of myelopathy in rats. ED$_{50}$ increased by 2–3 Gy.

Table 6.2 contains a list of rational innovative prevention strategies. Some of these are now being studied in vivo. Besides stimulation of endogenous cell regeneration, transplantation of glial progenitor cells or stem cells might be feasible. O-2A cells generated in vitro and transplanted into damaged parts of the central nervous system are capable of proliferation, migration, and development into differentiated oligodendrocytes (FRANKLIN and BLAKEMORE 1997). Whether this results in durable prevention of neurological complications needs yet to be examined. IJICHI et al. (1996) evaluated the influence of PDGF on stimulation of regeneration of O-2A progenitor cells after irradiation. They transplanted rat fibroblasts expressing PDGF-AA into the cisterna magna of rats. These cells migrated into the subarachnoid space of the cervical spinal cord. One week after injection, a significant increase in the number of O-2A progenitor colonies was observed, which persisted for at least 2 weeks. It remained unclear whether this increase was caused by increased proliferation or by migration of cells into the cervical spinal cord. REZVANI et al. (2001) transplanted neural stem cells after irradiation of rat spinal cord in order to prevent myelopathy. Initial data suggest that this strategy might be useful; however, their work needs to be expanded from immature to adult rats and to a broader range of radiation doses. Furthermore, long-term follow-up results have to be awaited.

Compared to these early data, a broader, but still limited experience exists with growth factor treatment. CNTF protected oligodendrocytes against toxicity of TNF-α in vitro (LOUIS et al. 1993). Yet, to our knowledge, studies of CNTF in radiation necrosis have not been published. IGF-1 was shown to ameliorate the neurological status in animal models of multiple sclerosis, where it increased the oligodendrocyte number and reduced the permeability of the blood–brain barrier (LIU et al. 1996). As already discussed, many data suggest possible involvement of several growth factors in the process of postradiation changes. Therefore, an animal model was developed in order to study the effects of either intrathecal or systemic administration of growth factors.

Table 6.2. Overview of emerging rational prevention strategies for radiation-induced central nervous system necrosis

Strategies in the early phase of irradiation	Strategies during the latent time after irradiation
Inhibition of radiation-induced apoptosis, e.g., administration of FGF-2, PDGF, or IGF-1	Vasoactive drugs or neovascularization, e.g., through VEGF
Radioprotective agents such as WR-2721 (amifostine) or N-acetyl-L-cysteine	Stem cell recruitment, e.g., through administration of growth factors
Cytokine inhibitors, kinase inhibitors, or proteasome inhibitors	Transplantation of stem cells or O-2A progenitor cells

FGF-2, basic fibroblast growth factor; IGF-1, insulin-like growth factor-1; VEGF, vascular endothelial growth factor; PDGF, platelet-derived growth factor.

6.8
Early Results of Growth Factor-Based Strategies

Our group has previously studied radiation myelopathy in adult Fisher F-344 rats, treated with ^{60}Co-gamma irradiation to the cervical spinal cord. The same model was used here. Continuous infusion of PDGF, FGF-2 or saline for 2 weeks either during or after radiotherapy was approved by the Institutional Animal Care and Use Committee. The animals were maintained and treated at the Department of Veterinary Medicine and Surgery, The University of Texas M. D. Anderson Cancer Center, Houston, TX, USA in accordance with US regulations and law. The rats were anesthetized by inhalation of halothane, as described in a previous publication (ANG et al. 1982). For the purpose of growth factor administration, a surgical technique was developed, where a dorsal midline incision was made over the caudal aspect of the skull and neck. A hole was drilled in the sagittal midline through the suture between the interparietal and occipital bone. A cannula produced by bending a 0.75-in., 23-gauge hypodermic stainless steel tubing at a 60° angle and cut to limit the depth to 6–6.5 mm was inserted along the rostral aspect of the occipital bone into the cisterna magna (Fig. 6.6). This route of application was chosen because a literature search did not result in conclusive data about blood–brain permeability for these growth factors. The external portion of the catheter was sutured to the dorsal cervical muscles. A polyethylene catheter connected this cannula with an osmotic Alzet pump (model 2ML1, Alza, Palo Alto, CA, USA), placed subcutaneously on the back along the dorsal midline. This type of pump contains 2 ml of fluid and delivers 10 μl/h for 7 days. In order to avoid extensive inactivation of proteins at body temperature over time, pumps were changed after 7 days. At this short surgical procedure, permeability of the catheter was checked by injection of saline. We also tested whether the pump was completely empty. The same procedures were performed after 14 days when the implanted material was removed in toto.

Follow-up was at 12 months. Rats were monitored every other day for development of paresis as a sign of spinal cord damage (clinical study endpoint). Two days after definitive paresis, rats were killed in a CO_2 chamber and prepared (formalin fixation, decalcification) for histopathological examination of HE-stained slides of the complete central nervous system. Thus, the diagnosis of radiation myelopathy was histologically verified. Rats suffering from severe intercurrent disease or treatment-induced tumors were also killed, as well as all remaining animals that completed the 12-month observation period. Initial experiments were performed with PDGF-BB (Chiron Corp., Emeryville, CA, USA) delivered at 35 μg per day over 2 weeks. This dose was determined as the maximum tolerable dose in a preliminary toxicity study that revealed mortality after 50 μg. The general range of doses was derived from published reports in a variety of other non-radiation-related conditions.

Infusion was given between two radiation fractions (16 Gy plus 14–20 Gy). Control animals received intrathecal saline. ED_{50} was 32.3 Gy (95% confidence interval, 31–33.1 Gy) in the control group. Median latency after 16 + 20 Gy was 143 days (95% confidence interval, 142–144 days). It was considerably shorter after treatment with PDGF (Fig. 6.7, $P=0.07$), probably resulting from cell-cycle-activating signals. Usually, many cell types undergo p53-induced G1 arrest after radiotherapy to allow for repair of treatment-induced lesions. By overriding this mechanism with high doses of PDGF, such cells might be forced to undergo apoptosis. There was no appreciable difference in histology of myelopathy, nor was there any other obvious abnormality in the central nervous system of PDGF-treated rats (NIEDER et al. 2000).

In a comparable setting, 2 weeks of FGF-2 (Chiron Corp., Emeryville, CA, USA) at 25 μg per day did not cause a significant acceleration or protection. These results have recently been published in greater detail (NIEDER et al. 2002). Perioperative death within 2 weeks from final surgery occurred in 29 of 182 animals (16%) treated during the first year, usually as a result of hematoma, infection, or damage to brain structures. The rate tended to decrease with increasing experience of the surgeons. Nineteen rats (10%) were found to have broken polyethylene catheters

Fig. 6.6. Lateral radiograph of a stainless steel cannula inserted into the cisterna magna of an adult F-344 rat

Fig. 6.7. Kaplan-Meier estimates of the risk of development of radiation myelopathy within 12 months of irradiation (PDGF vs saline, 30–36 Gy)

at second or third surgery. A median weight loss of 12% was measured between first and final surgery, which was completely recovered within 4–6 weeks. However, the saline groups had a median weight loss of 7% ($P=0.04$ in χ^2 test). No other acute or delayed toxicity was seen.

IGF-1 has been shown to cross the blood–brain barrier. Furthermore, subcutaneous injection every 12–24 h results in sufficient levels of the agent. Subcutaneous IGF-1 was delivered in a dose of 700 μg per injection concomitant to radiotherapy, as also described in a recent article (NIEDER et al. 2002). This treatment led to an increase in latent time; however, combining IGF-1 with intrathecal FGF-2 was even more effective as it actually decreased the incidence of radiation myelopathy (Fig. 6.8).

In summary, spinal cord protection by treatment with growth factors during radiotherapy appears feasible. At present, efforts continue to identify the optimum growth factor (or combination), dose level, and timing of administration in larger numbers of animals.

6.9
Conclusions

Currently, radiobiological principles and advanced treatment planning can be used to reduce radiation-induced central nervous system toxicity. The present dynamic pathogenetic model, which includes various effects of cytokines and growth factors, forms the basis of rational innovative prevention strategies, which are now being studied in vivo. A feasible technique of intrathecal administration of growth factors during or after radiotherapy of the cervical spinal cord in rats has been developed. Increasing experience of the treatment team reduced the surgical complication rate. We have shown that such treatment results in modulation of the dynamics of radiation myelopathy. However, the optimum growth factor-based approach has not been defined yet. Whether intrathecal treatment is mandatory is an open question. Further results of growth factor treatment will become available soon. Investigations are planned on the influence of these proteins on development, progression, and radiosensitivity of tumors as well, because such effects might counteract administration for normal tissue protection. Stem cell transplantation as well as pharmacological agents such as cytokine- or kinase-inhibitors might also be considered for evaluation. Noninvasive detection of early signs of radiation-induced central nervous system alterations which do not have clinical correlates at that time is still problematic (MOVSAS et al. 2001). Development of improved diagnostic methods such as MR spectroscopy or positron emission tomography might facilitate the evaluation of preventive strategies in preclinical models by looking at more complex endpoints than just presence or absence of radiation necrosis.

References

Akassoglou K, Bauer J, Kassiotis G et al (1998) Oligodendrocyte apoptosis and primary demyelination by local TNF/p55TNF receptor signaling in the central nervous system of transgenic mice: models for multiple sclerosis with primary oligodendrogliopathy. Am J Pathol 153:801–813

Fig. 6.8. Kaplan-Meier estimates of the risk of development of radiation myelopathy within 12 months of irradiation (IGF-1 plus FGF-2 (33 Gy) vs saline (32 and 34 Gy). (From NIEDER et al. 2002, with permission)

Ang KK, van der Kogel AJ, van der Schueren E (1982) Inhalation anaesthesia in experimental radiotherapy: a reliable and time-saving system for multifraction studies in a clinical department. Int J Radiat Oncol Biol Phys 8:145–148

Asahara T, Murohara T, Sullivan A et al (1997) Isolation of putative progenitor endothelial cells for angiogenesis. Science 275:964–967

Bar RS, Boes M, Dake BL et al (1988) Insulin, insulin-like growth factors and vascular endothelium. Am J Med 85 [Suppl 5A]:59–70

Bar BS, Boes M, Booth BA et al (1989) The effects of platelet-derived growth factor in cultured microvessel endothelial cells. Endocrinology 124:1841–1848

Baron W, de Jonge JC, de Vries H et al (1998) Regulation of oligodendrocyte differentiation: protein kinase C activation prevents differentiation of O-2A progenitor cells toward oligodendrocytes. Glia 22:121–129

Barres BA, Schmid R, Sendtner M et al (1993) Multiple extracellular signals are required for long-term oligodendrocyte survival. Development 118:283–295

Bartholdi D, Rubin BP, Schwab ME (1997) VEGF mRNA induction correlates with changes in the vascular architecture upon spinal cord damage in the rat. Eur J Neurosci 9:2549–2560

Bastaki M, Nelli EE, Dell'Era P et al (1997) Basic fibroblast growth factor-induced angiogenic phenotype in mouse endothelium. Arterioscler Thromb Vasc Biol 17:454–464

Belka C, Budach W, Kortmann RD et al (2001) Radiation induced CNS toxicity – molecular and cellular mechanisms. Br J Cancer 85:1233–1239

Benekou A, Bolaris S, Kazanis E et al (2001) In utero radiation-induced changes in growth factor levels in the developing rat brain. Int J Radiat Biol 77:83–93

Billis W, Fuks Z, Kolesnick R (1998) Signaling in and regulation of ionizing radiation-induced apoptosis in endothelial cells. Rec Prog Horm Res 53:85–93

Brüstle O, Jones KN, Learish RD et al (1999) Embryonic stem cell-derived glial precursors: a source of myelinating transplants. Science 285:754–756

Butt AM, Hornby MF, Ibrahim M et al (1997) PDGF-α receptor and myelin basic protein mRNAs are not coexpressed by oligodendrocytes in vivo: a double in situ hybridization study in the anterior medullary velum of the neonatal rat. Mol Cell Neurosci 8:311–322

Calver AR, Hall AC, Yu WP et al (1998) Oligodendrocyte population dynamics and the role of PDGF in vivo. Neuron 20:869–882

Cammer W (2000) Effects of TNFa on immature and mature oligodendrocytes and their progenitors in vitro. Brain Res 864:213–219

Chiang CS, McBride WH (1991) Radiation enhances tumor necrosis factor alpha production by murine brain cells. Brain Res 566:265–269

Chiang CS, McBride WH, Withers HR (1993) Radiation-induced astrocytic and microglial responses in mouse brain. Radiother Oncol 29:60–68

Chow BM, Li YQ, Wong CS (2000) Radiation-induced apoptosis in the adult central nervous system is p53-dependent. Cell Death Differ 7:712–720

Craig CG, Tropepe V, Morshead CM et al (1996) In vivo growth factor expansion of endogenous subependymal neural precursor cell populations in the adult mouse brain. J Neurosci 16:2649–2658

Daigle JL, Hong JH, Chiang CS, McBride WH (2001) The role of tumor necrosis factor signaling pathways in the response of murine brain to irradiation. Cancer Res 61:8859–8865

D'Angelo G, Struman J, Martial J et al (1995) Activation of mitogen-activated protein kinases by vascular endothelial growth factor and basic fibroblast growth factor in capillary endothelial cells is inhibited by the antiangiogenic factor 16-kDa N-terminal fragment of prolactin. Proc Natl Acad Sci U S A 92:6374–6378

D'Amore PA, Smith SR (1993) Growth factor effects on cells of the vascular wall: a survey. Growth Factors 8:61–75

Dewey WC, Ling CC, Meyn RE (1995) Radiation-induced apoptosis: relevance to radiotherapy. Int J Radiat Oncol Biol Phys 33:781–796

Edelberg JM, Aird WC, Wu W et al (1998) PDGF mediates cardiac microvascular communication. J Clin Invest 102:837–843

El-Agawami AY, Hopewell JW, Plowman PN et al (1996) Modulation of normal tissue responses to radiation. Br J Radiol 39:374–375

Ferrer I, Olive M, Blanco R et al (1995) Amoeboid microglial response following X-ray-induced apoptosis in the neonatal rat brain. Neurosci Lett 193:109–112

Fike JR, Gobbel GT, Marton LJ et al (1994) Radiation brain injury is reduced by the polyamine inhibitor α-difluoromethylornithine. Radiat Res 138:99–106

Franklin RJ, Blakemore WF (1997) Transplanting oligodendrocyte progenitors into the adult CNS. J Anat 190:23–33

Gangloff H, Haley TJ (1960) Effects of X-irradiation on spontaneous and evoked brain electrical activity in cats. Radiat Res 12:694–704

Ganter S, Northoff H, Mannel D et al (1992) Growth control of cultured microglia. J Neurosci Res 33:218–230

Giulian D, Ingleman JE (1988) Colony-stimulating factors as promoters of ameboid microglia. J Neurosci 8:4707–4717

Gobbel GT, Bellinzona M, Vogt AR et al (1998) Response of postmitotic neurons to x-irradiation: implications for the role of DNA damage in neuronal apoptosis. J Neurosci 18:147–155

Grothey A, Voigt W, Schober C et al (1999) The role of insulin-like growth factor I and its receptor in cell growth, transformation, apoptosis, and chemoresistance in solid tumors. J Cancer Res Clin Oncol 125:166–173

Gupta K, Kshirsagar S, Li W et al (1999) VEGF prevents apoptosis of human microvascular endothelial cells via opposing effects on MAPK/ERK and SAPK/JNK signaling. Exp Cell Res 247:495–504

Haimovitz-Friedman A, Vlodavsky I, Chaudhuri A et al (1991) Autocrine effects of fibroblast growth factor in repair of radiation damage in endothelial cells. Cancer Res 51:2552–2558

Haimovitz-Friedman A, Balaban N, McLoughlin M et al (1994) Protein kinase C mediates basic fibroblast growth factor protection of endothelial cells against radiation-induced apoptosis. Cancer Res 15:2591–2597

Hayashi T, Abe K, Itoyama Y (1998) Reduction of ischemic damage by application of vascular endothelial growth factor in rat brain after transient ischemia. J Cereb Blood Flow Metab 18:887–895

Heck S, Lezoualc'h F, Engert S et al (1999) Insulin-like growth factor-1-mediated neuroprotection against oxidative stress is associated with activation of nuclear factor kB. J Biol Chem 274:9828–9835

Hong JH, Chiang CS, Campbell IL et al (1995) Induction of acute phase gene expression by brain irradiation. Int J Radiat Oncol Biol Phys 33:619–626

Hopewell JW, Calvo W, Campling D et al (1989) Effects of radiation on the microvasculature. Front Radiat Ther Oncol 23: 85–95

Hopewell JW, van der Kogel AJ (1999) Pathophysiological mechanisms leading to the development of late radiation-induced damage to the central nervous system. Front Radiat Ther Oncol 33:265–275

Hopewell JW, van den Aardweg GJ, Morris GM et al (1994) Unsaturated lipids as modulators of radiation damage in normal tissues. In: Horrobin DF (ed) New approaches to cancer treatment. Churchill Communications Europe, London, pp 88–106

Hornsey S, Myers R, Coultas PG et al (1981) Turnover of proliferative cells in the spinal cord after X irradiation and its relation to time-dependent repair of radiation damage. Br J Radiol 54:1081–1085

Hornsey S, Myers R, Jenkinson T (1990) The reduction of radiation damage to the spinal cord by post-irradiation administration of vasoactive drugs. Int J Radiat Oncol Biol Phys 18:1437–1442

Hunter SF, Leavitt JA, Rodriguez M (1997) Direct observation of myelination in vivo in the mature human central nervous system. A model for the behaviour of oligodendrocyte progenitors and their progeny. Brain 120:2071–2082

Ijichi A, Noel F, Sakuma S et al (1996) Ex vivo gene delivery of platelet-derived growth factor increases O-2A progenitors in adult rat spinal cord. Gene Ther 3:389–395

Jin KL, Mao XO, Greenberg DA (2000) Vascular endothelial growth factor: direct neuroprotective effect in in vitro ischemia. Proc Natl Acad Sci U S A 97:10242–10247

Kamiryo T, Kassell NF, Thai QA et al (1996) Histological changes in the normal rat brain after gamma irradiation. Acta Neurochir (Wien) 138:451–459

Kavanaugh WM, Harsh GR, Starksen NF et al (1988) Transcriptional regulation of the A and B chain genes of platelet-derived growth factor in microvascular human endothelial cells. J Biol Chem 263:8470–8472

Kirsch M, Wilson JC, Black P (1997) Platelet-derived growth factor in human brain tumors. J Neuro Oncol 35: 289–301

Kondziolka D, Mori Y, Martinez AJ et al (1999) Beneficial effects of the radioprotectant 21-aminosteroid U-74389G in a radiosurgery rat malignant glioma model. Int J Radiat Oncol Biol Phys 44:179–184

Langley RE, Bump EA, Quartuccio SG et al (1997) Radiation-induced apoptosis in microvascular endothelial cells. Br J Cancer 75:666–672

Larocca JN, Farooq M, Norton WT (1997) Induction of oligodendrocyte apoptosis by C2-ceramide. Neurochem Res 22:529–534

Levine JM, Stincone F, Lee YS (1993) Development and differentiation of glial precursor cells in the rat cerebellum. Glia 7:307–321

Li YQ, Wong CS (1997) Radiation-induced apoptosis in the rat spinal cord: lack of equal effect per fraction. Int J Radiat Biol 71:413–420

Li YQ, Wong CS (1998) Apoptosis and its relationship with cell proliferation in the irradiated rat spinal cord. Int J Radiat Biol 74:405–417

Li YQ, Jay V, Wong CS (1996a) Oligodendrocytes in the adult rat spinal cord undergo radiation-induced apoptosis. Cancer Res 56:5417–5422

Li YQ, Guo YP, Jay V et al (1996b) Time course of radiation-induced apoptosis in the adult rat spinal cord. Radiother Oncol 39:35–42

Li YQ, Ballinger JR, Nordal RA et al (2001) Hypoxia in radiation-induced blood–spinal cord barrier breakdown. Cancer Res 61:3348–3354

Liu X, Yao DL, Webster HD (1996) Insulin-like growth factor-1 treatment reduces clinical deficits and lesion severity in acute demyelinating experimental autoimmune encephalomyelitis. Mult Scler 1:2–9

Louis JC, Magal E, Takayama S et al (1993) CNTF protection of oligodendrocytes against natural and tumor necrosis factor-induced death. Science 259:689–692

Maggirwar SB, Sarmiere PD, Dewhurst S et al (1998) Nerve growth factor-dependent activation of NF-kB contributes to survival of sympathetic neurons. J Neurosci 18: 10356–10365

McKay R (1997) Stem cells in the central nervous system. Science 276:66–71

Merrill JE (1991) Effects of interleukin-1 and tumor necrosis factor-alpha on astrocytes, microglia, oligodendrocytes and glial precursors in vitro. Dev Neurosci 13:130–137

Mildenberger M, Beach TG, McGeer EG et al (1990) An animal model of prophylactic cranial irradiation: histologic effects at acute, early and delayed stages. Int J Radiat Oncol Biol Phys 18:1051–1060

Morris GM, Coderre JA, Bywaters A et al (1996) Boron neutron capture irradiation of the rat spinal cord: histopathological evidence of a vascular-mediated pathogenesis. Radiat Res 146:313–320

Movsas B, Li BS, Babb JS et al (2001) Quantifying radiation therapy-induced brain injury with whole-brain proton MR spectroscopy: initial observations. Radiology 221: 327–331

Nakagawa M, Bellinzona M, Seilhan TM et al (1996) Microglial responses after focal radiation-induced injury are affected by alpha-difluoromethylornithine. Int J Radiat Oncol Biol Phys 36:113–123

Nieder C, Price RE, Rivera B et al (2000) Both early and delayed treatment with growth factors can modulate the development of radiation myelopathy (RM) in rats (abstract). Radiother Oncol 56 [Suppl 1]:S15

Nieder C, Price RE, Rivera B et al (2002) Experimental data for insulin-like growth factor-1 and basic fibroblast growth factor in prevention of radiation myelopathy (in German). Strahlenther Onkol 178:147–152

Noble M, Murray K, Stroobant P et al (1988) Platelet-derived growth factor promotes division and motility and inhibits premature differentiation of the oligodendrocyte/type-2 astrocyte progenitor cell. Nature 333:560–562

Noble M, Mayer-Proeschel M (1996) On the track of cell survival pharmaceuticals in the oligodendrocyte type-2 astrocyte lineage. Persp Dev Neurobiol 3:121–131

Okubo Y, Blakesley VA, Stannard B et al (1998) Insulin-like growth factor-1 inhibits the stress-activated protein kinase/c-Jun N-terminal kinase. J Biol Chem 273:25961–25966

Otero GC, Merrill JE (1994) Cytokine receptors on glial cells. Glia 11:117–128

Pan W, Kastin AJ (2000) Interactions of IGF-1 with the blood–brain barrier in vivo and in situ. Neuroendocrinology 72:171–178

Parrizas M, Saltiel AR, LeRoith D (1997) Insulin-like growth factor 1 inhibits apoptosis using the phosphatidylinositol 3'-kinase and mitogen-activated protein kinase pathways. J Biol Chem 272:154-161

Pellmar TC, Lepinski DL (1993) Gamma radiation (5-10 Gy) impairs neuronal function in the guinea pig hippocampus. Radiat Res 136:255-261

Pena LA, Fuks Z, Kolesnick RN (2000) Radiation-induced apoptosis of endothelial cells in the murine central nervous system: protection by fibroblast growth factor and sphingomyelinase deficiency. Cancer Res 60:321-327

Plotnikova D, Levitman MK, Shaposhnikova VV et al (1988) Protection of microvasculature in rat brain against late radiation injury by gammaphos. Int J Radiat Oncol Biol Phys 15:1197-1201

Proescholdt MA, Heiss JD, Walbridge S et al (1999) Vascular endothelial growth factor modulates vascular permeability and inflammation in rat brain. J Neuropathol Exp Neurol 58:613-627

Raff MC, Lillien LE, Richardson WD et al (1988) Platelet-derived growth factor from astrocytes drives the clock that times oligodendrocyte development in culture. Nature 333:562-565

Raff MC, Barres BA, Burne JF et al (1993) Programmed cell death and the control of cell survival: lessons from the nervous system. Science 262:695-700

Raju U, Gumin GJ, Tofilon PJ (1999) NFkB activity and target gene expression in the rat brain after one and two exposures to ionizing radiation. Radiat Oncol Invest 7:145-152

Raju U, Gumin GJ, Tofilon PJ (2000) Radiation-induced transcription factor activation in the rat cerebral cortex. Int J Radiat Biol 76:1045-1053

Rao MS (1999) Multipotent and restricted precursors in the central nervous system. Anat Rec 257:137-148

Redwine JM, Blinder KL, Armstrong RC (1997) In situ expression of fibroblast growth factor receptors by oligodendrocyte progenitors and oligodendrocytes in adult mouse central nervous system. J Neurosci Res 50:229-237

Rezvani M, Birds DA, Hodges H et al (2001) Modification of radiation myelopathy by the transplantation of neural stem cells in the rat. Radiat Res 156:408-412

Rosenstein JM, Mani N, Silverman WF et al (1998) Patterns of brain angiogenesis after vascular endothelial growth factor administration in vitro and in vivo. Proc Natl Acad Sci U S A 95:7086-7091

Roth NM, Sontag MR, Kiani MF (1999) Early effects of ionizing radiation on the microvascular networks in normal tissue. Radiat Res 151:270-277

Rubin P, Gash DM, Hansen JT et al (1994) Disruption of the blood-brain barrier as the primary effect of CNS irradiation. Radiother Oncol 31:51-60

Satoh J, Kastrukoff LF, Kim SU (1991) Cytokine-induced expression of intercellular adhesion molecule-1 (ICAM-1) in cultured human oligodendrocytes and astrocytes. J Neuropathol Exp Neurol 50:215-226

Scherer J, Schnitzer J (1994) Growth factor effects on the proliferation of different retinal glial cells in vitro. Brain Res Dev Brain Res 80:209-221

Scholz W (1934) Experimentelle Untersuchungen über die Einwirkung von Roentgenstrahlen auf das reife Gehirn (in German). Z Ges Neurol Psychiat 150:765

Schultheiss TE, Kun LE, Ang KK et al (1995) Radiation response of the central nervous system. Int J Radiat Oncol Biol Phys 31:1093-1112

Scolding N, Franklin R, Stevens S et al (1998) Oligodendrocyte progenitors are present in the normal adult human CNS and in the lesions of multiple sclerosis. Brain 121:2221-2228

Siegal T, Pfeffer MR (1995) Radiation-induced changes in the profile of spinal cord serotonin, prostaglandin synthesis, and vascular permeability. Int J Radiat Oncol Biol Phys 31:57-64

Siegal T, Pfeffer MR, Meltzer A et al (1996) Cellular and secretory mechanisms related to delayed radiation-induced microvessel dysfunction in the spinal cord of rats. Int J Radiat Oncol Biol Phys 36:649-659

Sims EC, Plowman PN (2001) Stereotactic radiosurgery XII. Large AVM and the failure of the radiation response modifier gamma linolenic acid to improve the therapeutic ratio. Br J Neurosurg 15:28-34

Slungaard A, Vercellotti GM, Walker G et al (1990) Tumor necrosis factor-alpha/cachectin stimulates eosinophil oxidant production and toxicity towards human endothelium. J Exp Med 171:2025-2041

Sondell M, Lundborg G, Kanje M (1999) Vascular endothelial growth factor has neurotrophic activity and stimulates axonal outgrowth, enhancing cell survival and Schwann cell proliferation in the peripheral nervous system. J Neurosci 5731-5740

Spence AM, Krohn KA, Edmondson SW et al (1986) Radioprotection in rat spinal cord with WR-2721 following cerebral lateral intraventricular injection. Int J Radiat Oncol Biol Phys 12:1479-1482

Spyridopoulos I, Brogi E, Kearney M et al (1997) Vascular endothelial growth factor inhibits endothelial cell apoptosis induced by tumor necrosis factor-α: balance between growth and death signals. J Mol Cell Cardiol 291:321-330

Stewart FA, van der Kogel AJ (1997) Proliferation and cellular organisation of normal tissues. In: Steel GG (ed) Basic clinical radiobiology, 2nd edn. Arnold, London, pp 24-29

Stone J, Itin A, Alon T et al (1995) Development of retinal vasculature is mediated by hypoxia-induced vascular endothelial growth factor (VEGF) expression by neuroglia. J Neurosci 15:4738-4747

Tada E, Yang C, Gobbel GT et al (1999) Long-term impairment of subependymal repopulation following damage by ionizing irradiation. Exp Neurol 160:66-77

Tamatani M, Che YH, Matsuzaki H et al (1999) Tumor necrosis factor induces Bcl-2 and Bcl-x expression through NFkB activation in primary hippocampal neurons. J Biol Chem 274:8531-8538

Tanaka J, Fujita H, Matsuda S et al (1997) Glucocorticoid- and mineralocorticoid receptors in microglial cells: the two receptors mediate differential effects of corticosteroids. Glia 20:23-37

Tanaka R, Miyasaka Y, Yada K, Ohwada T, Kameya T (1995) Basic fibroblast growth factor increases regional cerebral blood flow and reduces infarct size after experimental ischemia in a rat model. Stroke 26:2154-2158

Tofilon PJ, Fike JR (2000) The radioresponse of the central nervous system: a dynamic process. Radiat Res 153:357-370

Tsao MN, Li YQ, Lu G, et al (1999) Upregulation of vascular endothelial growth factor is associated with radiation-induced blood-spinal cord barrier breakdown. J Neuropathol Exp Neurol 58:1051-1060

Van der Kogel AJ (1986) Radiation-induced damage in the central nervous system: an interpretation of target cell responses. Br J Cancer 53 [Suppl 7]:207–217

Van der Maazen RW, Verhagen I, Kleiboer BJ et al (1992) Repopulation of O-2A progenitor cells after irradiation of the adult rat optic nerve analyzed by an in vitro clonogenic assay. Radiat Res 132:82–86

Vemuri GS, McMorris FA (1996) Oligodendrocytes and their precursors require phosphatidylinositol 3-kinase signaling for survival. Development 122:2529–2537

Vrdoljak E, Bill CA, Stephens LC et al (1992) Radiation-induced apoptosis of oligodendrocytes in vitro. Int J Radiat Biol 62:475–480

Witte L, Fuks Z, Haimovitz-Friedman A et al (1989) Effects of irradiation on the release of growth factors from cultured bovine, porcine, and human endothelial cells. Cancer Res 49:5066–5072

Wolswijk G, Noble M (1989) Identification of an adult-specific glial progenitor cell. Development 105:387–400

Wong D, Dorovini ZK (1992) Upregulation of intercellular adhesion molecule-1 (ICAM-1) expression in primary cultures of human brain microvessel endothelial cells by cytokines and lipopolysaccharide. J Neuroimmunol 39:11–21

Zhang FX, Hutchins JB (1997) Protein phosphorylation in response to PDGF stimulation in cultured neurons and astrocytes. Brain Res Dev Brain Res 99:216–225

7 Hematopoietic Tissue I: Response Modification by Erythropoietin

J. Dunst

CONTENTS

7.1 Physiological Role of Erythropoietin 89
7.2 Anemia in Patients Undergoing Radiotherapy 90
7.2.1 Frequency of Anemia 90
7.2.2 Pathophysiology of Anemia in Cancer Patients 90
7.2.3 Clinical Findings in Cancer-Related Anemia 91
7.3 Impact of Anemia on Survival 91
7.3.1 Prognostic Impact of Anemia 91
7.3.2 Hemoglobin Levels at the End of Radiotherapy are Most Important 92
7.3.3 Association Between Anemia and Tumor Hypoxia 93
7.4 Impact of Erythropoietin Treatment on Anemia 93
7.5 Impact of Erythropoietin on Tumor Hypoxia and Response to Radiotherapy 94
7.5.1 Impact of Erythropoietin on Tumor Hypoxia 94
7.5.2 Impact of Erythropoietin on Local Control and Survival: Experimental Data 94
7.5.3 Impact of Erythropoietin on Local Control and Survival: Clinical Data 94
7.5.4 Stimulation of Tumor Growth by Erythropoietin? 96
7.6 Impact of Erythropoietin on Normal Tissue Tolerance 96
7.7 Impact of Erythropoietin on Transfusion Requirements and Quality of Life in Patients Receiving Chemotherapy 97
7.8 Clinical Aspects of Erythropoietin Administration 97
7.8.1 Administration and Pharmacokinetics 97
7.8.2 Response and Response Prediction 98
7.8.3 Iron Substitution 98
7.8.4 Optimal Hemoglobin and Target Hemoglobin 98
7.8.5 Side Effects 98
7.9 Conclusions 99
References 99

J. Dunst, MD
Professor, Department of Radiotherapy, Martin-Luther-University Halle-Wittenberg, Dryanderstrasse 4, 06097 Halle, Germany

7.1 Physiological Role of Erythropoietin

Erythropoietin (EPO) has been identified as a 34-kDa glycoprotein hormone which controls red blood cell production. It is the only hematopoietic growth factor that is regulated by hypoxia.

Erythropoietin is not a typical growth factor like granulocyte colony-stimulating factor (G-CSF) or other colony-stimulating factors. Growth factors of granulopoiesis directly affect proliferation, maturation and differentiation of specific cell lines. In contrast, erythropoietin affects late erythroid progenitors (colony-forming unit erythroid, CFU-E) which, in the absence of erythropoietin, undergo apoptosis. Erythropoietin blocks apoptosis and thereby induces proliferation of CFU-E. Later stages of erythropoiesis (CFU-Es) can grow in the absence of EPO, but require other growth factors (Lacombe and Mayeux 2002).

EPO acts through a specific membrane receptor (EPOR). This receptor belongs to the cytokine receptor family and shows structural homology with other receptors, like receptors for interleukins (IL-2 to IL-7, IL9, IL-13, IL-15) and granulocyte-macrophage colony-stimulating factor (GM-CSF). The EPO-binding part of the receptor is a 66-kDa protein, possibly surrounded by other proteins. EPOR is present on erythroid cells (about one thousand receptors per cell) but has also been identified on a variety of non-erythroid cells, including megakaryocytes, endothelial cells, Leydig cells, embryonal stem cells, fetal liver, placenta, and neuronal cells. The binding of EPO to EPOR results in dimerization of the receptor with activation of downstream signaling pathways. These include rapid tyrosine phosphorylation of various proteins (for review see Lacombe and Mayeux 2002).

EPO is mainly produced in the kidney by interstitial cells in the kidney cortex. The main stimulus for EPO production is hypoxia. EPO production is controlled via a feedback mechanism which includes an oxygen sensor, probably a hem-containing flavoprotein. Hypoxia results in up-regulation of hypoxia-inducible factor HIF-1, which in a second step results in the up-regulation of a variety of secondary target genes, including the *EPO* gene. This hypoxia response seems to represent a common physiological mechanism in various tissues and has been demonstrated in a variety of animals, suggesting that the physiological mechanisms in response to tissue hypoxia have been highly conserved during evolution (BUNN and POYTON 1996). Under normoxic conditions, HIF-1 is rapidly ubiquinated and degraded. Under hypoxia, however, HIF-1 is stabilized and aggregates with hepatic nuclear factor (HNF-4). In EPO-producing cells, HIF-1 binds to an enhancer region of the *EPO* gene (BLANCHARD et al. 1993; BECK et al. 1993).

The kidney produces 80%–90% of EPO. Roughly 10%–20% of EPO stems from the liver. Other tissues only rarely express EPO-mRNA. Very recent results suggest that the function of EPO may extend beyond red cell production as EPO mRNA has been detected in astrocytes in response to tissue hypoxia and EPO receptors were found in the brain. EPO might be able to protect (possibly via inhibition of hypoxia-induced apoptosis) against experimental hypoxia and experimental brain injury in animals (CERAMI 2001; CERAMI et al. 2002). This neuroprotective potential is currently tested in clinical trials.

7.2
Anemia in Patients Undergoing Radiotherapy

7.2.1
Frequency of Anemia

In contrast to hematological malignancies, severe transfusion-requiring anemia is relatively uncommon in patients with solid tumors at diagnosis. Mild to moderate anemia, however, is frequently observed in patients undergoing radiotherapy. According to our own data, approximately 50%–60% of patients treated with curative intent for head and neck, cervical, esophageal or rectal cancer have hemoglobin (hb) levels in the normal range (>13 g/dl). Mild anemia (hb between 11 and 13 g/dl) is present in a further one-third of patients in all tumor sites. Moderate to severe anemia (hb between 9 and 11 g/dl) has been noted in roughly 15%–20% of patients with head and neck and cervical cancers, but was not observed in a smaller group of patients with esophageal and rectal cancers. Severe, transfusion-requiring anemia (hemoglobin below 9 g/dl) was noted only in a minority of patients, i.e., less than 1% of all patients and 4% of patients with cervical cancers (DUNST and MOLLS 2002a).

These findings are in accordance with data from the literature. In the first publication that has highlighted the impact of hemoglobin levels on treatment outcome, EVANS and BERGSJØ (1965) analyzed 880 patients with stage I–IV cancer of the cervix. The frequency of patients with a pretreatment hemoglobin below 11 g/dl was 25%. Anemia (hb <11 g/dl) increased with stage (13% in stage I, 21% in stage II, 34% in stage III, 73% in stage IV and 20% in patients treated postoperatively). GIRINSKI and co-workers analyzed 386 patients with cervical cancers from the Institute Gustave-Roussy at stage IIB (30%) or IIIB (70%). Of the entire group, 34 patients (9%) presented with a pretreatment hemoglobin of less than 10 g/dl; 42 patients (10%) received transfusions prior to (6% also during) treatment and an additional 56 patients (15%) were transfused during treatment (GIRINSKI et al. 1989). In an analysis by GROGAN and co-workers (1999) in patients with cervical cancers, 35% of all patients had a pretreatment hemoglobin below 12 g/dl.

Anemia is a frequent phenomenon in cancer patients undergoing radiotherapy. In a large prospective investigation by HARRISON and co-workers (2001), hemoglobin levels were analyzed in 574 random patients undergoing radiotherapy. Anemia (hb <12 g/dl) was present prior to treatment in 41% of all patients and this percentage increased during treatment to 54%. Pronounced anemia with hemoglobin levels below approximately 11 g/dl was mainly found in cervical and head and neck tumors. It is not likely that these differences result only from tumor bleeding because clinically relevant bleeding is rarely observed in most head and neck cancers and a prognostic impact of anemia has been demonstrated in early glottic cancers which do not bleed (CANADAY et al. 1999). However, the clinical observation of a higher frequency of tumor bleedings in patients with cervical cancers may contribute to pretreatment anemia in this cancer site.

7.2.2
Pathophysiology of Anemia in Cancer Patients

The anemia in cancer patients may result from several mechanisms. The main reasons are:
- Tumor-related anemia
  Most of the cancer patients who present at diagnosis with anemia have no obvious reason for their anemia. This type of anemia should therefore be

distinguished from bleeding anemia or therapy-induced anemia. From a pathophysiological point of view, tumor-related anemia resembles anemia in chronic inflammatory diseases (ACD) such as rheumatoid arthritis. It is characterized by reduced life-span of erythrocytes. Moreover, the serum levels of erythropoietin are lower in cancer-related anemia than bleeding anemia, suggesting that there is an insufficient response of erythropoietin because of immunological mechanisms. This finding also explains why cancer patients need higher doses of erythropoietin than patients with anemia from causes other than cancer. The pathophysiological mechanisms have recently been reviewed (NOWROUSIAN 2002).

- Therapy-induced anemia
Anemia may result from the hematological toxicity of chemotherapy and radiotherapy. With radiotherapy alone, the decrease in hemoglobin levels during a standard course of fractionated radiotherapy is small. After pelvic irradiation, an average decrease by about 1 g/dl after treatment occurs (GROGAN et al. 1999). In general, hb levels at the end of radiotherapy are lower than pretreatment hb levels (HARRISON et al. 2001)

- Anemia due to tumor bleeding
Bleeding is rarely the main reason for tumor anemia. Bleeding may be relevant in selected cancers only, mainly cervical cancers.

7.2.3
Clinical Findings in Cancer-Related Anemia

From a pathophysiological point of view, anemia in cancer patients resembles anemia in chronic inflammatory diseases such as rheumatoid arthritis. Laboratory work-up reveals normal values of mean corpuscular volume (MCV) and mean corpuscular hb concentration (MCHC) in most patients. Microcytic anemia (MCV <80 fl) occurs in about 14% of patients with solid cancers and anemia. The reticulocyte count is lowered, indicating hyporegenerative anemia. Serum iron levels, total iron binding capacity and transferrin saturation are lowered whereas serum ferritin and total amount of marrow iron are in the normal range. These findings support the assumption that cancer-related anemia does not result from an iron deficiency but from impaired mobilization of iron from storages (NOWROUSIAN 2002).

A further characteristic finding is the relatively low serum level of erythropoietin which is, with regard to the hb levels, lower than in anemic patients with blood loss (MILLER et al. 1990). These findings suggest that insufficient endogenous EPO production is a major causative factor (NOWROUSIAN 2002).

7.3
Impact of Anemia on Survival

7.3.1
Prognostic Impact of Anemia

Anemia has been demonstrated to be a significant and independent risk factor for survival and local control. A survey by GRAU and OVERGAARD (1998) analyzed 51 studies in the literature. Thirty-nine out of 51 studies with the vast majority of patients did indeed find an association between hemoglobin levels and local control or survival. A further analysis of 60 studies by CARO and co-workers (2001) supports the finding that anemic patients have an increased risk of mortality as compared to patients with normal hemoglobin levels (Table 7.1). Various other large analyses have supported these findings (KAPP et al. 1983; OVERGAARD 1988; FEIN et al. 1995; FROMMHOLD et al. 1998; LEE et al. 1998; GROGAN et al. 1999; RUDAT et al. 1999). From these data, a clear relationship between a decrease in hemoglobin and a decrease in local control and survival seems to exist. Our own data in cervical cancer also support this finding. In a multivariate prognostic model in locally advanced cervical cancers (FIGO stages IIB–IVA), anemia was the most important single prognostic factor for local control and survival (Fig. 7.1)

In summary, the data suggest that anemia has a significant prognostic impact in a variety of solid tumors and systemic malignancies. Anemia seems to represent an independent prognostic factor. This hypothesis is further supported by the fact that decreased hemoglobin levels are part of prognostic models, e.g., in bladder cancer or Hodgkin's disease (HANNISDAL et al. 1993; HASENCLEVER and DIEHL 1998).

Table 7.1. Impact of anemia on survival in patients with malignancies (From CARO et al. 2001, with permission)

Tumor site	Mean increase in mortality in patients with anemia as compared to normemic patients	Range
Head and neck	80%	37%–123%
Lymphomas	67%	30%–113%
Prostate	47%	27%–68%
Lung	67%	10%–129%
Total	65%	54%–77%

Fig. 7.1. Impact of hemoglobin levels prior to radiation therapy and during radiotherapy on survival in patients undergoing definitive radiotherapy for cervical cancers. Hb values give values prior to treatment at a radiation dose of 19.8 Gy. Anemia (hb <11 g/dl) during treatment was a significant risk factor irrespective of pretreatment hb levels. University of Halle, treatment period 1995–1999

7.3.2
Hemoglobin Levels at the End of Radiotherapy are most Important

Out of the variety of prospective and retrospective studies which have investigated the impact of anemia on outcome, most of the data refer to pretreatment hemoglobin levels, given that information on pretreatment factors is easily available even in retrospective analyses because a laboratory work-up is part of most staging procedures. There is less information on a possible impact of hemoglobin levels during treatment.

TARNAWSKI and co-workers (1997) analyzed prognostic factors in patients with head and neck cancers. They found that the hemoglobin levels at the end of radiotherapy in their analyses was the most powerful prognostic factor. Comparable findings have been reported by VAN ACHT and co-workers (1992). GROGAN and co-workers (1999) analyzed 450 patients with cervical cancers treated with definitive radiotherapy for locally advanced tumors. Patients with high hemoglobin levels at the end of treatment had a better prognosis than patients with low hb levels, irrespective of whether or not they had presented with high (n=228) or low pretreatment hemoglobin levels (n=25). In contrast, 222 patients had a low hb level at the end of treatment associated with poorer survival, irrespective of whether or not the patients had had a high (n=82) or low (n=140) pretreatment hb level. The average hb level during radiotherapy was also a significant prognostic factor. These data suggest that the hemoglobin during radiotherapy or at the end of radiotherapy may have an independent prognostic impact and may be more important than the pretreatment hb levels. The prognostic impact of pretreatment hb levels would then be best explained by the correlation of hb levels before and after treatment. Our own data in cervical cancer show identical findings (Fig. 7.2). The data are a strong argument in favor of correcting low hb levels during treatment. An impact of nadir hb levels during radiation therapy for local control and survival in cervical cancers was also found by LOGSDON and EIFEL (1999).

Another recent investigation has also found a significant impact of the nadir hemoglobin but not pretreatment hemoglobin on the response of locally advanced head and neck cancers treated with preoperative radiochemotherapy. WAGNER et al. (2000) treated 43 patients with an aggressive regimen of preoperative radiochemotherapy prior to planned resection in a phase II study. None of the patients had anemia prior to the start of treatment because only patients fit for surgery and fit for radiochemotherapy were included. The radiochemotherapy regimen produced profound anemia in a high proportion of patients at the end of treatment and the hemoglobin levels at the end of therapy were a significant prognostic factor for local control and survival, together with tumor size and histological response to radiochemotherapy.

Thus, the current data suggest that hemoglobin levels during a course of fractionated radiotherapy or even hemoglobin levels at the end of treatment may be at least as important or more crucial than pretreatment hemoglobin levels. The data are a strong argument for correcting anemia during radiotherapy. Furthermore, one randomized study has investigated the effect of transfusions in patients with cervical cancers (BUSH 1986). In this study, transfused

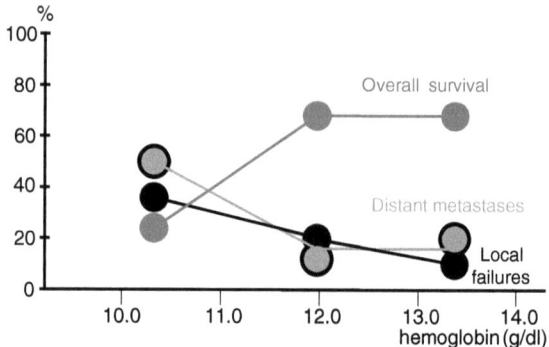

Fig. 7.2. Impact of pretreatment hemoglobin levels on local control, distant metastasis rate and overall survival: 87 patients with definitive radiotherapy for cervical cancers. University of Halle, treatment period 1995–1999

patients had a lower local failure rate than patients in the non-transfusion group. This study has, however, been criticized because the treatment groups were poorly balanced (FYLES et al. 2000).

7.3.3
Association Between Anemia and Tumor Hypoxia

The impact of anemia on tumor oxygenation has been investigated in several animal studies (KELLEHER et al. 1995, 1996; THEWS et al. 1998, 2001). Anemia was induced by treatment with carboplatin or by induction of hemorrhagic ascites. In all studies, nearly identical results were obtained. Anemic animals had significantly poorer oxygenated tumors than normemic animals. The median pO_2 level was lower and the frequency of hypoxic readings was higher in the presence of anemia. The correction of anemia was associated with an improvement in the oxygenation status (see Sect. 7.5.1, "Impact of Erythropoietin on Tumor Hypoxia").

We have recently analyzed the association between hemoglobin levels and oxygenation of normal and tumor tissue in 133 patients with head and neck cancers treated in our institutions from 1995 through 1999 (BECKER et al. 2000). It should be noted that none of these patients had severe anemia. The lowest hemoglobin level was 9.1 g/dl. Thirty-nine patients had a hemoglobin of at least 12 g/dl, 7 had mild anemia (12>hb ≥ 11 g/dl) and 10 had moderate anemia (11>hb ≥ 9.1 g/dl). Tumor oxygenation was measured by invasive pO_2 histography using the Eppendorf device within the tumor ($n=133$) and within corresponding normal tissue (contralateral sternocleidoid muscle, $n=69$). The patients were divided into three subgroups depending on their hemoglobin levels at the time of oxygenation measurement.

Figure 7.3 demonstrates that tumors were in general less well oxygenated than the normal tissue. A decrease in hemoglobin below 12 g/dl did not significantly impair oxygenation of normal tissue. However, tumor oxygenation was significantly poorer in patients with low hemoglobin levels than in patients with normal hemoglobin. In this investigation, nearly all patients with hb under 11 g/dl had poorly oxygenated tumors. In the same work, a multivariate analysis was performed to determine parameters that impact on tumor oxygenation. Tumor oxygenation was independent from stage (T and N category) or grading. Smoking had a significant impact. The strongest independent predictor for poor tumor oxygenation, however, was a low hb level at the time of oxygenation measurement. These findings have recently been supported in cervical and vulvar carcinomas by VAUPEL and co-workers (2002). They found significantly impaired tumor oxygenation if the hemoglobin was below the physiological range. Thus, there seems to be an optimal range of hemoglobin levels with regard to tumor tissue oxygenation, which is nearly identical to the physiological range.

The lack of effect from hemoglobin changes for the oxygenation of normal tissue over a broad range can be explained by the differences in the vascular network in tumors as compared to normal tissues. Normal tissues can compensate for a decrease in hemoglobin by an increase in perfusion. In contrast to normal tissues, malignant tumors cannot increase their perfusion rate. This is to be expected by the structure of tumor vessels, e.g., lack of smooth muscles and a chaotic network, which leads to a decreased intracapillary oxyhemoglobin saturation in malignant tumors as compared to normal tissue (MÜLLER-KLIESER et al. 1981; VAUPEL et al. 1989).

7.4
Impact of Erythropoietin Treatment on Anemia

Several recent investigations have proven that anemia in cancer patients who undergo radiotherapy or combined radiochemotherapy can effectively be treated by erythropoietin. A summary of the major trials in radiotherapy patients is provided in Table 7.2. All studies have shown that EPO is highly efficacious in correcting and preventing anemia in radiotherapy

Fig. 7.3. Impact of hemoglobin levels on oxygenation of normal tissue and tumors in 133 patients with head and neck cancers. Decreased hemoglobin levels had no significant impact on normal tissue oxygenation, but significantly worsened tumor oxygenation. Data from BECKER et al. (2000), with permission

Table 7.2. Dosage of rhEPO in prospective studies in radiotherapy patients. (Modified from HENKE (2002) with permission)

Author	rhEpo dose iron supplementation	Hb at start of study (g/dl)	Hb at end of study (g/dl)	Average hb increment per week (g/dl)	Target hb/% target hb reached
LAVEY and DEMPSEY (1993)	3×300 U/kg per week s.c. in week 1, then 2×150 U/kg + iron 325 mg t.i.d. p.o.	–	15.1	0.6	15 g/dl (65%)
DUSENBERY et al. (1994)	5×200 U/kg per week s.c. in weeks 1/2, then 3×200 U/kg + iron 325 mg t.i.d. p.o.	11.9	13.2	0.5	14 g/dl
SWEENEY et al. (1998)	5×200 U/kg per week s.c., reduce to 50% if target hb reached + iron 325 mg t.i.d. p.o.	11.4	13.6	0.41	15 g/dl (female 14 g/dl) (42%)
HENKE et al. (1999)	3×150 (300) U/kg per week i.v. (s.c.) + 800 mg Fe gluconate i.v. at start of treatment	12.1	14.6	0.7	15 g/dl (female 14 g/dl) (72%)

Hb, hemoglobin; *rhEPO*, recombinant human erythropoietin

patients. These data are in accordance with findings from prospective trials using EPO in patients with aggressive chemotherapy (Table 7.3)

7.5
Impact of Erythropoietin on Tumor Hypoxia and Response to Radiotherapy

7.5.1
Impact of Erythropoietin on Tumor Hypoxia

There are few reports in the literature looking at whether or not treatment of anemia impacts on tumor oxygenation. KELLEHER and co-workers (1995) investigated the effect of erythropoietin and transfusions on tumor oxygenation in an animal model. Both the use of erythropoietin and transfusions increased hb levels in anemic mice. This increase was associated with a significant improvement of tumor oxygenation in small tumors with a volume of less than 1.4 ml. The median pO_2 level increased with increasing hb and the frequency of hypoxic readings (with a $pO_2 < 5$ mmHg) decreased. However, oxygenation was not fully recovered and the oxygenation remained worse than in normemic animals. In tumors of a larger size (>1.4 ml volume), no impact of erythropoietin treatment on the oxygenation status was observed.

7.5.2
Impact of Erythropoietin on Local Control and Survival: Experimental Data

If one assumes that anemia decreases the local efficacy of radiotherapy via decreased tumor oxygenation, the most important question from a clinical point of view concerns whether or not correction of anemia impacts on radiosensitivity. In an experimental setting, THEWS and co-workers (1998) were able to demonstrate that treatment of anemia improves radiation response to a single fraction of 10 Gy. The time to regrowth of tumors was 4.5 days in anemic animals without erythropoietin treatment, 9.5 days in primarily anemic animals with erythropoietin treatment, and 12 days in nonanemic control animals (Fig. 7.4). The data have been confirmed (STÜBEN et al. 2001) and in a very recent experiment, the same group was able to demonstrate that erythropoietin is also able to fully restore the sensitivity of the tumor to treatment with cyclophosphamide (THEWS et al. 2001), which is a highly oxygen-dependent cytotoxic drug.

7.5.3
Impact of Erythropoietin on Local Control and Survival: Clinical Data

Further indirect evidence comes from clinical studies that have investigated the efficacy of erythropoietin or transfusions in radiotherapy patients. ANTONADOU and co-workers (1998) conducted a randomized study on pelvic cancers. The control group ($n=195$) was treated with radiotherapy and oral iron supplementation. In the investigative arm of the study, 190 patients received additional prophylactic erythropoietin during the whole course of radiotherapy. The group with erythropoietin had significantly higher hemoglobin levels at the end of radiotherapy (12.9±2.6 g/dl vs 10.7±2.5 g/dl, $p=0.0001$). This was associated with a significantly lower rate of local failures (22/190 vs 44/195, $p=0.007$, Table 7.4).

Table 7.3. Impact of rhEpo on transfusion requirements and quality of life in selected large studies of patients receiving myelosuppressive chemotherapy for hematological or nonhematological malignancies[a]

Author	Tumor type	No. of patients	Treatment	Effect of EPO
Prospective, nonrandomized studies				
Glaspy et al. (1997)	Non-myeloid malignancies	2030	Myelosuppressive chemotherapy	Increase in Hb, reduced need for transfusions
				QoL benefit for patients with hb increase
				QoL benefit independent of disease response
Demetri et al. (1998)	Non-myeloid malignancies	2289	Myelosuppressive chemotherapy	Increase in Hb, reduced need for transfusions
				QoL benefit for patients with hb increase
				Greatest benefit if hb increase >2 g/dl
Gabrilove et al. (2001)	Non-myeloid malignancies	2869	Myelosuppressive chemotherapy	Increase in Hb, reduced need for transfusions
				QoL benefit for patients with hb increase
				Greatest benefit if hb increase >2 g/dl
Prospective, randomized studies				
Glimelius et al. (1998)	GI/pancreatic tumors	100	Myelosuppressive non-platinum 5-FU-based chemotherapy	Increase in Hb, reduced need for transfusions
				QoL benefit for patients with hb increase
Littlewood et al. (2001)	Non-myeloid malignancies, solid tumors	375	Myelosuppressive non-platinum chemotherapy	Increase in Hb, reduced need for transfusions
				QoL benefit for patients with hb increase
Osterborg et al. (2002)	Myeloma, lymphoma	343	Myelosuppressive chemotherapy	Increase in Hb, reduced need for transfusions
				QoL benefit for patients with hb increase

QoL, Quality of life; *hb*, hemoglobin; *rhEPO*, recombinant human erythropoietin
[a] All studies have demonstrated comparable results

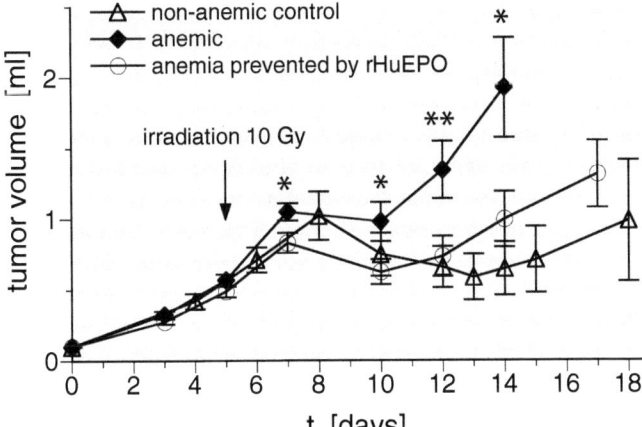

Fig. 7.4. Impact of treatment with erythropoietin on radiosensitivity of DS sarcoma in anemic rats. From Thews et al. (1998), with permission

Blohmer and co-workers (2002) have recently presented preliminary data from a randomized study in patients who received adjuvant therapy for high-risk cervical cancer. Patients with high risk for relapse after radical hysterectomy were treated with four courses of adjuvant chemotherapy (carboplatin plus ifosfamide) followed by external beam radiotherapy to the pelvis with 50 Gy in conventional fractionation. Patients in the investigational arm of this randomized study received the same treatment but also additional erythropoietin (three times weekly, 10,000 IU) for the whole treatment time unless the hb

Table 7.4. Impact of rhEPO on locoregional control in patients receiving radiotherapy for pelvic malignancies. Prospective, randomized trial (ANTONADOU et al. 1998). (From HENKE [2002], with permission)

Site	Stages	Actuarial 2-year locoregional control	
		XRT	XRT + rhEpo
Cervix	IIB, III	49/62 (79%)	55/58 (95%)
Endometrium	I, II	28/34 (82%)	34/36 (94%)
Bladder	T3, T4	28/40 (70%)	29/36 (81%)
Colorectum	B2, C	31/40 (77%)	32/38 (84%)
Prostate	B, C	15/19 (79%)	18/22 (82%)
All		151/195 (77%)	168/190 (88%) $p=0.007$

rhEPO, recombinant human erythropoietin; *XRT*, radiation therapy

increased to over 14 g/dl. In the investigational arm, the need for transfusions was significantly reduced. After a median follow-up of 30 months, patients treated with EPO experienced a significantly lower rate of failures than patients in the standard arm (11% vs 22%, $p=0.05$) (Table 7.5).

Further data have been published by LITTLEWOOD (2002). More than 500 patients with hematological malignancies and advanced or metastatic solid tumors with standard chemotherapies with or without EPO were included. The objective of the randomized study was to evaluate the impact of EPO on quality of life. Interestingly, patients in the EPO arm of the study had a longer median survival than patients in the control arm (Table 7.6). This effect was observed in patients with solid cancers as well as in patients with hematological malignancies although it was not significant. The impact of EPO on quality of life and reduction of the need for transfusions was proven in this study, but the sample size was insufficient to detect a small benefit in overall survival.

7.5.4
Stimulation of Tumor Growth by Erythropoietin?

EPO may theoretically impact on tumor growth in two ways: either directly via stimulation of tumor cells if they express EPO receptors or indirectly via improved tumor oxygenation after successful treatment of anemia.

EPO receptors are, as discussed in Sect. 7.1, rarely expressed in normal tissues. However, EPO receptors have been demonstrated on tumor cells in vitro in a variety of tumor cell lines (SELZER et al. 2000; WESTENFELDER and BARANOWSKI 2000; WESTPHAL et al. 2002). In a large investigation with various cell lines, however, administration of EPO did not result in increased proliferation in these cell lines and there was an increase in tyrosine kinase activity, suggesting that the EPO receptors in the tested tumor cell lines are functionally inactive and not necessary for tumor growth (WESTPHAL et al. 2002). In experimental models, treatment of anemic, tumor-bearing animals with EPO alone did not result in increased tumor growth (THEWS et al. 1998, 2001). However, EPO has been demonstrated to increase proliferation in some cytokine-dependent hematopoietic cell lines and in renal carcinoma cell lines (BERDEL et al. 1991; ROSTI et al. 1993; WESTENFELDER and BARANOWSKI 2000).

The question whether EPO treatment alone might impact on tumor growth in a clinical setting cannot be answered because this would require a study in which EPO would have to been administered without any other specific cancer treatment. All prospective studies using EPO for treatment of anemia have used EPO as additional treatment together with radiotherapy and/or chemotherapy. In none of these studies have poor results with EPO in terms of response or local control or survival been reported. The current data therefore suggest that EPO has no impact on tumor growth, at least in a setting where EPO is used as addendum to radio- and chemotherapy.

7.6
Impact of Erythropoietin on Normal Tissue Tolerance

If one assumes that the oxygenation of normal tissue is not impaired or is minimally impaired in case of mild to moderate anemia (in contrast to tumor tissue), an impact of anemia on the radiation tolerance of normal tissue is not to be expected. Therefore,

Table 7.5. Impact of rhEpo on the frequency of recurrences in patients receiving postoperative chemotherapy and subsequent radiation for high-risk cervical cancers. Prospective, randomized study. Median follow-up 35 months

Treatment group	n	Recurrences
Radical hysterectomy + 4 × ifosfamide/carboplatin + XRT	128	22%
Radical hysterectomy + 4 × ifosfamide/carboplatin + XRT + erythropoietin	128	11%, $p<0.05$

Table 7.6. Impact of rhEpo on survival in patients receiving non-platinum chemotherapy for hematological or nonhematological malignancies. Prospective, randomized, placebo-controlled trial.[a]

Treatment group	n	Died	Median survival
Whole study group			
Chemotherapy + placebo	124	82 (66%)	11 months
Chemotherapy + EPO	251	82 (66%)	17 months, $p=0.13$
Hematological malignancies			
Chemotherapy + placebo	58	30 (52%)	
Chemotherapy + EPO	115	54 (47%)	
Nonhematological malignancies			
Chemotherapy + placebo	66	52 (79%)	
Chemotherapy + EPO	136	101 (74%)	

[a] The primary study objective was to assess the impact of rhEpo on transfusion requirements and quality of life; the study was not designed to detect a survival benefit

an increase in acute or late normal tissue complications is unlikely. However, this question has so far not been clearly addressed in clinical studies.

In a recent large randomized study on advanced head and neck cancers treated with either accelerated hyperfractionated radiotherapy alone or radiotherapy plus simultaneous chemotherapy, hemoglobin was identified as a major prognostic factor for local control and survival. In this study, hb levels were not correlated with either acute or late complication rates (V. Budach 2002, personal communication). Moreover, the randomized studies with erythropoietin have so far not demonstrated an impact of EPO on acute side effects of chemotherapy or radiotherapy. In summary, the current data support the finding that EPO administration in anemic patients does not increase acute complication rates as long as the drug is used to increase low hb levels to the normal physiological range.

7.7
Impact of Erythropoietin on Transfusion Requirements and Quality of Life in Patients Receiving Chemotherapy

Several recent studies have clearly demonstrated that EPO can significantly increase hb levels and reduce the need for transfusions in patients receiving myelosuppressive chemotherapy (Table 7.3). Moreover, all of the studies addressing a possible impact on quality of life (QoL) found significant correlations between hb levels and QoL in cancer patients. Treating anemia with epoetin resulted in significant improvements in QoL in responding patients. The positive effect of EPO on QoL was present over a broad range of hb levels, suggesting that all patients with hb levels below the normal range may have some benefit from EPO if they respond with an increase in hb. The response was observed independent of the tumor response to chemotherapy in one study. In summary, the positive effect of EPO on transfusion needs and QoL is clearly proven.

7.8
Clinical Aspects of Erythropoietin Administration

7.8.1
Administration and Pharmacokinetics

Recombinant human erythropoietin (rhEPO, epoetin) is derived from CHO cells transfected with the human *EPO* gene. The protein part of rhEPO with 165 amino acids is identical to the human EPO, but differs with regard to the sugar chains. Two different forms of epoetin (epoetin-α and epoetin-β) are available on the market. They differ with regard to their carbohydrate side chains and are slightly different with regard to bioactivity and half-life. The peak plasma concentrations are reached immediately after i.v. and 9–29 h after s.c. injection. The serum half-life in normal adults is 4–11 h after i.v. and 9–29 h after s.c. administration. The peak plasma concentrations are 20 times higher after i.v. than s.c. injection. All pharmacokinetic studies have been conducted in healthy adults and patients with renal anemia (JELKMANN 2002).

A hyperglycosylated form of epoetin, the so-called novel erythropoiesis stimulating protein (NESP, darbepoetin alfa) has a larger carbohydrate portion and molecular mass (1 μg is equivalent to 200 U rhEPO). The half-life is significantly longer, about 25h after i.v. and 48.8 h after s.c. administration (MacDougall et al. 1999)

Compared to patients with renal anemia, cancer patients require higher doses due to a relative resistance to EPO. The standard dose of epoetin in patients with cancer is three times weekly 150 U per kg body weight (corresponding to about three times weekly 10,000 IU). The doses used in prospective studies in radiation oncology patients are listed in Table 7.1. Supplementary iron was used in all studies.

There is some evidence that a higher dose of 40,000 IU once weekly is comparably effective. Once weekly administration offers some advantages, especially for outpatients, and is increasingly used. NESP (darbepoetin) is routinely administered once weekly.

7.8.2
Response and Response Prediction

There are so far no parameters that clearly predict whether a patient will respond to erythropoietin or not. Patients with an increase in reticulocyte counts (>40,000/μl from baseline) and an increase in hb (≥0.5 g/dl) after 2 weeks of treatment have a high probability of response. In contrast, patients without an increase in hb despite high serum EPO levels (>100 mU/ml) have a high probability (>90%) of unresponsiveness (Ludwig et al. 1994; Beguin 2002). Several predictive algorithms have been proposed, but their clinical usefulness remains questionable.

In patients treated with standard radiotherapy or radiochemotherapy, the response rates (increase in hb) are high and lie in the range of 90%–100%. Depending on the pretreatment hb level, approximately 40%–70% of patients achieved the target hb (14 g/dl) in these studies. In patients undergoing more aggressive chemotherapy, the response rates were lower. The response is at least in part dose dependent. An increase in the dose of erythropoietin can improve the response. In patients with advanced metastatic disease, however, less than 50% respond to EPO.

An easy and cost-effective way to evaluate the response is to measure the increase in hb after 2 weeks of treatment with erythropoietin. In responding patients, the average increase in hb is about 0.5–1 g/dl hb per week, with a delay of roughly 10 days after starting treatment. If an increase in hb levels is observed after 2 weeks of treatment, the administration should continue in the same dosage. In case of insufficient response, the dose of erythropoietin can be doubled (three times weekly 20,000 IU) for a further 2 weeks of treatment.

7.8.3
Iron Substitution

The administration of iron as an addendum to the EPO treatment has been used in the vast majority of clinical studies. Patients with cancer-related anemia have a reduced availability of iron due to increased iron storage in macrophages, although the amount of total body iron is often in the normal range (Nowrousian 2002). Most of the clinical studies have used standard oral iron administration. According to the clinical data, this method of iron administration seems to be successful. Due to its lower toxicity, oral iron should therefore be preferred to intravenous iron substitution.

7.8.4
Optimal Hemoglobin and Target Hemoglobin

The question whether an optimal hb level exists with regard to response to radiotherapy or radiochemotherapy is currently investigated in prospective studies. Retrospective analyses suggest that the highest local control rates in patients undergoing definitive radiotherapy are achieved if the hb during and especially at the end of radiotherapy is in the normal range (Grogan et al. 1999; Dunst and Molls 2002b). Data on tumor oxygenation support this hypothesis (Becker et al. 2000; Vaupel et al. 2002). If EPO is administered in radiotherapy patients with the objective of improving response and local control, current data suggest that the hb level should at least be kept within the normal range (above 12 g/dl) or elevated up to 14 g/dl. This target hb level is also an optimal hb level with regard to improvement in quality of life. Higher hb levels should be avoided because of increasing side effects and because of impaired tumor oxygenation with high hb levels, probably because of rheological problems (Vaupel et al. 2002).

7.8.5
Side Effects

Erythropoietin administration has been associated with only minimal acute side effects in all studies. In four randomized studies, no difference in the incidence of adverse events between patients treated with EPO vs placebo was observed.

The main side effects include flu-like syndromes, skin rash, local reactions at the site of injection, bone pain, and headache. Hypertension and deep venous thrombosis have been observed in patients with significant elevation of hematocrit and hemoglobin. Hypertension, elevated hematocrit and electrolyte changes have been reported in patients with renal anemia after long-term use of epoetin.

Recently, the development of aplastic anemia after prolonged treatment with EPO has been described. This results from antibodies to recombinant erythropoietin and subsequent impairment of normal erythropoiesis. The risk is very low, although specific for erythropoietin. Most of the patients with aplastic anemia, however, had received prolonged EPO administration over years due to renal anemia. It is not clear whether the lower incidence of aplastic anemia in cancer patients is due to the shorter administration period (the most likely explanation) or the shorter survival in cancer patients. Most of the patients who have received EPO in prospective studies had advanced disease.

7.9
Conclusions

Human recombinant erythropoietin (rhEPO, epoetin alfa and beta, darbepoetin) can be used for prevention and treatment of anemia in cancer patients. The efficacy with regard to improvement of hb levels is high in patients undergoing standard radiotherapy or radiochemotherapy. A significant improvement in quality of life has been proven. Experimental data and preliminary data from clinical trials further suggest that the use of EPO might improve local control and survival. This extremely important issue is currently investigated in several large multicentric studies, mainly in head and neck and cervix cancer. Side effects of EPO occur infrequently and are in general mild and negligible. In summary, rhEPO is probably the most important currently available growth factor in radiation oncology.

References

Antonadou A, Cadarmakis E, Sarris G, Tzigounis T (1998) Effect of the administration of recombinant human erythropoietin in patients with pelvic malignancies during radiotherapy. Radiother Oncol 48 [Suppl 1]:S122

Beck I, Weinmann R, Caro J (1993) Characterization of hypoxia-responsive enhancer in the human erythropoietin gene shows presence of hypoxia-inducible 120-Kd nuclear DNA-binding protein in erythropoietin-producing and nonproducing cells. Blood 82:704–711

Becker A, Stadler P, Lavey R, Haensgen G, Kuhnt T, Lautenschlaeger C, Feldmann HJ, Molls M, Dunst J (2000) Severe anemia is associated with poor tumor oxygenation in head and neck squamous cell carcinoma. Int J Radiat Oncol Biol Phys 46:459–466

Beguin Y (2002) Predictive factors for response of anemia to recombinant human erythropoietin. In: Nowrousian MR (ed) Recombinant human erythropoietin (rhEPO) in clinical oncology. Springer, Vienna New York

Berdel WE, Oberberg D, Reufi B, Thiel E (1991) Studies on the role of recombinant erythropoietin in the growth regulation of human non-hematopoietic cells in vitro. Ann Hematol 63:5–8

Blanchard KL, Fandrey J, Goldberg MA (1993) Regulation of the erythropoietin gene. Stem Cells 11 [Suppl 1]:1–7

Blohmer JU, von Minckwitz G, Paepke S, Thomssen C, Kimmig R, Petry U, Würschmidt J, Pfisterer J, Lichtenegger W (2002) Sequential adjuvant chemo-radiotherapy with vs. without erythropoietin for patients with high-risk cervical cancer – second analysis of a prospective, randomized, open and controlled AGO- and NOGGO-intergroup study. Proc ASCO 21:206a

Bunn HF, Poyton RO (1996) Oxygen sensing and molecular adaption to hypoxia. Physiol Rev 76:839–885

Bush RS (1986) The significance of anemia in clinical radiation therapy. Int J Radiat Oncol Biol Phys 12:2047–2050

Canaday DJ, Regine WF, Mohiuddin M, Zollinger W, Machtay M, Schultz D, Rudoltz MS (1999) Significance of pretreatment hemoglobin levels in patients with T1 glottic cancer. Radiat Oncol Invest 7:42–48

Caro JJ, Salas M, Ward A, Goss G (2001) Anemia as an independent prognostic factor for survival in patients with cancer: a systematic, quantitative review. Cancer 91:2214–2221

Cerami A (2001) Beyond erythropoiesis: novel applications for recombinant erythropoietin. Semin Hematol 38 [Suppl 7]:33–39

Cerami A, Brins M, Ghezzi P, Cerami C, Itri LM (2002) Neuroprotective properties of epoetin alfa. Nephrol Dial Transplant 17 [Suppl 1]:8–12

Demetri GD, Kris M, Wade J et al (1998) Quality-of-life benefit in chemotherapy patients treated with epoetin alfa is independent of disease response or tumor type: results from a prospective community oncology study. Procrit Study Group. J Clin Oncol 16:3412–3425

Dunst J, Molls M (2002a) Incidence and impact of anemia in radiation oncology. In: Nowrousian MR (ed) Recombinant human erythropoietin (rhEPO) in clinical oncology. Springer, Vienna New York

Dunst J, Molls M (2002b) Relationship between anemia and tumor hypoxia. In: Nowrousian MR (ed) Recombinant human erythropoietin (rhEPO) in clinical oncology. Springer, Vienna New York

Dusenbery KE, McGuire WA, Holt PJ, Carson LF, Fowler JM, Twiggs LB, Potish RA (1994) Erythropoietin increases hemoglobin during radiation therapy for cervical cancer. Int J Radiat Oncol Biol Phys 29:1079–1084

Evans IC, Bergsjø P (1965) The influence of anemia on the results of radiotherapy in carcinoma of the cervix. Radiology 84:709–717

Fein DA, Lee WR, Hanlon AL, Ridge JA, Langer CJ, Curran WJ Jr, Coia LR (1995) Pretreatment hemoglobin level influences local control and survival of T1-T2 squamous cell carcinomas of the glottic larynx. J Clin Oncol 13:2077–2083

Frommhold H, Guttenberger R, Henke M (1998) The impact of blood hemoglobin content on the outcome of radiotherapy. The Freiburg experience. Strahlenther Onkol 174 [Suppl IV]:31–34

Fyles AW, Milosevic M, Pintilie M, Syed A, Hill RP (2000) Anemia, hypoxia and transfusion in patients with cervical cancer: a review. Radiother Oncol 57:13–19

Gabrilove JL, Cleeland CS, Livingston RB, Sarokhan B, Winer E, Einhorn LH (2001) Clinical evaluation of once-weekly dosing of epoetin alfa in chemotherapy patients: improvements in hemoglobin and quality of life are similar to three-times-weekly dosing. J Clin Oncol 19:2875–2882

Girinksi T, Pejovic-Lenfant MH, Bourhis J, Campana F, Cosset JM, Petit C, Malaise EP, Haie C, Gerbaulet A, Chassagne D (1989) Prognostic value of hemoglobin concentrations and blood transfusions in advanced carcinoma of the cervix treated by radiation therapy: results of a retrospective study of 386 patients. Int J Radiat Oncol Biol Phys 16:37–42

Glaspy J, Bukowski R, Steinberg D et al (1997) Impact of therapy with epoetin alfa on clinical outcomes in patients with nonmyeloid malignancies during cancer chemotherapy in community oncology practice. Procrit Study Group. J Clin Oncol 15:1218–1234

Glimelius B, Linne T, Hoffman K et al (1998) Epoetin beta in the treatment of anemia in patients with advanced gastrointestinal cancer. J Clin Oncol 16:434–440

Grau C, Overgaard J (1998) Significance of hemoglobin concentrations for treatment outcome. In: Molls M, Vaupel P (eds) Blood perfusion and microenvironment of human tumors. Implications for clinical radiooncology. Springer, Berlin Heidelberg New York, pp 101–112

Grogan M, Thomas GM, Melamed I, Wong FL (1999) The importance of maintaining high hemoglobin levels during radiation treatment of carcinoma of the cervix. Cancer 86:1531–1536

Hannisdal E, Fossa SD, Host H (1993) Blood tests and prognosis in bladder carcinomas treated with definitive radiotherapy. Radiother Oncol 27:117–122

Harrison L, Shasha D, Shiaova L, White C, Ramdeen B, Portenoy R (2001) Prevalence of anemia in cancer patients undergoing radiation therapy. Sem Oncol 28 [Suppl 8]:54–59

Hasenclever D, Diehl V (1998) A prognostic score for advanced Hodgkin's disease: International Prognostic Factors Project on Advanced Hodgkin's Disease. N Engl J Med 339:1506–1514

Henke M (2002) Clinical trials using rhEPO in radiation oncology. In: Nowrousian MR (ed) Recombinant human erythropoietin (rhEPO) in clinical oncology. Springer, Vienna New York

Henke M, Guttenberger R, Barke A, Pajonk F, Pötter R, Frommhold H (1999) Erythropoietin for patients undergoing radiotherapy: a pilot study. Radiother Oncol 50:185–190

Jelkmann W (2002) Pharmacology, pharmacokinetics and safety of rhEPO. In: Nowrousian MR (ed) Recombinant human erythropoietin (rhEPO) in clinical oncology. Springer, Vienna New York

Kapp DS, Fisher D, Gutierrez E, Kohorn IE, Schwartz PE (1983) Pretreatment prognostic factors in carcinoma of the uterine cervix: a multivariate analysis of the effect of age, stage, histology, and blood counts on survival. Int J Radiat Oncol Biol Phys 9:445–455

Kelleher DK, Matthiensen U, Thews O, Vaupel P (1995) Tumor oxygenation in anemic rats: effects of erythropoietin treatment versus red blood cell transfusion. Acta Oncol 34:379–384

Kelleher DK, Matthiensen U, Thews O, Vaupel P (1996) Blood flow, oxygenation and bioenergetic status of tumors after erythropoietin treatment in normal and anemic rats. Cancer Res 56:4728–4734

Lacombe C, Mayeux P (2002) Biology of erythropoietin. In: Nowrousian MR (ed) Recombinant human erythropoietin (rhEPO) in clinical oncology. Springer, Vienna New York

Lavey RS, Dempsey WH (1993) Erythropoietin increases hemoglobin in cancer patients during radiation therapy. Int J Radiat Oncol Biol Phys 27:1147–1152

Lee WR, Berkey B, Marcial V, Fu KK, Cooper JS, Vikram B, Coia L, Rotman M, Ortiz H (1998) Anemia is associated with decreased survival and increased locoregional failure in patients with locally advanced head and neck carcinoma: a secondary analysis of RTOG 85-27. Int J Radiat Oncol Biol Phys 42:1069–1075

Littlewood TJ (2002) Effect of rhEPO on survival in anemic cancer patients. In: Nowrousian MR (ed) Recombinant human erythropoietin (rhEPO) in clinical oncology. Springer, Vienna New York

Littlewood TJ, Bajetta E, Nortier JW et al (2001) Effects of epoetin alfa on hematologic parameters and quality of life in cancer patients receiving nonplatinum chemotherapy: results of a randomized, double-blind, placebo-controlled trial. J Clin Oncol 19:2865–2874

Logsdon MD, Eifel PJ (1999) FIGO IIIB squamous cell carcinoma of the cervix: an analysis of prognostic factors emphasizing the balance between external beam and intracavitary radiation therapy. Int J Radiat Oncol Biol Phys 43:763–775

Ludwig H, Fritz E, Leitgeb C, Pecherstorfer M, Samonigg L, Schuster J (1994) Prediction of response to erythropoietin treatment in chronic anemia of cancer. Blood 84:1056–1063

MacDougall IC, Gray SJ, Elston O, Breen C, Jenkins B, Browne J, Egrie J (1999) Pharmacokinetics of novel erythropoiesis stimulating protein compared to epoetin alfa in dialysis patients. J Am Soc Nephrol 10:2392–2395

Miller CB, Jones RJ, Piantadosi S, Abeloff MD, Spivak JL (1990) Decreased erythropoietin response in patients with the anemia of cancer. N Engl J Med 322:1689–1692

Müller-Klieser W, Vaupel P, Manz R, Schmidseder R (1981) Intracapillary oxyhemoglobin saturation in malignant tumors in humans. Int J Radiat Oncol Biol Phys 7:1397–1404

Nowrousian MR (2002) Pathophysiology of cancer-related anemia. In: Nowrousian MR (ed) Recombinant human erythropoietin (rhEPO) in clinical oncology. Springer, Vienna New York

Osterborg A, Brandberg Y, Molostova V et al (2002) Randomized, double-blind, placebo-controlled trial of recombinant human erythropoietin, epoetin beta, in hematologic malignancies. J Clin Oncol 20:2486–2494

Overgaard J (1988) The influence of hemoglobin concentrations on the response to radiotherapy. Scand J Clin Lab Invest 48:49–53

Rosti V, Pedrazzoli P, Ponchio L, Zibera C, Novella A, Lucotti C, Robustelli della Cunna G, Cazzola M (1993) Effect of recombinant human erythropoietin on the hematopoietic and nonhematopoietic malignant cell growth in vitro. Haematologica 78:208–212

Rudat V, Dietz A, Schramm O, Conradt C, Maier H, Flentje M, Wannenmacher M (1999) Prognostic impact of total tumor volume and hemoglobin concentration on the outcome of patients with advanced head and neck cancer after concomitant boost radiochemotherapy. Radiother Oncol 53:119–125

Selzer E, Wachek V, Kodym R, Schlagbauer-Wadl H, Schlegel W, Pehamberger H, Jansen B (2000) Erythropoietin receptor expression in human melanoma cells. Melanoma Res 10:421–426

Stüben G, Thews O, Poettgen C, Knuhmann K, Vaupel P, Stuschke M (2001) Recombinant human erythropoietin increases the radiosensitivity of xenografted human tumours in anaemic nude mice. J Cancer Res Clin Oncol 127:346–350

Sweeney PJ, Nicolae D, Ignacio L, Chen L, Roach M, Wara W, Marcus KC, Vijayakumar S (1998) Effect of subcutaneous recombinant human erythropoietin in cancer patients receiving radiotherapy: final report of a randomized, open-labelled phase II trial. Br J Cancer 77:1996–2002

Tarnawski R, Skladowski K, Maciejewski B (1997) Prognostic value of hemoglobin concentration in radiotherapy for cancer of the supraglottic larynx. Int J Radiat Oncol Biol Phys 38:1007–1011

Thews O, König R, Kelleher DK, Kutzner J, Vaupel P (1998) Enhanced radiosensitivity in experimental tumours following erythropoietin treatment of chemotherapy-induced anaemia. Br J Cancer 78:752–766

Thews O, Kelleher DK, Vaupel P (2001) Erythropoietin restores the anemia-induced reduction in cyclophosphamide cytotoxicity in rat tumors. Cancer Res 61:1358–1361

Van Acht MJ, Hermans J, Boks DE, Leer JW (1992) The prognostic value of hemoglobin and a decrease in hemoglobin during radiotherapy in laryngeal carcinoma. Radiother Oncol 23:229–235

Vaupel P, Kallinowski F, Okunieff P (1989) Blood flow, oxygen and nutrient supply, and metabolic environment of human tumors: a review. Cancer Res 49:6449–6465

Vaupel P, Thews O, Mayer A, Höckel S, Höckel M (2002) Oxygenation status of gynecological tumors: what is the optimal hemoglobin level? Strahlenther Onkol (in press)

Wagner W, Hermann R, Hartlapp J, Esser E, Christoph B, Müller M, Krech R, Koch O (2000) Prognostic value of hemoglobin concentrations in patients with advanced head and neck cancer treated with combined radio-chemotherapy and surgery. Strahlenther Onkol 176:73–80

Westenfelder C, Baranowski RL (2000) Erythropoietin stimulates proliferation of human renal carcinoma cells. Kidney Int 58:647–657

Westphal G, Niederberger L, Blum C, Wollman Y, Knoch TA, Rebel W, Debus J, Friedrich E (2002) Erythropoietin and G-CSF receptors in human tumor cells: expression and aspects regarding functionality. Tumori 88:150–159

8 Hematopoietic Tissue II: Role of Colony-Stimulating Factors

C. Nieder, B. Jeremic, T. Licht, and F. B. Zimmermann

CONTENTS

8.1 Introduction 103
8.2 Hematopoietic Cell Development 104
8.3 Radiosensitivity of the Bone Marrow 104
8.4 G-CSF and GM-CSF for Hematopoietic Recovery and Infection Prophylaxis in the Context of Chemotherapy 105
8.4.1 Leukemia Studies 105
8.4.2 Solid Tumors and Lymphomas 106
8.5 G-CSF and GM-CSF During Radiochemotherapy 106
8.6 Further Aspects of GM-CSF Functions 108
8.7 Aspects of M-CSF Functions 108
8.8 Aspects of Thrombopoietin Functions 108
8.9 Summary 109
References 109

8.1 Introduction

Colony-stimulating factors such as granulocyte colony-stimulating factor (G-CSF) and granulocyte-macrophage colony-stimulating factor (GM-CSF) have started to alter traditional patterns of supportive care both in radiation oncology and in medical oncology. After results of numerous clinical trials, these factors are being marketed to reduce both acute and late normal tissue toxicity, for example in hematopoietic and mucosal tissues in the context of chemotherapy, extended-field radiotherapy, combined modality treatment and autologous bone marrow transplantation. Furthermore, some studies address their use in cancer patients in the perioperative setting.

C. Nieder, MD; B. Jeremic, MD; F. B. Zimmermann, MD
Department of Radiation Oncology, Klinikum rechts der Isar, Technical University Munich, Ismaninger Strasse 22, 81675 Munich, Germany
T. Licht, MD
Department of Hematology and Medical Oncology, Klinikum rechts der Isar, Technical University Munich, Ismaninger Strasse 22, 81675 Munich, Germany

Myelosuppression continues to influence delivery and due to treatment interruption, perhaps outcome of oncological treatment. Both compromised dose intensity and impairment of quality of life, for example due to febrile infections and hospitalization, might be problematic. However, one must decide whether the risk of neutropenia associated with a particular treatment regimen warrants the use of colony-stimulating factors (CSFs). The cost of prevention or treatment of infectious complications might add substantially to the overall cost of cancer therapy in large numbers of patients with common malignancies. Therefore, the search for protective strategies should be accompanied by thorough evaluation of their cost-effectiveness. Cost analyses were reported in the 2000 update of recommendations for the use of hematopoietic colony-stimulating factors: evidence-based, clinical practice guidelines by the American Society of Clinical Oncology (ASCO; referred to as the ASCO guidelines in the following paragraphs; accessible at www.astro.org). They suggest that CSFs save money when the risk of febrile neutropenia is higher than 40%, which is not the case in routine chemotherapy and radiotherapy settings.

In recent years, increasing research on stem cell and progenitor cell biology has expanded our knowledge on the development of the hematopoietic compartments. The role of a large number of cytokines and growth factors has now been better defined, although the complex network of regulatory switches has not been completely uncovered yet. Nevertheless, based on experimental results, researchers were able to identify several possible targets for intervention. This chapter briefly summarizes current aspects from the radiation oncologist's point of view. There is a large body of literature available that expands this topic (Neta 1997; Neta et al. 1998), especially with focus on chemotherapy studies and infectious diseases (Hubel et al. 2002). The rapidly changing field of growth factor use in conjunction with stem cell transplantation, either in priming for mobilization or post-transplantation will not be addressed in this review.

8.2
Hematopoietic Cell Development

A complex regulatory network provides the basis for replication and differentiation of hematopoietic stem cells (Fig. 8.1) along lymphoid or myeloid lineages. Stem cells show features of long-term multilineage engraftment and high proliferative capacity, yet functional heterogeneity is present among such cells (GUENECHEA et al. 2001; HUTTMANN et al. 2001). Stem cells, which have the ability for extensive self-renewal, interact with a variety of other cell types, such as endothelial cells, adventitial cells, fibroblasts and macrophages, by communication pathways that involve cytokines and growth factors. Besides their location in the bone marrow, stem cells might also be present in the circulating blood and other organs such as the spleen, where a different microenvironment can be found. Bone marrow-derived stem cells showed the potential to differentiate into a variety of cell types. They might even be useful for regeneration of gastrointestinal epithelia (OKAMOTO et al. 2002). Under experimental circumstances, the spleen colony assay or the SCID repopulation assay can be used for in vivo assessment of hematopoietic stem cells. Primitive stem cells appear to be responsible for long-term hematopoiesis in mouse models, whereas more committed stem cells appear to be important for engraftment and rapid hematopoietic recovery. Human progenitor cells in the peripheral blood differ in some respects from their marrow counterparts. They are not cycling and show no propensity to differentiate while in the blood. Furthermore, expression of certain cell surface markers varies. After transplantation in vivo, the cells are capable of reconstituting short-term marrow hematopoiesis (MAUCH et al. 1995).

Fig. 8.1. CD-34 positive stem cells (From LÖFFLER and RASTETTER 1999, with permission). GOODELL et al. (1997) provided data on different primitive hematopoietic stem cells which are CD-34 negative

Granulocytes originate from stem cells in the bone marrow (simplified overview presented in Fig. 8.2), where they mature for up to 10 days before entering the blood circulation. Their half-life in the peripheral blood is in the range of 4–5 h. Neutropenia might result from chemotherapy, radiation therapy or replacement of normal bone marrow by infiltrating tumor cells. Absolute neutrophil counts below 1000/µl increase the risk of infection, whereas counts under 500/µl strongly correlate with severe infectious complications. Other risk factors such as monocytopenia or immunoglobulin deficiency might further increase the complication rate. G-CSF and GM-CSF might decrease the duration and severity of neutropenic episodes and the associated risk of infection.

Fibroblast growth factors are a complex family of mostly mitogenic proteins, which are involved in the differentiation of endothelial cells and fibroblasts, and wound repair. Basic fibroblast growth factor (bFGF) is expressed in cells of the bone marrow including stromal cells, and possibly cells from several hematopoietic cell lineages (ALLOUCHE and BIKFALVI 1995). The effects of single-dose as well as fractionated total body irradiation (TBI) might be counteracted by bFGF, which was shown to increase survival of irradiated mice due to accelerated recovery of bone marrow hematopoietic cells and peripheral blood cells of red and white lineage as well as platelets (DING et al. 1996, 1997). At present, no clinical data on the use of bFGF in humans after TBI are available.

8.3
Radiosensitivity of the Bone Marrow

The bone marrow is a highly radiosensitive tissue. Total dose, dose rate and volume influence the ultimate degree of injury. Peripheral blood cells respond with different kinetics. Lymphopenia occurs very rapidly after even modest radiation doses due to cell death in interphase. Neutropenia might occur in the first week, followed by thrombocytopenia in 2–3 weeks and anemia in 2–3 months. After localized radiation exposure of the bone marrow in rats, initial aplasia with extensive sinusoidal injury can be found. However, at 2 weeks the marrow regenerates to almost normal cellularity even after very high radiation doses (KNOSPE et al. 1966). Migration of circulating stem cells into aplastic regions is responsible for recovery. Later on, a delayed wave of aplasia and injury is observed after 1–3 months, again followed

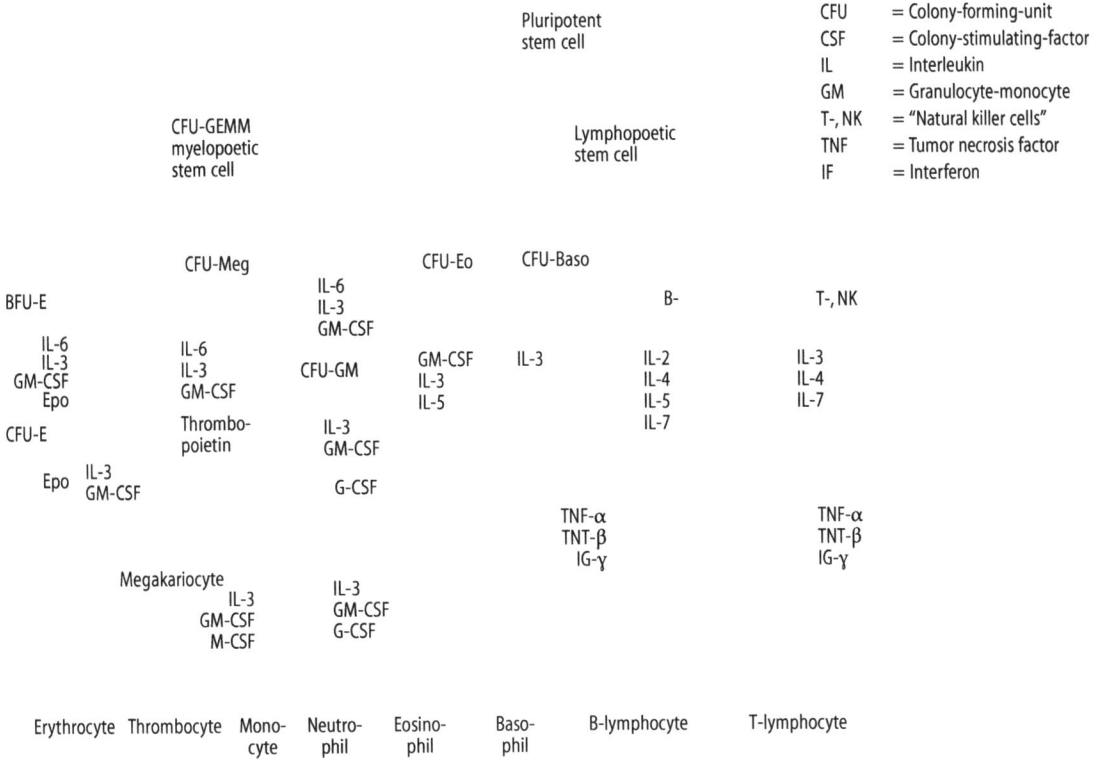

Fig. 8.2. Different hematopoietic cell lines (From LÖFFLER and RASTETTER 1999, with permission)

by regeneration. The amount of regeneration varies with dose (hypocellularity to aplasia). The delayed destruction of the sinusoid microcirculation causes such incomplete marrow recovery or marrow fibrosis. In humans, decreased marrow function may persist for several years following treatment. Historical data, for example, for mantle field irradiation of Hodgkin's disease with doses of 30–40 Gy, demonstrate that the bone marrow did not regenerate within the boundaries of the radiation field, whereas the unirradiated marrow became hyperactive to meet the increasing demand for hematopoiesis (SACKS et al. 1978; PARMENTIER et al. 1983). If large volumes of 50%–75% of the bone marrow were irradiated, in-field marrow regeneration could be observed in addition to activation of unexposed marrow and extension of functioning marrow into previously quiescent areas of the upper and lower extremities (or even spleen and liver). Bone marrow recovery usually requires a longer time than peripheral blood cell normalization. Chemotherapeutic agents tend to further exacerbate radiation-induced dysfunction. Occasionally, hypoplastic or myelodysplastic syndromes may be observed at late intervals.

8.4
G-CSF and GM-CSF for Hematopoietic Recovery and Infection Prophylaxis in the Context of Chemotherapy

8.4.1
Leukemia Studies

A number of placebo-controlled randomized clinical trials explored the use of G-CSF and GM-CSF in patients with acute myeloid leukemia and acute lymphoblastic leukemia (GODWIN et al. 1998; HEIL et al. 1997; HOWIECKI et al. 2002; OHNO et al. 1994; PUI et al. 1997; ROWE et al. 1995; STONE et al. 1995; WELTE et al. 1996). Despite differences in patient population, phase of the disease, treatment regimen and details of growth factor administration, a consistent significant reduction in the duration of severe neutropenia has been suggested. Fever, use of antibiotics and need for hospitalization were decreased as well. This might result in fewer chemotherapy delays. Administration of growth factors after chemotherapy improved survival in two rather small studies (HOWIECKI et al. 2002; ROWE et al. 1995). However, most studies did not find a difference in treatment outcome. There was no increase in refractory disease or leukemic relapse associated with growth factor treatment in these studies. According to the 2000 ASCO guidelines, CSF use can be considered after induction chemotherapy and after consolidation chemotherapy if benefits in terms of shortened hospitalization outweigh the costs.

8.4.2
Solid Tumors and Lymphomas

LYMAN et al. published a meta-analysis on G-CSF in dose-intensive cancer chemotherapy for solid tumors and lymphomas. Randomized trials in the prophylactic setting, i.e., before the onset of fever or neutropenia, were selected (LYMAN et al. 2002). Eight studies were included, five of which were double-blind and placebo-controlled. G-CSF treatment was associated with a reduced risk of febrile neutropenia (odds ratio, 0.38; statistically significant), documented infection (odds ratio, 0.51; statistically significant) and infection-related mortality (odds ratio, 0.6; not significant). Patients treated with G-CSF experienced significantly more bone pain (relative risk, 2.9). The 2000 ASCO guidelines state that CSFs do not provide a benefit in clinical outcome, such as improved survival in non-Hodgkin's lymphoma, Hodgkin's lymphoma, small cell lung cancer, germ cell tumors, and other malignancies. Therefore, use of CSFs should be reserved for high-risk patients for febrile neutropenia. Administration of CSFs to patients who previously experienced febrile neutropenia might be justified under certain circumstances, but chemotherapy dose reduction should be considered as the primary therapeutic option. In 2000, no recommendation was given to treat afebrile neutropenic patients with CSFs.

A meta-analysis of 11 eligible randomized clinical trials on use of G-CSF and GM-CSF in febrile neutropenic cancer patients was performed by BERGHMANS et al. Eventually, eight trials were analyzable (BERGHMANS et al. 2002). The relative risk of mortality from febrile neutropenia was 0.66 in the G-CSF and 0.97 in the GM-CSF group. Neither difference was statistically significant. The authors thus did not recommend the use of G-CSF or GM-CSF. This is in accordance with the 2000 ASCO guidelines for uncomplicated fever and neutropenia. Risk factors such as neutrophil counts lower than 100/µl, pneumonia, hypotension, sepsis syndrome, and invasive fungal infection may provide arguments for the use of CSFs in febrile neutropenic patients.

Issues regarding optimal timing and duration of CSF application and equivalent effectiveness of available CSFs on the market require additional clinical studies. Most recently, G-CSF has also been investigated together with the anti-CD20 monoclonal antibody rituximab in patients with indolent non-Hodgkin's lymphoma (KIMBY 2002). In a small study of 20 patients with relapsed disease, G-CSF plus rituximab increased the response duration compared to monotherapy, without significantly increased adverse events. G-CSF enhances antibody-dependent cell-mediated cytotoxicity by neutrophil granulocytes.

8.5
G-CSF and GM-CSF During Radiochemotherapy

BUNN et al. performed a multicenter phase III randomized trial where 230 patients with limited-stage small cell lung cancer treated with simultaneous chemoradiotherapy were included (BUNN et al. 1995). GM-CSF was given on days 4–18 of each of six cycles. These authors reported a significant increase in the frequency and duration of severe thrombocytopenia in the GM-CSF arm. Furthermore, more toxic deaths, days in hospital and nonhematological toxicity was observed after GM-CSF. Interestingly, white blood cell counts were higher after GM-CSF. However, grade IV leukopenia and neutropenia were similarly common. After GM-CSF, the rate of complete tumor remission was lower, but not significantly (36% and 44%, respectively). Survival was also somewhat shorter. The authors did not recommend the use of GM-CSF outside of experimental settings. They concluded that chest radiotherapy concurrent to cisplatin and etoposide does not induce a high enough rate of grade 4 hematological toxicity to justify prophylactic use of growth factors, even if they were effective.

LANGER et al. (1997) published a different trial. Thirty-five patients with stage III non-small cell lung cancer received two cycles of induction chemotherapy with paclitaxel and carboplatin separated by 3 weeks together with G-CSF from day 2–15 and 23–36. One group randomly received priming G-CSF for 5 days before day 1. On day 43, conventional radiotherapy with 30 fractions of 2 Gy was begun. Carboplatin and paclitaxel were given again on days 43 and 64 in escalated dose levels. No final evaluation of this trial has yet been published. Preliminary data do not allow firm conclusions about the usefulness of G-CSF in this setting.

The topical use of GM-CSF for oral mucositis from radiochemotherapy for advanced stage III and IV head and neck cancer was evaluated in a randomized study that was closed after 35 patients (SPRINZL et al. 2001). Regarding degree of oral mucositis, perception of pain, incidence of secondary infections, and hematological parameters, GM-CSF was not superior to conventional mouthwash in this setting. A different study from Finland included 40 head and neck cancer patients (MAKKONEN et al. 2000). Randomization was performed between GM-CSF s.c. plus sucralfate mouth washing or sucralfate alone. Again, no significant difference in the oral mucositis grade, oral pain, use of analgetics, and weight loss was found. Side effects in the GM-CSF group included skin reactions at the site of injection, fever (30%), bone pain (25%), and nausea.

Whereas hematological toxicity was mild, mucositis and skin reactions continued to be dose-limiting in a nonrandomized trial of concomitant radiochemotherapy for head and neck cancer (BROCKSTEIN et al. 2000). It included 54 patients, 25 with prior full-dose radiotherapy, who received 5-fluorouracil, hydroxyurea and paclitaxel together with two daily fractions of 1.5 Gy up to a median dose of 73 Gy and G-CSF. These more recent studies confirmed a previous summary of the literature published until the year 2000 (FUNG and FERRILL 2002). That review also did not find sufficient evidence confirming benefits of growth factor treatment, in this case GM-CSF, for oral mucositis, regardless of the mode of GM-CSF application or its time (prophylactic versus therapeutic).

G-CSF was further evaluated in 263 patients with stage III–IV head and neck cancer in a multicenter randomized trial (STAAR et al. 2001). Treatment was hyperfractionated accelerated simultaneous radiochemotherapy in arm A and hyperfractionated accelerated radiotherapy in arm B. In both arms, there was a second randomization for prophylactic use of G-CSF to prevent mucosal toxicity. Radiotherapy followed a concomitant boost concept up to 69.9 Gy (dose per fraction 1.8 and 1.5 Gy, respectively). In weeks 1 and 5, two cycles of 5-fluorouracil and carboplatin were administered. Subcutaneous G-CSF treatment was given on days 15–19. Patients with G-CSF showed reduced acute mucosal toxicities ($p=0.066$). Unfortunately, this statement is not supported by presentation of data in greater detail. However, in both treatment arms, G-CSF was associated with significantly worse local–regional control. This was more pronounced in the radiotherapy alone group. In multivariate analysis, inferior prognosis after G-CSF was confirmed. Although this was not endpoint of the study, the results do not encourage use of G-CSF in such settings.

These findings were not expected from a previous smaller trial that included the use of G-CSF (VOKES et al. 1994). They are, however, in accordance with in vitro studies in head and neck carcinoma cell lines, demonstrating expression of G-CSF receptor and a correlation of such expression with prognosis, possibly from enhanced invasive potential through matrix metalloproteinase 2 activation (CHEN et al. 1999; NODA et al. 1999; SUGIMOTO et al. 2001; SUNAGA et al. 2001; TSUZUKI et al. 1998). Despite some critical comments on study design and group sizes, these results do not encourage the use of G-CSF in radiotherapy-based treatment of oro- and hypopharyngeal head and neck tumors.

Comparable laboratory findings of expression of G-CSF and its receptor can be found for epithelial skin tumors (HIRAI et al. 2001), squamous cell carcinoma of the esophagus, both adenocarcinoma and lymphoma of the stomach (ICHIISHI et al. 2000; SUGIMOTO et al. 1999), colon carcinoma (BRETSCHER et al. 2000), osteosarcoma (THACKER et al. 1994), transitional cell carcinoma of the bladder (TACHIBANA et al. 1995) and ovarian carcinoma (MEROGI et al. 1997). In glial neoplasms, G-CSF, GM-CSF and/or their receptors were expressed in 22/22 tumors and derived cell cultures (MÜLLER et al. 1999). Expression correlated with higher tumor grade. In mouse mammary carcinoma, GM-CSF stimulated cell growth as well as activity of matrix metalloproteinase 2 and 9 in vitro (GABRI et al. 1999). From all these data, the question arises: do intensified treatment strategies based on addition of CSFs fail to show improved outcomes because stimulation of tumor cell proliferation and invasive potential counteract the possible increase in cell kill and prevent a net benefit in reducing the number of tumor cells? The 2000 ASCO guidelines recommend avoiding CSFs in patients receiving concomitant chemotherapy and radiotherapy. Their use may be considered under special circumstances in patients treated exclusively by radiotherapy, i.e., if prolonged delays in large field radiotherapy secondary to neutropenia are expected. However, extensive studies on this subject have not been published yet.

8.6
Further Aspects of GM-CSF Functions

Skin toxicity was assessed in two groups of patients irradiated for vulvar carcinoma by KOUVARIS et al. (2001). Thirty-seven woman applied steroid cream to irradiated skin areas during radiotherapy, whereas 24 woman used GM-CSF impregnated gauze after 20 Gy plus the same prescription of steroid cream. The score of skin reactions, the pain score and the time of radiotherapy interruption were significantly in favor of the GM-CSF group, where in addition healing time was significantly shorter. We could not identify additional studies on the subject of skin toxicity.

Intravesical infusion of GM-CSF was explored in order to improve radiation-induced bladder toxicity (DIAMANTOPOULOS et al. 2002). Thirty patients received 900 µg GM-CSF per day diluted in saline for 5 days. The solution was kept in the bladder for 60 min. The mean time from radiotherapy (60 Gy in 2-Gy-fractions) to GM-CSF treatment was 2 months. In a mean time of 3 days, 27 patients experienced symptom improvement. Three patients improved after a second course of GM-CSF, which was given 1 week later. Improvement was temporary in 33% of the patients (9–12 months) and stable for a longer time in 66%. The exact duration, however, has not been reported. The same holds true regarding the influence of this treatment on bladder tumor control.

Strategies of immune therapy-based gene therapy have explored the use of GM-CSF among various other cytokines (COLOMBO et al. 1991; DRANOFF et al. 1993). Clinical vaccination trials in renal cell carcinoma and melanoma patients have demonstrated limited responses with such treatment where irradiated tumor cells transduced with GM-CSF were reinfused to modulate the immune response (SIMONS et al. 1997). By use of GM-CSF and other cytokines, cultures from peripheral blood mononuclear cells can give rise to dendritic cells. The latter are potent antigen-presenting cells that are also being evaluated for the purpose of tumor immunotherapy (NESTLE et al. 1998). For more detailed descriptions on this subject, including clinical trial results, the reader is referred to a recent overview by BORRELLO and PARDOLL (2002).

GM-CSF apparently plays a role in regulation of surfactant homeostasis and lung host defense. Human pulmonary microvascular endothelial cells, which do not express GM-CSF at the transcriptional or protein level, can be stimulated in vitro by TNF-α and by IL-1β to release the cytokine (BURG et al. 2002). In knockout mice, targeted ablation of the *GM-CSF* gene or its receptor (–/– mice) resulted in pulmonary alveolar proteinosis but no hematological abnormalities (TRAPNELL and WHITSETT 2002). Alveolar macrophages from such mice were found to have reduced capacity for surfactant catabolism, cell adhesion, phagocytosis, and bacterial killing. They appeared to stop differentiation at an early stage. The changes were corrected by local expression of GM-CSF in the lung. Some data suggest that radiation exposure can increase GM-CSF protein levels from the mouse lung (FEDOROCKO et al. 2002). At present, the available information about GM-CSF functions in the lung is still preliminary. Whether modification of the GM-CSF pathway affects the radiation sensitivity of the lung has not been examined so far.

8.7
Aspects of Macrophage Colony-Stimulating Factor Functions

In contrast to G-CSF and GM-CSF, macrophage colony-stimulating factor (M-CSF) can not be used for stimulation of hematopoiesis. Its physiological role is different and mainly immunomodulatory. Thrombocytopenia might develop as dose-limiting toxicity in clinical trials (BUKOWSKI et al. 1994). In a porcine model of coronary artery balloon injury followed by intracoronary brachytherapy with 16 Gy at a 0.5-mm tissue depth (32-P balloon system), persistently increased levels of M-CSF were found in controls, but not in irradiated animals (FINKELSTEIN et al. 2002). Also, irradiated animals developed reduced neointimal proliferation during the observation time of 2 weeks, suggesting a possible role of inhibition of M-CSF expression after brachytherapy. The response of several tumors (B16 melanoma, Lewis lung carcinoma, renal cell carcinoma) to fractionated irradiation in animals can be enhanced by treatment with M-CSF as well as M-CSF plus IL-12 (TEICHER et al. 1996). A phase I trial combining M-CSF with a mouse monoclonal antibody against GD3 ganglioside in 19 patients with metastatic melanoma resulted in tumor regression in three cases and 2-year survival in six patients (MINASIAN et al. 1995).

8.8
Aspects of Thrombopoietin Functions

The role of recombinant thrombopoietin (TPO) for treatment of thrombocytopenia is currently under evaluation (MIYAZAKI 1998). This growth factor plays a pivotal role in the regulation of megakaryocytopoiesis and thrombopoiesis as well as early hematopoiesis (SITNICKA et al. 1996; BORGE et al. 1997). The effects of TPO on immature cell reconstitution after TBI were recently studied in rhesus monkeys. TPO facilitated the recovery of platelet counts and accelerated the recovery of immature CD34+ hematopoietic cells which represent progenitors of several bone marrow-derived cell lines (NEELIS et al. 1997a–c). In mice, TPO promoted the recovery of short-term repopulating stem cells at the relative expense of marrow-repopulating stem cells associated with long-term reconstitution (NEELIS et al. 1998). Such effects might prevent some of the lethal complications of TBI (MOUTHON et al. 2001). TPO might thus be administered in conjunction with G-CSF to facilitate simultaneous recovery of several cell lines involved in TBI-related syndromes.

Further experimental data suggest an additional role of TPO in proliferation of erythroid progenitors and their differentiation to mature erythroid cells (LIU et al. 1999). VAN DER MEEREN et al. studied the effect of recombinant human IL-11 administered after lethal TBI in mice (VAN DER MEEREN et al. 2002). If this moderately effective cytokine was administered along with TPO, survival of animals was increased significantly compared to either treatment alone. This could be explained by an interactive effect on hematopoietic reconstitution.

Pegylated recombinant murine megakaryocyte growth and development factor (MGDF), a truncated molecule related to TPO, injected intravenously immediately after a lethal regimen of carboplatin and TBI prevented death and enhanced hematopoietic recovery in a mouse model (ABUSHULLAIH et al. 2001). A comparable model was used by AKAHORI et al. They also reported reduced severity and duration of thrombocytopenia and anemia, which was more pronounced with early (day 1) rather than delayed treatment (AKAHORI et al. 1998).

8.9
Summary

With a focus on clinical recommendations outside of prospective trials, use of G-CSF or GM-CSF can be considered in leukemia patients after induction chemotherapy and after consolidation chemotherapy if benefits in terms of shortened hospitalization outweigh the costs. In solid tumors, CSFs might be administered to chemotherapy patients with neutropenic fever and risk factors. In the context of radiochemotherapy, the current data do not support the use of CSFs. Several interesting aspects of GM-CSF function have undergone preliminary study and need further exploration. The same holds true for M-CSF, where no meaningful clinical data could be identified. Thrombopoietin has also been investigated in experimental settings. Confirmatory clinical results are pending.

References

Abushullaih BA, Pestina TI, Srivastava DK et al (2001) A schedule of recombinant Mpl ligand is highly effective at preventing lethal myelosuppression in mice given carboplatin and radiation. Exp Hematol 29:1425–1431

Akahori H, Ozai M, Ida M et al (1998) Further examination of various administration protocols of pegylated recombinant human megakaryocyte growth and development factor on thrombocytopenia in myelosuppressed mice. Ther Apher 2: 58–64

Allouche M, Bikfalvi A (1995) The role of fibroblast growth factor-2 (FGF-2) in hematopoiesis. Prog Growth Factor Res 6:35–48

Berghmans T, Paesmans M, Lafitte JJ et al (2002) Therapeutic use of granulocyte and granulocyte-macrophage colony-stimulating factor in febrile neutropenic cancer patients. A systematic review of the literature with meta-analysis. Support Care Cancer 10:181–188

Borge OJ, Ramsfjell V, Cui L et al (1997) Ability of early acting cytokines to directly promote survival and suppress apoptosis of human primitive CD34+CD38– bone marrow cells with multilineage potential at the single-cell level: key role of thrombopoietin. Blood 90:2282–2292

Borrello I, Pardoll D (2002) GM-CSF-based cellular vaccines: a review of the clinical experience. Cytokine Growth Factor Rev 13:185–193

Bretscher V, Andreutii D, Neuville P et al (2000) GM-CSF expression by tumor cells correlates with aggressivity and with stroma reaction formation. J Submicrosc Cytol Pathol 32:525–533

Brockstein B, Haraf DJ, Stenson K et al (2000) A phase I–II study of concomitant chemoradiotherapy with paclitaxel (one-hour infusion), 5-fluorouracil and hydroxyurea with granulocyte colony-stimulating factor support for patients with poor prognosis head and neck cancer. Ann Oncol 11: 721–728

Bukowski RM, Budd GT, Gibbons JA et al (1994) Phase I trial of subcutaneous recombinant macrophage colony-stimulating factor: clinical and immunomodulatory effects. J Clin Oncol 12:97–106

Bunn BA Jr, Crowley J, Kelly K et al (1995) Chemoradiotherapy with or without granulocyte-macrophage colony-stimulating factor in the treatment of limited-stage small-cell lung cancer: a prospective phase III randomized study of the Southwest Oncology Group. J Clin Oncol 13:1632–1641

Burg J, Krump-Konvalinkova V, Bittinger F et al (2002) GM-CSF expression by human lung microvascular endothelial

cells: in vitro and in vivo findings. Am J Physiol Lung Cell Mol Physiol 283:L460–L467
Chen Z, Malhotra PS, Thomas GR et al (1999) Expression of proinflammatory and proangiogenic cytokines in patients with head and neck cancer. Clin Cancer Res 5:1369–1379
Colombo MP, Ferrari G, Stoppacciaro A et al (1991) Granulocyte monocyte colony stimulating factor gene transfer suppresses tumorigenicity of a murine adenocarcinoma in vivo. J Exp Med 173:889–897
Diamantopoulos J, Pliotas G, Karageorgis P (2002) Treatment of post-radiation cystitis with intravesical administration of GM-CSF (abstract). Radiother Oncol 64 [Suppl 1]:S306
Ding I, Huang K, Snyder ML et al (1996) Tumor growth and radiosensitivity in mice given myeloprotective doses of fibroblast growth factors. J Natl Cancer Inst 88:1399–1404
Ding I, Huang K, Wang X et al (1997) Radioprotection of hematopoietic tissue by fibroblast growth factors in fractionated radiation experiments. Acta Oncol 36:337–340
Dranoff G, Jaffee E, Lazenby A et al (1993) Vaccination with irradiated tumor cells engineered to secrete murine granulocyte-macrophage colony-stimulating factor stimulate potent specific and long lasting anti-tumor immunity. Proc Natl Acad Sci U S A 90:3539–3543
Fedorocko P, Egyed A, Vacek A (2002) Irradiation induces increased production of hemopoietic and proinflammatory cytokines in the mouse lung. Int J Radiat Biol 78:305–313
Finkelstein A, Makkar R, Doherty TM et al (2002) Increased expression of macrophage colony-stimulating factor after coronary artery balloon injury is inhibited by intracoronary brachytherapy. Circulation 105:2411–2415
Fung SM, Ferrill MJ (2002) Granulocyte-macrophage colony-stimulating factor and oral mucositis. Ann Pharmacother 36:517–520
Gabri MR, Menna PL, Scursoni AM et al (1999) Role of tumor-derived granulocyte-macrophage colony-stimulating factor in mice bearing a highly invasive and metastatic mammary carcinoma. Pathobiology 67:180–185
Godwin JE, Kopecky KJ, Head DR et al (1998) A double-blind placebo-controlled trial of granulocyte colony-stimulating factor in elderly patients with previously untreated acute myelogenous leukaemia: a Southwest Oncology Group Study. Blood 91:3607–3615
Goodell MA, Rosenzweig M, Kim H et al (1997) Dye efflux studies suggest that hematopoietic stem cells expressing low or undetectable levels of CD34 antigen exist in multiple species. Nat Med 3:1337–1345
Guenechea G, Gan OL, Dorrell C et al (2001) Distinct classes of human stem cells that differ in proliferative and self-renewal potential. Nat Immunol 2:75–82
Heil G, Hoelzer D, Sanz M et al (1997) A randomized, double blind, placebo-controlled, phase III study of Filgrastim in remission induction and consolidation therapy for adults with de novo acute myeloid leukaemia. Blood 90:4710–4718
Hirai K, Kumakiri M, Fujieda S et al (2001) Expression of granulocyte colony-stimulating factor and its receptor in epithelial skin tumors. J Dermatol Sci 25:179–188
Howiecki J, Giebel S, Krzemien S et al (2002) G-CSF administered in time-sequenced setting during remission induction and consolidation therapy of adult acute lymphoblastic leukemia has beneficial influence on early recovery and possibly improves long-term outcome: a randomized multicenter study. Leuk Lymph 43:315–325

Hubel K, Dale DC, Liles WC (2002) Therapeutic use of cytokines to modulate phagocyte function for the treatment of infectious diseases: current status of G-CSF, GM-CSF, M-CSF, and INF-gamma. J Infect Dis 185:1490–1501
Huttmann A, Liu SL, Boyd AW et al (2001) Functional heterogeneity within rhodamine123(lo) Hoechst33342(lo/sp) primitive hemopoietic stem cells revealed by pyronin. Exp Hematol 29:1109–1116
Ichiishi E, Yoshikawa T, Kogawa T et al (2000) Possible paracrine growth of adenocarcinoma of the stomach induced by granulocyte colony-stimulating factor produced by squamous cell carcinoma of the oesophagus. Gut 46:432–434
Kimby E (2002) Beyond immunochemotherapy: combinations of rituximab with cytokines interferon-alpha2a and granulocyte-macrophage colony-stimulating factor. Semin Oncol 29 [Suppl 6]:7–10
Knospe W, Blom J, Crosby W (1966) Regeneration of locally irradiated bone marrow I. Dose-dependent, long-term changes in the rat, with particular emphasis upon vascular and stromal reaction. Blood 28:1653–1668
Kouvaris JR, Kouloulias VE, Plantaniotis GA et al (2001) Dermatitis during radiation for vulvar carcinoma: prevention and treatment with granulocyte-macrophage colony-stimulating factor impregnated gauze. Wound Repair Regen 9:187–193
Langer CJ, Movsas B, Hudes R et al (1997) Induction paclitaxel and carboplatin followed by concurrent chemoradiotherapy in patients with unresectable, locally advanced non-small cell lung carcinoma. Semin Oncol 24 [Suppl 12]:89–95
Liu W, Wang M, Tang DC et al (1999) Thrombopoietin has a differentiative effect on late-stage human erythropoiesis. Br J Haematol 105:459–469
Löffler H, Rastetter J (1999) Atlas der klinischen Hämatologie, 5th edn (German). Springer, Berlin Heidelberg New York
Lyman GH, Kuderer NM, Djulbegovic B (2002) Prophylactic granulocyte colony-stimulating factor in patients receiving dose-intensive cancer chemotherapy: a meta-analysis. Am J Med 112:406–411
Makkonen TA, Minn H, Jekunen A (2000) Granulocyte macrophage colony-stimulating factor and sucralfate in prevention of radiation-induced mucositis: a prospective randomized study. Int J Radiat Oncol Biol Phys 46:525–534
Mauch P, Constine L, Greenberger J et al (1995) Hematopoietic stem cell compartment: acute and late effects of radiation therapy and chemotherapy. Int J Radiat Oncol Biol Phys 31:1319–1339
Merogi AJ, Marrogi AJ, Ramesh R et al (1997) Tumor-host interaction: analysis of cytokines, growth factors, and tumor-infiltrating lymphocytes in ovarian carcinomas. Hum Pathol 28:321–331
Minasian LM, Yao TJ, Steffens TA et al (1995) A phase I study of anti-GD3 ganglioside monoclonal antibody R24 and recombinant human macrophage-colony stimulating factor in patients with metastatic melanoma. Cancer 75:2251–2257
Miyazaki H (1998) Update on thrombopoietin in preclinical and clinical trials. Curr Opin Hematol 5:197–202
Mouthon MA, van der Meeren A, Vandamme M et al (2001) A single administration of thrombopoietin to lethally irradiated mice prevents the infectious and thrombotic events leading to mortality. Exp Hematol 29:30–40

Müller MM, Herold-Mende CC, Riede D et al (1999) Autocrine growth regulation by granulocyte macrophage colony-stimulating factor in human gliomas with tumor progression. Am J Pathol 155:1557–1567

Neelis KJ, Quingliang L, Thomas GR et al (1997a) Prevention of thrombocytopenia by thrombopoietin in myelosuppressed rhesus monkeys accompanied by prominent erythropoietic stimulation and iron depletion. Blood 90:58–63

Neelis KJ, Dubbelman YD, Quingliang L et al (1997b) Simultaneous TPO and G-CSF treatment of rhesus monkeys prevents thrombopenia, accelerates platelet and red cell reconstitution, alleviates neutropenia and promotes the recovery of immature bone marrow cells. Exp Hematol 25:1084–1093

Neelis KJ, Hartong SC, Egeland T et al (1997c) The efficacy of single-dose administration of thrombopoietin with coadministration of either granulocyte/macrophage or granulocyte colony-stimulating factor in myelosuppressed rhesus monkeys. Blood 90:2555–2564

Neelis KJ, Visser TP, Dimjati W et al (1998) A single dose of thrombopoietin early after myelosuppressive total body irradiation prevents pancytopenia by promoting short-term multilineage spleen repopulating cells at the transient expense of bone marrow repopulating cells. Blood 92:1586–1597

Nestle FO, Alijagic S, Gilliet M et al (1998) Vaccination of melanoma patients with peptide- or tumor lysate-pulsed dendritic cells. Nat Med 4:328–332

Neta R (1997) Modulation of radiation damage by cytokines. Stem Cells 15 [Suppl 2]:87–94

Neta R, Oppenheim JJ, Douches SD (1988) Interdependence of the radioprotective effects of human recombinant interleukin 1 alpha, tumor necrosis factor alpha, granulocyte colony-stimulating factor, and murine recombinant granulocyte-macrophage colony-stimulating factor. J Immunol 140:108–111

Noda I, Fujieda S, Ohtsubo T et al (1999) Granulocyte colony-stimulating factor enhances invasive potential of human head and neck carcinoma cell lines. Int J Cancer 80:78–84

Ohno R, Naoe T, Kanamaru A et al (1994) The Kohseisho Leukemia Study Group: a double blind controlled study of granulocyte colony stimulating factor started two days before induction chemotherapy in refractory acute myeloid leukaemia. Blood 83:2086–2092

Okamoto R, Yajima T, Yamazaki M et al (2002) Damaged epithelia regenerated by bone marrow-derived cells in the human gastrointestinal tract. Nature Med 8:1011–1017

Parmentier C, Morardet N, Tubiana M (1983) Late effects on human bone marrow after extended field radiotherapy. Int J Radiat Oncol Biol Phys 9:1303–1311

Pui CTL, Boyett JM, Hughes WT et al (1997) Human granulocyte colony-stimulating factor after induction chemotherapy in children with acute lymphoblastic leukaemia. N Engl J Med 336:1781–1787

Rowe JM, Andersen JW, Mazza JJ et al (1995) A randomized placebo-controlled phase III study of granulocyte-macrophage colony-stimulating factor in adult patients (>55 to 70 years of age) with acute myelogenous leukaemia: a study of the Eastern Cooperative Oncology Group. Blood 86:457–462

Sacks E, Goris M, Glatstein E et al (1978) Bone marrow regeneration following large field radiation. Influence of volume, age, dose, and time. Cancer 42:1057–1065

Simons JW, Jaffee EM, Weber CE et al (1997) Bioactivity of autologous irradiated renal cell carcinoma vaccines generated by ex vivo granulocyte-macrophage colony-stimulating factor gene transfer. Cancer Res 57:1537–1546

Sitnicka E, Lin N, Priestley GV et al (1996) The effect of thrombopoietin on the proliferation and differentiation of murine hematopoietic stem cells. Blood 87:4998–5005

Sprinzl GM, Galvan O, de Vries A et al (2001) Local application of granulocyte-macrophage colony stimulating factor for the treatment of oral mucositis. Eur J Cancer 37:2003–2009

Staar S, Rudat V, Stützer H et al (2001) Intensified hyperfractionated accelerated radiotherapy limits the additional benefit of simultaneous chemotherapy – results of a multicenter randomized German trial in advanced head and neck cancer. Int J Radiat Oncol Biol Phys 50:1161–1171

Stone RM, Berg DT, George SL et al (1995) Granulocyte-macrophage colony-stimulating factor after initial chemotherapy for elderly patients with primary acute myelogenous leukemia. N Engl J Med 332:1671–1677

Sugimoto M, Kajimura M, Hanai H et al (1999) G-CSF-producing gastric anaplastic large cell lymphoma complicating esophageal cancer. Dig Dis Sci 44:2035–2038

Sugimoto C, Fujieda S, Sunaga H et al (2001) Granulocyte colony-stimulating factor-mediated signalling regulates type IV collagenase activity in head and neck cancer cells. Int J Cancer 93:42–46

Sunaga H, Fujieda S, Tsuzuki H et al (2001) Expression of granulocyte colony-stimulating factor receptor and platelet-derived endothelial cell growth factor in oral and oropharyngeal precancerous lesions. Anticancer Res 21:2901–2906

Tachibana M, Miyakawa A, Tazaki H et al (1995) Autocrine growth of transitional cell carcinoma of the bladder induced by granulocyte-colony stimulating factor. Cancer Res 55:3438–3443

Teicher BA, Ara G, Menon K et al (1996) In vivo studies with interleukin-12 alone and in combination with monocyte colony-stimulating factor and/or fractionated radiation treatment. Int J Cancer 65:80–84

Thacker JD, Dedhar S, Hogge DE (1994) The effect of GM-CSF and G-CSF on the growth of human osteosarcoma cells in vitro and in vivo. Int J Cancer 56:236–243

Trapnell BC, Whitsett JA (2002) GM-CSF regulates pulmonary surfactant homeostasis and alveolar macrophage-mediated innate host defense. Annu Rev Physiol 64:775–802

Tsuzuki H, Fujieda S, Sunaga H et al (1998) Expression of granulocyte colony-stimulating factor receptor correlates with prognosis in oral and mesopharyngeal carcinoma. Cancer Res 58:794–800

Van der Meeren A, Mouthon MA, Gaugler MH et al (2002) Administration of recombinant human IL11 after supralethal radiation exposure promotes survival in mice: interactive effect with thrombopoietin. Radiat Res 157:642–649

Vokes EE, Haraf DJ, Mick R et al (1994) Intensified concomitant chemoradiotherapy with and without filgrastim for poor-prognostic head and neck cancer. J Clin Oncol 12:2351–2359

Welte K, Reiter A, Mempel K et al (1996) A randomized phase III study of the efficacy of granulocyte colony-stimulating factor in children with high-risk acute lymphoblastic leukaemia. Blood 87:3143–3150

9 Oral Mucosa: Response Modification by Keratinocyte Growth Factor

W. Dörr

CONTENTS

9.1 Introduction 113
9.1.1 Keratinocyte Growth Factor: Structure and Function 113
9.1.2 Response of Oral Mucosa to Irradiation 113
9.1.3 In-Vitro Effects of KGF 114
9.2 Tumour Effects of KGF 114
9.2.1 Studies in Tumour Cells in Vitro 114
9.2.2 In Vivo Studies 115
9.3 Modulation of Oral Mucosal Radio- or Chemotherapy Effects by KGF 115
9.3.1 Experimental Studies 116
9.3.2 Clinical Studies 118
9.4 Mechanisms of Reduction of Oral Mucositis by KGF 119
9.5 Conclusion 120
References 120

9.1 Introduction

9.1.1 Keratinocyte Growth Factor: Structure and Function

Keratinocyte growth factor (KGF) was first described in humans in 1989 (RUBIN et al. 1989) as a factor stimulating proliferation of epithelial cells. It is a heparin-binding member of the fibroblast growth factor group (FGF) family (FINCH et al. 1989) and is alternatively denoted as FGF-7.

Another factor with a structure and specificity to epithelial cell proliferation similar to that of KGF was called FGF-10, or KGF-2 (EMOTO et al. 1997). More recently, FGF-22 was cloned and found to be most similar to FGF-10 and FGF-7 (NAKATAKE et al. 2001).

KGF is exclusively synthesized by mesenchymal cells, particularly fibroblasts (Finch et al. 1995). The receptor KGFR, a tyrosine kinase that is encoded by the *fgfr-2* gene, is expressed solely on epithelial cells, in a variety of tissues. These include epidermis and hair follicles, oral and gastrointestinal epithelium, corneal epithelium, lung epithelium, urothelium, prostate epithelium, etc. (RUBIN et al. 1995;). KGF represents a paracrine mediator of mesenchymal-epithelial communication.

KGF induces a variety of responses in the epithelia, which include stimulation of epithelial proliferation, but also modification of migration and differentiation processes. Systemic administration of exogenous KGF to normal animals results in hyperproliferation of a variety of epithelia, eventually resulting in organ hyperplasia (RUBIN et al. 1995) and enhanced expression of tissue specific markers and organ function in a variety of systems (FARRELL et al. 2002).

During skin wound healing, KGF plays a predominant role. In experimental models a marked increase in dermal transcription activity was observed (WERNER et al. 1992, 1994, 1996; WERNER 1998). Topical application stimulated wound healing in animal models (STAIANO-COICO et al. 1993).

KGF has a pivotal role in ontogenetic processes, e.g. in gut (CHAILLER et al. 2000), ureter (QIAO et al. 2001), bladder urothelium (TASH et al. 2001), mammary gland (PEDCHENKO and IMAGAWA 2000), ovary (HSUEH et al. 2000) and lung (CHELLY et al. 1999; GRAEFF et al. 1999).

9.1.2 Response of Oral Mucosa to Irradiation

Oral mucosa represents a typical turnover tissue, with a clear hierarchy in the proliferative organization: under normal conditions, permanent cell loss at the surface, mainly based on mechanical but also on chemical stress, which is preceded by keratinocyte differentiation, is precisely balanced by continuous cell production. This takes place in the deeper, basal and suprabasal strata of the epithelium, which hence constitute the germinal layer of the tissue. Irradiation in mucosa, like in turnover tissues in general, results

---
W. Dörr, DVM, PhD
Medical Faculty Carl Gustav Carus, Technical University of Dresden, Fetscherstrasse 74, PF 58, 01307 Dresden, Germany

in an impairment of proliferation and cell production, which translates into a reduction in cellular supply to the postmitotic, functional cell layers. In contrast, the superficial cell loss is – over a wide dose range – independent of the administration of radiation, but is dependent on the physiological tissue turnover rate (DÖRR 2002a). Cells present at the time of radiation injury may undergo near normal differentiation (DÖRR et al. 1996; LIU et al. 1996).

After sufficient doses, with a threshold for conventional fractionation at about 20 Gy (VAN DER SCHUEREN et al. 1990), the radiation-induced perturbation of the equilibrium between cell production and loss eventually results in complete cellular depletion of the functional cell layers (DÖRR et al. 1994a; DÖRR 1997; DÖRR and OBEYESEKERE 2001). Clinically, this early radiation response manifests as focal or confluent denudation and ulceration, which is associated with a significant impairment of the epithelial barrier. It must be noted that the clinical grading of the symptoms of mucositis, which also include erythema and painful inflammatory changes, do not necessarily reflect the histological changes (DÖRR et al. 2002a).

Cells, which have already lost their unlimited proliferative capacity (clonogenicity) due to radiation injury, still can undergo a limited number of divisions, which are usually denoted as "abortive" divisions (DÖRR et al. 1994b; DÖRR 1997). This residual cell production is of major significance for the maintenance of the integrity of the epithelial barrier, and hence for the consequences of the radiation reaction for the patient. Abortive divisions, which occur even at high doses of radiation (DÖRR and KUMMERMEHR 1991; DÖRR et al. 1994a), also result in a prolongation of the latent time to ulceration in comparison to the tissue turnover time. The latter is about 5 days for various intraoral sites in normal human mucosa (DÖRR et al. 1995, 2002a). Similar turnover times were found for mouse lower tongue surface (DÖRR et al. 1994b; DÖRR and KUMMERMEHR 1991). The latent time to confluent mucositis, however, is 9 days after a threshold dose of 20 Gy for human intraoral mucosa (VAN DER SCHUEREN et al. 1990) and slightly longer for supraglottic mucosa (DENHAM et al. 1996). In excellent agreement with clinical data, ulceration of mouse tongue mucosa is observed after latent times of 10–11 days.

9.1.3
In-Vitro Effects of KGF

The effect of KGF on epithelial cells in vitro was investigated in a variety of studies. Stimulation of proliferation was demonstrated in rhesus monkey and human bronchial epithelial cells (MICHELSON et al. 1999; RUBIN et al. 1995), rat alveolar epithelial cells (PANOS et al. 1993), human mammary epithelial cells, human nasal epithelial cells (A. HILLE, unpublished data), embryonic mouse epidermal keratinocytes (RUBIN et al. 1995), neonatal human epidermal keratinocytes (SLONINA et al. 2001), murine skin keratinocytes (NING et al. 1998) and mouse oral mucosal keratinocytes (LACMANN et al. 1999). In in-vitro reconstituted mouse oral mucosa, an increase in epithelial thickness and cell numbers was found after treatment with KGF (LACMANN et al. 1999; DÖRR and LACMANN 2001; SANZ GARCIA et al. 2000).

Besides the stimulation of proliferation, KGF promotes differentiation processes (CHELLY et al. 1999; GIBBS et al. 2000; MARCHESE et al. 1990) and migration (PUTNINS et al. 1999; TSUBOI et al. 1993), as demonstrated in human keratinocytes and fetal alveolar epithelial cells.

Studies on normal human keratinocytes in vitro (SLONINA et al. 2001) showed that post-irradiation supplementation of the culture medium with KGF resulted in a significant increase in colony size, while colony numbers were unchanged. In studies on in-vitro reconstituted epithelium, treatment with KGF before and after single-dose radiation exposure as well as before and during fractionated irradiation resulted in a reduced radiation response, as assessed by cell numbers and epithelial thickness (DÖRR and LACMANN 2001).

These in vitro results and initial in-vivo studies in a variety of tissues rendered KGF a promising candidate for the modulation of radiation effects in oral mucosa.

9.2
Tumour Effects of KGF

A major prerequisite for the effective amelioration of acute oral mucosal reactions to radiotherapy or radiochemotherapy is selectivity. Hence, a number of studies on KGF effects on tumours, both in vitro and in vivo, have been performed.

9.2.1
Studies in Tumour Cells in Vitro

The expression of the receptor for KGF, KGFR, on epithelial tumour cells is variable. NING et al. (1998)

demonstrated by a RNase protection assay that KGFR was detectable in 7 out of 10 head and neck tumour cell lines. The level, quantitated as the ratio of KGFR to glyceraldehyde-3-phosphatase dehydrogenase (GAPDH) expression ranged between 0.3 and 12.3 (normal keratinocytes: 3.0). In six primary, low-passage tumour cell lines isolated from squamous cell carcinomas of head and neck or lung, HILLE et al. (2002) found detectable but low levels of KGFR mRNA.

Proliferative effects of KGF on squamous epithelial tumour cells in the studies by NING et al. (1998) were observed only in experiments with prolonged exposure (7 days) in four of the seven KGFR-positive cell lines and two KGFR-negative cell lines. The proliferative response, however, of normal keratinocytes was 24–70 times higher than that of the tumour cells. HILLE et al. (2002) found a significant proliferative response in only one out of eight primary tumour cell lines. In BeWo human choriocarcinoma cells, which are positive for KGFR, KGF stimulated the secretion of human chorionic gonadotropin (hCG), but did not affect proliferation (MATSUI et al. 2000).

Human salivary adenocarcinoma cells are normally KGFR-negative. Transfection with wild type KGFR reduced cell production (ZHANG et al. 2001), which was attributed by the authors to increased cell loss from the clonogenic compartment by stimulation of differentiation and apoptosis. This suggests that – in tumour cells expressing the receptor – even a growth inhibitory effect of KGF may be seen which, however, has not been demonstrated experimentally.

Prostate epithelial cells under conditions of benign hyperplasia of the prostate show increased expression of KGF, which is associated with increased proliferative activity (ROPIQUET et al. 1999). KGF transfection of immortalized prostate epithelial cells promoted migration as well as proliferation (ROPIQUET et al. 1999).

Clonogenic radiation survival was not affected by KGF in the four KGFR-positive cell lines (FaDu, Detroit562, SCC-9 and SCC-25) that displayed a proliferative response (see Sec. 9.1.2, Response of Oral Mucosa to Irradiation). Similarly, no systematic effect of KGF was observed in the other seven cell lines tested. The only significant changes were seen after exposure to 100 ng/ml KGF for 12 days, with a decrease in the shoulder of the cell survival curve (increased α/β ratio) in Detroit562 and SCC-25, and an increase in the shoulder (decreased α/β) in SCC-9 and HEp-2 (NING et al. 1998). In five primary tumour cell lines, HILLE et al. (2002) could not demonstrate an effect of KGF treatment (10–200 ng/ml, 3 days pre-irradiation) on clonogenic survival.

9.2.2
In Vivo Studies

KHT sarcomas, grown intramuscularly in C3H mice, were treated intra-tumorally with six daily doses of KGF-1, KGF-2 or FGF-2 (6 µg/mouse), and tumour weight, mitotic index and apoptotic index were determined at 1 day after the last injection (OKUNJEFF et al. 2001). Moreover, vasculature and oxygenation were assessed quantitatively after immunohistochemistry. The hypoxic volume decreased after treatment with KGF-2 and FGF-2. Median distances between perfused blood vessels and tumour cells, as well as between total vessels and angiogenic vessels, decreased after KGF-1 injections. A reduction in tumour growth independent of the apoptotic activity was seen after KGF-2 and FGF-2, while KGF-1 increased the apoptotic index.

Studies in human tumours xenografted into nude mice were performed with KGFR-positive squamous cell carcinomas FaDu, Detroit562 and A431. KGFR-negative murine B16 melanomas were grown in Balb/c mice (NING et al. 1998). Tumour growth delay was used as the endpoint and the results showed that KGF did not increase the growth rate of the tumours or interfere with the growth delay caused by radiotherapy. Unfortunately, no data are available for tumour cure and for clinically relevant fractionation protocols.

In summary, a variety of experiments did not yield evidence for increased cellular radiation tolerance of human cells in vitro in the presence of KGF. While no significant impact of KGF on proliferation has been observed in most tumours studied so far, systematic investigations into the effect of KGF on repopulation of clonogenic cells during fractionated radiation treatment at present are still lacking.

9.3
Modulation of Oral Mucosal Radio- or Chemotherapy Effects by KGF

Reviews of the in-vivo effect of KGF on radiation or chemotherapy-induced changes in a variety of experimental systems can be found in WERNER (1998), DANILENKO (1999) and FARRELL et al. (2002). This chapter focuses on modulation of changes in oral mucosa by KGF.

9.3.1
Experimental Studies

A first study on the effect of KGF on radiation-induced structural changes in the upper aerodigestive tract, i.e. tongue, buccal and oesophageal mucosa of mice, was performed by FARRELL et al. (1999). In normal mice, an increase in mucosal thickness by about a factor of 2 was observed after six daily injections of KGF at a dose of 5 mg/kg per injection. Also, keratohyaline granules, usually found in the functional layers, increased in number (~ ×1.4) and size (~ ×3.4). Desmosomes, i.e. intercellular adhesion complexes, showed an increase in length and density of intermediate filament insertions.

Interestingly, the excess number of cells induced by KGF treatment was removed from the epithelium by an apoptotic wave (DÖRR et al. 2000) with a maximum at 2 days after the last injection (Fig. 9.1). Normally, apoptosis is a very rare event in oral mucosa, with an apoptotic index around 0.1% in humans (BIRCHALL et al. 1995) and mice (DÖRR et al. 2000).

Single-dose irradiation with a dose of 12 Gy resulted in a 30%–40% decrease in epithelial thickness at 4 days after irradiation (FARRELL et al. 1999). Pre- or post-irradiation administration of KGF as well as a combination of both prevented the development of hypoplasia. The effect was most pronounced in mice that were treated with KGF after irradiation.

In mouse tongue mucosa, the mucoprotective effect of KGF was tested in combination with single-dose irradiation (DÖRR et al. 2000, 2001b). Mucosal ulceration was used as a quantal endpoint and full-dose response curves for the frequency of animals developing ulcer were generated to quantify the KGF effect. Pre-irradiation administration of KGF (daily, 5 mg/kg per injection) between days −4 and −2 or days −3 and −1 increased the ED50 values, i.e. the dose at which ulceration is expected in 50% of the animals, by a factor of 1.7 to 2.1, respectively (Fig. 9.2).

Administration of KGF on days 0 to +2, i.e. after irradiation, yielded an even more pronounced effect,

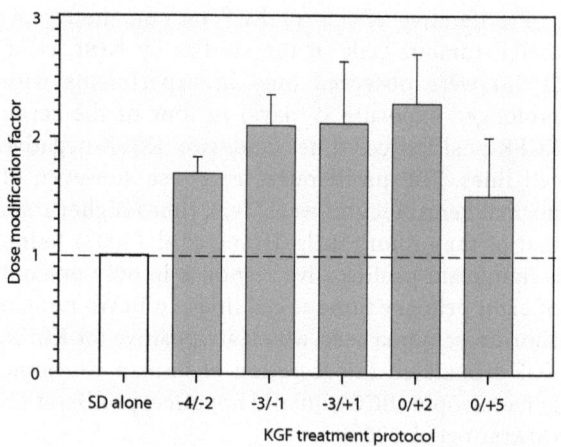

Fig. 9.2. Dose modification factors for single-dose irradiation. Based on the ED50 value for single-dose irradiation alone, dose modification factors were calculated from the ED50 values of the individual KGF treatment protocols. The experimental code gives the first and last day of injection of KGF at a dose of 5 mg/kg per day. Error bars were calculated from the standard deviation σ of the ED50 values

with an increase in ED50 by a factor of 2.3, while six post-irradiation treatments were less effective. Combined pre- and post-irradiation application of KGF (days −3 to +1) resulted in a dose modification factor (ED50 with KGF/ED50 in controls) of 2.1.

In the protocols with KGF treatment exclusively prior to irradiation, a slight increase in latent times before clinical manifestation of ulceration, i.e. complete mucosal denudation, from about 10 days to more than 11 days was found (DÖRR et al. 2000, 2001a, c). In contrast, post-irradiation administration of KGF resulted in a significant shortening of the latent time to 7–8 days in the pre- plus post-irradiation arm and to less than 7 days in the purely post-irradiation arms.

Radiochemotherapy studies with KGF in oral mucosa have so far been carried out only with single doses of radiation and chemotherapy, the latter consisting of cDDP, 5-FU or both (DÖRR et al. 2001). In this investigation, KGF was applied daily, either before or after radiochemotherapy (day −3 to −1, day +1 to +3), or both. For cDDP (30 min before irradiation),

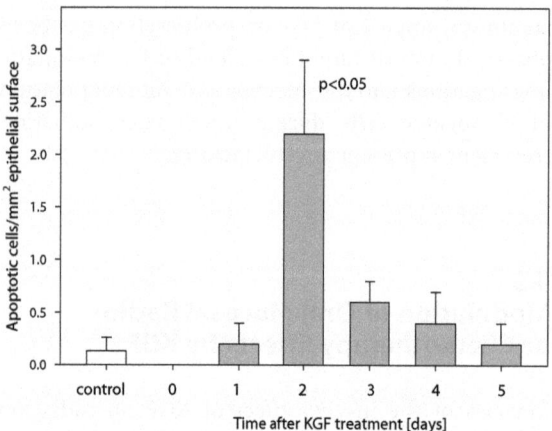

Fig. 9.1. Apoptotic activity (number of apoptotic cells) in mouse tongue mucosa after administration of rHuKGF (5 mg/kg per day subcutaneously) at days −2 to 0. Apoptoses were scored within three representative microscopic fields per animal. Error bars represent 1 SEM ($n=5$)

an increase in radiation ED50 values by a factor of 1.5–2.0 was found in the KGF arms. With 5-FU, KGF increased the ED50 by 1.9–2.7. With the combination of both drugs, dose modification by 1.6–1.7 was observed. Hence, the mucoprotective effect of KGF is maintained even if chemotherapy is added to the protocol, but no additional gain is achieved. However, fractionated radiochemotherapy studies are required to determine the efficacy of KGF treatment in a more clinically relevant scenario.

The efficacy of KGF in combination with daily fractionated irradiation was studied in mouse tongue mucosa, again analysing ulceration as the clinically relevant experimental endpoint (DÖRR et al. 2002b, c, d). Five fractions of 3 Gy were administered, followed by graded test doses after the weekend, i.e. on day 7. Hence differences in the test dose-effect curves reflect the effect of the KGF treatment. The growth factor was given daily before the onset of radiotherapy (days −4 to −2, −3 to −1), during irradiation (days 0 to +2, 0 to +4, over the weekend break (days +4 to +6) or in combinations (days −3 to +1, days +4 to +8).

Administration of KGF resulted in a significant increase in isoeffective radiation doses in all treatment protocols applied (DÖRR et al. 2002d). KGF administration *before* radiation treatment increased the ED50 values for test irradiation by a factor of 1.5 and 1.4 (Fig. 9.3). A more pronounced increase in ED50 values by a factor of 1.9 was observed when KGF was applied *during* radiation treatment. The maximum effect (×2.4) was seen after KGF injections during the weekend break. The protocols with injections on days −3 to +1 and +4 to +8 resulted in an increase in ED50 values by a factor of 1.6 and 2.1, respectively. In an additional experiment, single KGF injections of 5 mg/kg or 15 mg/kg were given on day −1 or +4. Single doses of 5 mg/kg were as effective as three injections. Administration of 15 mg/kg instead of 5 mg/kg increased the ED50 values further, with total dose modification by a factor of 2.5, suggesting a dose effect of KGF. In these experiments (DÖRR et al. 2002b, d), the time course of the mucosal response was largely independent of KGF application and protocol. Conversion of the changes in ED50 values into the number of dose fractions compensated by the KGF treatment reveals that with pre-irradiation administration 1–1.5 fractions, and in all other protocols about 3 fractions were counteracted by KGF. In the single-injection protocols, the resulting ED50 values were in the range of that for single-dose irradiation alone, indicating compensation of the entire fractionated radiation dose. Single doses of 15 mg/kg were even more effective, indicating that tissue tolerance was higher than even in previously untreated control animals.

A question that must be addressed is a potential interaction of KGF with repopulation processes, which in mouse tongue epithelium during daily fractionated irradiation do not start before the end of the first treatment week (DÖRR and KUMMERMEHR 1990; DÖRR 1994a, b, 1997; DÖRR and WEBER-FRISCH 1995). Therefore, an experimental series was initiated with 2 weeks of fractionation and test irradiation on day 14, i.e. after the second weekend (DÖRR et al. 2002). KGF in this study was administered either before and during radiotherapy (days −3 to −1 and +4, days −2 and +4, days −3 and +4, days −3, +4, +11) or exclusively during radiotherapy (days +4 to +6 and +11, days +5 and +11, days +4 and +11). These protocols hence included KGF administration during the period of effective repopulation in week 2.

The protocols with pre-treatment with KGF were all similarly effective, with dose modification factors of 2.1–2.2. With KGF given during radiotherapy, an increase in test ED50 values by a factor of 2.3–2.5 were achieved, indicating no impairment of repopulation processes. Again, single injections in all protocols were at least as effective as the treatment over 3 days. These data again indicate compensation, or even overcompensation, of the entire fractionated radiation dose by the KGF treatment.

Fig. 9.3. Dose modification factors for test irradiation after 5 × 3 Gy. Dose modification factors were calculated relative to the ED50 value for Top-up irradiation after 5 × 3 Gy. The experimental code at the abscissa gives the first and last day of daily injections of KGF at a dose of 5 mg/kg. For single-injection protocols, the dose is given in parentheses. Error bars were calculated from the standard deviations of the ED50 values

The dose effect of KGF was addressed in a further experimental series (Dörr et al. 2002). For this, five daily fractions of 3 Gy, followed by graded test doses on day 7 were combined with single injections of KGF on day −3 or +4. KGF doses tested range from 1 to 30 mg/kg. The preliminary data indicate of KGF dose effect up to doses of 15–20 mg/kg, and no further increase in mucoprotective efficacy at higher KGF doses.

One question of relevance for the design of clinical protocols with KGF was the effect on the time course of already manifest mucosal ulceration. Therefore, animals were irradiated with an effective single dose and KGF was applied daily (5 mg/kg) from the day of first diagnosis of ulceration (Dörr et al. 2002). In this study, a slight but significant increase in ulcer duration from 4.2±0.9 days in the placebo group to 4.8±0.8 days in the KGF arm ($P=0.02$) was observed (Dörr et al. 2002).

9.3.2
Clinical Studies

In human volunteers, the safety, pharmacokinetics and biological activity of rHuKGF, similar to that used in the mouse studies, was tested in a phase I study (Serdar et al. 1997). KGF was given as a single IV injection or daily for 3 days at doses between 0.2 and 20 μg/kg per day. Sixty-one healthy individuals were enrolled. The treatment was safe and well tolerated. Triphasic serum profiles were found, with rapid distribution, redistribution at 1–6 h, and log-linear elimination with a half-time of 4 h. No accumulation was seen. With Ki67 staining of buccal mucosal biopsies taken after 3 days of treatment, a dose-dependent increase of the labelling index was found. Moreover, an increase in mitotic figures was observed.

In a phase I/II trial in head and neck cancer patients (Brizel et al. 2001) were treated by radiochemotherapy with 1.25 Gy b.i.d. to a total dose 72.5 Gy in less than 7 weeks combined with 5-FU (1000 mg/m^2 per day, continuous infusion for 4 days) and bolus cisplatinum (100 mg/m^2, weeks 1 and 5), with a planned treatment break at week 4. Patients were randomized (1:3) to receive either placebo or rHuKGF (20–80 μg/kg) for 3 days before the onset of radiotherapy or once on day −3, and subsequently weekly injections to a total of 10 doses. Sixty patients were included in the study. Adverse effects of KGF treatment were mild to moderate, temporary skin flushing (8/46 patients, dose-dependent) and excess salivation (1/46 patients, 20 μg/kg) during the initial 3-day treatment period. One severe skin reaction in response to KGF injection occurred at 60 μg/kg. A transient, asymptomatic increase in serum lipase and amylase was observed in all patients after three rHuKGF injections. Similar flushing and amylase and lipase elevations in KGF-treated subjects were observed in other studies (Serdar et al. 1997; Durrant et al. 1999; Meropol et al. 2000; Spielberger et al. 2001; Clarke et al. 2001).

With regard to acute radiation effects in the head and neck cancer study (Brizel et al. 2001), the duration of mucositis (grade 3–4 RTOG/EORTC, 25–75 percentile) was shortened from 11 days (6–27) to 6.5 days (4–23), of grade 2–4 pharynx/oesophagus reactions from 40 days (15–58) to 22.8 days (23–56), and of salivary gland effects (grade 2–4) from 42.5 days (23–56) to 21.3 days (0–40). No significant differences were found at 1 year for actuarial loco-regional control, failure-free survival and overall survival. However, longer follow-up is required for definitive analysis. Moreover, the power of the study, with 60 patients only, appears insufficient for final conclusions.

No further clinical data are currently available on effects of KGF on radiation- or radiochemotherapy-induced oral mucositis. However, the mucoprotective efficacy of KGF was demonstrated for chemotherapy-induced oral mucositis, which is based on comparable mechanisms.

A phase I trial was conducted in 84 patients receiving mucotoxic chemotherapy (5-FU 425 mg/m^2 per day plus leucovorin 20 mg/m^2 per day for 5 days) for metastatic colorectal cancer (Meropol et al. 2000). In this randomized, double-blind placebo controlled study, KGF was given on day −3 to −1 before the onset of chemotherapy in doses between 1 and 60 μg/kg per day. Oral mucositis, grade 2–4, was observed in 67% of patients receiving placebo vs 43% in the KGF group ($P=0.06$). A minimum dose of 10 μg/kg/d was required to achieve an effect.

In a randomized phase II trial in 64 patients with advanced colorectal cancer (Clarke et al. 2001) receiving identical chemotherapy, rHuKGF or placebo was administered on days −3 to −1; the KGF dose was 40 μg/kg per day. The incidence of grade 2–4 mucositis was 78% in the placebo group ($n=36$) and 32% in the KGF-group ($n=28$, $P=0.001$). No differences in median survival were observed.

A further phase I dose-escalation study was performed in lymphoma patients treated with high-dose chemotherapy and transplantation of autologous peripheral blood progenitor cells (Durrant et al. 1999). A total of 234 patients were included in this study, which was designed as a randomized, placebo-controlled multicenter trial. Patients received rHuKGF either 3 days before or 3 days before and after BEAM (BCNU, etoposide, Ara-C, melphalan) at sequential dose levels between 5–80 µg/kg per day. In the placebo group, mucositis WHO grade 3–4 was observed in 22% and grade 2–4 in 51% of the patients; the mean duration in the latter group was 4.6±1.8 days. At a KGF dose of 60 µg/kg per day, the frequency of mucositis grade 2–4 was reduced to 13% with a mean duration of 0.8±0.5 days.

SPIELBERGER et al. (2001) performed a phase II study in patients with haematological malignancies subject to progenitor cell transplantation after 12 Gy total-body irradiation (TBI) followed by chemotherapy (etoposide or cyclophosphamide). The study randomized 129 patients to receive either rHuKGF (60 µg/kg per day) on days −3 to −1 before TBI, or placebo or rHuKGF on days −3 to −1 before and days +1 to +3 after TBI. The duration of mucositis (WHO grade 3–4) in the placebo group was 7.7 days, compared to 4 days in the pre- and post-irradiation KGF group ($P=0.001$) and to 5 days in the pre-irradiation group ($P=0.04$). This was also reflected by the functional consequences such as swallowing, drinking, eating, etc., and use of analgetics or parenteral nutrition.

In conclusion, KGF administration in cancer patients is, with the exception of skin reactions, safe at the doses tested so far. All studies revealed a positive effect on the manifestation of oral mucositis. With regard to the use of KGF for amelioration of oral mucosal reactions during radio- or radiochemotherapy of head and neck tumours, however, a sufficiently powered phase III trial would be desirable.

9.4
Mechanisms of Reduction of Oral Mucositis by KGF

The KGF treatment protocols in combination with fractionated radiotherapy tested so far are predominantly empirical, and need to be further optimized on the basis of the biological mechanisms underlying the mucoprotective efficacy of this growth factor. A discussion of these mechanisms at present, however, remains largely speculative, as not all effects have been identified so far. It is clear that keratinocyte proliferation is stimulated, but that also differentiation processes and organ and tissue function are significantly influenced.

One possible mechanism of KGF action is an increase in the number of epithelial stem cells due to stimulation of proliferation within the stem cell compartment. However, this would also require a switch of stem cell divisions from asymmetrical divisions (resulting in one stem cell and one differentiating daughter) to symmetrical divisions, with two stem cell daughters. Otherwise, no increase in stem cell numbers can be achieved (DÖRR 1997). An increased number of stem cells, present at the time of irradiation, would translate into an increase in radiation tolerance. This, in fact, has been observed in intestinal mucosa (POTTEN et al. 2000, 2001), where the number of crypts surviving cytotoxic treatment were increased after pre-irradiation administration of KGF. A similar mechanism may be involved in KGF effects in oral mucosa. Direct assessment of stem cell numbers is not possible in oral mucosa, like in most other tissues. However, it can be assumed that the radiation tolerance of the tissue reflects the stem cell number, and hence reduced radiation effects after KGF administration *prior to* irradiation may be associated with increased stem cell numbers. The efficacy of KGF administered *after* single dose irradiation illustrates that at least a part of the mucoprotective effect must be independent of an increased stem cell number in the epithelium.

Another potential mechanism is illustrated by the observation that, in mouse oral mucosa, an increase in latent time to ulceration is seen after pre-irradiation treatment with KGF. This was attributed to an increased total cell number, i.e. the sum of proliferating cells (including stem cells) and functional, differentiated cells, present at the time of irradiation. The consequence of the increased overall cellularity is that a longer time interval is required before all cells are lost at the normal rate. This, however, assumes that the excess cells are not removed by apoptosis, in contrast to the scenario without irradiation.

A third mechanism can be concluded from the finding that post-irradiation administration of KGF resulted in a significant shortening of the latent time to manifestation of ulcer. This can hypothetically be explained by changes in epithelial differentiation, resulting in an increased intraepithelial adhesion. Consequently, the cell may no longer be lost consecutively, but in entire squames of epithelium, which would accelerate cell loss. Histological studies suitable to identify these processes are currently performed.

As a working hypothesis, it can be assumed that KGF reduces cell loss by changes in differentiation, but also increases post-irradiation cell production by stimulation of abortive divisions. The latter represent the residual proliferative capacity of lethally damaged cells (DÖRR 1997). The combination of these two processes may result in a prolongation of the time before epithelial breakdown occurs, which is sufficiently long to allow the surviving (stem) cells to repopulate the tissue. Only in a few individual animals, where the epithelial adhesion is not sufficient, is the epithelium lost – presumably in squames – at time points earlier than normal (see above in this section). These hypotheses must be tested in extended histological studies, e.g. in mouse tongue epithelium, studies which are currently underway.

Assuming stimulation of abortive divisions, which normally are most effective during the irradiation-free weekend breaks (Dörr 1997; Dörr et al. 1995), administration of KGF at the end of the treatment weeks – before the onset of mucositis – should be most effective. This has been shown experimentally (Dörr et al. 2002).

If KGF is given at the time of manifest ulceration, no positive effect is observed in experimental models. This suggests that the efficacy of KGF is dependent on the presence of a sufficient number of cells – stem, transit or abortively dividing cells – able to proliferate. If the population is grossly depleted, no efficient stimulation of cell production is possible.

Single injections of KGF in mouse tongue mucosa were as effective as repeated injections with the same total dose. Hence, replacement of repeated injections by bolus treatment might be considered in clinical studies. Moreover, a clear dose effect of KGF was observed in the experimental studies for doses up to 15–20 mg/kg. Although minor side effects of KGF were observed in radio- and chemotherapy studies in the dose range of KGF administered so far, dose optimization for the prevention of oral mucositis may be possible.

Based on all these considerations, an effective combination of rHuKGF and fractionated radiotherapy could include administration before the onset of radiotherapy (to increase the total cell number and possibly the stem cell number), and administration at the end of treatment weeks 1, 2, and – if no gross mucositis is present – week 3.

9.5
Conclusion

In conclusion, it was demonstrated in a variety of studies that keratinocyte growth factor has a marked potential for reduction of radiation-induced mucositis. This could be shown for in-vitro systems as well as in experimental animals and – in a phase I study – in radiotherapy patients. Moreover, the mucoprotective effect was observed in a number of chemotherapy studies. The mechanisms underlying this effect deserve further investigation.

Selective sparing of normal mucosa and not of squamous cell carcinoma, which are the most frequent tumours in the head and neck region, might be expected, based on the data available so far. However, further preclinical studies, using established animal models and clinically relevant treatment protocols and endpoints, as well as clinical studies, are required. Furthermore, the efficacy of rHuKGF in conventional and unconventional radiotherapy and combined radiochemotherapy protocols must be demonstrated in well-designed and adequately powered phase III studies.

Moreover, clinical treatment protocols should be based on the mechanisms underlying the biological effects of KGF in untreated but also in irradiated tissue, and should be optimized with regard to frequency and timing of administration as well as dosage.

References

Birchall MA, Winterford CM, Allan DJ, Harmon BV (1995) Apoptosis in normal epithelium, premalignant and malignant lesions of the oropharynx and oral cavity: a preliminary study. Eur J Cancer B Oral Oncol 31B:380–383

Brizel DM, Herman T, Goffinet D, Sailer S, Agarwala S, Schwartz G, Venkatesan V, Cripps C, Meredith RF, Logan E, Yao B (2001) A phase I/II trial of escalating doses of recombinant human keratinocyte growth factor (rHuKGF) in head and neck cancer (HNC) patients receiving radiotherapy (RT) with concurrent chemotherapy (CCT) (abstract). Int J Radiat Oncol Biol Phys 51 [Suppl]:40

Chailler P, Basque JR, Corriveau L, Menard D (2000) Functional characterization of the keratinocyte growth factor system in human fetal gastrointestinal tract. Pediatr Res 48:504–510

Chelly N, Mouhieddine Gueddiche OB, Barlier Mur AM, Cahilley Heu B, Bourbon JR (1999) Keratinocyte growth factor enhances maturation of fetal rat lung type II cells. Am J Respir Cell Mol Biol 20:423–432

Clarke SJ, Abdi E, Davis ID, Schnell FM, Zalcberg JR, Gutheil J, Serdar C, Yao B, Heard R, Meropol N, Rosen LS (2001) Recombinant human keratinocyte growth factor (rHuKGF) prevents chemotherapy-induced mucositis in patients with advanced colorectal cancer: a randomized phase II trial. Proc ASCO 20:383a

Danilenko DM (1999) Preclinical and early clinical development of keratinocyte growth factor, an epithelial-specific tissue growth factor. Toxicol Pathol 27:64–71

Denham JW, Walker QJ, Lamb DS, Hamilton CS, O'Brien PC, Spry NA, Hindley A, Poulsen M, O'Brien M, Tripcony L (1996) Mucosal regeneration during radiotherapy. Radiother Oncol 41:109–118

Dörr W (1994) Repopulation in mouse oral mucosa: treatment splits. Radiother Oncol 33:139–147
Dörr W (1997) Three A's of repopulation during fractionated irradiation in squamous epithelia: asymmetry loss, acceleration of stem-cell divisions and abortive divisions. Int J Radiat Biol 72:635–643
Dörr W (2001) Modification of acute radio(chemo)therapy effects in squamous epithelia by keratinocyte growth factor (abstract). Radiother Oncol 60 [Suppl 2]:S8
Dörr W (2002) Akute Strahlenveränderungen der Gewebe. In: Bamberg M, Molls M, Sack H (eds) Radio-Onkologie, 5th edn. Zuckschwerdt, Munich (in press)
Dörr W, Kummermehr J (1990) Accelerated repopulation of mouse tongue epithelium during fractionated irradiations or following single doses. Radiother Oncol 17:249–259
Dörr W, Kummermehr J (1991) Proliferation kinetics of mouse tongue epithelium under normal conditions and following single-dose irradiation. Virchows Arch [B] 60:281–294
Dörr W, Lacmann A (2001) Effects of keratinocyte growth factor (KGF) on the radiation response of in vitro reconstituted oral mucosa (abstract). Cell Prolif 34:167
Dörr W, Weber-Frisch M (1995) Repopulation response of mouse oral mucosa during unconventional fractionation protocols. Radiother Oncol 37:230–236
Dörr W, Arui J, Beisker W, Schultz-Hector S (1994a) Cell kinetic studies in mouse tongue mucosa by autoradiographic, immunohistochemical, and flow cytometric techniques. Cell Prolif 27:321–332
Dörr W, Emmendörfer H, Haide E, Kummermehr J (1994b) Proliferation equivalent of "accelerated repopulation" in mouse oral mucosa. Int J Radiat Biol 66:157–167
Dörr W, Jakubec A, Kummermehr J, Herrmann T, Dölling-Jochem I, Eckelt U (1995) Effects of stimulated repopulation on oral mucositis during conventional radiotherapy. Radiother Oncol 37:100–107
Dörr W, Emmendörfer H, Weber-Frisch M (1996) Tissue kinetics in mouse tongue mucosa during daily fractionated radiotherapy. Cell Prolif 29:495–504
Dörr W, Brankovic K, Hartmann B (2000) Repopulation in mouse oral mucosa: changes in the effect of dose fractionation. Int J Radiat Biol 76:383–390
Dörr W, Obeyesekere MN (2001) A mathematical model for cell density and proliferation in squamous epithelium after single-dose irradiation. Int J Radiat Biol 77:497–505
Dörr W, Lacmann A, Noack R, Spekl K, Rex K, Farrell CL (2001a) Modulation of radiation effects in tissues by keratinocyte growth factor (KGF). In: Heinemann G, Müller W-U (eds) Strahlenbiologie und Strahlenschutz. Individuelle Strahlenempfindlichkeit und ihre Bedeutung für den Strahlenschutz, vol I. TÜV-Verlag, Cologne, pp 209–222
Dörr W, Noack R, Spekl K, Farrell CL (2001b) Modification of oral mucositis by keratinocyte growth factor: single radiation exposure. Int J Radiat Biol 77:341–347
Dörr W, Spekl K, Noack R, Farrell CL (2001c) Keratinocyte Growth Factor (rHuKGF) ameliorates oral mucositis (mouse) during fractionated irradiation (abstract). Int J Radiat Oncol Biol Phys 51 [Suppl 1]:129
Dörr W, Hamilton CS, Boyd T, Reed B, Denham JW (2002a) Radiation-induced changes in cellularity and proliferation in human oral mucosa. Int J Radiat Oncol Biol Phys 52: 911–917
Dörr W, Heider K, Reichel S, Spekl K (2002b) Modification of oral mucositis (mouse) by keratinocyte growth factor (KGF): effect of KGF treatment protocol. Int J Radiat Oncol Biol Phys [Suppl] (in press)
Dörr W, Spekl K, Farrell CL (2002c) The effect of keratinocyte growth factor on healing of manifest radiation ulcers in mouse tongue epithelium. Cell Prolif 35 (Suppl. 1):86–92
Dörr W, Spekl K, Farrell CL (2002d) Amelioration of acute oral mucositis by keratinocyte growth factor: fractionated irradiation (abstract). Int J Radiat Oncol Biol Phys 54:245
Durrant S, Pico JL, Schmitz N, Blaise D, Harousseau JL, Szer J, Boogaerts M, Finke J, Goldstone AH, Borkett K, Heard RG (1999) A phase 1 study of recombinant human keratinocyte growth factor (rHuKGF) in lymphoma patients receiving high-dose chemotherapy (HDC) with autologous peripheral blood progenitor cell transplantation (AutoPBPCT). Blood 4 [Suppl 1]:708a
Emoto H, Tagashira S, Mattei MG, Yamasaki M, Hashimoto G, Katsumata T, Negoro T, Nakatsuka M, Birnbaum D, Coulier F, Itoh N (1997) Structure and expression of human fibroblast growth factor-10. J Biol Chem 272:23191–23194
Farrell CL, Bready JV, Rex KL, Chen JN, DiPalma CR, Whitcomb KL, Yin S, Hill DC, Wiemann B, Starnes CO, Havill AM, Lu Z-N, Aukerman SL, Pierce GF, Thomason A, Potten CS, Ulich TR, Lacey DL (1998) Keratinocyte growth factor protects mice from chemotherapy and radiation-induced gastrointestinal injury and mortality. Cancer Res 58:933–939
Farrell CL, Rex KL, Kaufman SA, DiPalma CR, Chen N, Scully S, Lacey DL (1999) Effects of keratinocyte growth factor in the squamous epithelium of the upper aerodigestive tract of normal and irradiated mice. Int J Radiat Biol 75: 609–620
Farrell CL, Rex KL, Chen JN, Bready JV, DiPalma CR, Kaufman SA, Rattan A, Scully S, Lacey DL (2002) The effects of keratinocyte growth factor in preclinical models of mucositis. Cell Prolif 35 [Suppl 1]:1–8
Finch PW, Rubin JS, Miki T, Ron D, Aaronson SA (1989) Human KGF is FGF-related with properties of a paracrine effector of epithelial cell growth. Science 245:752–755
Finch PW, Cunha GR, Rubin JS, Wong J, Ron D (1995) Pattern of keratinocyte growth factor and keratinocyte growth factor receptor expression during mouse fetal development suggests a role in mediating morphogenetic mesenchymal-epithelial interactions. Dev Dyn 203:223–240
Gibbs S, Silva Ponto AN, Murli S, Huber M, Hohl D, Ponec M (2000) Epidermal growth factor and keratinocyte growth factor differentially regulate epidermal migration, growth, and differentiation. Wound Repair Regen 8:192–203
Graeff RW, Wang G, McGray PB (1999) KGF and FGF-10 stimulate liquid secretion in human fetal lung. Pediatr Res 46:523–529
Hsueh AJ, McGee EA, Hayashi M, Hsu SY (2000) Hormonal regulation of early follicle development in the rat ovary. Mol Cell Endocrinol 163:95–100
Lacmann A, Dörr W, Farrell CL (1999) Einfluss von Keratinozyten-Wachstumsfaktor (rhKGF) auf Keratinozyten in vitro (abstract). Strahlenther Onkol 175 Sondernr 1:57
Liu K, Kasper M, Trott KR (1996) Changes in keratinocyte differentiation during accelerated repopulation of the irradiated mouse epidermis. Int J Radiat Biol 69:763–769
Marchese C, Rubin J, Ron D, Faggioni A, Torrisi MR, Messina A, Frati L, Aaronson SA (1990) Human keratinocyte growth factor activity on proliferation and differentiation of human keratinocytes: differentiation response distinguishes KGF from EGF family. J Cell Physiol 144:326–332

Matsui H, Taga M, Kurogi K, Suyama K, Ohkouchi C, Minaguchi H (2000) Biological action of keratinocyte growth factor in BeWo cells, a human choriocarcinoma cell line. J Endocrinol Invest 23:19–22

Meropol NJ, Gutheil J, Pelley R, Rowinsky E, Rothenberg ML, Serdar CM, Yao B, Rosen L (2000) Keratinocyte growth factor (KGF) as a mucositis protectant: a randomized phase 1 trial (abstract). Proc ASCO 19:603a

Michelson PH, Tigue M, Panos RJ, Sporn PH (1999) Keratinocyte growth factor stimulates bronchial epithelial cell proliferation in vitro and in vivo. Am J Physiol 277:737–742

Nakatake Y, Hoshikawa M, Asaki T, Kassai Y, Itoh N (2001) Identification of a novel fibroblast growth factor, FGF-22, preferentially expressed in the inner root sheath of the hair follicle. Biochim Biophys Acta 1517:460–463

Ning S, Shui C, Khan WB, Benson W, Lacey DL, Knox SJ (1998) Effects of keratinocyte growth factor on the proliferation and radiation survival of human squamous cell carcinoma cell lines in vitro and in vivo. Int J Radiat Oncol Biol Phys 40:177–187

Okunjeff P, Li M, Liu W, Sun J, Fenton B, Zhang L, Ding I (2001) Keratinocyte growth factors radioprotect bowel and bone marrow but not KHT sarcoma. Am J Clin Oncol (CCT) 24:491–495

Panos RJ, Rubin JS, Csaky KG, Aaronson SA, Mason RJ (1993) Keratinocyte growth factor and hepatocyte growth factor/scatter factor are heparin-binding growth factors for alveolar type II cells in fibroblast-conditioned medium. J Clin Invest 92:969–977

Pedchenko VK, Imagawa W (2000) Estrogen treatment in vivo increases keratinocyte growth factor expression in the mammary gland. Endocrinology 165:39–49

Potten CS, Barthel D, Li YQ, Ohlrich R, Matthe B, Loeffler M (2000) Proliferation in murine epidermis after minor mechanical stimulation. Part 1. Sustained increase in keratinocyte production and migration. Cell Prolif 33:231–246

Potten CS, O'Shea JA, Farrell CL, Rex K, Booth C (2001) The effects of repeated doses of keratinocyte growth factor on cell proliferation in the cellular hierarchy of the crypts of the murine small intestine. Cell Growth Differ 12:265–275

Putnins EE, Firth JD, Lohachitranont A, Uitto VJ, Larjava H (1999) Keratinocyte growth factor (KGF) promotes keratinocyte cell attachment and migration on collagen and fibronectin. Cell Adhes Commun 7:211–221

Qiao J, Bush KT, Steer DL, Stuart RO, Sakurai H, Wachsman W, Nigam SK (2001) Multiple fibroblast growth factors support growth of the ureter bud but have different effects on branching morphogenesis. Mech Dev 109:123–135

Ropiquet F, Giri D, Lamb DJ, Itmann M (1999) FGF7 and FGF2 are increased in benign prostatic hyperplasia and are associated with increased proliferation. J Urol 162:595–599

Rubin JS, Osada J, Finch PW, Taylor W G., Rudikoff S, Aaronson SA (1989) Purification and characterization of a newly identified growth factor specific for epithelial cells. Proc Natl Acad Sci U S A 86:802–806

Rubin JS, Bottaro DP, Chedid M, Miki T, Ron D, Cunha GR, Finch PW (1995) Keratinocyte growth factor as a cytokine that mediates mesenchymal-epithelial interaction. EXS 74:191–214

Sanz Garcia S, Heredero SX, Hernandez IA, Pena PE, De Aledo BG, Hamann C (2000) Experimental model for local application of growth factors in studies of re-epithelialisation. Scand J Plast Reconstr Surg Hand Surg 34:199–206

Serdar CM, Heard R, Prathikanti R, Lau D, Danilenko D, Hunt T, Lacey D (1997) Safety, pharmacokinetics and biologic activity of rHuKGF in normal volunteers: results of a placebo-controlled randomized double-blind phase 1 study (abstract). Blood 90 [Suppl 1]:172a

Slonina D, Hoinkis C, Dörr W (2001) Effect of keratinocyte growth factor (rhKGF) on radiation survival and colony size of human epidermal keratinocytes in vitro. Radiatr Res 156:761–766

Spielberger RT, Stiff P, Emmanouilides C, Yanovich S, Bensinger W, Hedrick E, Noga S, Ziegler T, Keating A, Frankel S, Gentile T, Heard R, Yao B, Elhardt D (2001) Efficacy of recombinant human keratinocyte growth factor (rHuKGF) in reducing mucositis in patients with hematologic malignancies undergoing autologous peripheral blood progenitor cell transplantation (auto-PBPCT) after radiation-based conditioning-results of a phase 2 trial (abstract). Proc ASCO 20:7a

Staiano-Coico L, Krueger JG, Rubin JS, Dlimi S, Vallat VP, Valentino L, Fahey T III, Hawes A, Kingston G, Madden MR (1993) Human keratinocyte growth factor effects in a porcine model of epidermal wound healing. J Exp Med 178:856–878

Tash JA, David SG, Vaughan ED, Herzlinger DA (2001) Fibroblast growth factor-7 regulates stratification of the bladder urothelium. J Urol 166:2536–2541

Tsuboi R, Sato C, Kurita Y, Ron D, Rubin JS, Ogawa H (1993) Keratinocyte growth factor (FGF-7) stimulates migration and plasminogen activator activity of normal human keratinocytes. J Invest Dermatol 101:49–53

Van der Schueren E, Van den Bogaert W, Vanuytsel L, Van Limbergen E (1990) Radiotherapy by multiple fractions per day (MFD) in head and neck cancer: acute reactions of skin and mucosa. Int J Radiat Oncol Biol Phys 19:301–311

Werner S (1998). Keratinocyte growth factor: a unique player in epithelial repair processes. Cytokine Growth Factor Rev 9:153–165

Werner S, Peters KG, Longaker MT, Fuller-Pace F, Banda MJ, Williams LT (1992) Large induction of keratinocyte growth factor expression in the dermis during wound healing. Proc Natl Acad Sci U S A 89:6896–6900

Werner S, Smola H, Liao X, Longaker MT, Krieg T, Hofschneider PH, Williams LT (1994) The function of KGF in morphogenesis of epithelium and reepithelialization of wounds. Science 266:819–822

Werner S, Brauchle M, Madlener M, Wagner AD, Angermeyer K, Lauer U, Hofschneider PH, Gregor M (1996) Keratinocyte growth factor is highly overexpressed in inflammatory bowel disease. Am J Pathol 149:521–529

Zhang Y, Wang H, Toratani S, Sato JD, Kan M, McKeehan WL, Okamoto T (2001) Growth inhibition by keratinocyte growth factor receptor of human salivary adenocarcinoma cells through induction of differentiation and apoptosis. Proc Natl Acad Sci U S A 98:11336–11440

Part II: Malignancies

10 Role of Growth Factors in Tumor Growth and Progression of Gynecological Tumors

J. De Los Santos, J. Bonner, S. Goddard, and A. Fyles

CONTENTS

10.1 Introduction 125
10.2 Growth Factors 126
10.2.1 EGFR 126
10.2.1.1 EGFR and HPV 126
10.2.1.2 EGFR Detection Technique 127
10.2.1.3 EGFR's Role in Malignant Transformation 127
10.2.1.4 EGFR Overexpression and Prognosis 127
10.2.1.5 EGFR Blockade and Response to Radiation and Chemotherapy 129
10.2.2 VEGF 130
10.2.3 C-erbB-2/HER-2/*neu* 130
10.3 Human Papilloma Virus 131
10.4 Microenvironmental Factors 131
10.5 COX-2 131
10.6 Apoptosis-Related Proteins 132
10.6.1 Bcl-2 and Bax 132
10.7 Strategies for Response Modification 133
10.7.1 EGFR-Directed Therapy 133
10.7.2 VEGF 134
10.8 Strategies Targeting Tumor Microenvironment 134
10.9 COX-2 134
10.10 Conclusion 134
References 135

10.1 Introduction

The use of biologically-based prognostic factors to determine patient outcome and response to treatment has traditionally used immunohistochemical techniques for proteins expressed in archival fixed tissue. The increasing use of powerful genomic and proteomic techniques including array technology will increase our understanding of tumor behavior and specific therapeutic targets that may be exploited to individualize therapy and optimize treatment with radiation and chemotherapy. The development of biologically targeted therapy includes several recent successes including the development of HER2-*neu* targeting in breast cancer and the bcr-abl/c-kit antagonists in chronic myelogenous leukemia (CML) and gastrointestinal stromal tumors (GIST).

Tumor growth and progression is related not only to characteristics of the tumor, but also to those of the surrounding stroma. The importance of the vasculature in tumor response and metastasis is increasingly understood and offers great potential for therapy directed against new and existing blood vessels. The vascular compartment has particular importance for treatment with radiation due to its effects on vascular endothelium and the critical role of oxygenation in response to radiation.

Clinical trials of novel biological agents alone or with conventional chemotherapy and radiation will define the role for these agents in clinical practice. Thus an understanding of the role of growth factors in malignant response and progression will be critical to their expanding use. Studies frequently assess multiple markers from different pathways; therefore tables will be used to summarize the proportion of tumors with each marker, in order to illustrate the frequency of each. This chapter will review their impact in gynecological cancer, and suggest strategies for modification of radiation treatment response using biologically targeted therapies. This latter section will concentrate on cervix cancer since it is the predominant site for the use of definitive radiation and will highlight investigations in other gynecological sites.

J. De Los Santos, MD; J. Bonner, MD
Department of Radiation Oncology, University of Alabama at Birmingham, 1824 6th Avenue South, Birmingham, AL 35294, USA

S. Goddard, MD
Research Assistant, Department of Radiation Oncology, Princess Margaret Hospital, 610 University Avenue, Toronto, Ontario, M5G 2M9, Canada

A. Fyles, MD
Gynecologic Cancer Program Head, Department of Radiation Oncology, Princess Margaret Hospital, 610 University Avenue, Toronto, Ontario, M5G 2M9, Canada

10.2
Growth Factors

10.2.1
EGFR

Growth factor expression is frequently seen in epithelial tumors such as cervix cancer. The epithelial growth factor receptor (EGFR) or ErbB-1 is a 170,000-kDa transmembrane glycoprotein with three constituent parts: an extracellular ligand-binding domain, a transmembrane component, and an intracellular tyrosine kinase domain. It is one member of a family of four receptors, which also include HER2/ErbB-2, HER3/ErbB-3, and HER4/ErbB-4. Several ligands including epithelial growth factor (EGF), neuregulins, and tumor necrosis factor-alpha (TNF-α), activate the ligand-binding domain. Once bound, the receptor undergoes either homo- or heterodimerization and phosphorylation of the intracellular tyrosine kinase domain, leading to a signaling cascade with downstream effects that impact upon cellular proliferation, apoptosis, angiogenesis, invasion, metastases, and migration (Mendelson 2000). Moreover, these receptors may play an interdependent regulatory role regarding the activation or expression pattern of other receptors, as activation or overexpression of one member has been shown to change the expression of others (Sartor 2000).

Once activated, termination of the EGFR signal is accomplished through endocytosis of the receptor-ligand complex. The type of dimerization determines the strength and type of signal transduced, as well as how the receptors are processed following endocytosis (Yarden 2001). The heterodimerization of HER-2 with EGFR tends to decrease the rate of ligand dissociation as well as endocytosis, enhancing the strength of the signal as well as length of time of receptor activation. Additionally, heterodimerized receptors are recycled to the cell surface after endocytotic processing, further strengthening signal transduction, whereas EGFR homodimers are degraded.

10.2.1.1
EGFR and HPV

As noted above, any process that impairs the degradation of the receptor-ligand complex or promotes receptor recycling will enhance signal transduction by increasing the number of active receptors at the cell surface. Several viruses harness EGFR signaling for the purpose of replication, including Epstein-Barr virus (EBV), the hepatitis B virus and the human papilloma virus (HPV). With regards to gynecological malignancies, it appears that HPV E5 interacts with receptor processing by inhibiting an endosomal ATPase, blocking degradation of the activated receptor (Yarden 2001). Chapman et al. (1992) compared 47 colposcopically obtained biopsies from patients with squamous intraepithelial lesions (SIL) with 41 normal biopsies. The tissue was tested for HPV using Southern blot HPV DNA hybridization and a portion underwent immunohistochemical staining for EGFR. The authors looked at HPV type and correlated this with the degree of SIL. They demonstrated consistent EGFR expression in patients with SIL regardless of their HPV status. Although they found no correlation between EGFR expression and HPV status, there was a systematic progression in the pattern of EGFR staining that closely correlated with the grade of SIL. Low-grade lesions stained positive for EGFR in the lower third of the epithelium, whereas staining in higher-grade lesions extended into the upper two-thirds. Another study that specifically looked at HPV-positive lesions only, and studied them with immunohistochemistry for the presence of EGFR, found that 98% (95 out of 97 specimens) of the lesions expressed the receptor (Tervahauta et al. 1994). Mathur et al. (2001) tested one negative and two positive HPV cell lines and biopsies from women with normal epithelium, cervical intraepithelial neoplasia (CIN) I–III, and invasive cervical cancer with a semi-quantitative immunofluorescent assay to assess levels of both HPV-E6 and -E7 oncoproteins and EGFR. They found a significant correlation between HPV-E6, -E7, and EGFR levels, with the HPV negative cells expressing significantly lower levels ($p<0.001$) than those expressed in HPV positive cells. In the biopsy specimens, HPV-E6, -E7, and EGFR were negative in the controls and were significantly higher in the women with advanced CIN and cervical cancer as compared with controls ($p<0.001$). Linear regression analysis showed a positive correlation as well between HPV-E6, -E7, and EGFR levels ($p<0.001$), suggesting a potential relationship between the two. This work is further supported by a study by Akerman et al. (2001), where the individual roles these oncoproteins may play regarding EGFR expression and cell immortalization were investigated. They found that both the E6 and E7 proteins contributed to EGFR overexpression, but through separate mechanisms. Although the E6 protein could increase EGFR expression, it was unable alone to overcome mechanisms in place in normal cells that protect against increased EGFR signaling. This resistance was overcome with the addition of the E7 protein, which alone was unable to increase EGFR mRNA. Experiments have also showed an inhibitory effect of p53 on EGFR expression, and thus p53 inactivation by HPV-E6 may reverse the inhibition of EGFR, a finding which is also consistent with the finding that p53 mutations tend to occur more in patients with squamous cell carcinomas with HPV-negative lesions (GRANDIS et al. 1998). In summary, these data suggest a positive correlation between HPV and EGFR overexpression.

10.2.1.2
EGFR Detection Technique

Overexpression of EGFR occurs in cervical cancer but the incidence varies greatly, in part reflecting the technology used. It is thus worth mentioning the differences in accuracy in the technologies utilized widely for protein level detection, including immunohistochemistry (IHC) and ligand-binding assays (LBA). OWENS et al. (1992) tested 118 samples from 96 cases of ovarian carcinoma for the presence of EGFR, using both IHC and LBA. The LBA demonstrated a greater sensitivity by detecting EGFR in 47.5% of tumors as compared to 39.8% of tumors by IHC for a concordance rate of 69.5% that varied based on histology ($p<0.001$). The authors also noted that 13 cases that stained positive for EGFR by IHC stained negative by LBA, and recommended that the techniques be utilized together for maximal sensitivity. A second study from Japan also compared an EGFR LBA with IHC in patients with renal cell carcinoma and found an increased sensitivity of detection with the LBA (76% vs 52%) (YOSHIDA et al. 1997). Both of these techniques also have limitations. IHC provides reliable localization of EGFR, however limited quantitative information that can vary with the antibody and fixation technique. LBA, on the other hand, allows precise quantification of EGFR, but prevents histological analysis of the tissue. Neither approach can quantify EGFR per cell (PFEIFFER et al. 1998).

10.2.1.3
EGFR's Role in Malignant Transformation

Several groups have investigated downstream pathways correlated with EGFR overexpression that may contribute to a worse outcome in these patients. ALBINI et al. (1987) observed in vitro that the ability of proliferating cancer cells to form interconnecting cell clusters and cell extensions was associated with their metastatic potential in vivo. ALPER et al. (2001) investigated whether EGFR overexpression was correlated with an invasive phenotype and tried to define some of the mechanisms behind the pathogenesis of progression of ovarian carcinomas that overexpress EGFR. They compared an ovarian cancer cell line transfected with a vector containing EGFR antisense DNA with a cell line transfected with the vector alone for integrin expression, adhesion, matrix metalloprotease (MMP) activity, and ovarian cell migration. They found that the EGFR antisense cells were morphologically distinct from the control cells and had decreased adhesion to laminin-1, expression of the laminin-1 receptor α_6-integrin, and decreased matrix metalloprotease activity. CHEN et al. determined an association between EGFR overexpression and the presence of increased levels of ezrin, a membrane-actin cross-linking protein associated with functions of cell motility, invasion, and metastases in ovarian carcinomas (Z. CHEN et al. 2001). The authors were able to demonstrate ezrin membrane localization and the formation of pseudopodia in cells that were treated with either IL-1α or EGF, and utilizing Western blots showed significantly higher ezrin content in metastatic cells than in either nonmetastatic cancer cells or normal ovarian cells. These studies provide data supporting EGFR's role in tumor progression.

It is also unclear whether EGFR overexpression alone is solely responsible for enhanced tumorigenicity. Several receptor mutations have been identified in glioblastoma cell lines, and although these mutations have not yet been studied in gynecologic tumors, they may theoretically contribute to enhanced tumorigenicity in cells with normal or low levels of EGFR (BONNER et al. 2002).

10.2.1.4
EGFR Overexpression and Prognosis

The overexpression of EGFR has been demonstrated in up to 30% of epithelial malignancies, and has been shown to positively correlate with poor prognosis and resistance to various treatments in some malignancies (MENDELSON 2000; SARTOR 2000). As noted above, the incidence of EGFR overexpression and its prognostic relationship to gynecological malignancies has varied greatly in the literature. Using radioligand receptor binding, PFEIFFER et al. (1989) reported a significant increase in EGFR protein in cervical cancer specimens as compared with normal cervix epithelium (55±7 fmol/mg vs 7±1 fmol/mg, respectively, $p<0.05$). KIMMIG et al. (1997) reported 73% of cervical cancer specimens tested with two-color flow cytometry had more than

10,000 receptors/cell and 23% had greater than 30,000 receptors/cell. Using Elisa, KIM et al. (1996) reported over-expression of EGFR in 73% of cervical cancer. Using immunohistochemistry, KERSEMAEKERS et al. (1999) reported moderate to strong EGFR staining in 54% of tumors while KRISTENSEN et al. (1996) reported overexpression in 26% of cases.

Recently, overexpression of the epidermal growth factor receptor has been demonstrated in patients with both early as well as advanced disease, and has been associated with disease progression, tumor size (Kim), and a poor prognosis (PFEIFFER et al. 19898; KIM et al. 1996; KERSEMAEKERS et al. 1999; KRISTENSEN et al. 1996a; KIMMIG et al. 1997). In another recent study, however, SCAMBIA et al. (1998) failed to show a correlation with prognosis in a group of patients with more advanced disease and very aggressive therapy. Overexpression has also been demonstrated in both squamous cell histologies and adenocarcinoma, with one study in advanced (stages II, III, IV) cervical adenocarcinoma showing moderate to strong EGFR in 55% of cases (ALTAVILLA et al. 1996). A second study investigated the prognostic value of EGFR overexpression in 62 patients with stage IB/IIA squamous cell, adenocarcinoma, and adenosquamous histologies (HALE et al. 1993). Using an immunoperoxidase staining technique, 34% of cases stained positive, with squamous cell histology showing the greatest rate of positivity (50%) as compared to adenocarcinomas (19%) or adenosquamous carcinomas (33%). Among the three histologies, there was a significant correlation between positive staining and mortality ($p=0.003$). When analyzed separately by histology, the patients with adenosquamous cell carcinoma were the only group who retained a significant relationship between EGFR overexpression and increased mortality. This relationship was found for the overall group of patients with adenosquamous cell carcinoma ($p=0.005$) as well as the subpopulation of patients with negative nodes ($p<0.001$).

10.2.1.4.1
Endometrial Cancer

KHALIFA et al. (1994) retrospectively reviewed the pathology from 69 endometrial cancer patients, to determine the impact of EGFR overexpression on prognosis. EGFR was overexpressed in 34 (49%) of the tumors and was shown to be a statistically significant predictor of distant metastases on multivariate analysis. In this retrospective review, the patients whose tumors overexpressed EGFR had a threefold increase in their relative risk of death. In a prospective study of 74 cervical and 64 endometrial cancer patients, NAGAI et al. (2001) found EGFR expression in 57% and 60%, with mean levels of 18±38 fmol/mg and 9±42 fmol/mg of protein, respectively. They did not find a correlation between EGFR expression and clinicopathological findings, 5-year survival, or risk of death.

10.2.1.4.2
Vulvar Cancer

The prognostic significance of epidermal growth factor receptor has also been reviewed in patients with squamous cell carcinoma of the vulva. Sixty-one patients were reviewed in a study from the University of Oklahoma that investigated whether EGFR levels were correlated with the presence of metastases or overall survival (JOHNSON et al. 1997). There was a statistically significant increase in EGFR levels between primary tumors (67%) vs benign epithelium (31%), as well as between primary tumors (65%) and metastases from the same tumor (88%) in the 14 patients with lymph node metastases. Additionally, the risk of lymph node metastases was significantly greater for patients whose primary tumor had elevated EGFR levels of 90% or greater, and this translated into a significant disease-free survival difference of 25% vs 54% for those with 90% or more and less than 90% EGFR levels, respectively. In another study from China, the levels of TGF-α, EGF, and EGFR were quantified through immunohistochemical staining in a range of tissue from normal to dysplastic to invasive lesions (WU et al. 2001). Staining for TGF-α revealed a gradual increase in cytoplasmic staining intensity that paralleled the dysplastic tumor appearance, with faint immunoreactivity in normal and vulvar intraepithelial neoplasia (VIN) I-II specimens, increasing to intense immunoreactivity in patients with invasive squamous cell carcinoma. This was also observed in stains for EGF, with normal cells showing no cytoplasmic staining, and invasive lesions staining most intensely. The percentage of cases staining positive for EGFR was also significantly higher in invasive lesions (68%) than in VIN III (40%, $p<0.05$).

10.2.1.4.3
Ovarian Cancer

The EGF/ErbB receptors are present in normal ovarian epithelium, and play a crucial role in the normal development of ovarian follicles and in the ovarian surface epithelium (OSE) (MAIHLE et al. 2002;

DORAISWAMY et al. 2000). DORAISWAMY et al. (2000) postulated that dysregulation of OSE growth through aberrant growth factor gene expression was likely one of the factors promoting development and progression in ovarian cancer. The percentage of ovarian epithelial cancers reported to express high levels of the EGF receptors range from 33% to 100% (ALPER et al. 2001; HIWASA et al. 1992; SEWELL et al. 2002; SKIRNISDOTTIR et al. 2001). Additionally, 30% of ovarian cancers are associated with increased levels of the ligand, epithelial growth factor (SKIRNISDOTTIR et al. 2001). This overexpression of the receptor has been associated with a poorer prognosis, including an increase in disease recurrence and decreased survival (BERCHUCK et al. 1991). SKIRNISDOTTIR et al. (2001) found that both tumor grade and EGFR expression were independent prognostic factors for survival in patients with early-stage epithelial ovarian cancer, although there was no significant association between the two. An interesting finding from this study showed that the largest subset of tumors that were negative for both EGFR and HER-2/*neu* were the endometrioid and clear cell tumors. There was also no correlation between tumor grade and receptor positivity, although others have found a positive relationship (GOFF et al. 1996). MENDEN et al. (1995) did not find a positive relationship between EGFR and poor survival. Thus, as in cervical cancer, the impact of EGFR on prognosis remains controversial. It is unclear whether stage impacts on the percentage of ovarian epithelial specimens staining positive for EGFR. GOFF et al. (1996) found no difference between more advanced malignancies (stages III–IV) and earlier malignancies (stages I–II) in the degree of receptor positivity.

Thus the data supporting a prognostic correlation between EGFR overexpression and gynecological malignancies are mixed, although the preponderance of evidence would point towards a correlative relationship. Interestingly, two of the studies that found no relationship between its expression and clinicopathological features or survival did not use immunohistochemistry to quantify EGFR amount, but instead used a ligand-binding assay (SCAMBIA et al. 1998; NAGAI et al. 2001). One of these studies also did not find any detectable EGFR expression in normal cervical, endometrial, or ovarian tissue (NAGAI et al. 2001). These studies suggest that cervical cancer appears similar to other epithelial tumors as regards EGFR expression and behavior, although identifying optimal patients for therapy will likely require additional observations and correlations.

10.2.1.5
EGFR Blockade and Response to Radiation and Chemotherapy

Blockade of the EGF receptor has been shown both in vitro and in vivo to decrease proliferation of squamous cell lines, which overexpress the receptor (BONNER et al. 2000; MASUI et al. 1984; SATO et al. 1983; SALEH et al. 1999). The use of monoclonal antibodies to EGFR has also been shown in preclinical animal models to enhance the antitumor efficacy of radiation and chemotherapy (SARTOR 2000; MILAS et al. 2000; LAMMERING et al. 2001; BIANCO et al. 2000; SHIN et al. 2001; PENG 2001). The combination of EGFR inhibitors with radiation and/or chemotherapy are also tolerable in phase I and II trials in subjects with various tumor types. A phase I study combining increasing doses of C225 with curative radiation doses in patients with previously untreated head and neck cancer was completed at the University of Alabama (ROBERT et al. 2001). This study showed no enhancement of radiation toxicity and demonstrated impressive antitumor efficacy. It led to a pivotal phase III trial with randomization between radiation alone or radiation plus C225, which recently closed to accrual in March 2002. A wide variety of studies have shown the non-overlapping toxicities of C225 (skin rash) or protein kinase (PK) inhibitors (skin and diarrhea) with a variety of chemotherapy agents (MELLINGHOFF and SAWYERS 2000). SHIN et al. (2001) confirmed that C225 dose schedules of 400 mg/m^2 loading and 250 mg/m^2 weekly maintenance produced high levels of EGFR saturation without unusual side effects in combination with cis-platinum. Furthermore, it has been noted that the typical skin rash seen with anti-EGFR therapy may serve as a biological marker for skin and hair follicle EGFR blockade (ROBERT et al. 2001).

More importantly, synergism has been demonstrated when anti-EGFR agents have been combined with radiation, and phase Ib/IIa trials have shown acceptable toxicity. Squamous cell carcinoma xenografts in mice treated with concurrent radiation and the chimeric monoclonal antibody C225 demonstrated decreased proliferation and increased apoptosis, indicating a radiosensitizing effect (SATO et al. 1983; SALEH et al. 1999; MILAS et al. 2000; NASU et al. 2001). MILAS et al. (2000) also demonstrated that an enhancement in tumor radioresponse and curability as well as a decrease in recurrences could be achieved when C225 was given 6 h prior, and 3 and 6 days after radiation treatment in A431 tumor xenografts. A phase Ib–IIa trial of concurrent cetuximab and radiation for unresectable carcinoma of the head and neck (noted above) has since shown acceptable toxicity as well as promising response rates with 13 out of 15 evaluable patients achieving a complete response (ROBERT et al. 2001). In this trial, 15 evaluable patients were treated in five escalating dose cohorts. Nine patients experienced irradiation-related grade 3 or higher mucositis and five experienced cetuximab and/or irradiation-related grade 3 skin toxicity. No cetuximab dose delays were required and in general, the skin toxicities recovered during treatment or shortly thereafter to a grade 1 or 2 level. The initial results in phase I and II trials in other epithelial sites as well as the demonstration of EGFR overexpression in gynecological malignancies led to the initiation of receptor blockade therapy in gynecological tumors.

10.2.2
VEGF

Vascular endothelial growth factor (VEGF) is frequently up-regulated in cervix cancer, due to its relationship with hypoxia mediated by the HIF-1 transcription factor. LONCASTER et al. (2000) found VEGF expression to have independent impact on overall ($p=0.001$) and metastasis-free survival ($p=0.02$) but not on local control (Table 10.1). This suggests that VEGF may be less useful as a potentiator of radiation response, at least in cervix cancer. An independent effect of VEGF on disease-free and overall survival was also seen in a group of patients with early stage disease (CHENG et al. 2000).

In patients with ovarian cancer, VEGF overexpression is frequently seen and has been associated with poor survival in multivariate analysis, in addition to stage (SHEN et al. 2000). Serum VEGF also appears to have independent prognostic impact in addition to grade and stage (CHEN et al. 1999; TEMPFER et al. 1998), although this result was not confirmed in other trials (OEHLER and CAFFIER 2000; GADDUCCI et al. 1999).

Endometrial tumors exhibited VEGF overexpression in 39%–66% of cases (C.A. CHEN et al. 2001; YOKOYAMA et al. 2000). Similar to the results in ovarian cancer, there was a variable relationship between VEGF expression and outcome. GIATROMANOLAKI and HIRAI found significant effects in a multivariate analysis against overall and disease-free survival, and Chen found that VEGF overexpression correlated independently with recurrence (C.A. CHEN et al. 2001). YOKOYAMA found an independent correlation of the Flt-4 receptor but not for VEGF itself, whereas FINE et al. and SALVESEN and AKSLEN found no effect of VEGF or thrombospondin on outcome (YOKOYAMA et al. 2000; FINE et al. 2000; SALVESEN and AKSLEN 1999).

10.2.3
C-erbB-2/HER-2/neu

Positive staining for HER-2/neu has been shown in 18.9%–46.2% of patients with cervix tumors (NAKANO et al. 1996, 1997; NISHIOKA et al. 1999;

Table 10.1. Growth factors in gynecological tumors

Marker	Cut-off for survival analysis	Incidence of positivity	Sample size	Impact on survival
CerbB2 /HER-2/neu	Positivity: marked cell membrane or cytoplasmic staining	42.4% (NAKANO et al. 1997)	64	Worsened DFS ($p<0.01$)
	Definitive membranous staining & >10% of cells stained	33.6% (NISHIOKA et al. 1999)	107	Worsened ($p=0.019$)
	Marked cell membrane staining	46.2% (NAKANO et al. 1996)	52	Worsened ($p<0.025$)
	10%	18.9% (SKIRNISDOTTIR et al. 2001)	106	Cancer-specific survival: none ($p=0.5872$)
VEGF	Continuous Semi-quantitative 0–3	67% (LONCASTER et al. 2000)	100	Worsened OS in multivariate but not LC
	800 pg/mg protein	24% (CHENG et al. 2000)	135	Significant in multivariate analysis for DFS
HPV	Type 16/18	77% (TJALMA et al. 2001)	111	None ($p=0.246$)
		93.3% positive, 69% HPV16 (KRISTENSEN et al. 1996)	223	No effect of HPV positivity or of HPV type
	Any type	76.9% (ISHIKAWA et al. 2001)	52 (Stage IIIB)	No effect of HPV positivity

DFS, disease-free survival; *OS*, overall survival; *LC*, local control

SKIRNISDOTTIR et al. 2001) and has generally been associated with poorer survival in univariate analysis (Table 10.1). The lack of multivariate analyses limits the conclusions regarding the independent effects of HER-2/*neu* expression.

HER-2/*neu* was amplified (using fluorescence in situ hybridization [FISH]) in 40 of 61 patients with invasive ovarian cancer, but did not predict outcome in this series (Ross et al. 1999). These results are generally consistent with other studies in ovarian cancer although MEDEN et al. (1995) did report an independent effect of HER-2/*neu* expression on survival.

A number of studies have examined HER-2/*neu* expression in endometrial cancer and a small majority have found an independent effect on outcome (BERCHUCK et al. 1991; HETZEL et al. 1992).

10.3
Human Papilloma Virus

Oncogenic human papilloma virus subtypes are implicated in the development of virtually all cervix tumors. Using polymerase chain reaction (PCR) techniques, KRISTENSEN et al. (1996b) found evidence of HPV DNA in over 93% of specimens in 223 patients with cervix cancer, but no influence of HPV or its subtypes was found on prognosis (Table 10.1). This lack of effect on survival is consistent with other studies evaluating HPV subtypes 16 and 18 alone, and patients with Stage IIB tumors only (TJALMA et al. 2001; ISHIKAWA et al. 2001). Earlier studies suggesting an adverse effect of HPV negativity did not use multiple PCR primers and had a lower detection rate for HPV.

10.4
Microenvironmental Factors

Tumor cells exist in a microenvironment of extracellular matrix (ECM) characterized by stroma, interstitium and vascular compartments, each of which may have a profound effect on tumor behavior and treatment outcome. Epithelial–stromal interactions and vascular effects are mediated by growth factors and cytokines such as VEGF, fibroblast growth factors (FGF) etc.

Tumor angiogenesis is a necessary component for growth and progression, yet blood vessels in tumors are highly abnormal, less responsive to normal functional stimuli, resulting in erratic flow and leakiness of vessel walls. The consequence of these abnormalities is a tumor microenvironment characterized by heterogeneity in content of glucose, oxygen and other cellular nutrients as well as metabolic products such as lactic acid. Lactate levels have been demonstrated to be a prognostic factor in patients with cervix cancer, as well as head and neck tumors (WALENTA et al. 2000).

Hypoxia is a characteristic of many cancers and is frequently seen in cervix tumors (HOCKEL et al. 1993). Hypoxia has been assessed with extrinsic nitroimidazole markers such as pimonidazole and EF-5, invasive polarographic electrodes and, more recently, intrinsic markers such as HIF-1 and carbonic anhydrase IX (CA-IX). CA-IX is also involved in pH homeostasis and so may be a multifunctional marker of microenvironmental characteristics.

In patients with cervix cancer, hypoxia has consistently been found to have prognostic power for patients treated surgically (HOCKEL et al. 1996) and by radiation (HOCKEL et al. 1996; KNOCKE et al. 1999; FYLES et al. 2002). In multivariate analysis, it has added to stage, tumor size and nodal status in defining treatment results.

HIF-1 expression has been correlated with hypoxia in cervical cancer xenografts (VUKOVIC et al. 2001) and has shown a relationship with outcome in patients with early disease (BIRNER et al. 2000). In contrast, in patients with more advanced tumors, no relationship with survival was found (HAUGLAND et al. 2002).

CA-IX is a HIF-1 responsive transmembrane glycoprotein that appears to correlate with hypoxia (LONCASTER et al. 2001; OLIVE et al. 2001). In clinical studies CA-IX overexpression has been associated with worse survival in multivariate analysis (Table 10.2). Further studies will be required to determine whether it may be as effective a marker as hypoxia measured using polarographic electrodes.

10.5
COX-2

Cyclooxygenase-2 (COX-2) is an inducible enzyme required in the conversion of prostaglandins (PGs) from arachidonic acid. Overexpression of COX-2 has been linked to promotion of tumorigenesis, resistance to apoptosis, and abnormal cell cycle regulation. Data in the literature show a link between COX-2 activity and hypoxia-induced angiogenesis in cancer. Prostaglandin E_2 (PGE_2) is a major COX-2-derived

Table 10.2. Microenvironmental factors in gynecological cancer

Marker	Cut-off for survival analysis	Incidence of positivity	Mean labeling index	Median labeling index	Sample size	Impact on survival
COX-2	10% of cells	50% (Gaffney et al. 2001)			24	Worsened ($p=0.0126$)
HP5	50%		47% (Fyles et al. 2002)	48% (Fyles et al. 2002)	106	Worsened PFS ($p=0.004$); MV analysis: significant only in node-negative group ($p=0.007$), not in node-positive ($p=0.18$)
	Median		28% (Knocke et al. 1999)	22% (Knocke et al. 1999)	59	Worsened DFS ($p<0.02$)
	None			55% (Sheridan et al. 2000)	42	
PO_2	Median		18 (Knocke et al. 1999)	10 (Knocke et al. 1999)	59	Worsened DFS ($p<0.02$)
	None		14 (Fyles et al. 2002)	5 (Fyles et al. 2002)	106	
	Median of pooled values =10 mmHg	45% (Hockel et al. 1993)			33	Worsened survival; UV: ($p=0.027$); MV: not significant
	None			4 (Sheridan et al. 2000)	42	
	Median of pooled values =10 mmHg	51% (Hockel et al. 1996)			42	Borderline significance for survival ($p=0.0638$); significant for DFS ($p=0.0350$)
	1%	71% (Loncaster et al. 2001)			130	DFS: worsened ($p=0.0041$); metastasis-free survival: worsened ($p=0.0049$)
CA-IX	10%	35% (Skirnisdottir et al. 2001)			106	Worsened cancer-specific survival ($p=0.0233$), also significant on MV: $p=0.0183$
Lactate	Median (Walenta et al. 2000)		8.3		34	Worsened ($p=0.0015$)

PFS, progression-free survival; *MV*, multivariate analysis; *DFS*, disease-free survival; *UV*, univariate analysis

product, and has also been shown to be a stimulator of angiogenesis. COX-2 is highly expressed in a large number of human tumors, including prostate, non-small cell lung cancer, skin cancer, and squamous cell carcinoma of the head and neck (Chan et al. 1999; Tucker et al. 1999; Komhoff et al. 2000; Yoshimura et al. 2000; Higashi et al. 2000). COX-2 expression has also been found to be increased in cervix cancers. Ryu et al. (2000) studied stage IB cervical cancer patients, treated with primary surgery, and found a significantly increased expression of COX-2 with lymph node or parametrial involvement. They suggested that the expression of COX-2 in these patients may down-regulate apoptotic processes and enhance tumor invasion and metastasis. Gaffney has demonstrated that 12/24 patients had 10% or greater staining for COX-2 and that COX-2 overexpression had prognostic effect for survival (Gaffney et al. 2001).

10.6
Apoptosis-Related Proteins

10.6.1
Bcl-2 and Bax

Apoptosis is an active process that, in the normal organism, maintains homeostasis between proliferative and growth-inhibitory signals. Cancer cells are defective in genes that control apoptosis, resulting in survival of cells with DNA damage that would normally undergo destruction. Bcl-2 is one of several cell death proteases whose overexpression prevents initiation of apoptosis. In vivo, bcl-2 associates with the pro-apoptotic protein bax to control the apoptotic threshold. P53 also appears to play a role as a promoter of bax and down-regulator of bcl-2.

In cervix cancer, bcl-2 protein expression is seen in 6%–68% of cells, using cut-offs for positivity of 1%–30%. Bcl-2 overexpression appears to be associated with a better prognosis in two studies, but had no effect in another (Table 10.3). Bax expression is also quite variable, occurring in 13%–83% of tumors, but with no apparent prognostic effect.

10.7
Strategies for Response Modification

Modification of radiation response using modulators of growth factors, apoptotic thresholds and microenvironmental features offers the potential to customize therapy based on tumor and individual patient characteristics.

10.7.1
EGFR-Directed Therapy

Chapter 15 deals with EGFR and radiation response in detail; therefore the role of EGF in gynecological cancer will be dealt with briefly. The data to document that EGFR is an important molecular target for anti-tumor drug development is extensive and well summarized in several recent reviews (MENDELSON 2000; BONNER et al. 2002; ARTEAGA 2001; BASELGA 2001; CIARDIELLO and TORTORA 2001). Therapeutically, preclinical trials showed that treatment with either the mouse monoclonal antibody against the EGF receptor, m225, or the chimeric antibody, C225, had antitumor activity against ovarian cell lines (PENG 2001). A combined in vitro/in vivo study of the EGFR-targeted tyrosine kinase inhibitor ZD 1839 has additionally shown growth inhibition of up to 50% in ovarian cancer cell lines expressing EGFR levels to varying degrees with and without the simultaneous administration of TGF-α (SEWELL et al. 2002). In this latter report, one cell line with no detectable EGFR protein showed no growth stimulation in response to TGF-α as well as no significant growth inhibition to ZD 1839. The in vivo portion evaluated growth inhibition of a xenograft model at two levels: 50 mg/kg per day and 200 mg/kg per day. Growth inhibition occurred in a dose-dependent fashion, with the higher dose producing a greater than 50% inhibition at the end of the treatment period lasting until sacrifice 31 days after treatment. The lower dose produced a smaller effect yet significant growth inhibition at 17 days, which reversed prior to sacrifice.

Phase I and II trials of EGFR-targeted therapy alone have produced a low to moderate frequency of objective responses (5%–20%) in advanced stages of disease including cancer of the head and neck, lung, ovary, and colon. Recent studies suggest that the most beneficial role of anti-EGFR therapy may be the use of this treatment in combination with other anticancer treatments. Researchers at the University of Alabama demonstrated that a monoclonal antibody to EGFR (C225) plus radiation produced an enhanced rate of complete remission, prolongation of tumor doubling time and prolongation of survival as compared to radiation alone in a mouse A431 model (SALEH et al. 1999). Similar effects were reported in A431 tumors by MILAS et al. (2000) while others reported C225 enhancement of radiation effects in head and neck and colon cancer models. In regards to anti-EGFR enhancement of chemotherapy effects in animal models, MENDELSOHN (2000) has recently summarized his series of studies. Benefits were seen in combination with cis-platinum, adriamycin and paclitaxel while CIARDIELLO and TOTTORA (2001)

Table 10.3. Apoptotic proteins in gynecological cancer

Marker	Cut-off for survival analysis	Incidence of positivity	Sample size	Impact on survival
Bax	>5% of cells	47% (MUKHERJEE et al. 2001)	78 IIIB only	
	>70% of cells	20% (CRAWFORD et al. 1998)	44	None ($p=0.47$)
	>10% of cells	13% (HARIMA et al. 2000)	37	
	>30% of cells	22.7% (HARIMA et al. 1998)	44	None ($p=0.55$)
	>1% of cells	15% (OHNO et al. 1998)	20	
	>10% of cells	83% (TJALMA et al. 2001)	111	None
Bcl2	>5% of cells	8% (MUKHERJEE et al. 2001)	78 IIIB only	
	>10% of cells	34% (CRAWFORD et al. 1998)	44	Improved ($p=0.03$)
	>10% of cells	35% (HARIMA et al. 2000)	37	
	>30% of cells	61.4% (HARIMA et al. 1998)	44	None ($p=0.09$)
	>1% of cells	15% (OHNO et al. 1998)	20	
	>5% of cells	68% (TJALMA et al. 2001)	111	Improved ($p<0.001$)

reported benefit with topotecan. BURNS et al. (2000) reported a dramatic effect of C225 in combination with gemcitabine utilizing an orthotopic pancreatic cancer model. Inhibition of tumor growth, metastases and angiogenesis was demonstrated. Thus, EGFR blockade enhances radiation and a broad array of chemotherapy agents in several EGFR-positive tumor models. Multiple phase III combined modality trials in common tumors are in progress. Ongoing studies utilizing EGFR blockade along with concurrent chemotherapy and/or radiation for high-risk gynecological malignancies has exciting prospects in improving the therapeutic ratio.

10.7.2
VEGF

A detailed review of therapy directed against VEGF and other angiogenic growth factors will be found in Chap. 14. VEGF receptor tyrosine kinase inhibitors have shown activity in animal models of ovarian cancer. XU et al. (2000) demonstrated reduction in ascites formation in one of two cell lines, mediated by a decrease in vascular permeability. GORSKI et al. (1999) determined that the effect of VEGF neutralizing antibodies in several cell lines was due to inhibition of radiation-induced VEGF production rather than effects on tumor radiosensitivity. There has been limited clinical activity reported in gynecological cancers although studies are ongoing.

10.8
Strategies Targeting Tumor Microenvironment

Measures to improve tumor oxygenation have included increased oxygen delivery using carbogen, blood transfusion and, more recently, erythropoietin. Although improvements in tumor oxygenation may be seen (AQUINO-PARSONS et al. 2000), it is not yet clear that improvements in tumor control and survival necessarily follow. This may be related to the heterogeneity of response to these agents, where a critical subpopulation of tumor cells are resistant and result in treatment failure. Efforts to overcome resistance related to transient blood flow (for example, using nicotinamide in combination with carbogen, ARCON) or drugs specifically directed against hypoxic cells (tirapazamine and cisplatin), or using vascular targeting agents such as the combretastatins are in progress.

In gynecological cancer, randomized trials are evaluating erythropoietin in cervix cancer as an alternative to transfusion. Although anemia has a demonstrated prognostic effect in clinical studies of cervix cancer, its relationship to hypoxia is not at all clear (FYLES et al. 2000). An alternative hypothesis suggests that anemia is a surrogate for tumor size and response to therapy, and that oxygen delivery is maintained by multiple homeostatic mechanisms such as shifts in the hemoglobin dissociation curve.

Novel approaches include the use of nonpathogenic clostridium bacteria to deliver drugs or secrete therapeutic proteins such as cytosine deaminase (NUYTS et al. 2002). Furthermore, protein expression may be controlled by a radiation-inducible promoter, resulting in exquisite spatial and temporal specificity. In a similar vein, hypoxia-inducible activation of a prodrug or its activating enzyme has been modeled in vitro and in vivo (SHIBATA et al. 2002; PATTERSON et al. 2002).

10.9
COX-2

Current trials in cervix cancer are evaluating COX-2 inhibitors such as celecoxib in combination with chemoradiotherapy (more detail can also be found in Chap. 18). At Princess Margaret Hospital we have treated 15 patients with celecoxib 400 mg twice daily for 2 weeks prior to and during standard chemoradiotherapy for patients with cervix cancer. Preliminary results indicate that toxicity is acceptable and positive effects on tumor oxygenation having been observed with 4 of 10 measurable patients showing a decrease in hypoxic fraction.

10.10
Conclusion

Growth factors and characteristics of the tumor microenvironment clearly have an important role in epithelial gynecological cancers. Future studies will better characterize the most important markers and assays and assess relationships between markers. Examples might include interactions between HIF-responsive proteins such as VEGF and CA-IX and microenvironmental assays of hypoxia and lactate. At present, the best characterized markers appear to be microenvironmental, in terms of independent prognostic ability. Future work will concentrate on the critical genes and proteins responsible for resistance associated with the hypoxic phenotype, in order to identify new therapeutic targets.

Clinical trials of response-modifying agents are just beginning in gynecological cancer. Biologically targeted therapies, particularly in combination with radiation therapy, offer the prospect of customized treatment selection based on analysis of the individual tumor characteristics, thereby increasing tumor kill while minimizing toxicity.

References

Akerman GS, Tolleson WH, Brown KL et al (2001) Human papillomavirus type 16 E6 and E7 cooperate to increase epidermal growth factor receptor (EGFR) mRNA levels, overcoming mechanisms by which excessive EGFR signaling shortens the life span of normal human keratinocytes. Cancer Res 61:3837–3843

Albini A, Iwamoto Y, Kleinman HK et al (1987) A rapid in vitro assay for quantitating the invasive potential of tumor cells. Cancer Res 47:3239–3245

Alper O, Bergmann-Leitner ES, Bennet TA et al (2001) Epidermal growth factor receptor signaling and the invasive phenotype of ovarian carcinoma cells. J Natl Cancer Inst 93:1375–1384

Altavilla G, Castellan L, Wabersich J et al (1996) Prognostic significance of epidermal growth factor receptor (EGFR) and c-erbB-2 protein overexpression in adenocarcinoma of the uterine cervix. Eur J Gynaecol Oncol 17:267–270

Aquino-Parsons C, Green A, Minchinton AI (2000) Oxygen tension in primary gynaecological tumours: the influence of carbon dioxide concentration. Radiother Oncol 57:45–51

Arteaga CL (2001) The epidermal growth factor receptor: from mutant oncogene in nonhuman cancers to therapeutic target in human neoplasia. J Clin Oncol 19 [Suppl]: 32S–40S

Baselga J (2001) Targeting the epidermal growth factor receptor: a clinical reality. J Clin Oncol 19 [Suppl]:41S–44S

Berchuck A, Rodriguez GC, Kamel A et al (1991) Epidermal growth factor receptor expression in normal ovarian epithelium and ovarian cancer. I. Correlation of receptor expression with prognostic factors in patients with ovarian cancer. Am J Obstet Gynecol 164:669–674

Berchuck A, Rodriguez G, Kinney RB et al (1991) Overexpression of HER-2/neu in endometrial cancer is associated with advanced stage disease. Am J Obstet Gynecol 164:15–21

Bianco C, Bianco R, Tortora G et al (2000) Antitumor activity of combined treatment of human cancer cells with ionizing radiation and anti-epidermal growth factor receptor monoclonal antibody C225 plus type I protein kinase A antisense oligonucleotide. Clin Cancer Res 6:4343–4350

Birner P, Schindl M, Obermair A et al (2000) Overexpression of hypoxia-inducible factor 1alpha is a marker for an unfavorable prognosis in early-stage invasive cervical cancer. Cancer Res 60:4693–4696

Bonner JA, Raisch KP, Trummell HQ et al (2000) Enhanced apoptosis with combination C225/radiation treatment serves as the impetus for clinical investigation in head and neck cancers. J Clin Oncol 18 [Suppl]:47S–53S

Bonner JA, De Los Santos J, Waksal HW et al (2002) Epidermal growth factor receptor as a therapeutic target in head and neck cancer. Semin Radiat Oncol 12 [Suppl 2]:11–20

Burns CJ, Harbison MT, Davis DW et al (2000) Epidermal growth factor receptor blockade with C225 plus gemcitabine results in regression of human pancreatic carcinoma growing orthotopically in nude mice by antiangiogenic mechanisms. Clin Cancer Res 6:1936–1948

Chan G, Boyle JO, Yang EK, et al (1999) Cyclooxygenase-2 expression is up-regulated in squamous cell carcinoma of the head and neck. Cancer Res 59:991–994

Chapman WB, Lorincz AT, Willett GD et al (1992) Epidermal growth factor receptor expression and the presence of human papillomavirus in cervical squamous intraepithelial lesions. Int J Gynecol Pathol 11:221–226

Chen CA, Cheng WF, Lee CN et al (1999) Serum vascular endothelial growth factor in epithelial ovarian neoplasms: correlation with patient survival. Gynecol Oncol 74:235–240

Chen CA, Cheng WF, Lee CN et al (2001) Cytosol vascular endothelial growth factor in endometrial carcinoma: correlation with disease-free survival. Gynecol Oncol 80:207–212

Chen Z, Fadiel A, Feng Y et al (2001) Ovarian epithelial carcinoma tyrosine phosphorylation, cell proliferation, and ezrin translocation are stimulated by interleukin 1alpha and epidermal growth factor. Cancer 92:3068–3075

Cheng WF, Chen CA, Lee CN et al (2000) Vascular endothelial growth factor and prognosis of cervical carcinoma. Obstet Gynecol 96:721–726

Ciardiello F, Tortora G (2001) A novel approach in the treatment of cancer: targeting the epidermal growth factor receptor. Clin Cancer Res 7:2958–2970

Crawford RA, Caldwell C, Iles RK et al (1998) Prognostic significance of the bcl-2 apoptotic family of proteins in primary and recurrent cervical cancer. Br J Cancer 78:210–214

Doraiswamy V, Parrott JA, Skinner MK (2000) Expression and action of transforming growth factor alpha in normal ovarian surface epithelium and ovarian cancer. Biol Reprod 63:789–796

Fine BA, Valente PT, Feinstein GI, Dey T (2000) VEGF, flt-1, and KDR/flk-1 as prognostic indicators in endometrial carcinoma. Gynecol Oncol 76:33–39

Fyles AW, Milosevic M, Pintilie M et al (2000) Anemia, hypoxia and transfusion in patients with cervix cancer: a review. Radiother Oncol 57:13–19

Fyles AW, Milosevic M, Hedley D et al (2002) Tumor hypoxia has independent predictor impact only in patients with node-negative cervix cancer. J Clin Oncol 20:680–687

Gadducci A, Ferdeghini M, Fanucchi A et al (1999) Serum preoperative vascular endothelial growth factor (VEGF) in epithelial ovarian cancer: relationship with prognostic variables and clinical outcome. Anticancer Res 19:1401–1405

Gaffney DK, Holden J, Davis M et al (2001) Elevated cyclooxygenase-2 expression correlates with diminished survival in carcinoma of the cervix treated with radiotherapy. Int J Radiat Oncol Biol Phys 49:1213–1217

Goff BA, Shy K, Greer BE et al (1996) Overexpression and relationships of HER-2/neu, epidermal growth factor receptor, p53, Ki-67, and tumor necrosis factor alpha in epithelial ovarian cancer. Eur J Gynaecol Oncol 17:487–492

Gorski DH, Beckett MA, Jaskowiak NT et al (1999) Blockage of the vascular endothelial growth factor stress response increases the antitumor effects of ionizing radiation. Cancer Res 59:3374–3378

Grandis JR, Zeng Q, Drenning SD, Tweardy DJ (1998) Normalization of EGFR mRNA levels following restoration of wild-type p53 in a head and neck squamous cell carcinoma cell line. Int J Oncol 13:375–378

Hale RJ, Buckley CH, Gullick WJ et al (1993) Prognostic value of epidermal growth factor receptor expression in cervical carcinoma. J Clin Pathol 46:149–153

Harima Y, Harima K, Shikata N et al (1998) Bax and Bcl-2 expressions predict response to radiotherapy in human cervical cancer. J Cancer Res Clin Oncol 124:503–510

Harima Y, Nagata K, Harima K et al (2000) Bax and Bcl-2 protein expression following radiation therapy versus radiation plus thermoradiotherapy in stage IIIB cervical carcinoma. Cancer 88:132–138

Haugland HK, Vukovic V, Pintillie M et al (2002) Expression of hypoxia-inducible factor-1alpha in cervical carcinomas: correlation with tumor oxygenation. Int J Radiat Oncol Biol Phys 53:854–861

Hetzel DJ, Wilson TO, Keeney GL et al (1992) HER-2/neu expression: a major prognostic factor in endometrial cancer. Gynecol Oncol 47:179–185

Higashi Y, Kanekura T, Kanzaki T (2000) Enhanced expression of cyclooxygenase (COX)-2 in human skin epidermal cancer cells: evidence for growth suppression by inhibiting COX-2 expression. Int J Cancer 86:667–671

Hiwasa T, Hirono M, Suzuki M, Tanaka T (1992) Expression and localization of epidermal growth factor receptors and ras oncogene products in gynecologic tumors. Eur J Gynaecol Oncol 13:241–245

Hockel M, Vorndran B, Schlenger K et al (1993) Tumor oxygenation: a new predictive parameter in locally advanced cancer of the uterine cervix. Gynecol Oncol 51:141–149

Hockel M, Schlenger K, Aral B et al (1996) Association between tumor hypoxia and malignant progression in advanced cancer of the uterine cervix. Cancer Res 56:4509–4515

Ishikawa H, Mitsuhashi N, Sakurai H et al (2001) The effects of p53 status and human papillomavirus infection on the clinical outcome of patients with stage IIIB cervical carcinoma treated with radiation therapy alone. Cancer 91:80–89

Johnson GA, Mannel R, Khalifa M et al (1997) Epidermal growth factor receptor in vulvar malignancies and its relationship to metastasis and patient survival. Gynecol Oncol 65:425–429

Kersemaekers AM, Fleuren GJ, Kenter GG et al (1999) Oncogene alterations in carcinomas of the uterine cervix: overexpression of the epidermal growth factor receptor is associated with poor prognosis. Clin Cancer Res 5:577–586

Khalifa MA, Abdoh AA, Mannel RS et al (1994) Prognostic utility of epidermal growth factor receptor overexpression in endometrial adenocarcinoma. Cancer 73:370–376

Kim JW, Kim YT, Kim DK et al (1996) Expression of epidermal growth factor receptor in carcinoma of the cervix. Gynecol Oncol 60:283–287

Kimmig R, Pfeiffer D, Landsmann H, Hepp H (1997) Quantitative determination of the epidermal growth factor receptor in cervical cancer and normal cervical epithelium by 2-color flow cytometry: evidence for down-regulation in cervical cancer. Int J Cancer 74:365–373

Knocke TH, Weitmann HD, Feldmann HJ et al (1999) Intratumoral pO2-measurements as predictive assay in the treatment of carcinoma of the uterine cervix. Radiother Oncol 53:99–104

Komhoff M, Guan Y, Shappell HW et al (2000) Enhanced expression of cyclooxygenase-2 in high-grade human transitional cell bladder carcinomas. Am J Pathol 157:29–35

Kristensen GB, Holm R, Abeler VM, Trope CG (1996a) Evaluation of the prognostic significance of cathepsin D, epidermal growth factor receptor, and c-erbB-2 in early cervical squamous cell carcinoma. An immunohistochemical study. Cancer 78:433–440

Kristensen GB, Karlsen F, Jenkins A et al (1996b) Human papilloma virus has no prognostic significance in cervical carcinoma. Eur J Cancer 32A:1349–1353

Lammering G, Hewit TH, Hawkins WT et al (2001) Epidermal growth factor receptor as a genetic therapy target for carcinoma cell radiosensitization. J Natl Cancer Inst 93: 921–929

Loncaster JA, Cooper RA, Longue JP et al (2000) Vascular endothelial growth factor (VEGF) expression is a prognostic factor for radiotherapy outcome in advanced carcinoma of the cervix. Br J Cancer 83:620–625

Loncaster JA, Harris AL, Davidson SE et al (2001) Carbonic anhydrase (CA IX) expression, a potential new intrinsic marker of hypoxia: correlations with tumor oxygen measurements and prognosis in locally advanced carcinoma of the cervix. Cancer Res 61:6394–6399

Maihle NJ, Baron AT, Barrette BA et al (2002) EGF/ErbB receptor family in ovarian cancer. Cancer Treat Res 107:247–258

Masui H, Kawamoto T, Sato JD et al (1984) Growth inhibition of human tumor cells in athymic mice by anti-epidermal growth factor receptor monoclonal antibodies. Cancer Res 44:1002–1007

Mathur SPMathur RS, Rust PF, Young RC (2001) Human papilloma virus (HPV)-E6/E7 and epidermal growth factor receptor (EGF-R) protein levels in cervical cancer and cervical intraepithelial neoplasia (CIN). Am J Reprod Immunol 46:280–287

Meden H, Marx D, Raab T et al (1995) EGF-R and overexpression of the oncogene c-erbB-2 in ovarian cancer: immunohistochemical findings and prognostic value. J Obstet Gynaecol 21:167–178

Mellinghoff I, Sawyers C (2000) Kinase inhibitor therapy in cancer. Princ Pract Oncol 14:1–11

Mendelson J (2000) Blockade of receptors for growth factors: an anticancer therapy – the fourth annual Joseph H Burchenal American Association of Cancer Research Clinical Research Award Lecture. Clin Cancer Res 6:747–753

Milas L, Mason K, Hunter N et al (2000) In vivo enhancement of tumor radioresponse by C225 antiepidermal growth factor receptor antibody. Clin Cancer Res 6:701–708

Mukherjee G, Freeman A, Moore R et al (2001) Biologic factors and response to radiotherapy in carcinoma of the cervix. Int J Gynecol Cancer 11:187–193

Nagai N, Oshita T, Fujii T et al (2001) Are DNA ploidy and epidermal growth factor receptor prognostic factors for untreated ovarian cancer? A prospective study. Am J Clin Oncol 24:215–221

Nakano T, Oka K, Ishikawa A, Morita S (1997) Correlation of cervical carcinoma c-erb B-2 oncogene with cell proliferation parameters in patients treated with radiation therapy for cervical carcinoma. Cancer 79:513–520

Nakano T, Oka K, Taniguchi N (1996) Manganese superoxide dismutase expression correlates with p53 status and local

recurrence of cervical carcinoma treated with radiation therapy. Cancer Res 56:2771-2775
Nasu S, Ang KK, Fan Z, Milas L (2001) C225 antiepidermal growth factor receptor antibody enhances tumor radiocurability. Int J Radiat Oncol Biol Phys 51:474-477
Nishioka T, West CM, Gupta N et al (1999) Prognostic significance of c-erbB-2 protein expression in carcinoma of the cervix treated with radiotherapy. J Cancer Res Clin Oncol 125:96-100
Nuyts S, Van Mellaert L, Theys J et al (2002) Clostridium spores for tumor-specific drug delivery. Anticancer Drugs 13:115-125
Oehler MK, Caffier H (2000) Prognostic relevance of serum vascular endothelial growth factor in ovarian cancer. Anticancer Res 20:5109-5112
Ohno T, Nakano T, Niibe Y, Tsujii H, Oka K (1998) Bax protein expression correlates with radiation-induced apoptosis in radiation therapy for cervical carcinoma. Cancer 83:103-110
Olive PL, Aquino-Parsons C, MacPhail SH et al (2001) Carbonic anhydrase 9 as an endogenous marker for hypoxic cells in cervical cancer. Cancer Res 61:8924-8929
Owens OJ, Stewart C, Leake RE, McNicol AM (1992) A comparison of biochemical and immunohistochemical assessment of EGFR expression in ovarian cancer. Anticancer Res 12:1455-1458
Patterson AV, Williams KJ, Cowen RL et al (2002) Oxygen-sensitive enzyme-prodrug gene therapy for the eradication of radiation-resistant solid tumours. Gene Ther 9:946-954
Peng D (2001) Epidermal growth factor: a potential target for cancer therapy. Fellow Reporter 6:31-34
Pfeiffer D, Stellwag B, Pfeiffer A et al (1989) Clinical implications of the epidermal growth factor receptor in the squamous cell carcinoma of the uterine cervix. Gynecol Oncol 33:146-150
Pfeiffer D, Kimmig R, Herrmann J et al (1998) Epidermal-growth-factor receptor correlates negatively with cell density in cervical squamous epithelium and is down-regulated in cancers of the human uterus. Int J Cancer 79:49-55
Robert F, Ezekiel MP, Spencer SA et al (2001) Phase I study of anti-epidermal growth factor receptor antibody cetuximab in combination with radiation therapy in patients with advanced head and neck cancer. J Clin Oncol 19:3234-3243
Ross JS, Yang F, Kallakury BV et al (1999) HER-2/neu oncogene amplification by fluorescence in situ hybridization in epithelial tumors of the ovary. See comments. Am J Clin Pathol 111:299-301; 10078102, comment in: Am J Clin Pathol 2000, 113:905-906; 10874893. Am J Clin Pathol 1999, 111:311-316
Ryu HS, Chang KH, Yang HW et al (2000) High cyclooxygenase-2 expression in stage IB cervical cancer with lymph node metastasis or parametrial invasion. Gynecol Oncol 76:320-325
Saleh MN, Raisch KP, Stackhouse MA et al (1999) Combined modality therapy of A431 human epidermoid cancer using anti-EGFr antibody C225 and radiation. Cancer Biother Radiopharm 14:451-463
Salvesen HB, Akslen LA (1999) Significance of tumour-associated macrophages, vascular endothelial growth factor and thrombospondin-1 expression for tumour angiogenesis and prognosis in endometrial carcinomas. Int J Cancer 84:538-543
Sartor CI (2000) Biological modifiers as potential radiosensitizers: targeting the epidermal growth factor receptor family. Semin Oncol 27 [Suppl 11]:15-20; discussion 92-100
Sato JD, Kawamoto T, Le AD et al (1983) Biological effects in vitro of monoclonal antibodies to human epidermal growth factor receptors. Mol Biol Med 1:511-529
Scambia G, Ferrandina G, Distefano M et al (1998) Epidermal growth factor receptor (EGFR) is not related to the prognosis of cervical cancer. Cancer Lett 123:135-139
Sewell JM, Macleod KG, Ritchie A et al (2002) Targeting the EGF receptor in ovarian cancer with the tyrosine kinase inhibitor ZD 1839 ("Iressa"). Br J Cancer 86:456-462
Shen GH, Ghazizadeh M, Kawanami O et al (2000) Prognostic significance of vascular endothelial growth factor expression in human ovarian carcinoma. Br J Cancer 83:196-203
Sheridan MT, West CM, Cooper RA et al (2000) Pretreatment apoptosis in carcinoma of the cervix correlates with changes in tumour oxygenation during radiotherapy. Br J Cancer 82:1177-1182
Shibata T, Giaccia AJ, Brown JM (2002) Hypoxia-inducible regulation of a prodrug-activating enzyme for tumor-specific gene therapy. Neoplasia 4:40-48
Shin DM, Donato NJ, Perez-Soler R et al (2001) Epidermal growth factor receptor-targeted therapy with C225 and cisplatin in patients with head and neck cancer. Clin Cancer Res 7:1204-1213
Skirnisdottir I, Sorbe B, Seidal T (2001) The growth factor receptors HER-2/neu and EGFR, their relationship, and their effects on the prognosis in early stage (FIGO I-II) epithelial ovarian carcinoma. Int J Gynecol Cancer 11:119-129
Tempfer C, Obermair A, Hefler L et al (1998) Vascular endothelial growth factor serum concentrations in ovarian cancer. Obstet Gynecol 92:360-363
Tervahauta A, Syrjanen S, Syrjanen K (1994) Epidermal growth factor receptor, c-erbB-2 proto-oncogene and estrogen receptor expression in human papillomavirus lesions of the uterine cervix. Int J Gynecol Pathol 13:234-240
Tjalma WA, Weyler JJ, Bogers JJ et al (2001) The importance of biological factors (bcl-2, bax, p53, PCNA, MI, HPV and angiogenesis) in invasive cervical cancer. Eur J Obstet Gynecol Reprod Biol 97:223-230
Tucker ON, Dannenberg AJ, Yang EK et al (1999) Cyclooxygenase-2 expression is up-regulated in human pancreatic cancer. Cancer Res 59:987-990
Vukovic V, Haugland HK, Nicklee T et al (2001) Hypoxia-inducible factor-1alpha is an intrinsic marker for hypoxia in cervical cancer xenografts. Cancer Res 61:7394-7398
Walenta S, Wetterling M, Lehrke M et al (2000) High lactate levels predict likelihood of metastases, tumor recurrence, and restricted patient survival in human cervical cancers. Cancer Res 60:916-921
Wu X, Xin Y, Yao J et al (2001) Expression of epithelial growth factor receptor and its two ligands, transforming growth factor-alpha and epithelial growth factor, in normal and neoplastic squamous cells in the vulva: an immunohistochemical study. Med Electron Microsc 34:179-184
Xu L, Yoneda J, Herrera C et al (2000) Inhibition of malignant ascites and growth of human ovarian carcinoma by oral administration of a potent inhibitor of the vascular endothelial growth factor receptor tyrosine kinases. Int J Oncol 16:445-454
Yarden Y (2001) The EGFR family and its ligands in human

cancer. Signalling mechanisms and therapeutic opportunities. Eur J Cancer 37 [Suppl 4]:S3–S8

Yokoyama Y, Sato S, Futagami M et al (2000) Prognostic significance of vascular endothelial growth factor and its receptors in endometrial carcinoma. Gynecol Oncol 77:413–418

Yoshida K, Hosoya Y, Sumi S et al (1997) Studies of the expression of epidermal growth factor receptor in human renal cell carcinoma: a comparison of immunohistochemical method versus ligand binding assay. Oncology 54:220–225

Yoshimura R, Sano H, Masuda C et al (2000) Expression of cyclooxygenase-2 in prostate carcinoma. Cancer 89:589–596

11 Growth Factor Expression in Central Nervous System Tumours

C. Nieder, N. Andratschke and J. Schlegel

CONTENTS

11.1 Introduction 139
11.2 Activation of Oncogenes and Role of Related Growth Factors 140
11.3 Targeting the Tumour Angiogenesis 140
11.4 Growth Factors in Astrocytic and Oligodendroglial Gliomas 141
11.5 Growth Factors in Ependymomas 141
11.6 Growth Factors in Meningeomas 142
11.7 Growth Factors in Pituitary Adenomas 142
11.8 Growth Factors in Medulloblastomas 142
11.9 Growth Factors in Vestibular Nerve Schwannomas 142
11.10 Summary and Discussion 143
11.11 Perspectives 143
References 144

11.1 Introduction

Central nervous system (CNS) tumour pathogenesis probably is a multi-step process in which tumour suppressor gene inactivation and oncogene activation and overexpression play a part, along with alterations in cell cycle progression, abnormalities in signal transduction pathways, glial cell invasion, and angiogenesis (Nagane et al. 1997; Ueki et al. 2002). The role of growth factors in this process has increasingly been studied over the last few years. This chapter summarizes the available data, usually derived from adult patients, and discusses their limitations as well as their potential influence on future therapeutic strategies. One of the most common types of brain tumours, malignant gliomas, may arise via a number of apparently distinct molecular pathways, illustrated in Table 11.1. For example, glioblastoma multiforme (GBM) can be divided into at least two distinct genetic subsets: those characterized by *p53* mutations and allelic loss of chromosome *17p* in the absence of epidermal growth factor receptor (*EGFR*) gene amplification, and those with *EGFR* gene amplification but no *p53* mutations or chromosome *17p* loss. Tumours with *p53* mutations occur primarily in younger patients and those with *EGFR* gene amplification arise primarily in older patients (Louis 1996). Molecular classification of gliomas is a major challenge in the effort to improve therapeutic decisions.

C. Nieder, MD
Department of Radiation Oncology, Klinikum rechts der Isar, Technical University Munich, Ismaninger Strasse 22, 81675 Munich, Germany
N. Andratschke, MD
Department of Experimental Radiation Oncology, The University of Texas M.D. Anderson Cancer Center, Box 66, 1515 Holcombe Blvd., Houston, TX 77030, USA
J. Schlegel, MD
Department of Pathology, Klinikum rechts der Isar, Technical University Munich, Ismaninger Strasse 22, 81675 Munich, Germany

Table 11.1. Simplified scheme of genetic events in the development of gliomas

Oncogenes and growth factors	Astrocyte ↓	Tumour suppressor genes and cell cycle regulators
	↓	LOH 17 p (p53), LOH 10q (*DMBT1*)
	Grade II astrocytoma	
EGFR	↓	LOH 9q (p15, p16), LOH 13q (pRb)
MDM2	↓	LOH 19q, LOH 18q (*DCC*)
PDGF, bFGF, VEGF	↓	CDK-4, cyclin D-1, p27^{Kip1}
	Anaplastic astrocytoma	
TGF-β	↓	LOH 10q (*MMAC/PTEN*)
	Glioblastoma multiforme	

LOH, loss of heterozygosity; *EGFR*, epidermal growth factor receptor; *PDGF*, platelet-derived growth factor; *bFGF*, basic fibroblast growth factor; *VEGF*, vascular endothelial growth factor; *CDK-4*, cyclin-dependent kinase-4; *TGF-β*, transforming growth factor-b. From Andratschke et al. (2001), with permission

11.2
Activation of Oncogenes and Role of Related Growth Factors

In human primary GBM, amplification of the *EGFR* gene coding for the EGF receptor on chromosome *7p* can be observed in approximately 40% of patients (Hiesiger et al. 1993; Schlegel et al. 1994a; Zhu et al. 1996). The rate appears to be lower in anaplastic astrocytomas (Smith et al. 2001). The *EGFR* gene was first identified as the homologous cellular gene to the viral *v-erbB* oncogene of avian erythroblastosis virus and belongs to the ERBB family of receptor tyrosine kinases (RTK). Normal signal transduction by RTKs is mediated after ligand binding through receptor oligomerization and consecutive transphosphorylation. After binding of its cognate ligands EGF or transforming growth factor α (TGF-α), different *EGFR*-dependent intracellular pathways, including the mitogen-activated protein (MAP) kinase cascade and the phosphatidyinositol-3'-kinase pathway, are activated. *EGFR* overexpression in GBM may be associated with more aggressive clinical behaviour and treatment resistance (Hiesiger et al. 1993; Schlegel et al. 1994b; Barker et al. 2001; Chakravarti et al. 2001; Muracciole et al. 2002), especially in *p53* wild type cases (Simmons et al. 2001). Numerous strategies are currently being investigated to specifically inhibit the overexpression and activation of the EGF receptor, using tyrosine kinase inhibitors, antibodies, immunoconjugates, or antisense technology.

Transforming growth factor β (TGF-β) apparently plays a physiological role (termination of the glial proliferative response to injury and/or cytokine-induced stimulation) within the brain (Jennings and Pietenpol 1998). However, this inhibitory role is converted to that of a progression factor among GBM, where platelet-derived growth factor (PDGF) serves as the principal mediator of TGF-β's growth stimulatory effect. The exact mechanism of conversion, which might involve the loss of a putative tumour suppressor gene, which mediates TGF-β's inhibition of growth, or the enhancement of an active oncogenic pathway, remains to be determined. Dhandapani et al. suggested that basic fibroblast growth factor (bFGF) can induce the release of TGF-β1 from C6 glioma cells, but not from rat cortical astrocytes in vitro (Dhandapani et al. 2002). A different study reported that TGF-β induces the expression of matrix metalloproteinase-2, thus promoting glioma invasion (Wick et al. 2001). Experimental therapeutic strategies against TGF-β have been reported already (Fakhrai et al. 1996). A recent study in 28 patients with GBM did not find a correlation between plasma TGF-β and survival (Hulshof et al. 2001).

Insulin-like growth factor-1 (IGF-1) is crucially involved in normal growth and development, but can also function as a growth factor in a variety of tumours such as gliomas. Inhibition of IGF-1 expression has been shown to enhance immune response and subcutaneous injection of IGF-1 antisense-transfected C6 glioma cells induced the regression of pre-established wild type gliomas in a rat model (Trojan et al. 1993). Recently, a pilot study of anti-sense oligodeoxynucleotide directed against the IGF-1 receptor was reported. Ex vivo treatment of autologous glioma cells induced apoptosis and a host response. Among 12 patients with malignant astrocytomas, 8 responded for 2–27 weeks (Andrews et al. 2001).

Overexpression of another important growth factor receptor (platelet-derived growth factor receptor α, PDGFR-α) appears to be an early event in glioma pathogenesis and is present in most grades of tumours (Bogler et al. 1995). Up-regulation of PDGF (existing in three isoforms: AA, AB, BB) has also been described, especially in endothelial cells localized specifically within the tumour. PDGFR-α exhibits high affinity to both the A and B chains of PDGF, whereas the β receptor exclusively binds to the PDGF-B chain (PDGF-B is encoded by the *c-sis* gene). Accumulating evidence suggests an important role of PDGF ligands and receptors in the vascularization of gliomas (Morrison 1999). Thus, inhibition of signal transduction could influence tumour progression.

Up-regulation of vascular endothelial growth factor (VEGF) transcription is frequently found in human brain tumours and probably regulated by both tissue hypoxia and acidic pH (Fukumura et al. 2001). VEGF has also been associated with brain oedema, because it can increase vascular permeability (Bjerkvig et al. 1997). Van der Valk et al. (1997) examined 86 gliomas: the higher the grade, the more growth factors and the more positive cells were found.

11.3
Targeting the Tumour Angiogenesis

Angiogenesis is a fundamental process of tumour growth. Through complex mechanisms of autocrine and paracrine stimulation, the growth and invasiveness of GBM depends on vascular neoformation, promoted by, for example, PDGF, bFGF, and VEGF

(PLATE and RISAU 1995). Antisense-mediated inactivation of VEGF effectively inhibited angiogenesis and tumorigenesis of GBM cells (SALEH et al. 1996). VEGF monoclonal antibodies inhibited growth of GBM in nude mice when administered either at the time of tumour inoculum or after tumour was established (KIM et al. 1993). The density of vessels was decreased in antibody-treated tumours and the magnitude of response was greater in more rapidly proliferating, more angiogenesis-dependent tumours (KIM et al. 1993). In addition, GBM contains both tumour cells and blood vessels which are relatively resistant to radiotherapy. Blocking the binding of VEGF to its receptor Flk-1 on the tumour endothelium by administration of receptor antagonists might revert GBM tumour models to a radiation-sensitive phenotype (GENG et al. 2001). Further in-vitro data suggest that inhibition of the FGF signalling pathways may also represent a promising therapeutic strategy (AUGUSTE et al. 2001).

11.4
Growth Factors in Astrocytic and Oligodendroglial Gliomas

PDGF-related genes are rarely amplified in astrocytomas in contrast to the more common EGF-receptor amplification found in high-grade tumours (SMITH et al. 2000). Yet their products are often overexpressed. Most astrocytoma cell lines and resection specimens overexpress at least one PDGF chain and its respective receptor. In surgical specimens, all malignant astrocytomas, and to a lesser extent low-grade astrocytomas, overexpressed PDGF-A and PDGFR-α as compared to normal glia. PDGF-B and PDGFR-β were also present in most of the tumours (GUHA et al. 1995). A different study identified PDGFR-β transcripts in 24 out of 29 gliomas (83%), with higher levels in glioblastomas compared to lower-grade astrocytomas (MAURO et al. 1991). Some authors reported preferential expression of PDGF-AA and PDGFR-α in tumour cells and of PDGF-BB and PDGFR-β in proliferating endothelial cells within the tumour. Accumulating evidence suggests that PDGF autocrine loops represent an early event in the pathogenesis of malignant astrocytomas.

The majority of astrocytomas appear immunoreactive for VEGF, for example, 77% in the series by NISHIKAWA et al. (1999). OEHRING et al. presented immunohistochemical data on VEGF expression in a larger series of 162 astrocytomas. Grade II astrocytomas expressed VEGF in 37%, grade III tumours in 67%, and glioblastomas in 64%. VEGF was not an independent prognostic factor for survival in multivariate analysis (OEHRING et al. 1999). Comparable results were found in 91 oligodendrogliomas, where VEGF expression correlated with survival in univariate analysis only, because of its dependence on histological grade (KORSHUNOV and GOLANOV 2000). In a different study, however, oligodendrogliomas and the oligodendroglial component of mixed gliomas showed no VEGF immunoreactivity at all (PIETSCH et al. 1997). ABDULRAUF et al. (1998) investigated 74 adult patients with supratentorial fibrillary low-grade astrocytoma. Immunoreactivity for VEGF was correlated with shorter survival in uni- and multivariate analyses (5.3 vs 11.2 years) and with a greater chance of malignant transformation. Microvessel density also influenced survival. In contrast, bFGF and EGF were not correlated with either of these endpoints.

FRIEND et al. examined a panel of five immortalized glioma cell lines. All of these expressed mRNA for growth hormone (GH) receptor and IGF-1 receptor. Two expressed IGF-2 receptor, yet none of them was positive for either IGF-1 or IGF-2. IGF-1 stimulated mitogenesis (measured by (3)H-thymidine uptake) in two cell lines (FRIEND et al. 2001). Data from 39 human glioma showed that expression of IGF-1 and IGF-1R correlated with histopathological grade and Ki-67 indices. Increased levels were also found in reactive astrocytes at the tumour margins (HIRANO et al. 1999). Interesting data suggest that besides growth factors, the plasminogen activator system might be useful to characterize subgroups of glioma patients with different prognoses, adding information to features such as histological grade and necrosis. In this study of 59 patients, low levels of plasminogen activator inhibitor type 1 (PAI-1) characterized patients with favourable survival despite of high-grade tumours (MURACCIOLE et al. 2002).

11.5
Growth Factors in Ependymomas

Recent data indicate that polypeptide growth factor and receptor expression might also contribute to ependymoma tumorigenesis. Expression of the EGF receptor is a constant feature in the majority of ependymal tumours (HALL et al. 1990). Most interestingly, it has been shown recently that EGF receptor expression in ependymomas seems to correlate with activation of the anti-apoptotic PI3K pathway rather than the proliferative MAPK cascade (HERZOG and SCHLEGEL 2001). One small series of five ependymomas also reported expression of each PDGF isoform and receptor in all cases (BLACK et al. 1996).

11.6
Growth Factors in Meningeomas

NAGASHIMA et al. (2001) showed that more than 80% of meningeomas expressed PDGF-BB protein and c-sis mRNA, regardless of the histological grade. The expression of PDGF and its receptors was evaluated by immunohistochemistry and in situ hybridization in another series of 61 meningeomas. Almost all expressed PDGF-BB and PDGFR-β, with higher intensity in atypical meningeomas. There was also a correlation between the proliferative activity, measured by proliferating cell nuclear antigen labelling index, and the overexpression of PDGF-BB and PDGFR-β. PDGF-AA was demonstrated in 49%. Only two tumours expressed PDGFR-α (YANG and XU 2001). Virtually all meningeoma samples examined by BLACK et al. expressed PDGFR-β as well as PDGF-A and PDGF-B chain mRNA. Cells from 10 human meningeoma incubated with PDGF-BB responded with a significant growth-stimulating effect (BLACK et al. 1994).

CHRISTOV et al. studied the expression of vascular permeability factor (VPF)/VEGF in 60 meningeomas. Thirty of these were further evaluated for flt-1 expression. VPF/VEGF immunoreactivity was mainly observed in vessel endothelium and in a total of 65% of tumours (CHRISTOV et al. 1999). An even higher rate of 15 of 19 cases (79%) was recorded by NISHIKAWA et al. (1999). A different group of authors reported a significant correlation between meningeoma grade and VEGF content in 69 human tumours. Atypical meningeomas had twofold higher, malignant meningeomas 10-fold higher content than benign meningeomas. VEGF did not correlate with vascularity or invasiveness. Contradictory data, i.e. lack of correlation between VEGF expression and grade of malignancy, have also been published (PIETSCH et al. 1997).

BFGF, hepatocyte growth factor/scatter factor and placenta growth factor did not show any association with one of these three tumour features. Endothelial chemotaxis and capillary-like tube formation in vitro were induced by meningeoma extracts and were most effectively blocked by addition of antibodies against bFGF, followed by VEGF-antibodies (LAMSZUS et al. 2000). Expression of members of the ERBB family of RTKs seems to play an important role in meningeoma tumorigenesis. It has been shown that the EGF receptor is expressed in the majority of meningeomas and that high expression might correlate with a more aggressive growth behaviour and higher recurrence rates. It has also been shown that the ERBB2 receptor (also known as HER2 or NEU) is constitutively expressed in human meningeomas (SCHLEGEL et al. 1993).

11.7
Growth Factors in Pituitary Adenomas

We identified two studies, one restricted to the role of PDGF and one to VEGF. All 34 pituitary adenomas investigated by Northern blot analysis expressed the PDGF-A and -B subunits. Ninety-four per cent expressed PDGFR-β and 44% expressed PDGFR-α (LEON et al. 1994). The normal anterior pituitary expressed all of the PDGF subunits and receptor subunits as well, indicating that PDGF does not play a pathophysiological role in pituitary adenomas. All 15 pituitary adenomas studied by NISHIKAWA et al. (1999) expressed VEGF.

11.8
Growth Factors in Medulloblastomas

In one study, medulloblastomas expressed predominantly PDGFR-α (SMITS et al. 1996). Another one, however, detected just transcripts for PDGFR-β and the PDGF-A ligand (BLACK et al. 1996). The literature did not contain further studies for review.

11.9
Growth Factors in Vestibular Nerve Schwannomas

Obviously, the expression of growth factors and their receptors has not been studied systematically yet. Cell cultures from nine vestibular nerve schwannomas were examined for the effects of TGF-β and bFGF on DNA synthesis. TGF-β but not bFGF stimulated DNA synthesis. A combination of both growth factors resulted in a much greater mitogenic response than produced by TGF-β alone (WEERDA et al. 1998).

One of the most stimulating findings in experimental tumorigenesis of the nervous system was the discovery of the *neu* oncogene. It is the rat homologue of the human *ErbB2* gene (also called *c-neu* or *HER-2*) and was first identified by gene transfer experiments in chemically induced Schwann cell tumours of BD-IX rats (SCHECHTER et al. 1984). The *neu* gene encodes a RTK which is structurally related to the EGF receptor. In experimental neurinomas the neu gene becomes activated to a dominant oncogene by a single T→A transversion in the coding region of the transmembrane domain of the receptor molecule, which is invariably detected in rat schwannomas both in vivo and in vitro (NIKITIN et al. 1991). An amino acid substitution of glutamic acid for valine (V664E) in the NEU protein caused by the point mutation is thought to be responsible for stable oligomerization of receptor complexes. Receptor oligomers containing mutated NEU proteins exhibit constitutive phosphorylation indicating receptor activation. Not only mutation but also overexpression of a structurally unaltered but highly expressed copy of the human *ErbB2* gene transfected into NIH3T3 cells caused their malignant transformation. Interestingly, the transformed phenotype of cells carrying *ErbB2/ neu* genes activated by mutation or overexpression is invariably associated with receptor activation. In human Schwann cell tumours, a constitutive expression of ERBB2 receptors has also been shown (SCHLEGEL et al. 1998).

11.10
Summary and Discussion

In GBM, amplification of the *EGFR* gene can be observed in approximately 40% of patients. After binding of its cognate ligands EGF or TGF-a, different EGFR-dependent intracellular pathways, including the MAP kinase cascade and the PI-3-K pathway, are activated. *EGFR* overexpression in GBM may be associated with more aggressive clinical behaviour and treatment resistance. Accumulating experimental and clinical evidence suggests an important role of PDGF and VEGF ligands and receptors in the vascularization of several brain tumour types. Through complex mechanisms of autocrine and paracrine stimulation, the growth and invasiveness of, for example, GBM depends on vascular neoformation, promoted by growth factors. Overexpression of an important growth factor receptor (PDGFR-α) appears to be an early event in glioma pathogenesis and is present in most grades of tumours (BOGLER et al. 1995). Up-regulation of PDGF has also been described, not only in tumour but also in endothelial cells localized specifically within the tumour (KIRSCH et al. 1997). At least 60%–80% of astrocytic gliomas overexpress PDGF or VEGF. Whether one of these factors independently influences survival can not be judged at this time. In the light of conflicting results, further research on this subject is needed.

At least 80% of meningeomas express some form of PDGF, whereas 65%–80% express VEGF. Data on correlation with histological grading are contradictory. Expression of members of the ERBB family of RTKs seems to play an important role in meningeoma tumorigenesis. It has been shown that the EGF receptor is expressed in the majority of meningeomas and that high expression might correlate with a more aggressive growth behaviour. Pituitary adenoma show immunostaining for either PDGF or VEGF ligands or receptors in all cases. Very limited data exist on different other types of brain tumours, precluding any definitive statement.

It must be noted that techniques for assessing the expression of growth factors and their receptors vary widely. The most common technique used is immunohistochemistry. However, different methods have been reported, including non-uniform cut-off values, etc. Therefore, results may vary because of different antibodies, variations in incubation and antigen fixation techniques, and subjectivity in scoring. Ideally, especially when examining prognostic factors, future studies should involve large numbers of specimens derived from patients treated with identical regimens. The method of assessment should be as reproducible and accurate as possible.

11.11
Perspectives

Recent experimental data indicate that inhibition of the VEGF, FGF, and IGF-1 signalling pathways may represent promising therapeutic strategies. Some inhibitory agents have now entered clinical trials. It is, however, interesting to note that the same growth factors, i.e. PDGF, bFGF, VEGF, and IGF-1, appear promising for prevention of radiation-induced normal tissue damage (NIEDER et al. 1999, 2002a). Studies have consistently described that administration of growth factors concomitant to radiotherapy (CNS and other tissues) yielded better results than delayed treatment (DING et al. 1996; OKUNIEFF et al.

1998; Pena et al. 2000; Paris et al. 2001; Nieder et al. 2002a, b). In conjunction with single-dose radiotherapy, e.g. radiosurgery, growth factor administration would last approximately 48 h. A drawback of concomitant growth factor treatment might be exposure of malignant tumours which are to be sterilized effectively by radiotherapy. If administration of growth factors protects tumour cells and normal tissues to a comparable degree, no therapeutic gain can be obtained.

Data regarding the effect of short-term growth factor treatment on established macroscopic tumours are scarce. Ding et al. used three different mouse tumour models (sarcoma and squamous cell carcinoma) to evaluate the impact of intravenous bFGF on tumour growth and radiosensitivity. Their data did not support the hypothesis that bFGF treatment of these transplanted tumours immediately before radiotherapy might have a detrimental effect on tumour growth and radiation-induced tumour growth delay (Ding et al. 1996). Yet CNS tumours have not been studied so far. Black et al. (1994) published in vitro results of growth stimulation of meningeoma cells exposed to PDGF. Cultures contained 1, 3, or 6 ng/ml of PDGF-BB for 48 h. A concentration of 3 ng/ml led to a maximum stimulation of cell division. However, since 1/3 of the tumours were stimulated by PDGF and all but one expressed PDGFR-β, the relationship of stimulation by PDGF-BB to receptor expression is not uniform. Certainly, more experimental data need to be generated before an alternative therapeutic strategy of radiotherapy dose escalation with administration of growth factors for the purpose of CNS protection can be considered.

References

Abdulrauf SI, Edvardsen K, Ho KL et al (1998) Vascular endothelial growth factor expression and vascular density as prognostic markers of survival in patients with low-grade astrocytoma. J Neurosurg 88:513–520

Andratschke N, Grosu AL, Molls M et al (2001) Perspectives in the treatment of malignant gliomas in adults. Anticancer Res 21:3541–3550

Andrews DW, Resnicoff M, Flanders AE et al (2001) Results of a pilot study involving the use of an antisense oligodeoxynucleotide directed against the insulin-like growth factor type I receptor in malignant astrocytomas. J Clin Oncol 19:2189–2200

Auguste P, Gursel DB, Lemiere S et al (2001) Inhibition of fibroblast growth factor/fibroblast growth factor receptor activity in glioma cells impedes tumor growth by both angiogenesis-dependent and -independent mechanisms. Cancer Res 61:1717–1726

Barker FG Jr, Simmons ML, Chang SM et al (2001) EGFR overexpression and radiation response in glioblastoma multiforme. Int J Radiat Oncol Biol Phys 51:410–418

Bjerkvig R, Lund-Johansen M, Edvardsen K (1997) Tumor cell invasion and angiogenesis in the central nervous system. Curr Opin Oncol 9:223–229

Black PM, Carroll R, Glowacka D et al (1994) Platelet-derived growth factor expression and stimulation in human meningeomas. J Neurosurg 81:388–393

Black P, Carroll RS, Glowacka D (1996) Expression of platelet-derived growth factor transcripts in medulloblastomas and ependymomas. Pediatr Neurosurg 24:74–78

Bogler O, Huang HJ, Kleihues P et al (1995) The p53 gene and its role in human brain tumors. Glia 15:308–327

Chakravarti A, Delaney MA, Noll E et al (2001) Prognostic and pathologic significance of quantitative protein expression profiling in human gliomas. Clin Cancer Res 7:2387–2395

Christov C, Lechapt-Zalcman E, Adle-Biassette H et al (1999) Vascular permeability factor/vascular endothelial growth factor (VPF/VEGF) and its receptor flt-1 in microcystic meningiomas. Acta Neuropathol (Berl) 98:414–420

Dhandapani KM, Wade MF, Mahesh VB et al (2002) Basic fibroblast growth factor induces TGF-beta release in an isoform and glioma-specific manner. Neuroreport 13:239–241

Ding I, Huang K, Snyder ML et al (1996) Tumor growth and radiosensitivity in mice given myeloprotective doses of fibroblast growth factors. J Natl Cancer Inst 88:1399–1404

Fakhrai H, Dorigo O, Shawler DL et al (1996) Eradication of established intracranial rat gliomas by transforming growth factor β antisense gene therapy. Proc Natl Acad Sci U S A 93:2909–2914

Friend KE, Khandwala HM, Flyvbjerg A et al (2001) Growth hormone and insulin-like growth factor-1: effects on the growth of glioma cell lines. Growth Horm IGF Res 11:84–91

Fukumura D, Xu L, Chen Y et al (2001) Hypoxia and acidosis independently up-regulate vascular endothelial growth factor transcription in brain tumours in vivo. Cancer Res 61:6020–6024

Geng L, Donnelly E, McMahon G et al (2001) Inhibition of vascular endothelial growth factor receptor signaling leads to reversal of tumor resistance to radiotherapy. Cancer Res 61:2413–2419

Guha A, Dashner K, Black PM et al (1995) Expression of PDGF and PDGF receptors in human astrocytoma operation specimens supports the existence of an autocrine loop. Int J Cancer 60:168–173

Hall WA, Merrill MJ, Walbridge S et al (1990) Epidermal growth factor receptors on ependymomas and other brain tumors. J Neurosurg 72:641–646

Herzog C, Schlegel J (2001) EGF receptor mediated signaling pathways in human ependymomas (abstract). Acta Neuropathol (Wien) 102:527

Hiesiger EM, Hayes RL, Pierz DM et al (1993) Prognostic relevance of epidermal growth factor receptor and c-neu/erbB2 expression in glioblastomas. J Neurooncol 16:93–104

Hirano H, Lopes MB, Laws ER et al (1999) Insulin-like growth factor-1 content and pattern of expression correlates with histopathologic grade in diffusely infiltrating astrocytomas. Neurooncology 1:109–119

Hulshof MC, Sminia P, Barten-van Rijbroek AD et al (2001) Prognostic value of plasma transforming growth factor-

beta in patients with glioblastoma multiforme. Oncol Rep 8:1107–1110
Jennings MT, Pietenpol JA (1998) The role of transforming growth factor β in glioma progression. J Neurooncol 36:123–140
Kim KJ, Li B, Winer J et al (1993) Inhibition of vascular endothelial growth factor-induced angiogenesis suppresses tumour growth in vivo. Nature 362:841–844
Kirsch M, Wilson JC, Black P (1997) Platelet-derived growth factor in human brain tumors. J Neurooncol 35:289–301
Korshunov A, Golanov A (2000) The prognostic significance of vascular endothelial growth factor immunoexpression in oligodendroglioma. J Neurooncol 48:13–19
Lamszus K, Lengler U, Schmidt NO et al (2000) Vascular endothelial growth factor, hepatocyte growth factor/scatter factor, basic fibroblast growth factor, and placenta growth factor in human menigeomas and their relation to angiogenesis and malignancy. Neurosurgery 46:938–947
Leon SP, Carroll RS, Dashner K et al (1994) Messenger ribonucleic acid expression of platelet-derived growth factor subunits and receptors in pituitary adenomas. J Clin Endocrinol Metab 79:51–55
Louis DN (1996) Clinicopatho-genetic subsets of glioblastoma multiforme: from both sides now (editorial). Brain Pathol 6:223–224
Mauro A, Bulfone A, Turco E et al (1991) Coexpression of platelet-derived growth factor (PDGF) B chain and PDGF B-type receptor in human gliomas. Childs Nerv Syst 7:432–436
Morrison RS (1999) Growth factor-mediated signaling pathways. In: Berger MS, Wilson CB (eds) The gliomas. Saunders, Philadelphia, pp 52–63
Muracciole X, Romain S, Dufour H et al (2002) PAI-1 and EGFR expression in adult glioma tumors: toward a molecular prognostic classification. Int J Radiat Oncol Biol Phys 52:592–598
Nagane M, Huang HJ, Cavenee WK (1997) Advances in the molecular genetics of gliomas. Curr Opin Oncol 9:215–222
Nagashima G, Aoyagi M, Yamamoto S et al (2001) Involvement of disregulated c myc but not c sis/PDGF in atypical and anaplastic meningeomas. Clin Neurol Neurosurg 103:13–18
Nieder C, Ataman F, Price RE et al (1999) Radiation myelopathy: new perspective on an old problem. Radiat Oncol Invest 7:193–203
Nieder C, Price RE, Rivera B et al (2002a) Experimental data for insulin-like growth factor-1 and basic fibroblast growth factor in prevention of radiation myelopathy (in German). Strahlenther Onkol 178:147–152
Nieder C, Andratschke N, Price RE et al (2002b) Innovative prevention strategies for radiation necrosis of the central nervous system. Anticancer Res 22:1017–1023
Nishikawa R, Cheng SY, Nagashima R et al (1999) Expression of vascular endothelial growth factor in human brain tumors. Acta Neuropathol (Berl) 97:429–432
Nikitin AYU, Ballering LA, Lyons J, Rajewsky MF (1991) Early mutation of the neu (erbB-2) gene during ethylnitrosourea-induced oncogenesis in the rat Schwann cell lineage. Proc Natl Acad Sci U S A 88:9939–9943
Oehring RD, Miletic M, Valter MM et al (1999) Vascular endothelial growth factor in astrocytic gliomas – a prognostic factor? J Neurooncol 45:117–125
Okunieff P, Mester M, Wang J et al (1998) In vivo radioprotective effects of angiogenic growth factors on the small bowel of C3H mice. Radiat Res 150:204–211
Paris F, Fuks Z, Kang A et al (2001) Endothelial apoptosis as the primary lesion initiating intestinal radiation damage in mice. Science 293:293–297
Pena LA, Fuks Z, Kolesnick RN (2000) Radiation-induced apoptosis of endothelial cells in the murine central nervous system: protection by fibroblast growth factor and sphingomyelinase deficiency. Cancer Res 60:321–327
Pietsch T, Valter MM, Wolf HK et al (1997) Expression and distribution of vascular endothelial growth factor protein in human brain tumors. Acta Neuropathol (Berl) 93:109–117
Plate K, Risau W (1995) Angiogenesis in malignant glioma. Glia 15:339–347
Saleh M, Stacker SA, Wilks AF (1996) Inhibition of growth of C6 glioma cells in vivo by expression of antisense vascular endothelial growth factor sequence. Cancer Res 56:393–401
Schechter AL, Stern DF, Vaidyanathan L, Decker SJ, Drebin JA, Greene MI, Weinberg RA (1984) The neu oncogene: an erb-B-related gene encoding a 185,000-Mr tumour antigen. Nature 312:513–516
Schlegel J, Ullrich B, Stumm G et al (1993) Expression of the c-erbB-2 encoded oncoprotein and progesterone receptor in human meningioma. Acta Neuropathol (Berl) 86:474–479
Schlegel J, Stumm G, Brändle K et al (1994a) Amplification and differential expression of oncogenes of the erbB-gene family in human glioblastoma. J Neurooncol 2:201–207
Schlegel J, Merdes A, Stumm G et al (1994b) Amplification of the epidermal growth factor receptor gene correlates with different growth behaviour in human glioblastoma. Int J Cancer 56:72–77
Schlegel J, Muenkel K, Trenkle T et al (1998) Expression of the ERBB2/neu and neurofibromatosis type 1 gene products in reactive and neoplastic Schwann cell proliferation. Int J Oncol 13:1281–1284
Simmons ML. Lamborn KR, Takahashi M et al (2001) Analysis of complex relationships between age, p53, epidermal growth factor receptor, and survival in glioblastoma patients. Cancer Res 61:1122–1128
Smith JS, Wang XY, Qian J et al (2000) Amplification of the platelet-derived growth factor receptor-A (PDGFRA) gene occurs in oligodendrogliomas with grade IV anaplastic features. J Neuropathol Exp Neurol 59:495–503
Smith JS, Tachibana I, Passe SM et al (2001) PTEN mutation, EGFR amplification, and outcome in patients with anaplastic astrocytoma and glioblastoma multiforme. J Natl Cancer Inst 93:1246–1256
Smits A, van Grieken D, Hartman M et al (1996) Coexpression of platelet-derived growth factor alpha and beta receptors on medulloblastomas and other primitive neuroectodermal tumors is consistent with an immature stem cell and neuronal derivation. Lab Invest 74:188–198
Trojan J, Johnson TR, Rudin SD et al (1993) Treatment and prevention of rat glioblastoma by immunogenic C6 cells expressing antisense insulin-like growth factor-1 RNA. Science 259:94–97
Ueki K, Nishikawa R, Nakazato Y et al (2002) Correlation of histology and molecular genetic analysis of 1p, 19q, 10q, TP53, EGFR, CDK4, and CDKN2 A in 91 astrocytic and oligodendroglial tumors. Clin Cancer Res 8:196–201
Van der Valk P, Lindeman J, Kamphorst W (1997) Growth factor profiles of human gliomas. Ann Oncol 8:1023–1029

Weerda HG, Gamberger TI, Siegner A et al (1998) Effects of transforming growth factor-beta1 and basic fibroblast growth factor on proliferation of cell cultures derived from human vestibular nerve schwannoma. Acta Otolaryngol 118:337–343

Wick W, Platten M, Weller M (2001) Glioma cell invasion: regulation of metalloproteinase activity by TGF-beta. J Neurooncol 53:177–185

Yang SY, Xu GM (2001) Expression of PDGF and its receptors as well as their relationship to proliferating activity and apoptosis of meningeomas in human meningeomas. J Clin Neurosci 8 [Suppl 1]:49–53

Zhu A, Shaeffer J, Leslie S et al (1996) Epidermal growth factor receptor: an independent predictor of survival in astrocytic tumors given definitive irradiation. Int J Radiat Oncol Biol Phys 34:809–815

12 Role of Growth Factors and Biological Response Modifiers in Lung, Head and Neck and Gastrointestinal Tumors

G. Stüben and M. Stuschke

CONTENTS

12.1 Lung Tumors 147
12.2 Head and Neck Tumors 150
12.3 Gastrointestinal Tumors 151
     References 153

The role of growth factors in tumor growth and progression and their usefulness as prognostic and/or predictive factors is a topic of great interest which is reflected by an increasing number of publications over the last few years. These data are briefly summarized in this chapter for a variety of tumors, followed by a discussion of therapeutic approaches that are not covered elsewhere in this book.

The concept of immunotherapy of proliferative disease is still in the phase of active development, involving new technology and a vast range of biological approaches. Virtually any agent capable of altering the host–tumor relationship in favor of the host can be considered as a biological response modifier.

However, in view of the increasing interest in altered fractionation schedules and combined radiochemotherapy of lung, head and neck and gastrointestinal tumors, only limited data on the use of biological modifiers of the radiation response of these tumors are available. Most of the published trials are phase I/II studies, usually with small numbers of patients. A notable exception to this are the ongoing and planned head and neck (Henke et al. 1999) and lung (Scagliotti and Novello 2001) trials with the use of erythropoietin as potential radiosensitizer. The available preclinical and clinical data on this strategy are discussed in detail in Chap. 7, "Hematopoietic Tissue I: Response Modificationb yE rythropoietin".

Already numerous aspects of the standard treatments of lung, head and neck and gastrointestinal tumors are subject to intense scientific discussion. The large number of substances potentially acting as biological modifiers of radiosensitivity lead to several possible combination schedules with the standard treatments. Therefore, only selected aspects of the available data can be discussed.

Biological response modifiers (BRM) are a new class of antineoplastic agents that target the pathways tumor cells use to circumvent normal growth regulation, and may inhibit signals that protect tumor cells from radiation damage, thus acting as radiosensitizers (Sartor 2000). Therefore, an increased tumor cell response to irradiation might be observed, despite of the lack of direct cytotoxicity of these drugs. A possible synergistic effect of biological modifiers with radiation treatment is the basis and subject of ongoing studies.

12.1 Lung Tumors

An analysis of 60 squamous cell carcinoma specimens for immunohistochemical expression of epidermal growth factor receptor (EGFR), transforming growth factor-α (TGF-α) and erbB-2 showed higher expression of these three targets than in 60 specimens of normal bronchial epithelium (Piyathilake et al. 2002). Precancerous lesions showed intermediate expression of EGFR and TGF-α. The localization of EGFR in the cytoplasm, but not in the membrane, was significantly related to decreased overall survival. This might be an indication of the prognostic importance of trafficking of the EGFR between the Golgi apparatus and cell membranes. Data on immunohistochemical expression of HER-2/neu protein in specimens of resected non-small cell lung cancer (NSCLC) stage I–IIIA were reported by Selvaggi et al. (2002). From a total of 130 specimens, 16% were positive. No correlation with stage or histol-

---

G. Stüben, MD
Klinik für Strahlentherapie und Radiologische Onkologie der Universität Essen, Hufelandstrasse 55, 45122 Essen, Germany
M. Stuschke, MD
Professor, Klinik für Strahlentherapie und Radiologische Onkologie der Universität Essen, Hufelandstrasse 55, 45122 Essen, Germany

ogy was found. By using a cut-off of greater than 5% expression for definition of positivity, HER-2/neu was associated with impaired survival. This finding was also observed by HAN et al. (2002) who examined 85 stage I NSCLC patients (29% overexpressed HER-2/neu in immunohistochemical evaluation). Additional expression of p53 was associated with even worse outcome. Vascular endothelial growth factor (VEGF) might be expressed by a large number of NSCLCs. TAKAHAMA et al. (1998) detected VEGF in 64 of 74 adenocarcinomas (86.5%), 38 of 67 squamous cell carcinomas (57%) and four of four large cell carcinomas. Well-differentiated tumors had a higher degree of immunohistochemical positivity. VEGF expression did not correlate with tumor size or stage. SHOU et al. (2001) investigated the immunohistochemical expression of platelet-derived growth factor (PDGF), basic fibroblast growth factor (bFGF) and VEGF in 119 NSCLCs. VEGF expression was significantly associated with local invasion, lymph node involvement, pathological stage and lymphatic permeation. PDGF was related to lymph node involvement. Expression of VEGF and bFGF were associated with decreased overall survival. VOLM et al. (1999) investigated the immunohistochemically determined expression of PDGF, bFGF and VEGF in 168 non-small cell lung carcinomas stage I–IIIA. PDGF was expressed in 50%, VEGF in 59% and bFGF in 67%. These factors were not significantly correlated to the risk of lymph node metastases determined in pathology specimens. However, if all factors were negative only 43% of patients had lymph node metastases. With one positive factor, this figure increased to 53%, with two positive factors to 68% and with all three factors positive to 73%. In 80 lung adenocarcinomas with maximum diameter of 2cm that were treated by resection immunohistochemical staining showed VEGF positivity in 40% and bFGF positivity in 52.5% (ITO et al. 2002). There was some indication for decreased overall survival of patients with VEGF- or bFGF-positive tumors. However, VEGF expression was not prognostic in multivariate analysis for overall survival in 47 patients with resected stage I adenocarcinoma (MINAMI et al. 2002).

Serum levels of VEGF and bFGF were evaluated preoperatively in operable patients with NSCLC by BRATTSTROM et al. (2002). Fifty-eight patients were examined by use of enzyme-linked immunosorbent assays (ELISA). VEGF level was a significant prognostic factor in univariate tests, but associated with tumor volume. However, bFGF remained significant in a multivariate analysis. JOENSUU et al. (2002) also evaluated serum bFGF before treatment by ELISA. They studied 138 cases of NSCLC and 46 cases of small cell lung cancer (SCLC). A bFGF level greater than 3.4 pg/ml (highest tertile) was associated with poor overall survival (relative risk, 1.6). A multivariate analysis confirmed this prognostic influence in NSCLC patients. Further data failed to show a role of serum VEGF as an independent prognostic factor in 118 patients with NSCLC stage I–IV (LAACK et al. 2002). This study suggested that matrix metalloproteinase-9 might serve as a prognostic marker. Serum levels of insulin-like growth factor-1 (IGF-1) appear to be reduced in patients with lung cancer (LEE et al. 1999). NSCLC patients had lower levels than SCLC patients in this small study ($n=41$). Prognostic and predictive value were not reported. A recent review by JUNKER (2001) summarizes further data on limited stage NSCLC and concludes that single angiogenesis parameters might not have sufficient selectivity to serve as an exclusive discriminator for adjuvant treatment. Combining several parameters might better define subgroups of patients with high risk for distant relapse. In SCLC, data on serum VEGF levels were collected in 70 patients by MALL et al. (2002). There was a good correlation with advanced tumor stage, superior to the correlation of stage with albumin, lactate dehydrogenase or neuron-specific enolase. Seventy-five surgically treated SCLC patients were examined for the prognostic impact of VEGF (immunohistochemistry) by FONTANINI et al. (2001). VEGF expression was significantly correlated to overall survival in multivariate analysis. Almost 30% of 193 specimens from patients with extensive-stage SCLC were immunohistochemically positive for HER-2/neu overexpression (POTTI et al. 2002). This patient group showed decreased survival and multivariate testing confirmed an independent influence of HER-2/neu. The potential pitfalls of studies evaluating the role of biological markers as prognostic and predictive factors, for example variations in immunohistochemistry protocols and cut-off values, and poorly defined inclusion criteria resulting in large heterogeneity with regard to therapeutic modalities as well as tumor stage, histological types, etc., have recently been highlighted by THAMES et al. (2002) and NIEDER et al. (2001), who evaluated the influence of p53 on therapeutic outcome in a variety of tumors.

Most available studies on the use of biological modifiers in the treatment of lung cancer concentrate on SCLC. At the time of diagnosis of SCLC, a major proportion of patients suffer from (micro-) metastasized disease. The early disseminated nature of SCLC has led to the use of chemotherapy as the main therapeutic modality at all tumor stages (KRISTENSEN et al. 1996). Radiotherapy alone plays no relevant role in the treatment of SCLC. Therefore, most studies on biological response modifiers concentrate on chemotherapy-induced myelosuppression. In order to reduce the risk and costs of neutropenic fever colony-stimulating factors such as granulocyte-colony stimulating factor (G-CSF) have been evaluated for clinical usefulness. G-CSF has been shown to decrease the duration and severity of chemotherapy-induced myelotoxicity (CRAWFORD et al. 1991), thereby keeping the chemotherapy dose intensity high (BRONCHUD et al. 1987; CRAWFORD et al. 1991; MASUDA et al. 1992; PACCAGNELLA et al. 1993). In addition, granulocyte-macrophage-colony stimulating factor (GM-CSF) was introduced into the clinic with the aim of reducing neutropenia after chemotherapy (ANTMAN et al. 1988). However, the data on a possible reduction in the incidence of severe infections are conflicting (ANDERSON et al. 1991; ANTMAN et al. 1988; PACCAGNELLA et al. 1993). Clear evidence of an improvement in response rate or survival for SCLC patients with either G-CSF or GM-CSF is still lacking (KRISTENSEN et al. 1996).

Based on experimental data (CRAWFORD et al. 1991), an interferon alpha (IFN-α) maintenance therapy for SCLC patients was experimented (MASUDA et al. 1992). More than 400 patients received chemotherapy based on cyclophosphamide, vincristine and etoposide followed by a split course of radiotherapy. A subsequent randomization divided the patients into three groups: a control group (receiving no further treatment), a group treated with maintenance chemotherapy (six cycles) and a further group treated with 6 months of low-dose IFN-α. No significant difference in survival between the three groups was observed. Similar results were obtained in a randomized SWOG (Southwest Oncology Group) trial (KELLY et al. 1995). Responders to initial chemotherapy received IFN-α as maintenance treatment. This treatment was poorly tolerated (fatigue, malaise, lethargy) and no improvement in local control or survival could be demonstrated. A further randomized trial on IFN-α (MATTSON et al. 1992) reported no prolongation of median survival, although a trend towards improvement in survival for patients with limited disease was observed.

Interferon gamma (IFN-γ) has been tested by the Cancer and Leukemia Group B in SCLC patients who have responded to chemotherapy (BITRAN et al. 1995). Patients who achieved complete or partial response (CR or PR) after chemotherapy with cisplatin, doxorubicin, cyclophosphamide, and etoposide received 0.2 mg IFN-γ subcutaneously daily. The objective response rate was 6.7%. The North Central Cancer Treatment Group confirmed the low activity of IFN-γ in SCLC in a randomized phase III study (JETT et al. 1994). Patients who achieved CR after six cycles of chemotherapy were randomized to observation or IFN-γ treatment, which consisted of 4 million units subcutaneously every day for 6 months. Time to progression and survival were slightly inferior in the IFN-γ-arm, although the differences to the control arm were not statistically significant.

In summary, the available data give no convincing evidence that interferons have a substantial role in the treatment of SCLC (GHAEMMAGHAMI and JETT 1998).

Only limited data on the effects of biological response modifiers on NSCLC are available with sufficient numbers of patients on relevant endpoints such as survival. An exception to this are the studies on bestatin (ubenimex), a low molecular biological response modifier (an antibiotic of microbial origin that inhibits certain aminopeptidases), which was shown to have some immunomodulatory and antineoplastic effects (UMEZAWA et al. 1976). The drug was added to the treatment of lung cancer in randomized trials (YASUMITSU et al. 1990). In a complex study design, bestatin was given postoperatively to patients with NSCLC for as long as possible. The treatment design differed for adenocarcinoma and squamous/large cell carcinoma. Radiotherapy was basically given with a low tumor dose of 40 Gy to all stage III squamous cell and large cell carcinoma and to incurable operated cases. An interim analysis (YASUMITSU et al. 1990), based on 155 patients (72 with squamous cell carcinoma, 66 with adenocarcinoma, and 15 with other types of cancer), gave evidence for improved survival in the bestatin-treated group only for patients with squamous cell carcinoma. The 5-year survival rate for all stages was 58.3% for the bestatin group ($n=36$) and 36.8% for the control group ($n=34$). As no significant differences in survival were observed for the subset of stages II and III squamous cell carcinoma, stage I and curatively operated cases mainly contributed to the survival benefit found in the bestatin group. No significant benefit in the other tumor histologies was observed after bestatin treatment. A study of the EUROPEAN LUNG CANCER STUDY GROUP on the use of bestatin as adjuvant treatment in operated stage I and stage II non-small cell lung cancer (MOURITZEN 1990) showed a trend in favor of bestatin in terms of disease-free survival, but the trend was far from significant. No serious side effects have been reported. A further randomized trial on inoperable lung cancer (TAKADA et al. 1990) found no statistically significant difference in response rate or survival between the 113 patients treated by bestatin combination therapy and controls ($n=114$).

Based on promising data of phase I/II trials testing β-interferon in combination with radiotherapy in patients with advanced NSCLC, the Radiation Therapy Oncology Group (RTOG) initiated a phase III trial (BRADLEY et al. 2002). This multicenter trial accrued 123 patients with histologically confirmed stage IIIA or IIIB non-small-cell lung cancer. The β-interferon was given 30 min before radiation therapy for a total of nine doses. Irradiation was delivered at 2 Gy per fraction, 5 days a week, for a total of 60 Gy. The 1-year survival rate for the radiation-alone arm was 44% and 42% for the combined (β-interferon/radiation) arm. Grade 3 and 4 acute toxicities were significantly higher in the β-interferon arm. Only 76% of all patients completed β-interferon, as the acute toxicity resulted in non-compliance of patients. In summary, this controlled phase III trial failed to confirm the efficacy of β-interferon in patients receiving definitive radiotherapy for locally advanced NSCLC.

At present, studies concentrate on biological staging models (discussed in detail in O'BYRNE et al. 2001) as a basis for development of novel targeted therapeutic agents for treatment of micrometastatic and macroscopic NSCLC. As major potential targets for these efforts, hypoxia, angiogenesis, angiogenic and epidermal growth factors (RABEN et al. 2002), erb family receptors, matrix metalloproteinases, E-cadherin-regulation, p53 tumor suppressor gene alterations (ZALCMAN et al. 2000), p21 protein expression (BENNETT et al. 1998), TGF-b1 regulation (BENNETT et al. 1998), interleukin-6 (DE VITA et al. 1998) and interleukin-10 serum levels (DE VITA et al. 2000) are under investigation. Data on these promising molecular targeted therapies are rapidly evolving.

12.2
Head and Neck Tumors

Overexpression of EGFR was evaluated by immunohistochemical staining in a series of 38 patients by GUPTA et al. (2002). Ninety-seven percent of the specimens were strongly positive for EGFR. Experimental data from this group suggest that signaling from EGFR to phosphatidylinositol-3-kinase can lead to radioresistance. However, not all clinical data support this hypothesis. AEBERSOLD et al. (2002) published a series of 95 patients with oropharyngeal cancer treated by curative radiotherapy, with biopsies evaluated by immunohistochemical staining for EGFR, TGF-α and PDGF. None of these was predictive for radioresponse and none was of prognostic value. The only correlation was found between development of distant metastases and expression of PDGF-B (found in 54% of cases). KHAN et al. (2002) evaluated 56 patients with cancer of the oral cavity or oropharynx, stage III or IV, treated with resection plus adjuvant radiotherapy. Immunohistochemistry showed HER-2/neu overexpression in 17% without correlation to stage, grade, survival or disease-free survival. However, HER-2/neu did correlate with VEGF expression. Only four cases were amplified for HER-2/neu by fluorescence in situ hybridization (FISH). Three of these developed disease relapse. MINETA et al. (2002) examined immunohistochemical VEGF expression in 109 patients with squamous cell carcinoma of the tongue. High expression of VEGF was found in 63% and correlated with Ki-67 and p53 overexpression. VEGF overexpression also correlated with advanced stage III/IV disease. In multivariate analysis, VEGF expression and stage grouping independently predicted relapse-free survival. A different study of 52 patients, which was not limited to tongue cancer, identified lymph node metastases, tumor vascularization, COX-2 protein expression and PgE(2) tumor levels as significant multivariate prognostic factors for overall survival (GALLO et al. 2002). VEGF expression was less important in this study. Also, the results of 22 glottic squamous cell carcinoma (T_1 and T_{2a}) treated by radiotherapy showed no correlation of radioresistance and immunohistochemical expression of VEGF or VEGF-C (HOMER et al. 2001).

There is some evidence suggesting that the VEGF staining pattern might be associated with outcome in papillary thyroid cancer, where expression was detected in 98% of patients but with a different pattern (LENNARD et al. 2001). Diffuse, intense expression of VEGF was an unfavorable prognostic indicator.

Due to the nutritional status and smoking and drinking habits of patients with advanced head and neck tumors, many patients have a depressed immune system. The necessary nonsurgical treatment of these tumors consists mainly of radiotherapy, combined radiochemotherapy or chemotherapy alone. All these treatments might worsen the function of the immune system (WANEBO et al. 1975; YOSHIDA et al. 1997), as most chemotherapies lead to myelosuppression and radiotherapy usually leads to mucositis, resulting in a more severely deteriorated nutritional status of patients. Additionally, the tumor burden itself has a major impact on patients' immunological status. Therefore, some approaches focus on the recovery of immunological deterioration and maintenance of the immunity of patients with advanced head and neck tumors by treatment with biological response modifiers (YOSHIDA et al. 1997). As a parameter of immunological competence and as markers of efficacy of treatment with BRM several immunological parameters such as lymphocyte count, CD4, CD8, CD11, CD16, CD57, and NK cell activity are under investigation. In a study with β-1,3-glucan-possessing biological response modifiers (sizofiran and lentinan) as adjuvant treatment of patients with head and neck tumors, a prolonged survival in patients with stages III and IV tumors was observed. This corresponded to a more rapid recovery of lymphocyte count, CD8+ cells and peripheral blood NK cell activity in the BRM group of patients.

However, the two treatment groups consisted of a limited number of patients (55 patients in total) and the study investigated tumors of different anatomical origin within the groups. No detailed information of the treatment (besides the biological response modifiers) was given and salvage treatment was performed when local recurrences were observed. Therefore, the potential impact of the investigated biological response modifiers sizofiran and lentinan on survival remains to be proven in additional studies.

Further new approaches attempt to target the EGFR family as biological modifiers with the potential to improve radiosensitivity (SARTOR 2000). EGFR overexpression is sometimes associated with radioresistance in human head and neck tumors (MAURIZI et al. 1996). Therefore, inhibitors of EGFR activation may cause radiosensitization (SARTOR 2000). Indeed, monoclonal antibodies that inhibit EGFR-overexpressing head and neck cancer cell lines lead to significant radiosensitization (HUANG et al. 1999; HARARI and HUANG 2002). The potential mechanisms of radiosensitization by the EGFR family were recently discussed in detail (SARTOR 2000). Cell cycle alterations, interference with DNA damage repair and abrogation or attenuation of signals required for survival during cell cycle arrest are the most relevant mechanisms with potential to improve radiosensitivity. Evidence is increasing that these factors are related (SARTOR 2000). The clinical application of these mechanisms is in an early phase. First, clinical data on an inhibitory antibody of EGFR, C225, showed a clinical complete response in 13 of 16 patients with advanced unresectable head and neck tumors after radiotherapy plus C225 (ROBERT et al. 2001). Further studies including phase III trials with this interesting approach are underway (SARTOR 2000).

As pointed out recently (SARTOR 2000), the trial design of investigations involving biological modifiers of radiation response requires that new and unique issues surrounding these substances be considered. Traditionally, the highest tolerable dose of new cytotoxic agents, either alone or in combination with other substances, is assessed with dose-escalating studies. The resulting dose is then used as the basis for future studies. In view of the usually relatively low or selective toxicity of many biological agents, the maximum tolerated dose may not be the best determinant of the most effective dose. In fact, dose escalation may be counterproductive if at higher dose levels a biological agent loses its selectivity for tumor cells (SARTOR 2000). The biologically most effective dose, however, can usually not be determined, as markers that indicate that the targeted pathway is inhibited effectively are not available at present. Further research on the underlying mechanisms and pathways will help to design clinical trials with the best possible chance of success in terms of highest possible radiosensitization and tolerable side effects.

12.3
Gastrointestinal Tumors

Adenocarcinoma associated with Barrett's esophagus might show amplified HER-2/neu in 19% (FISH analysis by BRIEN et al. 2000), which might also correlate with survival. Immunohistochemical expression of EGFR or HER-2/neu was not associated with survival in a series of 117 patients with squamous cell carcinoma treated with resection (WANG et al. 1999). In adenocarcinoma, the addition of the antibody Herceptin to radiochemotherapy is the subject of ongoing clinical trials (H. SAFRAN, personal communication). In a small study of 56 patients undergoing preoperative radiochemotherapy for esophageal cancer, 21 preoperative biopsy specimens were examined for VEGF expression (IMDAHL et al. 2002). Tumor samples from patients who achieved a complete response showed significantly lower VEGF expression than samples from other patients. SHIMADA et al. (2002) investigated biopsy specimens from 52 patients with squamous cell cancer treated with radiochemotherapy. Patients either underwent surgery or additional radiotherapy after reassessment. By immunohistochemical staining, 44% were positive for VEGF. VEGF expression was significantly associated with unfavorable clinical response and 5-year survival rate. Multivariate analysis confirmed the prognostic value of VEGF expression.

Pretreatment serum level of VEGF was evaluated by ELISA in 96 patients with squamous cell carcinoma of the esophagus and in 24 healthy controls (SHIMADA et al. 2001). VEGF was significantly elevated in cancer patients and correlated to tumor size, tumor depth, stage and lymph node and distant metastases. Responders to radiochemotherapy had significantly lower VEGF levels than nonresponders. Survival was significantly shorter in patients with high VEGF levels, in both uni- and multivariate analyses.

In gastric cancer, preoperative serum VEGF levels (ELISA) were significantly higher than in controls ($n=58$ vs 61) and correlated with disease stage, depth of tumor invasion and presence of distant metastases (KARAYIANNAKIS et al. 2002). Furthermore, VEGF level significantly influenced survival in multivariate analysis. Immunohistochemical staining for VEGF might also be commonly seen, e.g., with 50% positive cases in a recent study (LIU et al. 2001). The latter group also demonstrated a decrease in the growth of tumor xenografts in nude mice with lowered VEGF levels.

In colon cancer, expression of the HER-2 oncoprotein occurs very infrequently (ARNAOUT et al. 1992). Experimental data indicate a role for serum IGF-1 in tumor development and metastasis, partly through expression of VEGF in such tumors (WU et al. 2002). Serum VEGF levels in patients with colorectal cancer were measured before surgery in a small study of 33 patients by NAKAYAMA et al. (2002). A nonsignificant trend was observed for correlation of high levels with advanced disease and more aggressive behavior during follow-up. Substantially more information can be derived from the paper by WERTHER et al. (2000). They studied VEGF levels in serum from 91 healthy blood donors and 614 patients with colorectal cancer scheduled to receive primary resection. Cancer patients had significantly higher VEGF levels. Dukes stage D patients had higher values than stage A, B or C patients, who had comparable values. Colon cancer patients had higher values than rectal cancer patients. Overall survival was significantly shorter with VEGF levels greater than 465 pg/ml (upper limit of the 95th percentile in healthy blood donors). Seventy-nine patients were studied by CASCINU et al. (2002), all of whom were node-positive and treated by surgery plus adjuvant radiochemotherapy. Immunohistochemically detected VEGF expression was significantly correlated with development of distant metastases and shorter event-free survival. LANDRISCINA et al. (1998) performed ELISA measurements of VEGF and bFGF in 35 patients with colorectal cancer. They used intestinal biopsies and blood samples from ten healthy subjects as controls: bFGF was significantly lower in tumors, whereas VEGF was up-regulated. Both factors were increased in mesenteric blood. VEGF, but not bFGF, tumor and serum levels were significantly correlated with disease stage. EGFR was positive in only a few colorectal cancers in the small study ($n=30$) by DI CARLO et al. (2001). In a different data set, EGFR expression did not predict development of metastases after curative resection of rectal cancer ($n=64$, GUNTHER et al. 2002).

FRIESS et al. (1999) examined mRNA expression for EGFR, c-erbB2 and c-erbB3 in 80 patients with pancreatic cancer. Expression was enhanced 2.5- to 5.2-fold compared to normal pancreatic tissues. Immunostaining scores were also significantly higher. HER-2/neu was evaluated by immunohistochemical analysis in 154 patients with pancreatic adenocarcinoma (SAFRAN et al. 2001). Twenty-one percent of specimens were positive. However, only 27% of the positive cases had gene amplification by FISH. KNOLL et al. (2001) reported that 47% of resected pancreatic carcinoma coexpressed VEGF and EGF. The impact of VEGF on recurrence-free survival after curative resection was recently studied in 70 patients with ductal adenocarcinoma (NIEDERGETHMANN et al. 2002). Immunoreactivity was 89% and positive mRNA signals were found in the cytoplasm of carcinoma and endothelial cells in 81%. VEGF expression significantly correlated with microvessel density. Furthermore, VEGF expression was an independent predictor of recurrence in multivariate analysis. Comparable results were obtained by SEO et al. (2000) in 142 resected cases of ductal adenocarcinoma (93% positive for VEGF by immunohistochemistry, significant correlation with microvessel density). However, in that study VEGF expression was associated with both development of liver metastases and shorter survival.

In view of potential modification of radiation response, most available studies concentrate on esophageal and gastric cancer. Japanese trials focused on the potential radiosensitization of advanced esophageal cancer by OK-432 (MUKAI et al. 1992), a lyophilized powder of *Streptococcus pyogenes* A3. The substance was injected locally by endoscopy and the tumor lesions were irradiated to total doses ranging from 50.2 to 66 Gy. Thirty patients without distant metastases completed the protocol and were evaluable for a sufficient follow-up period. All patients had biopsy-proven squamous cell carcinoma and were inoperable or refused surgery. The median follow-up was 16 months. Most patients developed high fever after the OK-432 treatment; other severe side effects were not reported. The overall survival of patients was 29% at 3 years, complete response was obtained in 22 of 30 patients. This was considered to be better than comparable historical controls. Accelerated repair of tissue after tumor shrinkage by attracted effector cells was postulated as a possible mechanism of action of the drug (MUKAI et al. 1992).

Recently, the results of preoperative intratumoral injection of OK-432 for gastric cancer were reported (GOCHI et al. 2001). In a multi-institutional randomized trial, 370 patients who had undergone curative resection for gastric cancer were enrolled in the study and followed up for 10 years postoperatively. OK-432 was endoscopically injected into the tumor prior to surgery. Multivariate analysis of survival revealed no improved survival and disease-free survival rates for the OK-432 patients. However, the subset of patients with stage IIIA and IIIB disease seemed to benefit from the preoperative intratumoral injections of OK-432, especially in the presence of moderate lymph node involvement (pN_2) and tumor-infiltrating lymphocytes (TILs). Therefore, a micro-metastasis-eliminating effect in lymph nodes was postulated as major mechanism of action (GOCHI et al. 2001). This effect might be of interest in further studies in combination with radiation.

At present, the available data give no convincing evidence to warrant any of the biological modifiers being proposed as a significant part of a standard radiation treatment protocol of lung, head and neck or gastrointestinal tumors. However, several possible mechanisms may lead to a relevant radiosensitization, which might result in improved treatment results in the near future.

Our increasing knowledge of the biological basis and molecular mechanisms of the current anticancer therapies provides new opportunities to identify and design further biological response modifiers aiming at reduced toxicity or enhanced efficacy of our present treatment strategies.

References

Aebersold DM, Froehlich SC, Jonczy M et al (2002) Expression of transforming growth factor-alpha, epidermal growth factor receptor and platelet-derived growth factors A and B in oropharyngeal cancers treated by curative radiation therapy. Radiother Oncol 63:275–283

Anderson H, Gurney H, Thatcher N et al (1991) Recombinant human GM-CSF in small cell lung cancer: a phase I/II study. Rec Res Cancer Res 121:155–161

Antman KS, Griffin JD, Elias A et al (1988) Effect of recombinant human granulocyte-macrophage colony-stimulating factor on chemotherapy-induced myelosuppression. N Engl J Med 319:593–598

Arnaout AH, Dawson PM, Soomro S et al (1992) HER2 (c-erbB-2) oncoprotein expression in colorectal adenocarcinoma: an immunohistochemical study using three different antibodies. J Clin Pathol 45:726–727

Bennett WP, el-Deiry WS, Rush WL et al (1998) p21waf1/cip1 and transforming growth factor beta 1 protein expression correlate with survival in non-small cell lung cancer. Clin Cancer Res 4:1499–1506

Bitran JD, Green M, Perry M et al (1995) A phase II study of recombinant interferon-gamma following combination chemotherapy for patients with extensive small cell lung cancer. CALGB. Am J Clin Oncol 18:67–70

Bradley JD, Scott CB, Paris KJ et al (2002) A phase III comparison of radiation therapy with or without recombinant beta-interferon for poor-risk patients with locally advanced non-small-cell lung cancer (RTOG 93-04). Int J Radiat Oncol Biol Phys 52:1173–1179

Brattstrom D, Bergqvist M, Hesselius P et al (2002) Elevated preoperative serum levels of angiogenic cytokines correlate to larger primary tumors and poorer survival in non-small cell lung cancer patients. Lung Cancer 37:57–63

Brien TP, Odze RD, Sheehan CE et al (2000) HER-2/neu gene amplification by FISH predicts poor survival in Barrett's esophagus-associated adenocarcinoma. Hum Pathol 31:35–39

Bronchud MH, Scarffe JH, Thatcher N et al (1987) Phase I/II study of recombinant human granulocyte colony-stimulating factor in patients receiving intensive chemotherapy for small cell lung cancer. Br J Cancer 56:809–813

Cascinu S, Graziano F, Catalano V et al (2002) An analysis of p53, BAX and vascular endothelial growth factor expression in node-positive rectal cancer. Br J Cancer 86:744–749

Crawford J, Ozer H, Stoller R et al (1991) Reduction by granulocyte colony-stimulating factor of fever and neutropenia induced by chemotherapy in patients with small-cell lung cancer. N Engl J Med 325:164–170

De Vita F, Orditura M, Auriemma A et al (1998) Serum levels of interleukin-6 as a prognostic factor in advanced non-small cell lung cancer. Oncol Rep 5:649–652

De Vita F, Orditura M, Galizia G et al (2000) Serum interleukin-10 levels as a prognostic factor in advanced non-small cell lung cancer patients. Chest 117:365–373

Di Carlo A, Mariano A, D'Alessandro V et al (2001) Evaluation of epidermal growth factor receptor, carcinoembryonic antigen and Lewis carbohydrate antigens in human colorectal and liver neoplasias. Oncol Rep 8:387–392

Fontanini G, Faviana P, Lucchi M et al (2001) A high vascular count and overexpression of vascular endothelial growth factor are associated with unfavourable prognosis

in operated small cell lung carcinomas. Br J Cancer 86: 558–563
Friess H, Wang L, Zhu Z et al (1999) Growth factor receptors are differentially expressed in cancers of the papilla of Vater and pancreas. Ann Surg 230:767–774
Gallo O, Masini E, Bianchi B et al (2002) Prognostic significance of cyclooxygenase-2 pathway and angiogenesis in head and neck squamous cell carcinoma. Hum Pathol 33: 708–714
Ghaemmaghami M, Jett JR (1998) New agents in the treatment of small cell lung cancer. Chest 113:86S–91S
Gochi A, Orita K, Fuchimoto S et al (2001) The prognostic advantage of preoperative intratumoral injection of OK-432 for gastric cancer patients. Br J Cancer 84:443–451
Gunther K, Dworak O, Remke S et al (2002) Prediction of distant metastases after curative surgery for rectal cancer. J Surg Res 103:68–78
Gupta AK, McKenna WG, Weber CN (2002) Local recurrence in head and neck cancer: relationship to radiation resistance and signal transduction. Clin Cancer Res 8:885–892
Han H, Landreneau RJ, Santucci TS et al (2002) Prognostic value of immunohistochemical expression of p53, HER-2/neu, and bcl-2 in stage I non-small cell lung cancer. Hum Pathol 33:105–110
Harari PM, Huang SM (2002) Epidermal growth factor receptor modulation of radiation response: preclinical and clinical development. Semin Radiat Oncol 12:21–26
Henke M, Guttenberger R, Barke A et al (1999) Erythropoietin for patients undergoing radiotherapy: a pilot study. Radiother Oncol 50:185–190
Homer JJ, Greenman J, Stafford ND (2001) The expression of vascular endothelial growth factor (VEGF) and VEGF-C in early laryngeal cancer: relationship with radioresistance. Clin Otolaryngol 26:498–504
Huang SM, Bock JM, Harari PM (1999) Epidermal growth factor receptor blockade with C225 modulates proliferation, apoptosis, and radiosensitivity in squamous cell carcinomas of the head and neck. Cancer Res 59:1935–1940
Imdahl A, Bognar G, Schulte-Monting J et al (2002) Predictive factors for response to neoadjuvant therapy in patients with oesophageal cancer. Eur J Cardiothorac Surg 21: 657–663
Ito H, Oshita F, Kameda Y et al (2002) Expression of vascular endothelial growth factor and basic fibroblast growth factor in small adenocarcinomas. Oncol Rep 9:119–123
Jett JR, Maksymiuk AW, Su JQ et al (1994) Phase III trial of recombinant interferon gamma in complete responders with small-cell lung cancer. J Clin Oncol 12:2321–2326
Joensuu H, Anttonen A, Eriksson M et al (2002) Soluble syndecan-1 and serum basic fibroblast growth factor are new prognostic factors in lung cancer. Cancer Res 62: 5210–5217
Junker K (2001) Prognostic factors in stage I/II non-small cell lung cancer. Lung Cancer 33 [Suppl 1]:S17–S24
Karayiannakis AJ, Syrigos KN, Polychronidis A et al (2002) Circulating VEGF levels in the serum of gastric cancer patients: correlation with pathological variables, patient survival, and tumor surgery. Ann Surg 236:37–42
Kelly K, Crowley JJ, Bunn PA Jr et al (1995) Role of recombinant interferon alfa-2a maintenance in patients with limited-stage small-cell lung cancer responding to concurrent chemoradiation: a Southwest Oncology Group study. J Clin Oncol 13:2924–2930

Khan AJ, King BL, Smith BD et al (2002) Characterization of the HER-2/neu oncogene by immunohistochemical and fluorescence in situ hybridization analysis in oral and oropharyngeal squamous cell carcinoma. Clin Cancer Res 8:540–548
Knoll MR, Rudnitzki D, Sturm J et al (2001) Correlation of postoperative survival and angiogenic growth factors in pancreatic carcinoma. Hepatogastroenterology 48: 1162–1165
Kristensen CA, Jensen PB, Poulsen HS et al (1996) Small cell lung cancer: biological and therapeutic aspects. Crit Rev Oncol Hematol 22:27–60
Laack E, Kohler A, Kugler C et al (2002) Pretreatment serum levels of matrix metalloproteinase-9 and vascular endothelial growth factor in non-small cell lung cancer. Ann Oncol 13:1550–1557
Landriscina M, Cassano A, Ratto C et al (1998) Quantitative analysis of basic fibroblast growth factor and vascular endothelial growth factor in human colorectal cancer. Br J Cancer 78:765–770
Lee DY, Kim SJ, Lee YC (1999) Serum insulin-like growth factor (IGF)-1 and IGF-binding proteins in lung cancer patients. J Korean Med Sci 14:401–404
Lennard CM, Patel A, Wilson J et al (2001) Intensity of vascular endothelial growth factor expression is associated with increased risk of recurrence and decreased disease-free survival in papillary thyroid cancer. Surgery 129:552–558
Liu DH, Zhang XY, Fan DM et al (2001) Expression of vascular endothelial growth factor and its role in oncogenesis of human gastric carcinoma. World J Gastroenterol 7: 500–505
Mall JW, Schwenk W, Philipp AW et al (2002) Serum vascular endothelial growth factor levels correlate better with tumor stage in small cell lung cancer than albumin, neuron-specific enolase or lactate dehydrogenase. Respirology 7: 99–102
Masuda N, Fukuoka M, Furuse K (1992) CODE chemotherapy with or without recombinant human granulocyte colony-stimulating factor in extensive-stage small cell lung cancer. Oncology 49 [Suppl 1]:19–24
Mattson K, Niiranen A, Pyrhonen S et al (1992) Natural interferon alfa as maintenance therapy for small cell lung cancer. Eur J Cancer 28A:1387–1391
Maurizi M, Almadori G, Ferrandina G et al (1996) Prognostic significance of epidermal growth factor receptor in laryngeal squamous cell carcinoma. Br J Cancer 74: 1253–1257
Minami K, Saito Y, Imamura H et al (2002) Prognostic significance of p53, Ki-67, VEGF and Glut-1 in resected stage I adenocarcinomas of the lung. Lung Cancer 38:51–55
Mineta H, Miura K, Ogino T et al (2002) Vascular endothelial growth factor (VEGF) expression correlates with p53 and ki-67 expressions in tongue squamous cell carcinoma. Anticancer Res 22:1039–1044
Mouritzen C (1990) Bestatin as adjuvant treatment in operated stage I and stage II non-small cell lung cancer. European Lung Cancer Study Group. Acta Oncol 29:817–820
Mukai M, Morita S, Tsunemoto H (1992) Combination therapy of local administration of OK-432 and radiation for esophageal cancer. Int J Radiat Oncol Biol Phys 22:1047–1050
Nakayama Y, Sato T, Shibao K et al (2002) Prognostic value of plasma vascular endothelial growth factor in patients with colorectal cancer. Anticancer Res 22:2437–2442

Nieder C, Petersen S, Petersen C et al (2001) The challenge of p53 as prognostic and predictive factor in Hodgkin's or non-Hodgkin's lymphoma. Ann Hematol 80:2–8

Niedergethmann M, Hildenbrand R, Wostbrock B et al (2002) High expression of vascular endothelial growth factor predicts early recurrence and poor prognosis after curative resection for ductal adenocarcinoma of the pancreas. Pancreas 25:122–129

O'Byrne KJ, Cox G, Swinson D et al (2001) Towards a biological staging model for operable non-small cell lung cancer. Lung Cancer 34 [Suppl 2]:S83–S89

Paccagnella A, Favaretto A, Riccardi A et al (1993) Granulocyte-macrophage colony-stimulating factor increases dose intensity of chemotherapy in small cell lung cancer. Relationship between clinical results, peripheral blood cell modifications, and bone marrow kinetics. Cancer 72:697–706

Piyathilake CJ, Frost AR, Manne U et al (2002) Differential expression of growth factors in squamous cell carcinoma and precancerous lesions of the lung. Clin Cancer Res 8:734–744

Potti A, Willardson J, Forseen C et al (2002) Predictive role of HER-2/neu overexpression and clinical features at initial presentation in patients with extensive stage small cell lung cancer. Lung Cancer 36:257–261

Raben D, Helfrich BA, Chan D et al (2002) ZD1839, a selective epidermal growth factor receptor tyrosine kinase inhibitor, alone and in combination with radiation and chemotherapy as a new therapeutic strategy in non-small cell lung cancer. Semin Oncol 29:37–46

Robert F, Ezekiel MP, Spencer SA et al (2001) Phase I study of anti-epidermal growth factor receptor antibody cetuximab in combination with radiation therapy in patients with advanced head and neck cancer. J Clin Oncol 19:3234–3243

Safran H, Steinhoff M, Mangray S et al (2001) Overexpression of the HER-2/neu oncogene in pancreatic adenocarcinoma. Am J Clin Oncol 24:496–499

Sartor CI (2000) Biological modifiers as potential radiosensitizers: targeting the epidermal growth factor receptor family. Semin Oncol 27:15–20

Scagliotti GV, Novello S (2001) Role of erythropoietin in the treatment of lung cancer associated anaemia. Lung Cancer 34 [Suppl 4]:S91–S94

Selvaggi G, Scagliotti GV, Torri V et al (2002) HER-2/neu overexpression in patients with radically resected non-small cell lung carcinoma. Impact on long-term survival. Cancer 94:2669–2674

Seo Y, Baba H, Fukuda T et al (2000) High expression of vascular endothelial growth factor is associated with liver metastases and a poor prognosis for patients with ductal pancreatic adenocarcinoma. Cancer 88:2239–2245

Shimada H, Takeda A, Nabeya Y et al (2001) Clinical significance of serum vascular endothelial growth factor in esophageal squamous cell carcinoma. Cancer 92:663–669

Shimada H, Hoshino T, Okazumi S et al (2002) Expression of angiogenic factors predicts response to chemoradiotherapy and prognosis of oesophageal squamous cell carcinoma. Br J Cancer 86:552–557

Shou Y, Hirano T, Gong Y et al (2001) Influence of angiogenetic factors and matrix metalloproteinases upon tumour progression in non-small cell lung cancer. Br J Cancer 85:1706–1712

Takada M, Fukuoka M, Negoro S et al (1990) Combination therapy with bestatin in inoperable lung cancer. A randomized trial. Acta Oncol 29:821–825

Takahama M, Tsutsumi M, Tsujiuchi T et al (1998) Frequent expression of the vascular endothelial growth factor in human non-small cell lung cancers. Jpn J Clin Oncol 28:176–181

Thames HD, Petersen C, Petersen S et al (2002) Immunohistochemically detected p53 mutations in epithelial tumors and results of treatment with chemotherapy and radiotherapy. A treatment-specific overview of the clinical data. Strahlenther Onkol 178:411–421

Umezawa H, Aoyagi T, Suda H et al (1976) Bestatin, an inhibitor of aminopeptidase B, produced by actinomycetes. J Antibiot (Tokyo) 29:97–99

Volm M, Koomägi R, Mattern J (1999) PD-ECGF, bFGF, and VEGF expression in non-small cell lung carcinomas and their association with lymph node metastasis. Anticancer Res 19:651–656

Wanebo HJ, Jun MY, Strong EW et al (1975) T-cell deficiency in patients with squamous cell cancer of the head and neck. Am J Surg 130:445–451

Wang LS, Chow KC, Chi KH et al (1999) Prognosis of esophageal squamous cell carcinoma: analysis of clinicopathological and biological factors. Am J Gastroenterol 94:1933–1940

Werther K, Christensen IJ, Brunner N et al (2000) Soluble vascular endothelial growth factor levels in patients with primary colorectal carcinoma. Eur J Surg Oncol 26:657–662

Wu Y, Yakar S, Zhao L et al (2002) Circulating insulin-like growth factor-1 levels regulate colon cancer growth and metastasis. Cancer Res 62:1030–1035

Yasumitsu T, Ohshima S, Nakano N et al (1990) Bestatin in resected lung cancer. A randomized clinical trial. Acta Oncol 29:827–831

Yoshida T, Saeki T, Aoyama Y et al (1997) Treatment of head and neck cancers with BRMs – prolongation of survival. Biotherapy 10:115–120

Zalcman G, Tredaniel J, Schlichtholz B et al (2000) Prognostic significance of serum p53 antibodies in patients with limited-stage small cell lung cancer. Int J Cancer 89:81–86

13 Role of Signaling Pathway Modification

O. Riesterer, M. Pruschy, and S. Bodis

CONTENTS

13.1 Advantages and Disadvantages of Current Radiotherapy 157
13.1.1 Intensity Modulated Radiotherapy 157
13.1.2 Functional and Molecular Imaging 158
13.1.3 The Radiobiological Approach 158
13.2 Why Do We Need a Broad Therapeutic Window? 159
13.2.1 Radiosensitizers and Radioprotectors Used So Far 160
13.3 The New Age of Signal Transduction 162
13.3.1 Active Versus Passive Mode of Cell Death 162
13.3.2 Active Versus Passive Mode of Treatment Resistance 164
13.3.3 Conflicting Signals 165
13.4 Ionizing Radiation and Signaling 165
13.4.1 DNA-Damage-Induced Signaling 165
13.4.2 Non-DNA-Damage-Induced Signaling 167
13.4.2.1 Receptor Tyrosine Kinases 167
13.4.2.2 The Sphingomyelin Pathway 168
13.5 Pharmacological Signaling Modification in Combination with Ionizing Radiation 169
13.5.1 Signaling Modification in Active Mode of Cell Death: p53 169
13.5.2 Signaling Modification in Active Mode of Treatment Resistance: PI3K/Akt Pathway 172
13.6 Outlook 173
References 174

more, in patients presenting with locoregional disease, some are cured whereas in others disease recurs and progresses either locally and/or systemically. Some tumors are controlled with high probability by low doses of radiation (e.g., seminomas, lymphomas), others are controlled by moderate to high radiation doses (e.g., breast and prostate adenocarcinomas) and still others will progress even after treatment with high radiation doses, exceeding normal tissue tolerance (e.g., glioblastoma, melanoma). The reason for failure to cure may include treatment-related factors (e.g., metastases out of treatment volume, large volume, unfavorable location) or tumor-related factors (e.g., radiation-resistant tumor cells, limited tolerance of the surrounding normal tissue, hypoxic tumor cells) (Jung and Dritschilo 1996). Research for improvement of radiotherapy focuses on physical and biological aspects: with the improvement of radiation technology (e.g., intensity-modulated radiation therapy [IMRT]) and the introduction of novel imaging techniques (e.g., PET), the control of treatment-related factors has increased. Modern radiobiology focuses on the modulation of molecular processes, thereby overcoming inherent radiation resistance of the tumor cell.

13.1
Advantages and Disadvantages of Current Radiotherapy

A unique aspect of ionizing radiation as a therapeutic tool is the locoregional application of the cytotoxic therapy without systemic toxicity. However, there are several limitations to the efficacy of radiation treatment: ionizing radiation is mainly effective for the treatment of cancers that have not spread. Further-

13.1.1
Intensity Modulated Radiotherapy

Over the last 20 years, major changes in clinical radiotherapy came predominantly from innovative techniques. Recent important technical advances include CT simulation, 3D conformal radiotherapy and IMRT. Especially IMRT has evoked great enthusiasm among clinicians for the treatment precision allowing dose escalation and fractionation modulation. In pilot clinical studies it was suggested that IMRT can reduce toxicity (e.g., treatment of head and neck cancer with IMRT can reduce xerostomia by sparing salivary glands), without reduction of tumor control (Eisbruch et al. 2001; Chao et al. 2001). However, IMRT has technical as well as biological limitations (Goff-

O. Riesterer, MD; M. Pruschy, PhD; S. Bodis, MD
Laboratory for Molecular Radiobiology, Department Radiation Oncology, University Hospital Zurich, 8091 Zurich, Switzerland

man and Glatstein 2002), for example, treatment fields with narrow margins require that these fields essentially cover the target. However, currently available imaging techniques (CT, MRI, PET or the fusion of PET and CT) in many cases cannot accurately identify the macroscopic and microscopic tumor extension. Moreover, new techniques for real-time verification of the patient position during treatment have to be developed to control significant patient and organ movements. IMRT is used in some patients to reduce toxicity of critical structures such as the salivary glands. However for biological reasons, it does also potentially increase normal tissue toxicity in comparison to classic radiotherapy because it results in much larger volumes of normal tissue exposure. This could increase the risk of radiation-induced malignancies, especially in pediatric patients, because modest doses of radiation (e.g., at the radiation field edges) have been reported to induce cancers in the young after long latencies (Ron et al. 1988a,b, 1995). Furthermore, IMRT significantly increases total body exposure due to extended treatment duration. We have to acknowledge that current data on the long-term effect of very high radiation doses on neighboring normal tissues or normal structures such as nerves and vessels are still not comprehensive enough. It is of some concern that it can take years to see the full impact of hypofractionated irradiation, especially in neuronal tissue (Johansson et al. 2000). Major biological limitations of IMRT are inherent radiation resistance of tumor cells and occult metastasis. Radiation oncologists like to assume that the higher the administered dose the better the tumor control. However, the survival curve for selected tumors such as glioblastoma is probably so shallow that curative doses are difficult to achieve due to normal tissue tolerance. Large tumors might be controlled by very large doses of IMRT, but with their enormous potential for metastasis, any local therapy may have little impact on prolonging survival.

13.1.2
Functional and Molecular Imaging

A major challenge of IMRT is the identification of the critical target for dose escalation. Beside the tumor outline on a radiological image, possible future targets are those that are defined by the unique biology of the tumor, the stroma and normal tissue (Coleman 2002).

Tumors are heterogeneous structures that contain hypoxic and normoxic areas, invasive cancer, or in-situ cancer, normal tissue such as vasculature and stroma, and cells representing the host response of the tumor such as immune cells and the inflammatory reaction. These compartments characterize the specific microenvironment of a tumor that may be substantially different from tumor cells studied and grown in clonogenic cultures (Coleman 2002; Hanahan and Weinberg 2000). Some of the biological subunits of a tumor might benefit from the higher tumor doses that can be delivered with IMRT (Coleman 2002). The concept of a biological treatment volume (or a biological treatment boost) was recently described (Ling et al. 2000) and the tools for biological target definition such as functional and molecular imaging techniques are already being developed. Imaging modalities (e.g., PET) can roughly discriminate cancer from normal tissue based on metabolic differences (glucose uptake). Pilot studies with new PET tracers show that this technique can not only identify and delineate the tumor within anatomical structures but it can also identify metabolic subregions in the tumor such as hypoxic tumor areas (Bentzen et al. 2000). Accordingly, magnetic resonance techniques can also pinpoint hypoxic subregions within the tumor (Stubbs 1999). By fusing functional and molecular images with CT, dose escalation with IMRT to the hypoxic compartment of the tumor becomes feasible. Thereby one of the major biological limitations of radiotherapy, the radioresistance of the hypoxic tumor fraction, might be overcome.

13.1.3
The Radiobiological Approach

In parallel to the physical improvement of clinical radiotherapy during the last century, radiobiological concepts were developed to understand the clinical response to fractionated ionizing radiation on the cellular and molecular level. In the last 50 years, clonogenic cell survival assays were optimized to describe the cellular response to irradiation. Cell survival curves allowed a dose-dependent determination of radiation sensitivity in established tumor cell lines and normal cells. Different mathematical models were created to describe the characteristics of these survival curves and to classify tumor cells as radiosensitive or radioresistant. For example, radiosensitivity can be defined by the terminal slope of the survival curve after exposure of cells to graded doses of ionizing radiation (single hit, multitarget model) or by integrating the area under the curve (linear quadratic equation; α/β model). Another possible parameter is the surviving fraction after exposure to 2 Gy (SF2). Applying these concepts to tumor cell lines allowed for their classification into categories that are relatively sensitive or relatively resistant to ionizing radiation exposure (HALL 2000; JUNG and DRITSCHILO 1996).

From the clinical point of view, ionizing radiation is a locally applied cancer therapy that exerts local side effects whereas chemotherapy is applied systemically and has systemic side effects. On the contrary, on the cellular level the effect of ionizing radiation is more complex (systemic targeting) than the effect of modern molecular-defined chemotherapy that selectively targets specific receptors and signal transduction pathways in cancer cells (local targeting). The major mechanism of radiation-induced cell death is DNA damage. However, over the last decade radiobiological research elucidated that ionizing radiation as a stress response also targets a complex network of signal transduction pathways downstream of DNA damage or independent of DNA damage. Some of these pathways mediate the cytoprotective and cytotoxic responses of cell survival and cell death (SCHMIDT-ULLRICH et al. 2000) and therefore are interesting targets to modulate the radiation effect. In nearly all human tumors these signaling pathways are deregulated by mutations in oncogenes or tumor suppressor genes (HANAHAN and WEINBERG 2000) and the genetic profile of a cancer cell might decide over treatment resistance or treatment response. An example of a gene that can predict the response of a cell to ionizing radiation is p53. Cells with aberrant p53 have a number of altered phenotypes, including loss of the G1 cell cycle checkpoint and a diminished ability to undergo apoptosis after irradiation (GIACCA and KASTAN 1998; KINZLER and VOGELSTEIN 1996; PRUSCHY et al. 2001; LOWE et at. 1994) (see Sect. 13.3.2, "Active Versus Passive Mode of Treatment Resistance").

The cellular molecular response to ionizing radiation on the level of signal transduction pathways is an important step in developing molecular radiosensitizers, i.e., molecular defined pharmacological agents that interact with ionizing radiation on the signal transduction level. In the last few years, the knowledge in this field of research has dramatically increased and a lot of molecular-defined treatment strategies have been developed. Preclinical studies showed that some of the strategies that were first tested alone and in combination with classic cytotoxic chemotherapy also have radiosensitizing properties. Given that over the past decade, the most impressive gains in local tumor control have not been achieved with larger doses of ionizing radiation but with radiation given with concomitant chemotherapy, combined treatment modality with ionizing radiation and the novel class of molecular-defined compounds might be a highly promising approach to improve clinical radiotherapy.

In this chapter we will focus on the basic principles of interaction between ionizing radiation and signal transduction pathways in cancer cells and how the radiation effect can be increased by modulating these pathways with molecular defined compounds. In the other chapters of this volume the current most promising compounds will be discussed in detail.

13.2
Why Do We Need a Broad Therapeutic Window?

Local failure is the cause of 40%–60% of cancer deaths (WASSERMAN et al. 1997). It is likely that more patients could be cured if radiotherapy was delivered with higher doses to the tumor. However, in the clinical situation the dose delivered to a tumor is often not determined by the radiosensitivity of the tumor but by the surrounding normal tissue tolerance. Further dose escalation would drastically increase the risk of irreversible side effects. The ratio of the treatment effect to the tumor compared to the treatment effect to normal tissues is called the therapeutic index (TI). The TI is defined as the width between the sigmoid-shaped curves of tumor cure and normal tissue toxicity, when the probabilities for both are plotted against the radiation dose (Fig. 13.1a). In this model, the steepness of the effective range of tumor cure emphasizes the importance of small increases in the medium dose range. However, in the medium dose range the risk of normal tissue toxicity also increases dramatically. The ideal approach to improve radiotherapy should increase the radiation effect on the tumor and decrease the radiation effect on normal tissue. In the graph (Fig. 13.1a) both curves would be shifted apart as could be achieved by dose fractionation. Dividing a dose into a number of fractions spares normal tissues because of the repair of sublethal damage between dose fractions and cellular repopulation. At the same time, fractionation improves tumor response because of reoxygenation and reassortment (HALL 2000). Recent physical improvements such as conformal treatment and IMRT further widen the therapeutic index. However, they do not increase the radiation effect on the tumor but tailor the radiation beam in a way that the normal tissue can be spared and toxicity is reduced (tumor

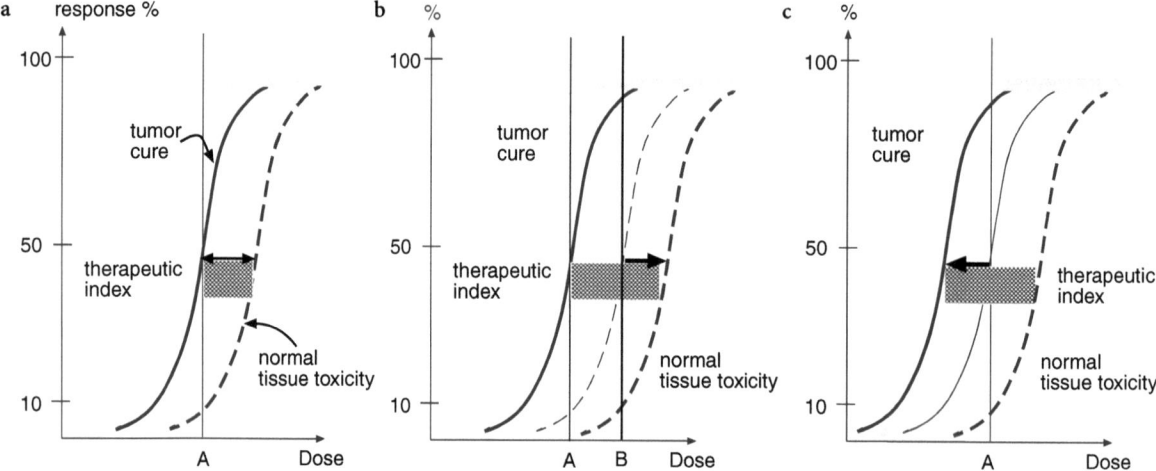

Fig. 13.1a–c. The Therapeutic Index. **a** Therapeutic index for treatment with radiation alone. Radiation with *dose A* implies specific probabilities for tumor cure and normal tissue toxicity (e.g., 50% cure vs <10% toxicity). **b** If radiation is combined with radioprotectors, the radiation dose can be increased (*dose B*) because normal tissue toxicity is reduced (curve for normal tissue toxicity shifted to the right) **c** If radiation is combined with radiosensitizers, the probability for tumor cure increases (curve for tumor cure shifted to the left). Radioprotectors and radiosensitizers both increase the therapeutic index

cure curve not changed, normal tissue toxicity curve shifted to the right; see Fig. 13.1b). Another approach to modify the therapeutic index of radiotherapy is to combine radiotherapy with pharmacological agents (e.g., tumor-selective radiosensitizers and/or normal tissue-specific radioprotectors). Generally, four ways of interaction between pharmacological agents and ionizing radiation can be distinguished: toxicity independence, additive interaction (spatial cooperation), radiosensitization (synergistic interaction) and radioprotection (Steel and Peckham 1979). Toxicity independence means that full doses of the two treatment modalities do not increase the severity of toxicities of either treatment alone. An example for the opposite, interactive toxicity (toxicity dependence), is the radiation recall reaction, which is an erythema in the radiation field in patients who have received radiotherapy and who subsequently receive chemotherapy with doxorubicin, paclitaxel or gemcitabine. The initial rationale of combining traditional chemotherapeutic agents with ionizing radiation has been additive interaction, which implies that both treatments act independently and have no interaction on the cellular level, for example, radiotherapy locally eradicates the tumor and chemotherapy eradicates systemic metastases or ionizing radiation is used only to treat sites not reached by the drug (e.g., brain metastases). In the last few years this concept has changed and for some cytotoxic drugs the mode of interaction with ionizing radiation may be described as synergistic interaction or radiosensitization. In this regard, synergism could be understood as a biological effect that is greater than would be expected from the addition of the effects of the component agents (Hall 2000).

13.2.1
Radiosensitizers and Radioprotectors Used So Far

The classic approach to describing the radiosensitivity of tumors to fractionated radiotherapy includes the 4 Rs of radiotherapy: repair of sublethal damage, reassortment of cells within the cell cycle, repopulation and reoxygenation. This model is still valid even though in modern radiobiology the term radiosensitive is mostly used to describe the intrinsic radiosensitivity of specific tumor cells or tumor cell lines, which is determined by the genetic profile consisting of specific mutations in oncogenes and/or tumor suppressor genes. Quantification of cellular radiosensitivity is still performed by in vitro assays and is described by distinct shapes of the survival curve. Moreover, cellular radiation sensitivity can be linked to the different cell cycle phases with a high sensitivity at the G2-M transition, intermediate sensitivity in G1 and early S-phase, and low sensitivity in late S-phase. The reason for differential radiosensitivity during the cell cycle is not completely understood on the molecular level but might be due to an insufficient capacity to repair IR-induced DNA damage in the G2-M phase of the cell cycle.

Intrinsic radiosensitivity can be increased by pharmacological agents (radiosensitizers) that interact with ionizing radiation on the molecular level. Many traditional chemotherapeutic agents interact with ionizing radiation by affecting DNA synthesis or function and therefore increase radiation-induced DNA damage or affect DNA repair (e.g., cis-platinum, gemcitabine, 5-fluorouracil). Other mechanisms of radiosensitization are reported for the taxanes that arrest cells in the G2-M phase of the cell cycle and interact with signal transduction pathways, for example, paclitaxel can induce p53-independent apoptosis in cancer cells (Pruschy et al. 2001; O'Connor et al. 1997). However, from the radiobiological point of view, cytotoxic drugs are not ideal radiosensitizers because of their lack of tumor cell selectivity and extensive toxicity. Radiosensitizers should increase local tumor control without increasing early and late side effects of ionizing radiation (Fig. 13.1c, tumor cure curve shifted to the left). Another goal is the eradication of micrometastases. During decades of research, agents were developed and tested with the focus on IR and its direct and deleterious damage of DNA. The halogenated pyrimidines, 5-iododeoxyuridine (IUdR) and 5-bromodeoxyuridine (BUdR) are similar to the DNA precursor thymidine, having a halogen substituted in place of the methyl group. Because of the similarity, these compounds are incorporated into the DNA instead of thymidine decreasing the stability of DNA. Radiosensitization with halogenated pyrimidines highly depends on the amount of DNA incorporation, which can be up-regulated by the concomitant application of 5-FU. Great efforts were undertaken to transfer this group of compounds to the clinic. A clinical obstacle was that halogenated pyrimidines must be applied by intra-arterial infusion because the liver would dehalogenate the drug. Pilot clinical studies with halogenated pyrimidines were done in patients with gliomas, which are rapidly growing tumors that are surrounded by slowly growing or nongrowing brain tissue. The only randomized phase III study ever done (RTOG 94-04) comparing radiation therapy with or without BUdR in patients with gliomas, with all patients receiving adjuvant PCV chemotherapy, was closed early because of a lack of benefit using BUdR. A similar mechanism of radiosensitization as for halogenated pyrimidines is reported for ribonucleotide reductase inhibitors such as 2', 2'-Difluoro-2'deoxycytidine (gemcitabine) that deplete deoxynucleoside triphosphates required for DNA synthesis (Kinsella et al. 1984; E.M. Miller et al. 1992; L.S. Miller et al. 1992; Lawrence et al. 1999; Sun et al. 1997).

Another class of compounds targets a major tumor-related aspect. In general, the response of cells to IR strongly depends on oxygen. Hypoxia confers radioresistance to a wide range of cells irrespective of the genetic background (Brown and Giaccia 1998; Brown 1999; Overgaard 1989). The mechanism behind this phenomenon is that oxygen chemically interacts with IR-induced DNA radicals and thereby fixes these lesions and renders them irreparable. In a hypoxic environment, these DNA radicals can be restored by cellular-abundant molecular hydrogen donors. Beside a long history of physical approaches (e.g., application of hyperbaric oxygen), many chemical approaches were developed during the last 2 decades to overcome hypoxia by the replacement of oxygen with other electron-affinic compounds that react with the free electron of the IR-induced DNA radical. Monofunctional 2-nitroimidazole and bi-functional alkylating derivatives were tested but these approaches often failed due to nonspecific neurotoxicity (misonidazole) or lack of a significant overall benefit (misonidazole and etanidazole). Recently, the combination of radiotherapy and a newer and less toxic agent, nimorazole, showed a significant improvement in local tumor control and a trend for improved survival in a randomized double-blind phase III trial (Overgaard et al. 1998). A meta-analysis by Overgaard (1995) included 10,703 cases entered into 83 randomized controlled trials and showed an overall improvement in local tumor control of 4.6% ($p=0.0001$) and in survival of 2.8% ($p=0.005$) for different approaches to overcome hypoxia (Overgaard 1994, 1995). In addition, bioreductive drugs such as tirapazamine are now under clinical investigation that exploit hypoxia as a selective environment for the generation of hypoxic cytotoxins. Combined treatment with tirapazamine and ionizing radiation probably has a supra-additive tumor-killing effect due to complementary cytotoxicity (Brown 1999, 2001; Overgaard 1989; Rauth et al. 1998). The use of tirapazamine is currently being tested in clinical phase I and II studies.

Protection from acute and late toxicity has long been of interest to radiation oncologists. Radioprotectors are chemicals that reduce the biological effects of ionizing radiation. The ideal radioprotector for the clinical use should selectively protect normal tissues and hence permit radiation dose escalation (Fig. 13.1b, normal tissue toxicity curve shifted to the right). Furthermore, the ideal radioprotector could work as well as a chemoprotector and protect normal tissue against the side effects of chemotherapy given concomitantly with ionizing radiation. The identification of important signal transduction pathways that mediate cytotoxicity and cytoprotection revealed potential molecular targets for radioprotection. However, research in the molecular era still focuses on radiosensitizers and the search for molecular radioprotectors is still in the beginning stages. For decades research in this field concentrated mainly on one compound: amifostine, also known as Ethyol or WR-2721, is an organic thiophosphate with cytoprotective capability against ionizing radiation and chemotherapeutic agents. Amifostine, a free thiol, acts as a potential scavenger of oxygen-free radicals induced by ionizing radiation. Several randomized studies have found a significant reduction of xerostomia, mucositis, fibrosis and dysphagia in patients with head and neck cancer (BUNTZEL et al. 2002; BRIZEL et al. 2000) and significant reduction of severe esophagitis and pneumonitis in patients with non-small cell lung cancer (KOMAKI et al. 2002; ANTONADOU 2002). Another group of potential radioprotectors used so far only in preclinical settings are the nitroxides, which showed radioprotective effects in a concentration-dependent fashion (HAHN et al. 2000). The mechanism of differential radioprotection of nitroxides is the differential bioreduction, which occurs to a greater extent in the tumor than in normal tissues (HAHN et al. 1997; KUPPUSAMY et al. 1998). A major clinical limitation of nitroxides is their systemic toxicity when administered at high concentrations (HAHN et al. 2000). As already mentioned, a more innovative approach for radioprotection is to selectively inhibit proteins and genes that confer radiosensitivity, for instance, inhibition of p53 with pifithrin could be beneficial for many patients because p53 is inactivated in about 50% of all human cancers. In patients with p53-deficient tumors, pifithrin would selectively protect only the normal tissue cells but not the tumor cells (KOMAROV et al. 1999). As already discussed, physical inventions such as conformal treatment or IMRT from the biological point of view have radioprotective properties as well and their effectiveness might be compared with pharmacological agents in clinical studies in the near future.

13.3
The New Age of Signal Transduction

On the molecular level, cell function is regulated by a complex network of intracellular and extracellular signal transduction pathways. A major focus in biomedical research over the past 10 or 15 years has been the identification and characterization of the components that make up such signaling pathways. We are now beginning to understand how such pathways are controlled, communicate with each other and, most importantly, what goes wrong in disease states. Cancer is a disease of dysregulated growth control (cancer cells that grow when they should not and do not die, that is, undergo apoptosis, when they should). Mutant proteins derived from mutated growth control genes (oncogenes, tumor suppressor genes) and the DNA repair machinery are often components of the signaling pathways that regulate cell growth, survival, motility, etc. Aberrant signaling also allows cancer cells to maintain oxygen and nutrient supply by induction of angiogenesis and invade adjacent and distant tissues. The aberrant capabilities of cancer cells were described as the hallmarks of cancer (HANAHAN and WEINBERG 2000).

A great deal of excitement has recently been raised by the development of a specific inhibitor of the BcrAbl kinase (Gleevac/Glivac, formerly STI-571). This kinase is constitutively active in chronic myelocytic leukemia (CML) cells as a result of the specific chromosome 9/22 reciprocal translocation that generates the BcrAbl fusion gene (Philadelphia chromosome). Unlike in most epithelial tumors, in the case of CML probably only this single genetic abnormality causes the disease. Accordingly, inhibition of the BcrAbl fusion kinase drastically increased response rates in patients. However, a high frequency of relapse is reported for chronic and advanced disease because of drug resistance associated with either mutations or amplification of the *BrcAbl* gene (LA ROSEE et al. 2002). In contrast to CML, most solid tumors are induced by more than one mutation and treatment with only a single drug may not control or cure these tumors. Therefore, combination therapy may be required for prolonged tumor control in many cases (COLEMAN 2002).

13.3.1
Active Versus Passive Mode of Cell Death

The prevailing cell death mechanism for tumor cells by ionizing radiation is postmitotic or reproductive cell death. Unrepaired or misrepaired DNA double-strand breaks are the critical lesion leading to cell inactivation during mitosis. Damaged cells do not necessarily die immediately but may undergo several cycles of cell division before reaching a critical level of genomic instability. Recent data indicate that programmed cell death (apoptosis) might also be an important factor for radiation-induced cell death and radiosensitivity in specific tumors (VERHEIJ and BARTELINK 2000). Ultimately, the apoptotic program is executed by distinct caspases. Two pathways leading to caspase activation have been characterized (Fig. 13.2) (GREEN 2000; WANG 2001). The extrinsic pathway is initiated by ligation of transmembrane death receptors (CD95, TNF receptor, and Trail receptor) to activate initiator caspases (caspase 8 and 10), which in turn cleave and activate effector caspases (e.g., caspase 3 and 7). The intrinsic pathway requires disruption of the mitochondrial membrane potential and the release of cytochrome C. Cytochrome C functions with apoptosis-protein-associated factor (Apaf) to induce activation of caspase 9, thereby also activating the downstream effector caspases. Mitochondrial membrane permeabilization is regulated by the opposing actions of pro- and anti-apoptotic Bcl-2 family members. There is considerable cross talk between the extrinsic and the intrinsic pathways. For example, caspase 8 can activate Bid, which then facilitates cytochrome C release. In some cell lines, this amplifies the apoptotic signal following death receptor activation. Conversely, activators of the intrinsic pathway can sensitize the cell to extrinsic death ligands (JOHNSTONE et al. 2002 and references therein; PRUSCHY et al. 2001).

Typical examples of cells that display strong apoptotic responses upon irradiation are those from the lymphoid and myeloid lineage and epithelial cells located in the intestinal crypts and salivary glands (HENDRY and POTTEN 1982; STEPHENS et al. 1991; RADFORD and MURPHY 1994). In a recent report it has been shown that in the progression of gastrointestinal damage upon whole body irradiation of mice microvascular endothelial cell apoptosis plays an important role (PARIS et al. 2001). This concept of endothelial cells as an important target of ionizing radiation might as well be valid for human tumors because endothelial apoptosis was reported to precede tumor cell apoptosis by 3–5 days after antiangiogenic cancer therapy (BROWDER et al. 2000). Evidence for the importance of apoptosis in the endothelial radiation response has been gained because growth factors affect both radiation-induced apoptosis and clonogenic cell survival, for example, basic fibroblast growth factor (bFGF) inhibits radiation-induced gastrointestinal syndrome and endothelial apoptosis in vivo and in vitro (PARIS et al. 2001; FUKS et al. 1994; HAIMOVITZ-FRIEDMAN et al. 1994a).

Decreased radiosensitivity has also been observed in epithelial cancer cells in the presence of epidermal growth factor (EGF), which serves as an important regulator of cellular proliferation but also contributes to protect cells from radiation damage. Clonogenic survival increases in EGF-stimulated cells (BALABAN et al. 1996), whereas antibodies against the EGF receptor sensitize cells to radiation by inducing apoptosis in vitro (HARARI and HUANG 2001; BALABAN et al. 1996). Another line of evidence for the importance of apoptosis is provided by studies showing that overexpression of apoptosis-promoting or apoptosis-suppressing genes modify radiation-induced cell survival and radiosensitivity. For instance, cells that are made resistant to radiation-induced apoptosis, either by overexpression of Bcl-2 or inactivation of p53, show an increase in clonogenic cell survival (SENTMAN et al. 1991; LOWE et al. 1994; STRASSER et al. 1994). However, many experiments

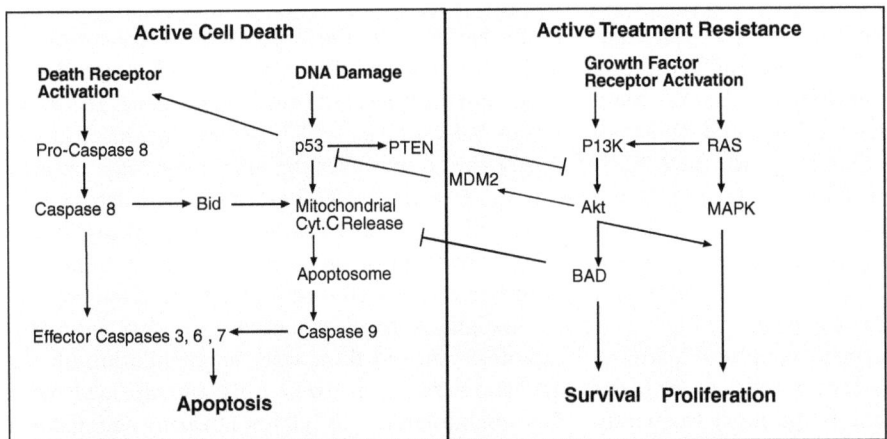

Fig. 13.2. Signaling pathways mediating active cell death and active treatment resistance. Cellular stress (e.g., ionizing radiation) might simultaneously induce death signaling (e.g., via DNA damage) and increase treatment resistance (e.g., via growth factor activation). Different cross-talks (e.g., via PTEN, MDM2 or BAD) exist between conflicting pathways and mutations of the corresponding genes might decide over the balance

in apoptosis research have been performed with normal cells transformed with dominant oncogenes and the results have been extrapolated to human malignancies. Whether treatment-induced tumor cell apoptosis is an important predictive factor for tumor eradication in solid human malignancies is not yet definitively elucidated. This is both due to a lack of good preclinical experimental models and the difficulty in documenting tumor cell apoptosis in solid human malignancies. Intercellular and cell matrix interactions, including angiogenesis, are critical for solid-tumor cell survival and thus, apoptosis in solid tumors has to be investigated in the more complex background of the cellular microenvironment.

13.3.2
Active Versus Passive Mode of Treatment Resistance

As a sensor of cellular stress, p53 is a critical initiator of the intrinsic apoptotic pathway. The sensor of DNA damage, ATM, phosphorylates and stabilizes p53 directly, and inhibits MDM2-mediated degradation of p53 (KHANNA and JACKSON 2001). P53 can initiate apoptosis by transcriptionally activating pro-apoptotic Bcl-2 family members (e.g. Bax, Bak, PUMA and Noxa), thereby inducing mitochondrial cytochrome C release and, at the same time, by repressing anti-apoptotic Bcl-2 proteins (Bcl-2, Bcl-xl) and inhibitor of apoptosis proteins (IAPs) (surviving) (BARTKE et al. 2001; HOFFMAN et al. 2002; RYAN et al. 2001; WU et al. 2001). P53 can also activate other genes that may contribute to apoptosis including *PTEN*, *Apaf-1*, and genes that lead to an increase of reactive oxygen species (ROS) (MORONI et al. 2001; STAMBOLIC et al. 2001; RYAN et al. 2001). In addition, p53 can transcriptionally activate both CD95 and Trail Receptor 2 (TrailR2/DR5), thereby sensitizing cells to death receptor-mediated apoptosis (HERR and DEBATIN 2001; RYAN et al. 2001). P53 may also have transcription-independent activities that potentiate cell death (RYAN et al. 2001). Therefore, p53 functions as a master regulator of the apoptotic program, capable of coordinating the process at multiple levels via several mechanisms (JOHNSTONE et al. 2002).

Disruption of the intrinsic apoptotic pathway is extremely common in cancer cells. Indeed, the p53 tumor suppressor gene is the most frequently mutated tumor suppressor gene in human tumors known so far. Loss of p53 function can disable apoptosis, accelerating tumor development in transgenic mice (RYAN et al. 2001; ATTARDI and JACKS 1999) and confer resistance to ionizing radiation (LOWE 1994). In thymocytes derived from mice homozygously negative (−/−) for p53, radiation and other types of DNA damage fail to induce apoptosis (CLARKE et al. 1993; LOWE et al. 1993). Furthermore, small intestinal epithelial cells from p53-$^{-/-}$ mice were radioresistant, with no apoptotic death observed between 4 h and 8 h after 8-Gy irradiation, a dose and time frame where apoptosis is readily seen in normal crypt cells (MERRITT et al. 1994; CLARKE et al. 1994). Although p53 plays a significant role in apoptosis induced by irradiation and other stimuli, apoptosis may also be p53-independent under certain conditions; for example, although p53-$^{-/-}$ thymocytes are resistant to radiation-induced apoptosis, they remain sensitive to dexamethasone-induced apoptosis (CLARKE et al. 1994). In small intestinal epithelial cells derived from p53-$^{-/-}$ mice, delayed G_2/M-associated p53-independent apoptosis occurred following irradiation (MERRIT et al. 1997). Although loss of p53 in these mice completely abrogated the early wave of apoptosis, there was a wave of apoptosis in the small intestine at 24 h and 40 h in the p53-$^{-/-}$ animals irradiated with 8 Gy. In this model, early apoptosis was shown to be p53-dependent, whereas late apoptosis was shown to be p53-independent.

Disruption of apoptotic pathways by mutated tumor suppressor genes such as *p53* is one way in which cancer cells become treatment-resistant. Another determinant of a more active mode of treatment resistance is increased survival signaling initiated by activated oncogenes (e.g., *Ras*), growth factor stimulation or activation of survival pathways as a stress response upon cytotoxic therapies (e.g., ionizing radiation) (Fig. 13.2). *Ras* is the most frequently mutated oncogene in human tumors and oncogenic mutations lead to the expression of constitutively active Ras protein. The frequency of mutated *Ras* genes and the type of the mutated *Ras* gene (*H-Ras, K-Ras* or *N-Ras*) varies widely depending on the tumor type. *K-Ras* is, however, the most frequently mutated *Ras* gene, with the highest incidence detected in pancreatic (90%) and sporadic colorectal carcinoma (50%). Overexpression or transformation of human or rodent cells with the oncogene *Ras* not only results in malignant transformation but also increases radioresistance in these cells; and inhibition of *Ras* activation radiosensitizes cells transformed with Ras and human tumor cell lines bearing endogenous mutations of *Ras* (GUPTA et al. 2001 and references therein). Different pharmacological compounds such as farnesyltransferase inhibitors inhibit Ras processing. They are currently under clinical investigation, as discussed by other authors in this volume. In recent years, a second pathway downstream of RTKs (sometimes via Ras) that involves phosphatidylinositol 3-kinase (PI3K) and Akt has come onto stage and is thought to be an important regulator of mammalian cell proliferation and survival. Several components of the PI3K/Akt pathway are dysregulated in a wide spectrum of human cancers. Both elevated PI3K and Akt activities have been identified in various tumor types due to amplified gene copy numbers and this pathway has been linked not only to apoptosis suppression but also to oncogenesis. Mutations of *PTEN* (which acts as a PI3K signaling antagonist) also often correlate with an apoptosis-resistant tumor phenotype (ZUNDEL et al. 2000; DAVIES et al. 1998; BELLACOSA et al. 1995). Different therapeutic strategies that target the PI3K/Akt pathway are now in development (VIVANCO and SAWYERS 2002).

13.3.3
Conflicting Signals

The cellular stress response generally depends on the balance of conflicting signaling pathways. Critical for the decision to undergo cell death is the balance between signaling pathways that mediate active cell death (e.g., the intrinsic apoptotic pathway) or active treatment resistance (e.g., the PI3K/Akt pathway). Both pathways might be activated at the same time (e.g., irradiation activates the intrinsic apoptotic pathway by inducing DNA damage and the PI3K/Akt pathway by directly activating the EGF receptor, see Sect. 13.4.2.1, "Receptor Tyrosine Kinases"). Furthermore, there is a considerable cross-talk between potentially conflicting pathways that consists of stimulatory and inhibitory feedback loops. A fascinating example for such cross-talk between the intrinsic apoptotic pathway and the PI3K/Akt survival pathway via PTEN and MDM2 has recently been revealed (Fig. 13.2). The survival protein Akt induces degradation (inhibition) of the pro-apoptotic protein p53 via phosphorylation of MDM2. Phosphorylated MDM2 translocates more efficiently to the nucleus, where it can bind p53, resulting in enhanced p53 degradation (MAYO and DONNER 2001; ZHOU et al. 2001). A self-regulatory interaction between p53 and Akt is indicated by the finding that p53 can positively regulate the PTEN promoter, which leads to inhibition of PI3K and Akt (STAMBOLIC et al. 2001). In normal cells the balance might depend on additional factors such as the amount of DNA damage (radiation dose) or on interactions with other pathways that are not yet elucidated. In cancer cells, mutations of the tumor suppressor genes *p53* and/or *PTEN* and mutations of the oncogenes *Akt* and *MDM2* that decide on the balance are often prevalent.

13.4
Ionizing Radiation and Signaling

The predominant mechanism by which IR induces cell death in mammalian cells is thought to be the reproductive mode of cell death: DNA single- and double-strand breaks are produced by incident photons, electrons or by radiation-induced free radicals. While single-strand breaks can be repaired efficiently by the endogenous repair machinery, remaining residual or misrepaired strand breaks (most often double-strand breaks) induce genetic instability, increased frequency of mutations or chromosomal aberrations that eventually lead to postmitotic cell death. However- the cellular radiation response to radiation is more complex than simply DNA damage repair. It is now evident that DNA damage by irradiation induces a complex network of inter- and intracellular signaling that can lead either to cell cycle arrest and induction of the DNA repair machinery or to programmed cell death in distinct cells. Evidence for the involvement of radiation-induced DNA double-stranded breaks in apoptosis was provided by experiments utilizing metabolic incorporation of 125I-labeled 5-iodo-2'-deoxyuridine ([125I]dURd). [125I]dURd replaces thymidine in DNA and when targeted to DNA produces DNA double-stranded breaks, eventually resulting in apoptotic cell death. But ionizing radiation not only induces signaling pathway modifications upon DNA damage, it also induces specific signaling pathway modifications at the cell membrane (e.g., growth factor activation) or in the cytoplasm independent of DNA damage (Fig. 13.3). Mutations or pharmacological modulation of key elements of this complex regulatory network of signal transduction cascades can dramatically change the radiation response of tumor cells, for example from DNA repair to cell death, and thus change their biologic radiosensitivity.

13.4.1
DNA-Damage-Induced Signaling

The DNA damage response pathway is characterized by the presence of a sensor that recognizes DNA

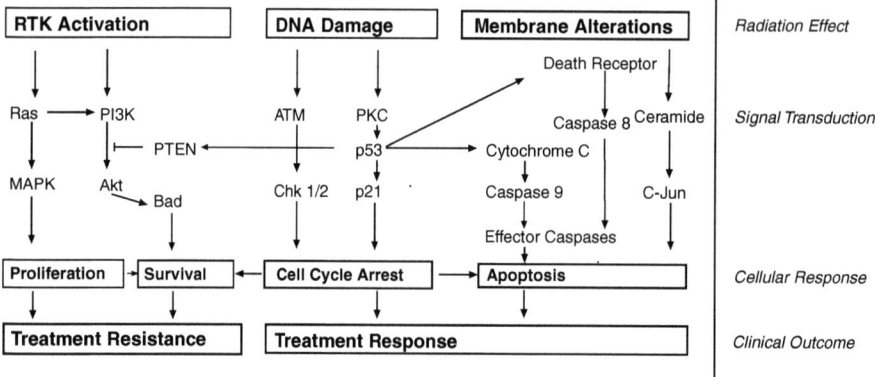

Fig. 13.3. Radiation-induced DNA-damage-dependent and DNA-damage-independent signaling. A complex network of signal transduction pathways leads to either treatment resistance or treatment response according to the genetic profile of a cancer cell

damage and transmits signals to a series of downstream effector molecules to activate signaling mechanisms for cell cycle arrest, induction of DNA repair, or apoptosis. A well-characterized response upon DNA damage is the cell cycle arrest to provide time for DNA repair, thus preventing mutations from being propagated. Cell cycle arrest occurs predominantly at the G1-S transition, but also in G2 phase before mitosis. In both cases, the cell cycle arrest is mediated by inhibition of cyclin-dependent-kinase (cdk)-cyclin complexes, which regulate both the G_1-S and the G_2-M checkpoints (HALL 2000). Indirect evidence for the importance of cell cycle checkpoints for the maintenance of genomic stability is provided by genetic disorders such as A-T (ataxia telangiectasia), which is associated with checkpoint deficiencies. The ATM (ataxia-telangiectasia-mutated) protein kinase, which is mutated in A-T, and the related ATR (A-T- and Rad3-related) protein kinase are both critical components in complex signaling networks, collectively referred to as replication and DNA damage checkpoints (ZHOU and ELLEDGE 2000). ATM is primarily activated by ionizing radiation, whereas ATR responds to a wider spectrum of DNA lesions. Activation of ATM results in subsequent phosphorylation of multiple downstream proteins that collectively regulate the repair and arrest functions of different checkpoint pathways. Although these signaling pathways are incompletely understood, the best characterized ATM-dependent functions involve the cell cycle arrest in response to DNA damage. ATM directly phosphorylates p53 and inhibits MDM2-dependent degradation of p53, allowing p53 to accumulate in the cell. Activated p53 increases the expression of multiple gene products, including the $p21^{cip1/waf1}$ protein. Binding of p21 to the G1 cyclin-dependent kinase complex inhibits their activity and prevents G1-to-S-phase progression upon DNA damage. Thus in A-T cells, loss of ATM function results in a delayed and attenuated accumulation of p53 upon ionizing radiation and abrogation of the IR-inducible G1 arrest. In contrast to the G1 arrest, the G2-M cell cycle arrest is probably controlled in a p53-independent way. Activation of ATM and ATR by ionizing radiation leads to phosphorylation of Chk2 and Chk1, respectively. Activated Chk2 and Chk1 phosphorylate cdc25C (mitosis-promoting-phosphatase), which leads to activation of the CyclinB1/Cdk1 complex and results in a G2 arrest (KHANNA et al. 2001; SARKARIA and ESHLEMAN 2001).

ATM also regulates key proteins of DNA repair such as the BRCA1 breast cancer susceptibility gene product. Heterozygous germline mutations of the *BRCA1* gene in women result in a greater than 75% lifetime risk for developing breast or ovarian malignancies, and approximately half of hereditary breast cancers are associated with loss of BRCA1 function (EASTON et al. 1995). Although the function of BRCA1 is not well understood, several lines of evidence indicate that it might function in DNA repair. In support of this assumption, cells lacking functional BRCA1 are hypersensitive to IR, and the radiation sensitivity of a BRCA1 mutant breast cancer cell line (HCC1937) is restored to normal levels by expression of normal levels of BRCA1 in these cells. In response to DNA damage, ATM, ATR, and Chk2 all phosphorylate BRCA1 on distinct amino acid residues that are important for BRCA1 function, and mutation of any one of these phosphorylation sites prevents BRCA1 from restoring the normal radiation sensitivity of HCC1937 cells (CORTEZ et al. 1999; LEE et al. 2000; TIBBETTS et al. 2000). The implications of these findings for breast radiotherapy in patients with a *BRCA1* mutation are not yet clear.

13.4.2
Non-DNA-Damage-Induced Signaling

It has long been known that radiation and free radicals can alter membrane proteins and lipids (LAVIN 1998 and references therein). However, the biological significance remained uncertain for a long time. More recently, it could be shown that ionizing radiation can induce specific signal transduction pathways at the level of the cell membrane and the cytoplasm as a stress response upon membrane alterations and membrane receptor activation.

13.4.2.1
Receptor Tyrosine Kinases

Receptor tyrosine kinases (RTKs) make up a group of receptors that are critically involved in human cancer (ZWICK et al. 2001). Examples of receptor tyrosine kinases are the insulin receptor, the epithelial growth factor receptor (EGFR) family and the vascular endothelial growth factor receptor (VEGFR) family. Ionizing radiation can stimulate RTKs, e.g., the EGF receptor family, by induction of autophosphorylation of the receptor. RTKs are interesting targets for radiosensitization, because aberrant signaling by RTKs in the form of constitutive activation of RTKs as well as receptor activation by autocrine and paracrine growth factor loops are critically involved in many human cancers. Constitutive activation of RTKs, which has been shown to be important for malignant transformation and tumor proliferation, can occur by several mechanisms such as gene amplification, overexpression or mutations (KOLIBABA and DRUKER 1997). Somatic and germline mutations, which are associated with distinct inherited and spontaneous human cancer syndromes, have been observed in at least ten different RTK families (ROBERTSON et al. 2000). These alterations mostly result in a constitutive active RTK, as reported for the RTK HER2/*neu* (PENUEL et al. 2001). Activation of autocrine growth factor loops is another mechanism for aberrant growth factor signaling and has been described for EGFR and the insulin-like growth factor receptor (IGF-IR) family (DERYNCK et al. 1987; KALEKO et al. 1990). This potential mechanism of activation occurs when elevated levels of both growth factor receptor and its ligand are expressed concomitantly, as reported for many solid tumors (SALOMON et al. 1995).

Ionizing radiation can directly activate specific RTKs such as the EGFR family (ErbB1-4) (BOWERS et al. 2001; SCHMIDT-ULLRICH et al. 2000; BALABAN et al. 1996). Similar effects of stimulation by IR and growth factors (GF), for example, activation of the pro-proliferative mitogen-activated protein kinase (MAPK) have been postulated so far for ErbB1. However, recently distinct ErbB response profiles after exposure to GF or IR have been reported in mammary carcinoma cell lines differing in their ErbB expression profile (BOWERS et al. 2001). In autocrine growth-related mammary carcinoma cells, at least one of the ErbB receptors with GF-binding specificity and an active kinase domain, such as ErbB1 or ErbB4, are dominantly expressed. Treatment of these cells with GF such as EGF (ErbB1-specific) and heregulin (ErbB4-specific) results in hierarchic transactivations of ErbB2 or ErbB3, respectively, dependent on GF-binding specificity. In contrast, IR activates all ErbB species (ErbB1-4), reflecting the specific expression profile of the cell. Moreover, downstream effects are different when IR is combined with different specific inhibitors of the ErbB family. In combination with a specific ErbB1 and ErbB4 inhibitor (Tyrphostin, AG 1478), MAPK activation is completely inhibited whereas selective inhibition of ErbB2 with Tyrphostin AG825 in combination with IR caused an enhanced MAPK response, simulating an amplified ErbB1 (or ErbB4) response. These data indicate that ErbB2 is a modulator of ErbB1 (or 4) function, leading to different MAPK response profiles upon GF or IR exposure (BOWERS et al. 2001).

Specifically, EGFR (ErbB1) is a promising target for radiosensitization as was shown in several preclinical studies. The rationale for targeting EGFR is based on the concept that EGFR signaling strongly promotes cell proliferation via MAPK. Many clinical phase I–III trials are currently under way with different ErbB1 targeting agents (monoclonal antibodies, e.g., C225 [Cetuximab]), and receptor tyrosine kinase inhibitors (e.g., ZD1839, [Iressa]), either alone or in combination with cytotoxic therapies such as IR. Although aberrant EGFR signaling is not described for endothelial cells, a direct effect of EGFR inhibition on endothelial cells and angiogenesis is discussed (MENDELSOHN 2001; BRUNS et al. 2000).

A well-known paracrine growth factor loop is the pro-angiogenic interaction between tumor cells and endothelial cells upon hypoxic stress (e.g., irradiation). Irradiation targets both tumor cells and endothelial cells and as part of a stress response enhances the expression of VEGF in the tumor tissue. VEGF is secreted from the tumor cells and binds specifically to the VEGF receptor on endothelial cells, protecting endothelial cells from radiation damage. With the help of this paracrine growth factor loop, the tumor cells not only promote angiogenesis and endothelial survival but also indirectly promote tumor cell survival by building up new supplies with oxygen and nutrition. VEGF receptor inhibitors down-regulate the VEGF-dependent proliferative activity of the tumor microvasculature, concomitantly block the enhanced VEGF-mediated survival processes in response to irradiation and might thereby lead to a cooperative effect (GENG et al. 2001; GORSKI et al. 1999).

13.4.2.2
The Sphingomyelin Pathway

The sphingomyelin (SM) pathway is a ubiquitous, evolutionarily conserved signaling system. Ceramide has been implicated as a mediator of the apoptotic response following exposure to a variety of stimuli, including tumor necrosis factor (TNF), Fas ligand, exposure to glucocorticoids and ionizing radiation (PENA et al. 1997). Radiation-induced damage of the cell membrane generates ceramide via catabolism of SM by either neutral or acid sphingomyelinase, or by de novo synthesis by ceramide synthase. In the radiation response, ceramide serves as a second messenger in initiating apoptosis, while some of its metabolites (e.g., sphingosine-1-phosphate, S 1-P) block apoptosis. In certain cells, such as endothelial, lymphoid and hematopoietic cells, ceramide can mediate apoptosis (LIN et al. 2000). The studies of HAIMOVITZ-FRIEDMAN et al. (1994b) provided the first evidence that generation of ceramide might initiate signaling of apoptosis. Irradiation of bovine aortic endothelial cells (BAEC) induced rapid hydrolysis of SM to generate ceramide, and analogs of ceramide mimicked the effect of radiation to signal for apoptosis. Other studies indicate that the p53 dependence of ceramide-induced apoptosis might be cell-type specific. Acid sphingomyelinase (ASMase) knockout mice do not display SM hydrolysis to ceramide or endothelial apoptosis in the lung upon irradiation. Alternately, p53 knockout animals manifest normal ceramide generation and apoptosis in the lung after total body ionizing radiation, even though apoptosis in the thymus is abrogated (SANTANA et al. 1996). In contrast, ceramide-induced apoptosis is p53 dependent in genetically defined (p53 wild type or p53-deficient) mouse fibrosarcoma cells (PRUSCHY et al. 1999).

The c-Jun kinase (JNK) cascade was reported to mediate pro-apoptotic signals downstream of ceramide in BAEC and in a human monomyelocytic cell line (U937 cells). Overexpression of dominant negative mutants of kinases of the JNK cascade blocked apoptosis in response to radiation and ceramide analogs. JNK induces apoptosis presumably via transcriptional regulation of unknown genes (VERHEIJ et al. 1996). Another mechanism of ceramide-mediated apoptosis is inhibition of the survival stress response of irradiated cells. Ceramide was reported to inactivate directly PI3K (ZUNDEL and GIACCIA 1998) or mediate inhibition of PKB/Akt via ceramide-activated protein phosphatases (CAPPs) (SALINAS et al. 2000).

Some data provided evidence that ATM reciprocally regulates the activity of ceramide synthase and consequently apoptosis after radiation exposure. In some cell lines, DNA damage-induced apoptosis is normally inhibited by ATM. EBV-immortalized B cell lines from six AT patients with different mutations exhibited radiation-induced ceramide synthase activation, ceramide generation, and apoptosis, whereas three lines from normal patients failed to manifest these responses. Stable transfection of wild type ATM cDNA reversed these events in the mutant lines, while anti-sense inactivation of ATM in normal B cells conferred this AT phenotype. The pro-apoptotic ceramide signal may be also counterbalanced by an anti-apoptotic signal mediated via protein kinase C (PKC). Activation of PKC by phorbol esters blocked radiation-induced ceramide generation and apoptosis in several different cell types (WARD 1994; SANTANA et al. 1995; ALLAN-YORKE et al. 1998; CHMURA et al. 1996a,b).

A great body of evidence implies that endothelial cells use ceramide generation for induction of apoptosis in response to radiation and other stresses. The vulnerability of the endothelium to stress appears related to the abundance of ASMase in endothelium (20 times as much as in other cell types, MARATHE et al. 1998). Whole-lung irradiated C3H/HeJ mice manifest lethal inflammatory pneumonitis within 1–6 months, depending on the radiation dose used. The first pathological change in the irradiated mouse lung is widespread endothelial apoptosis within 4–10 h after exposure (FUKS et al. 1995). Evidence that endothelial apoptosis is relevant to the development of inflammatory radiation pneumonitis was derived from studies using bFGF. Pretreatment with bFGF renders mice resistant to endothelial apoptosis and inflammatory radiation pneumonitis. Moreover, endothelial apoptosis in the lung is preceded by ceramide elevation, which occurred from 0.5 to 2 h, peaking at twice the control (SANTANA et al. 1996). In a recent report, radiation-induced gastrointestinal tract damage (GI syndrome) after whole-body-irradiation of mice was prevented when endothelial cell apoptosis was inhibited by intravenous application of bFGF and genetically by deletion of the ASMase gene, confirming the importance of endothelial apoptosis for radiation toxicity syndromes (Paris et al. 2001). This concept of endothelial cells as important or even as primary target of ionizing radiation might as well be valid for human tumors considering the fact that there is an intensive communication between tumor cells and endothelial cells by means of various paracrine growth factor loops (e.g., VEGF) and because endothelial apoptosis was reported to precede tumor cell apoptosis by 3–5 days after antiangiogenic cancer therapy (Browder et al. 2000).

13.5
Pharmacological Signaling Modification in Combination with Ionizing Radiation

In the last few years, the knowledge on the signal transduction processes making up the radiation response of eukaryotic cells to ionizing radiation has dramatically expanded. The availability of chemical agents that modulate these signaling processes in the active mode of cell death and the active mode of treatment resistance has increased tremendously and is beyond the scope of this review. Some of the most promising classes of compounds nowadays are discussed by other authors in this volume. However, to elucidate the objectives and the complexity of signal transduction modification, an example will be given to show how specific inhibitors of the protein kinase C simultaneously modulate the apoptotic response and a major radioresistance pathway in tumor cells. Furthermore, not only the mode of radiosensitization of different PKC inhibitors varies according to the p53 status, but also the apoptotic response is mediated over different pathways dependent on the cell lines used.

13.5.1
Signaling Modification in Active Mode of Cell Death: p53

The state of the tumor suppressor p53 is pivotal for the response of tumor cells to irradiation. Mutations in the p53 gene are involved in acquired and intrinsic treatment resistance in human tumors and render tumor cells refractory to many anticancer therapies (Giaccia and Kastan 1998; Kinzler and Vogelstein 1996). After irradiation, p53 is activated and induces a crucial block to cell cycle progression, providing enough time for sufficient DNA repair prior to deleterious DNA replication in S phase. On the other hand, apoptosis may arise through p53-mediated signal transduction cascades, leading to the activation of the apoptotic machinery. Radioresistance of tumor cells devoid of p53 may be a consequence of a diminished ability to undergo apoptosis in vitro and in vivo (Lowe et al. 1993, 1994). Thus, treatment strategies that combine with ionizing radiation to restore p53 function are interesting strategies for cancer treatment. In the last few years, a great deal of effort has focused on *p53* gene replacement for cancer. Current approaches use several methods of delivery, including adenoviral vectors, retroviral vectors, herpes vectors and nonviral vectors. In addition, studies combining *p53* gene replacement with DNA-damaging agents such as cisplatin and ionizing radiation indicate synergy in terms of induction of apoptosis (Roth et al. 2001). Preclinical studies of *p53* gene therapy in combination with ionizing radiation indicated that gene delivery of *p53* to p53-deficient tumor cells, both in vitro and in vivo, increases their sensitivity to radiation (Spitz et al. 1996). In a phase II clinical trial, 17 patients with localized non-small cell lung cancer (NSCLC) were treated with adenoviral-mediated *p53* gene transfer in conjunction with radiation therapy. Safety data indicated that this combination has an acceptable safety profile. The major side effects were pneumothoraces after drug application. The results of this study were encouraging, with a 1-year survival rate of 56% and a local response rate at the injection site of 53% (Swisher et al. 1999).

Another treatment strategy is to bypass the p53-dependent death pathway and induce p53-independent cell killing. Of more than ten cytotoxic agents tested, only one compound namely Taxol displayed a largely p53-independent antitumor effect alone and in combination with ionizing radiation (Blagosklonny and Fojo 1999; Pruschy et al. 2001). However, as already discussed, Taxol is not an ideal radiosensitizer because of the relatively small therapeutic index (extensive toxicity). A p53-independent radiosensitizing effect has also been reported for several inhibitors of the PKC family of serine/threonine kinases.

Members of the PKC family function as transducers for various lipid second messengers in the regulation, transduction and propagation of cell proliferative stimuli. The identification of protein kinase C as a target for radiosensitization goes back to the observation that PKC activation is functionally related to the induction of tumor necrosis factor (TNF) and immediate early genes such as *EGR-1*, *c-jun* and *c-fos*, mainly investigated in tumor cells of hematopoietic origin (HALLAHAN et al. 1991a-c; SHERMAN et al. 1991). Moreover, radiation-induced PKC activation limits the production of ceramide from the hydrolysis of sphingomyelin and rescues cells from IR-mediated apoptosis (KOLESNICK 1994; HAIMOVITZ-FRIEDMAN et al. 1994a). In addition, inhibition of PKC and subsequent ceramide production was reported to alter the expression and function of antiapoptotic proteins (CHMURA et al. 1996a,b) and to activate caspases (CED3/CPP32 proteases), which are required for IR-mediated apoptosis. However, release of the apoptotic second messenger ceramide as mediator of IR-induced apoptosis might be relevant only in some cells, while in others ceramide may only serve as a co-signal or does not play a role in the death response (SANTANA et al. 1996; HAIMOVITZ-FRIEDMAN et al. 1994a,b, 1997).

Based on these rationales, different classes of PKC inhibitors were tested as radiosensitizing compounds (HAIMOVITZ-FRIEDMAN et al. 1994a; KIM et al. 1992; HALLAHAN et al. 1992). One of these compounds, PKC412 [*N*-benzoyl staurosporine (formerly called CGP-41251)], is a staurosporine-related drug that is currently under clinical investigation for its anticancer activity. PKC 412 is a competitive inhibitor of ATP, binding to the PKC isoforms α, β, and γ. It shows a broad antiproliferative activity against different tumor types in vitro and in vivo, but more important, PKC412 also significantly enhances the antitumor activity of 5-FU, cis- and carboplatinum, doxorubicin, vinblastine and Taxol against solid tumors that do not show a response against single treatment with PKC412 alone. Interestingly, PKC412 also has the potential to revert the multidrug-resistant phenotype in cancer cells and thus makes it an interesting candidate for combined treatment modalities such as reversing the cytotoxic drug resistance towards adriamycin. The tumor growth control effect in vivo is further enhanced by inhibition of ligand-induced autophosphorylation of the VEGF receptor tyrosine kinase, resulting in an additional antiangiogenic effect by PKC 412 (GESCHER et al. 1998; FABBRO et al. 1999). Recently it was reported that PKC412 is also a highly active inhibitor of the FLT3 tyrosine kinases. Constitutively activating FLT3 receptor mutations have been found in 35% of patients with acute myeloblastic leukemia (AML) and PKC412 is a candidate for testing as an antileukemia agent in AML patients with mutant FLT3 receptors (WEISBERG et al. 2002). Depending on the cellular genetic background and the treatment conditions, PKC412 exerts different cellular responses and mechanisms of radiosensitization. Treatment of glioblastoma cells and other tumor cell types with PKC412 in the 0.5–1 µM range resulted in a pronounced G2-M arrest (BEGEMANN et al. 1996, 1998; IKEGAMI et al. 1996) and a cooperative decrease in clonogenic survival (BEGEMANN et al. 1998). The same authors showed that PKC412 directly inhibits cdc2- and cdk2-associated kinase activities, implying that it is not the PKC inhibitory function of PKC412 that is responsible for the cell cycle modulatory effect. However, treatment with a low concentration of PKC412 that does not affect cell cycle distribution (0.2 µM) by itself results in G2 arrest and supra-additive loss of clonogenicity when applied in combination with clinically relevant doses of IR in p53-deficient cells (ZAUGG et al. 2001). Moreover, in a genetically defined tumor cell system, a p53-dependent mode of cell death in vitro and in vivo was investigated when PKC412 was applied in combination with IR. PKC412 sensitized both p53-wild-type and p53-deficient *E1A/ras* oncogene-transformed murine embryo fibroblasts for treatment with ionizing radiation (Fig. 13.4a). In p53 wild-type cells, combined treatment drastically induced apoptotic cell death whereas no apoptosis induction could be observed in p53-deficient cells in clonogenic assays (Fig. 13.4b) and in histological tumor sections (ZAUGG et al. 2001; PRUSCHY et al. 2001). Further, in p53 wild-type cells, combined treatment resulted in cooperative cytochrome C release, drastically activating the caspase 9/caspase 3 apoptotic pathway, but was completely absent in p53-deficient isogenic tumor cells. A strict requirement for this specific apoptotic pathway by PKC412/IR-induced cell kill in p53 wild-type cells was revealed by comparing oncogene-transformed caspase-9 wild-type and caspase-9-deficient embryo fibroblasts (ROCHA et al. 2000). The same authors also showed that a clinically relevant fractionated treatment schedule of IR (4+3 Gy) in combination with PKC412 displays a promising combined tumor control effect against p53-deficient mouse embryo fibroblasts (Fig. 13.5a) and p53-mutated human SW480 colon adenocarcinoma xenografts (data not shown). Likewise in another report, chelerythrine, a selective ATP-independent inhibitor of α, β PKC isoforms, radiosensitized p53-deficient SQ-20B human head and neck squamous cancer cells both in cellular and animal xenograft studies (Fig. 13.5b; CHMURA et al. 1997). IR treatment alone did not induce apoptosis in p53-deficient radioresistant SQ-20B cells but combined treatment supra-additively increased the fraction of apoptotic tumor cells in vivo, suggesting that Chelerythrine also lowers an apoptotic threshold for IR-induced apoptosis and tumor cell

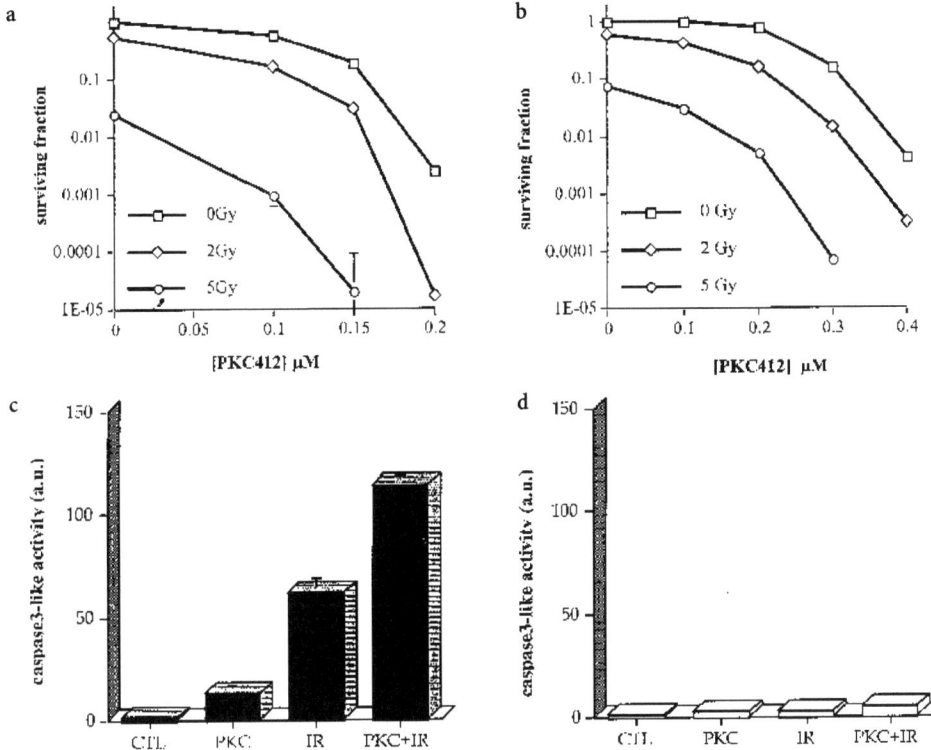

Fig. 13.4a-d. P53-dependent mechanism of radiosensitization of PKC412 on E1A/ras-transformed murine embryo fibroblasts (MEFs). A: Single-seeded p53 +/+ (a) and p53 -/- (b) transformed MEFs were treated with increasing doses of PKC412 and IR. PKC412 radiosensitizes both, p53 +/+ (a) and p53 -/- (b) cells. B: The mechanism of radiosensitization in p53 +/+ cells is apoptosis induction (c), whereas in p53 -/- cells no apoptosis induction can be detected (d) (caspase-3-like activity assay as apoptotic read out) (ZAUGG et al. 2001, with permission)

Fig. 13.5a-c. The effect of RT and PKC412 alone or combined on the growth of p53 -/- E1A/ras transformed murine MEFs (A) and human p53-mutated colon adenocarcinoma xenografts (B) in nude mice. Treatment on 4 consecutive days (3 Gy, 100 mg/kg PKC412 alone or combined) was started after tumors reached a minimal volume of 150 mm^3 (day 14) (ZAUGG et al. 2001, with permission). Likewise, the PKC-Inhibitor, Chelerythrine, radiosensitized p53-deficient SQ-20B human head and neck squamous cancer cells in animal xenograft studies (C, CHMURA et al. 1997, with permission) but, in contrast to PKC412, induced p53-independent apoptosis (data not shown) killing (CHMURA et al. 1997). Interestingly, both compounds, PKC412 and chelerythrine, displayed different mechanisms of radiosensitizing p53-dysfunctional tumor cells, either G2 arrest or apoptosis induction, respectively. However, ZAUGG et al. (2001) did not investigate whether ceramide was also generated after combined treatment with PKC412 and IR in the p53-deficient tumor cells that underwent G2 arrest and whether the ceramide-dependent apoptotic pathway was interrupted by further mutations downstream of ceramide in these cells.

13.5.2
Signaling Modification in Active Mode of Treatment Resistance: PI3K/Akt Pathway

Activated oncogenes are major determinants in increasing tumor cell resistance to radiation. Overexpression or transformation of rodent or human cells with the oncogene *Ras* in many cases results in cell lines that are substantially more resistant to radiation than the parental cells (GUPTA et al. 2001; MILLER et al. 1993; MCKENNA et al. 1990; LING and ENDLICH 1989). Moreover, inhibition of *Ras* activation radiosensitizes both rodent cells transfected with *Ras* (BERNHARD et al. 1996) and human tumor cell lines bearing endogenous mutations of *Ras* (MILLER et al. 1993; BERNHARD et al. 1998). Different pharmacological compounds that inhibit Ras processing such as farnesyltransferase inhibitors are currently under clinical investigation, as discussed by other authors in this volume. Furthermore, the identification of signaling pathways downstream of Ras is of considerable interest because these pathways are potential targets for even more selective manipulation of radiosensitivity in tumor cells with *Ras* mutations. The most extensively investigated Ras signaling pathways are the Ras-to-MAPK (mitogen-activated protein kinase) and the phosphatidylinositide 3-kinase (PI3K)/Akt signal transduction pathways. In a recent report, the authors outlined that the PI3K/Akt and not the Ras-to-MAPK pathway is the major determinant of cellular resistance to apoptotic stress stimuli: the PI3K inhibitor LY294002 radiosensitized cells bearing mutant *Ras* oncogenes, but the survival of cells bearing wild-type Ras was not affected. Inhibition of the PI3K downstream target p70S6K by rapamycin,

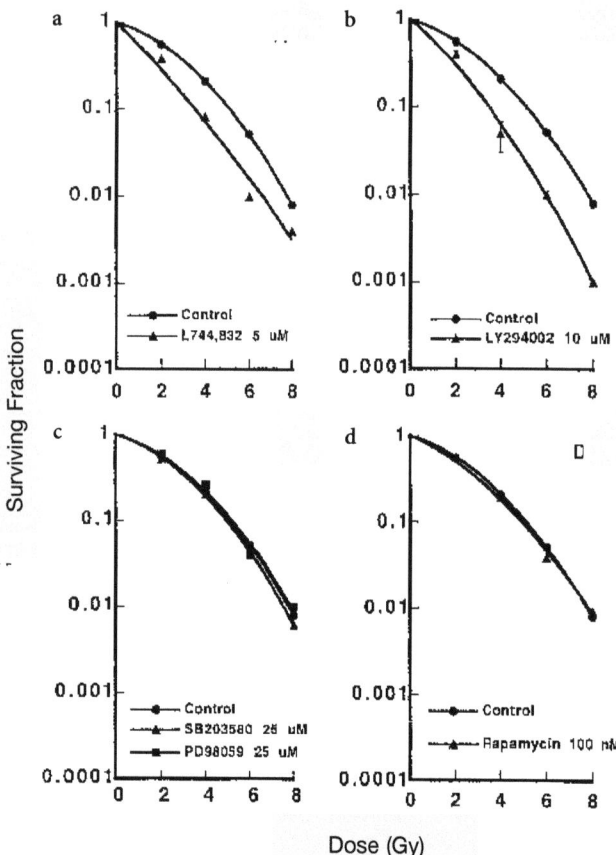

Fig. 13.6a–d. Clonogenic survival in T24 cells after treatment with inhibitors of the Ras signal transduction pathway. Survival after treatment with *A*, FTI L744,832 (▲); *B*, LY294002 (▲); *C*, SB203580 (▲), PD98059 (■); and *D*, rapamycin (▲). The control curve (●) in all of the panels is the same. The error bars are shown and, if not visible, were contained within the point of the graph. (GUPTA et al. 2001, with permission)

the RAF-MEK-MAPK pathway with PD98059, or the Ras-MEK kinase p38 pathway with SB203580 had no effect on radiation survival in cells with oncogenic Ras (Fig. 13.6). Moreover, expression of active PI3K in cells with wild-type Ras resulted in increased radiation resistance that could be inhibited with LY294002 (GUPTA et al. 2001). The importance of the PI3K/Akt pathway as mediator of radioresistance is further supported by the fact that EGF, which plays a critical role in cell proliferation, mediated through the MAPK pathway, also activates the PI3K/Akt pathway (GUPTA et al. 2001; OKANO et al. 2000). An association between EGFR and clinical radioresistance has been reported in patients with head and neck cancers (MAURIZI et al. 1996) and astrocytic gliomas (ZHU et al. 1996). Upon activation, the PI3K/Akt pathway controls several downstream targets involved in apoptosis regulation, glucose transport and glycogen synthesis (e.g., the bcl-2 family member Bad, caspase 9 and the transcription factor cross-talk, glycogen synthase kinase 3). Different cross-talks exist in other growth promoting and cell survival signaling pathways, but the exact mechanism of their regulation is still under investigation (DOWNWARD 1998; KENNEDY et al. 1997, 1999; ZUNDEL and GIACCIA 1998). Both elevated PI3K and Akt activities have been identified in various tumor types due to amplified gene copy numbers and this pathway has been linked not only to apoptosis suppression but also to oncogenesis. Further inactivating mutations of the lipid phosphatase and tumor suppressor PTEN that acts as a PI3K signaling antagonist also often correlate with an apoptosis-resistant tumor phenotype (ZUNDEL et al. 2000; DAVIES et al. 1998; BELLACOSA et al. 1995).

Interestingly, dose-dependent down-regulation of the PI3K/Akt pathway by PKC412 (0–1 µM) correlates with decreased proliferative activity and activation of the apoptotic machinery. Different mechanisms might exist for PKC412-dependent down-regulation of this pathway. At elevated antiproliferative concentrations, PKC412 directly inhibits 3'phosphoinositide-dependent protein kinase 1 (PDK1), the kinase mediating the stimulatory signal from PI3K to Akt (HILL et al. 2001). On the other hand, low concentration of PKC412 that has only a minimal antiproliferative effect by itself, but strongly sensitizes for IR, also down-regulates Akt activity, presumably through inhibition of a different upstream interacting target. Whether a specific PKC isoform is responsible for this is not known so far. Nevertheless, other clinically nonrelevant inhibitory compounds such as the PI3K inhibitor LY294002 also show that overcoming an intrinsic treatment threshold by the inhibition of this PI3K/Akt pathway is an important concept to sensitize tumor cells for IR (TENZER et al. 2001; BELLACOSA et al. 1995).

13.6
Outlook

Novel technology such as IMRT further tailors the radiation beam and increases the therapeutic index by an optimized sparing of normal surrounding tissue. However, it does not overcome intrinsic radioresistance. Ionizing radiation not only induces DNA damage but also as a stress response activates a complex network of signal transduction pathways within tumor cells and normal tissue cells. With the knowledge of the proteins and genes that make up these pathways, a multitude of targets has been revealed that allow modulating the radiation effect in the cell. It is now becoming feasible to lower the intrinsic radioresistance of tumor cells by modulating signaling pathways of active cell death, active treatment resistance or DNA repair or even to increase the intrinsic radioresistance of the surrounding normal tissue. In addition, a significant amount of highly promising signal transduction targets are located outside of tumor cells in the microenvironment that co-influence the response to ionizing radiation and combined treatment modality (e.g., endothelial cells, growth factor loops, matrix metalloproteinases, etc.). The complexity of the entire signal transduction network of cancer cells and their microenvironment is far from clear and many cancer cells do not respond to treatment with even highly selective molecular compounds by simply using redundant signaling pathways or activating escape mechanisms.

The first generation of molecular-defined radiosensitizers are currently being investigated in clinical phase I–III studies. The trend for the future might be to use molecular compounds even more selectively and especially based on the molecular profile of the tumor and/or the surrounding normal tissue of every single patient. The tools for molecular profiling such as gene arrays or protein arrays are currently being investigated. As it becomes increasingly evident that signal transduction processes are highly complex, in the future even a designed cocktail of molecular defined compounds might be used to modulate the effect of ionizing radiation. However such "extra-large" cocktails might lose specificity and could be accompanied by prohibitive costs.

Given that over the past decade the most impressive gains in local tumor control have been obtained with the combination of traditional chemotherapy and ionizing radiation, combined treatment modality with ionizing radiation and the novel generation of molecular defined compounds is a highly promising approach for further improvements of clinical radiation oncology and it is to be anticipated that molecular radiobiology in the future will also help to improve patient cure rates.

Acknowledgements. We thank W. Gillies McKenna and Ralph R. Weichselbaum for permission to present their data and Karin Bühler for preparing the illustrations.

References

Allan-Yorke J, Record M, de Preval C et al (1998) Distinct pathways for tumor necrosis factor alpha and ceramides in human cytomegalovirus infection. J Virol 72:2316–2322

Antonadou D (2002) Radiotherapy or chemotherapy followed by radiotherapy with or without amifostine in locally advanced lung cancer. Semin Radiat Oncol 12:50–58

Attardi LD, Jacks T (1999) The role of p53 in tumour suppression: lessons from mouse models. Cell Mol Life Sci 55:48–63

Balaban N, Moni J, Shannon M et al (1996) The effect of ionizing radiation on signal transduction: antibodies to EGF receptor sensitize A431 cells to radiation. Biochim Biophys Acta 1314:147–156

Bartke T, Siegmund D, Peters N et al (2001) p53 upregulates cFLIP, inhibits transcription of NF-kappaB-regulated genes and induces caspase-8-independent cell death in DLD-1 cells. Oncogene 20:571–580

Begemann M, Kashimawo SA, Choi YA et al (1996) Inhibition of the growth of glioblastomas by CGP 41251, an inhibitor of protein kinase C, and by a phorbol ester tumor promoter. Clin Cancer Res 2:1017–1030

Begemann M, Kashimawo SA, Heitjan DF et al (1998) Treatment of human glioblastoma cells with the staurosporine derivative CGP 41251 inhibits CDC2 and CDK2 kinase activity and increases radiation sensitivity. Anticancer Res 18:2275–2282

Bellacosa A, de Feo D, Godwin AK et al (1995) Molecular alterations of the AKT2 oncogene in ovarian and breast carcinomas. Int J Cancer 64:280–285

Bentzen L, Keiding S, Horsman MR et al (2000) Feasibility of detecting hypoxia in experimental mouse tumours with 18F-fluorinated tracers and positron emission tomography – a study evaluating [18F]Fluoro-2-deoxy-D-glucose. Acta Oncol 39:629–637

Bernhard EJ, Kao G, Cox AD et al (1996) The farnesyltransferase inhibitor FTI-277 radiosensitizes H-ras-transformed rat embryo fibroblasts. Cancer Res 56:1727–1730

Bernhard EJ, McKenna WG, Hamilton AD et al (1998) Inhibiting Ras prenylation increases the radiosensitivity of human tumor cell lines with activating mutations of ras oncogenes. Cancer Res 58:1754–1761

Blagosklonny MV and Fojo T (1999) Molecular effects of paclitaxel: myths and reality (a critical review). Int J Cancer 83:151–156

Bowers G, Reardon D, Hewitt T et al (2001) The relative role of ErbB1-4 receptor tyrosine kinases in radiation signal transduction responses of human carcinoma cells. Oncogene 20:1388–1397

Brizel DM, Wasserman TH, Henke M et al (2000) Phase III randomized trial of amifostine as a radioprotector in head and neck cancer. J Clin Oncol 18:3339–3345

Browder T, Butterfield CE, Kraling BM et al (2000) Antiangiogenic scheduling of chemotherapy improves efficacy against experimental drug-resistant cancer. Cancer Res 60:1878–1886

Brown JM, Giaccia AJ (1998) The unique physiology of solid tumors: opportunities (and problems) for cancer therapy. Cancer Res 58:1408–1416

Brown JM (1999) The hypoxic cell: a target for selective cancer therapy – eighteenth Bruce F. Cain Memorial Award lecture. Cancer Res 59:5863–5870

Brown JM (2001) Therapeutic targets in radiotherapy. Int J Radiat Oncol Biol Phys 49:319–326

Bruns CJ, Solorzano CC, Harbison MT et al (2000) Blockade of the epidermal growth factor receptor signaling by a novel tyrosine kinase inhibitor leads to apoptosis of endothelial cells and therapy of human pancreatic carcinoma. Cancer Res 60:2926–2935

Buntzel J, Glatzel M, Kuttner K et al (2002) Amifostine in simultaneous radiochemotherapy of advanced head and neck cancer. Semin Radiat Oncol 12:4–13

Chao KS, Deasy JO, Markman J et al (2001) A prospective study of salivary function sparing in patients with head and-neck cancers receiving intensity-modulated or three-dimensional radiation therapy: initial results. Int J Radiat Oncol Biol Phys 49:907–916

Chmura SJ, Nodzenski E, Weichselbaum RR et al (1996a) Protein kinase C inhibition induces apoptosis and ceramide production through activation of a neutral sphingomyelinase. Cancer Res 56:2711–2714

Chmura SJ, Nodzenski E, Crane MA et al (1996b) Cross-talk between ceramide and PKC activity in the control of apoptosis in WEHI-231. Adv Exp Med Biol 406:39–55

Chmura SJ, Mauceri HJ, Advani S et al (1997) Decreasing the apoptotic threshold of tumor cells through protein kinase C inhibition and sphingomyelinase activation increases tumor killing by ionizing radiation. Cancer Res 57:4340–4347

Clarke AR, Purdie CA, Harrison DJ et al (1993) Thymocyte apoptosis induced by p53-dependent and -independent pathways. Nature 362:849–852

Clarke AR, Gledhill S, Hooper ML et al (1994) p53 dependence of early apoptotic and proliferative responses within the mouse intestinal epithelium following gamma-irradiation. Oncogene 9:1767–1773

Coleman CN (2002) Radiation oncology – linking technology and biology in the treatment of cancer. Acta Oncol 41:6–13

Cortez D, Wang Y, Qin J et al (1999) Requirement of ATM-dependent phosphorylation of BRCA1 in the DNA damage response to double-strand breaks. Science 286:1162–1166

Davies MA, Lu Y, Sano T et al (1998) Adenoviral transgene expression of MMAC/PTEN in human glioma cells inhibits Akt activation and induces anoikis. Cancer Res 58:5285–5290

Derynck R, Goeddel DV, Ullrich A et al (1987) Synthesis of messenger RNAs for transforming growth factors alpha and beta and the epidermal growth factor receptor by human tumors. Cancer Res 47:707–712

Downward J (1998) Ras signalling and apoptosis. Curr Opin Genet Dev 8:49–54

Easton DF, Ford D, Bishop DT (1995) Breast and ovarian cancer incidence in BRCA1-mutation carriers. Breast Cancer Linkage Consortium. Am J Hum Genet 56:265–271

Eisbruch A, Kim HM, Terrell JE et al (2001) Xerostomia and its predictors following parotid-sparing irradiation of head-and-neck cancer. Int J Radiat Oncol Biol Phys 50:695–704

Fabbro D, Buchdunger E, Wood J et al (1999) Inhibitors of protein kinases: CGP 41251, a protein kinase inhibitor with potential as an anticancer agent. Pharmacol Ther 82:293–301

Fuks Z, Persaud RS, Alfieri A et al (1994) Basic fibroblast growth factor protects endothelial cells against radiation-induced programmed cell death in vitro and in vivo. Cancer Res 54:2582–2590

Fuks Z, Alfieri A, Haimovitz-Friedman A et al (1995) Intravenous basic fibroblast growth factor protects the lung but not mediastinal organs against radiation-induced apoptosis in vivo. Cancer J Sci Am 1:62

Geng L, Donnelly E, McMahon G, Lin PC, Sierra-Rivers E, Oshinka H, Hallahan DE (2001) Inhibition of vascular endothelial growth factor receptor signaling leads to reversal of tumor resistance to radiotherapy. Cancer Res 61:2413–2419

Gescher A (1998) Analogs of staurosporine: potential anticancer drugs? Gen Pharmacol 31:721–728

Giaccia AJ, Kastan MB (1998) The complexity of p53 modulation: emerging patterns from divergent signals. Genes Dev 12:2973–2983

Goffman TE, Glatstein E (2002) Intensity-modulated radiation therapy. Radiat Res 158:115–117

Gorski D, Beckett M, Jaskowiak N et al (1999) Blockage of the vascular endothelial growth factor stress response increases the antitumor effects of ionising radiation. Cancer Res 59:3374–3378

Green DR (2000) Apoptotic pathways: paper wraps stone blunts scissors. Cell 102:1–4

Gupta AK, Bakanauskas VJ, Cerniglia GJ et al (2001) The Ras radiation resistance pathway. Cancer Res 61:4278–4282

Hahn SM, Mitchell JB, Shacter E (1997) Tempol inhibits neutrophil and hydrogen peroxide-mediated DNA damage. Free Radic Biol Med 23:879–884

Hahn SM, Krishna MC, DeLuca AM et al (2000) Evaluation of the hydroxylamine Tempol-H as an in vivo radioprotector. Free Radic Biol Med 28:953–958

Haimovitz-Friedman A, Kan CC, Ehleiter D et al (1994a) Ionizing radiation acts on cellular membranes to generate ceramide and initiate apoptosis. J Exp Med 180:525–535

Haimovitz-Friedman A, Balaban N, McLoughlin M et al (1994b) Protein kinase C mediates basic fibroblast growth factor protection of endothelial cells against radiation-induced apoptosis. Cancer Res 54:2591–2597

Haimovitz-Friedman A, Kolesnick RN, Fuks Z (1997) Ceramide signaling in apoptosis. Br Med Bull 53:539–553

Hall EJ (2000) Radiobiology for the radiologist. Lippincott Williams and Wilkins, Philadelphia

Hanahan DE, Weinberg RA (2000) The hallmarks of cancer. Cell 100:57–70

Hallahan DE, Sukhatme VP, Sherman ML et al (1991a) Protein kinase C mediates x-ray inducibility of nuclear signal transducers EGR1 and JUN. Proc Natl Acad Sci U S A 88:2156–2160

Hallahan DE, Virudachalam S, Sherman ML et al (1991b) Tumor necrosis factor gene expression is mediated by protein kinase C following activation by ionizing radiation. Cancer Res 51:4565–4569

Hallahan DE, Virudachalam S, Beckett M et al (1991c) Mechanisms of X-ray-mediated protooncogene c-jun expression in radiation-induced human sarcoma cell lines. Int J Radiat Oncol Biol Phys 21:1677–1681

Hallahan DE, Virudachalam S, Schwartz JL et al (1992) Inhibition of protein kinases sensitizes human tumor cells to ionizing radiation. Radiat Res 129:345–350

Harari PM, Huang SM (2001) Radiation response modification following molecular inhibition of epidermal growth factor receptor signaling. Semin Radiat Oncol 11:281–289

Hendry JH, Potten CS (1982) Intestinal cell radiosensitivity: a comparison for cell death assayed by apoptosis or by a loss of clonogenicity. Int J Radiat Biol Relat Stud Phys Chem Med 42:621–628

Herr I, Debatin KM (2001) Cellular stress response and apoptosis in cancer therapy. Blood 98:2603–2614

Hess C, Vuong V, Hegyi I et al (2001) Effect of VEGF receptor inhibitor PTK787/ZK222584 [correction of ZK222548] combined with ionizing radiation on endothelial cells and tumour growth. Br J Cancer 85:2010–2016

Hill MM, Andjelkovic M, Brazil DP et al (2001) Insulin-stimulated protein kinase B phosphorylation on Ser-473 is independent of its activity and occurs through a staurosporine-insensitive kinase. J Biol Chem 276:25643–25646

Hoffman WH, Biade S, Zilfou JT et al (2002) Transcriptional repression of the anti-apoptotic surviving gene by wild type p53. J Biol Chem 277:3247–3257

Ikegami Y, Yano S, Nakao K (1996) Effects of the new selective protein kinase C inhibitor 4'-N-benzoyl staurosporine on cell cycle distribution and growth inhibition in human small cell lung cancer cells. Arzneimittelforschung 46:201–204

Johansson S, Svensson H, Denekamp J (2000) Timescale of evolution of late radiation injury after postoperative radiotherapy of breast cancer patients. Int J Radiat Oncol Biol Phys 48:745–750

Johnstone RW, Ruefli AA, Lowe SW (2002) Apoptosis: a link between cancer genetics and chemotherapy. Cell 108:153–164

Jung M, Dritschilo A (1996) Signal transduction and cellular responses to ionizing radiation. Semin Radiat Oncol 6:268–272

Kaleko M, Rutter WJ, Miller AD (1990) Overexpression of the human insulinlike growth factor I receptor promotes ligand-dependent neoplastic transformation. Mol Cell Biol 10:464–473

Kennedy SG, Wagner AJ, Conzen SD et al (1997) The PI 3-kinase/Akt signaling pathway delivers an anti-apoptotic signal. Genes Dev 11:701–713

Kennedy SG, Kandel ES, Cross TK et al (1999) Akt/protein kinase B inhibits cell death by preventing the release of cytochrome c from mitochondria. Mol Cell Biol 19:5800–5810

Khanna KK, Jackson SP (2001) DNA double-strand breaks: signaling, repair and the cancer connection. Nat Genet 27:247–254

Khanna KK, Lavin MF, Jackson SP et al (2001) ATM, a central controller of cellular responses to DNA damage. Cell Death Differ 8:1052–1065

Kim CY, Giaccia AJ, Strulovici B et al (1992) Differential expression of protein kinase C epsilon protein in lung cancer cell lines by ionising radiation. Br J Cancer 66:844–849

Kinsella TJ, Mitchell JB, Russo A et al (1984) The use of halogenated thymidine analogs as clinical radiosensitizers: rationale, current status, and future prospects: non-hypoxic cell sensitizers. Int J Radiat Oncol Biol Phys 10:1399–1406

Kinzler KW, Vogelstein B (1996) Life (and death) in a malignant tumour. Nature 379:19–20

Kolesnick R (1994) Signal transduction through the sphingomyelin pathway. Mol Chem Neuropathol 21:287–297

Kolibaba KS, Druker BJ (1997) Protein tyrosine kinases and cancer. Biochim Biophys Acta 1333:F217–F248

Komaki R, Lee JS, Kaplan B et al (2002) Randomized phase III study of chemoradiation with or without amifostine for patients with favorable performance status inoperable stage II–III non-small cell lung cancer: preliminary results. Semin Radiat Oncol 12:46–49

Komarov PG, Komarova EA, Kondratov RV et al (1999) A chemical inhibitor of p53 that protects mice from the side effects of cancer therapy. Science 285:1733–1737

Kuppusamy P, Wang P, Shankar RA et al (1998) In vivo topical EPR spectroscopy and imaging of nitroxide free radicals and polynitroxyl-albumin. Magn Reson Med 40:806–811

La Rosee P, O'Dwyer ME, Druker BJ (2002) Insights from pre-clinical studies for new combination treatment regimens with the Bcr-Abl kinase inhibitor imatinib mesylate (Gleevec/Glivec) in chronic myelogenous leukemia: a translational perspective. Leukemia 16:1213–1219

Lavin MF (1998) Radiation-induced cell death and its implications in human disease. In: Kumar S (ed) Apoptosis: mechanisms and role in disease. Springer, Berlin Heidelberg New York, pp 213–232

Lawrence TS, Eisbruch A, McGinn CJ et al (1999) Radiosensitization by gemcitabine. Oncology (Huntingt) 13:55–60

Lee JS, Collins KM, Brown AL et al (2000) hCds1-mediated phosphorylation of BRCA1 regulates the DNA damage response. Nature 404:201–204

Lin X, Fuks Z, Kolesnick R (2000) Ceramide mediates radiation-induced death of endothelium. Crit Care Med 28: N87–N93

Ling CC, Endlich B (1989) Radioresistance induced by oncogenic transformation. Radiat Res 120:267–279

Ling CC, Humm J, Larson S et al (2000) Towards multidimensional radiotherapy (MD-CRT): biological imaging and biological conformality. Int J Radiat Oncol Biol Phys 47: 551–560

Lowe SW, Schmitt EM, Smith SW et al (1993) p53 is required for radiation-induced apoptosis in mouse thymocytes. Nature 362:847–849

Lowe SW, Bodis S, McClatchey A et al (1994) p53 status and the efficacy of cancer therapy in vivo. Science 266:807–810

Marathe S, Schissel SL, Yellin MJ et al (1998) Human vascular endothelial cells are a rich and regulatable source of secretory sphingomyelinase. Implications for early atherogenesis and ceramide-mediated cell signaling. J Biol Chem 273:4081–4088

Maurizi M, Almadori G, Ferrandina G et al (1996) Prognostic significance of epidermal growth factor receptor in laryngeal squamous cell carcinoma. Br J Cancer 74: 1253–1257

Mayo LD, Donner DB (2001) A phosphatidylinositol 3-kinase/Akt pathway promotes translocation of Mdm2 from the cytoplasm to the nucleus. Proc Natl Acad Sci U S A 98: 11598–11603

McKenna WG, Weiss MC, Bakanauskas VJ et al (1990) The role of the H-ras oncogene in radiation resistance and metastasis. Int J Radiat Oncol Biol Phys 18:849–859

Mendelsohn J (2001) The epidermal growth factor receptor as a target for cancer therapy. Endocr Relat Cancer 8:3–9

Merritt AJ, Potten CS, Kemp CJ et al (1994) The role of p53 in spontaneous and radiation-induced apoptosis in the gastrointestinal tract of normal and p53-deficient mice. Cancer Res 54:614–617

Merritt AJ, Allen TD, Potten CS et al (1997) Apoptosis in small intestinal epithelial from p53-null mice: evidence for a delayed, p53-independent G2/M-associated cell death after gamma irradiation. Oncogene 14:2759–2766

Miller LS, Lombardo TW, Fowler SC (1992) Time of day effects on a human force discrimination task. Physiol Behav 52: 839–841

Miller EM, Fowler JF, Kinsella TJ (1992) Linear-quadratic analysis of radiosensitization by halogenated pyrimidines. II. Radiosensitization of human colon cancer cells by bromodeoxyuridine. Radiat Res 131:90–97

Miller AC, Kariko K, Myers CE et al (1993) Increased radioresistance of EJras-transformed human osteosarcoma cells and its modulation by lovastatin, an inhibitor of p21ras isoprenylation. Int J Cancer 53:302–307

Moroni MC, Hickman ES, Denchi EL et al (2001) Apaf-1 is a transcriptional target for E2F and p53. Nat Cell Biol 3: 552–558

O'Connor PM, Jackman J, Bae I et al (1997) Characterization of the p53 tumor suppressor pathway in cell lines of the National Cancer Institute anticancer drug screen and correlations with the growth-inhibitory potency of 123 anticancer agents. Cancer Res 57:4285–4300

Okano J, Gaslightwala I, Birnbaum MJ et al (2000) Akt/protein kinase B isoforms are differentially regulated by epidermal growth factor stimulation. J Biol Chem 275:30934–30942

Overgaard J (1989) Sensitization of hypoxic tumour cells – clinical experience. Int J Radiat Biol 56:801–811

Overgaard J (1994) Clinical evaluation of nitroimidazoles as modifiers of hypoxia in solid tumors. Oncol Res 6:509–518

Overgaard J (1995) Modification of hypoxia-from Gotwald Schwarz to nicotinamide: have we learned the lesson? Danish Cancer Society. In: Kogelnik HD (ed) Progress in radiation oncology V. International proceedings division. Bologna, Italy, pp 469–475

Overgaard J, Hansen HS, Overgaard M et al (1998) A randomized double-blind phase III study of nimorazole as a hypoxic radiosensitizer of primary radiotherapy in supraglottic larynx and pharynx carcinoma. Results of the Danish Head and Neck Cancer Study (DAHANCA) Protocol 5-85. Radiother Oncol 46:135–146

Paris F, Fuks Z, Kang A et al (2001) Endothelial apoptosis as the primary lesion initiating intestinal radiation damage in mice. Science 293:293–297

Pena LA, Fuks Z, Kolesnick R (1997) Stress-induced apoptosis and the sphingomyelin pathway. Biochem Pharmacol 53: 615–621

Penuel E, Schaefer G, Akita RW et al (2001) Structural requirements for ErbB2 transactivation. Semin Oncol 28:36–42

Pruschy M, Resch H, Shi YQ et al (1999) Ceramide triggers p53-dependent apoptosis in genetically defined fibrosarcoma tumour cells. Br J Cancer 80:693–698

Pruschy M, Rocha S, Zaugg K et al (2001) Key targets for the execution of radiation-induced tumor cell apoptosis: the role of p53 and caspases. Int J Radiat Oncol Biol Phys 49: 561–567

Radford IR, Murphy TK (1994) Radiation response of mouse lymphoid and myeloid cell lines, part III. Different signals can lead to apoptosis and may influence sensitivity to killing by DNA double-strand breakage. Int J Radiat Biol 65: 229–239

Rauth AM, Melo T, Misra V (1998) Bioreductive therapies: an overview of drugs and their mechanisms of action. Int J Radiat Oncol Biol Phys 42:755–762

Robertson SC, Tynan JA, Donoghue DJ (2000) RTK mutations and human syndromes when good receptors turn bad. Trends Genet 16:265–271

Rocha S, Soengas MS, Lowe SW et al (2000) Protein kinase C inhibitor and irradiation-induced apoptosis: relevance of the cytochrome c-mediated caspase-9 death pathway. Cell Growth Differ 11:491–499

Ron E, Modan B, Boice JD Jr et al (1988a) Tumors of the brain and nervous system after radiotherapy in childhood. N Engl J Med 319:1033–1039

Ron E, Modan B, Boice JD Jr (1988b) Mortality after radiotherapy for ringworm of the scalp. Am J Epidemiol 127: 713–725

Ron E, Lubin JH, Shore RE et al (1995) Thyroid cancer after exposure to external radiation: a pooled analysis of seven studies. Radiat Res 141:259–277

Roth JA, Grammer SF, Swisher SG et al (2001) Gene therapy approaches for the management of non-small cell lung cancer. Semin Oncol 28:50–56

Ryan KM, Phillips AC, Vousden KH (2001) Regulation and function of the p53 tumor suppressor protein. Curr Opin Cell Biol 13:332–337

Salinas M, Lopez-Valdaliso R, Martin D et al (2000) Inhibition of PKB/Akt1 by C2-ceramide involves activation of ceramide-activated protein phosphatase in PC12 cells. Mol Cell Neurosci 15:156–169

Salomon DS, Brandt R, Ciardiello F et al (1995) Epidermal growth factor-related peptides and their receptors in human malignancies. Crit Rev Oncol Hematol 19: 183–232

Santana P, Llanes L, Hernandez I et al (1995) Ceramide mediates tumor necrosis factor effects on P450-aromatase activity in cultured granulosa cells. Endocrinology 136:2345–2348

Santana P, Pena LA, Haimovitz-Friedman A et al (1996) Acid sphingomyelinase-deficient human lymphoblasts and mice are defective in radiation-induced apoptosis. Cell 86:189–199

Sarkaria JN, Eshleman JS (2001) ATM as a target for novel radiosensitizers. Semin Radiat Oncol 11:316–327

Schmidt-Ullrich RK, Dent P, Grant S et al (2000) Signal transduction and cellular radiation responses. Radiat Res 153: 245–257

Sentman CL, Shutter JR, Hockenbery D et al (1991) Bcl-2 inhibits multiple forms of apoptosis but not negative selection in thymocytes. Cell 67:879–888

Sherman ML, Datta R, Hallahan DE et al (1991) Regulation of tumor necrosis factor gene expression by ionizing radiation in human myeloid leukemia cells and peripheral blood monocytes. J Clin Invest 87:1794–1797

Spitz FR, Nguyen D, Skibber JM et al (1996) Adenoviral-mediated wild-type p53 gene expression sensitizes colorectal cancer cells to ionizing radiation. Clin Cancer Res 2: 1665–1671

Stambolic V, MacPherson D, Sas D et al (2001) Regulation of PTEN transcription by p53. Mol Cell 8:317–325

Steel GG, Peckham MJ (1979) Exploitable mechanisms in combined radiotherapy–chemotherapy: the concept of additivity. Int J Radiat Oncol Biol Phys 5:85–91

Stephens LC, Ang KK, Schultheiss TE et al (1991) Apoptosis in irradiated murine tumors. Radiat Res 127:308–316

Strasser A, Harris AW, Jacks T et al (1994) DNA damage can induce apoptosis in proliferating lymphoid cells via p53-independent mechanisms inhibitable by Bcl-2. Cell 79: 329–339

Stubbs M (1999) Application of magnetic resonance techniques for imaging tumour physiology. Acta Oncol 38: 845–853

Sun LQ, Li YX, Guillou L et al (1997) Antitumor and radiosensitizing effects of (E)-2'-deoxy-2'-(fluoromethylene) cytidine, a novel inhibitor of ribonucleoside diphosphate reductase, on human colon carcinoma xenografts in nude mice. Cancer Res 57:4023–4028

Swisher SG, Roth JA, Nemunaitis J et al (1999) Adenovirus-mediated p53 gene transfer in advanced non-small-cell lung cancer. J Natl Cancer Inst 91:763–771

Tenzer A, Zingg D, Rocha S et al (2001) The phosphatidylinositide 3'-kinase/Akt survival pathway is a target for the anticancer and radiosensitizing agent PKC412, an inhibitor of protein kinase C. Cancer Res 61:8203–8210

Tibbetts RS, Cortez D, Brumbaugh KM et al (2000) Functional interactions between BRCA1 and the checkpoint kinase ATR during genotoxic stress. Genes Dev 14:2989–3002

Verheij M, Bose R, Lin XH et al (1996) Requirement for ceramide-initiated SAPK/JNK signalling in stress-induced apoptosis. Nature 380:75–79

Verheij M, Bartelink H (2000) Radiation-induced apoptosis. Cell Tissue Res 301:133–142

Vivanco I, Sawyers CL (2002) The phosphatidylinositol 3-kinase AKT pathway in human cancer. Nat Rev Cancer 2:489–501

Wang X (2001) The expanding role of mitochondria in apoptosis. Genes Dev 15:2922–2933

Ward JF (1994) The complexity of DNA damage: relevance to biological consequences. Int J Radiat Biol 66:427–432

Wasserman TH, Chapman JD, Coleman CN et al (1997) Chemical modifiers of radiation. In: Perez CA, Brady LW (eds) Principles and practice of radiation oncology. Lippincott-Raven, Philadelphia, pp 685–704

Weisberg E, Boulton C, Kelly LM et al (2002) Inhibition of mutant FLT3 receptors in leukemia cells by the small molecule tyrosine kinase inhibitor PKC412. Cancer Cell 1:433–443

Wu Y, Mehew JW, Heckman CA et al (2001) Negative regulation of bcl-2 expression by p53 in hematopoietic cells. Oncogene 20:240–251

Zaugg K, Rocha S, Resch H et al (2001) Differential p53-dependent mechanism of radiosensitization in vitro and in vivo by the protein kinase C-specific inhibitor PKC412. Cancer Res 61:732–738

Zhou BB, Elledge SJ (2000) The DNA damage response: putting checkpoints in perspective. Nature 408:433–439

Zhou BP, Liao Y, Xia W et al (2001) HER-2/neu induces p53 ubiquitination via Akt-mediated MDM2 phosphorylation. Nat Cell Biol 3:973–982

Zhu A, Shaeffer J, Leslie S et al (1996) Epidermal growth factor receptor: an independent predictor of survival in astrocytic tumors given definitive irradiation. Int J Radiat Oncol Biol Phys 34:809–815

Zundel W, Giaccia A (1998) Inhibition of the anti-apoptotic PI(3)K/Akt/Bad pathway by stress. Genes Dev 12: 1941–1946

Zundel W, Schindler C, Haas-Kogan D et al (2000) Loss of PTEN facilitates HIF-1-mediated gene expression. Genes Dev 14:391–396

Zwick E, Bange J, Ullrich A (2001) Receptor tyrosine kinase signalling as a target for cancer intervention strategies. Endocr Relat Cancer 8:161–173

14 Anti-VEGF Strategies in Combination with Radiotherapy

D. ZIPS and M. BAUMANN

CONTENTS

14.1 Introduction *179*
14.2 VEGFs in Tumor Angiogenesis *179*
14.3 Anti-VEGF Strategies *180*
14.4 Combination of Anti-VEGF Strategies with Radiotherapy *181*
14.4.1 Anti-VEGF Strategies and Irradiation of Experimental Tumors *181*
14.4.2 Mechanisms Underlying the Enhanced Effect of Anti-VEGF Agents When Combined with Irradiation *182*
14.4.3 Impact of Anti-VEGF Strategies on Radiobiological Hypoxia *184*
14.4.4 Sequencing of Anti-VEGF Strategies Combined with Radiotherapy *184*
14.4.5 Side Effects of Anti-VEGF Compounds Combined with Radiotherapy *185*
14.4.6 Conclusions *185*
References *185*

14.1 Introduction

Formation of new blood vessels, i.e. angiogenesis, is essential for the development and growth of solid tumors (FOLKMAN 1971, 1986, 1995). Tumor angiogenesis results from an imbalance between pro-angiogenic factors, e.g. vascular endothelial growth factor (VEGF), fibroblast growth factor (FGF) and platelet-derived growth factor (PDGF), and endogenous anti-angiogenic factors such as angiostatin and endostatin (FOLKMAN 1995; O'REILLY et al. 1996, 1997; ENDRICH and VAUPEL 1998; FERRARA and ALITALO 1999; CARMELIET and JAIN 2000; KERBEL 2000; YAN-

COPOULOS et al. 2000). Extensive experimental data indicate that application of either inhibitors of pro-angiogenic factors or administration of endogenous anti-angiogenic factors reduce the formation of new blood vessels. As a result, tumors grow at a slower rate or even shrink. However, in most cases no permanent tumor control can be achieved. In theory, the combination of anti-angiogenic strategies with cytotoxic agents such as chemotherapy or irradiation represents a promising approach to increasing treatment efficacy in solid tumors (FOLKMAN 1971; TEICHER et al. 1992; DENEKAMP 1993; FOLKMAN 1995; SIEMANN et al. 2000; KOUKOURAKIS 2001; ROSEN 2002).

Angiogenesis is not restricted to tumors but can also be found in many other physiological and pathological conditions, e.g., normal growth, pregnancy, menstrual cycle, wound healing, proliferative retinopathies, rheumatoid arthritis and inflammation (for review see FOLKMAN 1995; CARMELIET and JAIN 2000). Hence, effects on physiological angiogenesis have to be considered when anti-angiogenic treatment is applied to patients. Even if in the majority of adult cancer patients angiogenesis might be confined to tumor and metastases, inhibition of angiogenesis in combination with chemotherapy or irradiation may be associated with increased normal tissue reactions or increased resistance of the tumor to therapy. Therefore the therapeutic ratio of anti-angiogenic strategies in combination with radiotherapy needs to be thoroughly determined for translation of this approach into clinical practice.

14.2 VEGFs in Tumor Angiogenesis

The vascular endothelial growth factors (VEGFs) are potent and specific mitogens for endothelial cells and key mediators of tumor angiogenesis (for review see DVORAK et al. 1995; KERBEL et al. 1998; FERRARA 1999; CARMELIET 2000; CARMELIET and COLLEN 2000; CARMELIET and JAIN 2000; KARKKAINEN and

D. ZIPS, MD
Klinik und Poliklinik für Strahlentherapie und Radioonkologie, Universitätsklinikum Carl Gustav Carus, Dresden
M. BAUMANN, MD, PhD
Experimentelles Zentrum, Medizinische Fakultät Carl Gustav Carus der Technischen Universität Dresden, Fetscherstrasse 74, 01307 Dresden

Petrova 2000; Kerbel 2000; Veikkola et al. 2000; Yancopoulos et al. 2000). The VEGFs represent a family of distinct proteins, i.e., VEGF (VEGF-A), VEGF-B, VEGF-C, VEGF-D, VEGF-E, and isoforms (e.g., $VEGF_{121}$ and $VEGF_{165}$). VEGF expression can be demonstrated in the vast majority of tumors and is usually elevated above normal tissue levels. Until tumors reach a volume of about 1 mm^3, tumor cells are supplied by diffusion from the surrounding tissues (Folkman 1971; Ausprunk and Folkman 1977; Folkman 1986). At larger volumes, impaired supply with oxygen and nutrients and accumulation of metabolites occur in the tumor. This is accompanied by important changes in the tumor micromilieu, e.g., hypoxia, hypoglycemia and acidosis, which result in up-regulated production and release of VEGF and other angiogenic factors by the tumor cells. In addition to environmental factors, other triggers such as mechanical stress, immune/inflammatory responses, and genetic alterations (e.g., activation of oncogenes or deletion of tumor-suppressor genes that control production of angiogenesis regulators) may influence the expression of VEGF (Kerbel et al. 1998; Okada et al. 1998; Carmeliet and Jain 2000). Secreted VEGFs bind to specific receptors (VEGFR-1/Flt-1, VEGFR-2/KDR, VEGFR-3/Flt-4), which are almost exclusively expressed on the surface of endothelial cells (Jakeman et al. 1992; Veikkola et al. 2000; Yancopoulos et al. 2000). Based on studies of endothelial cell lines, VEGFR-2 is currently considered as a major receptor transducing the effects of VEGF into endothelial cells (Karkkainen and Petrova 2000). Within the families of VEGFs and VEGFRs, ligand affinity and receptor properties are variable (for details see Karkkainen and Petrova 2000; Veikkola et al. 2000). VEGFRs consist of distinct structural elements, most importantly an extracellular immunoglobulin-like binding domain and an intracellular tyrosine kinase domain. Binding of VEGF is followed by receptor dimerization, tyrosine kinase activation, autophosphorylation and eventually in activation of a complex cascade of intracellular pathways (Guo et al. 1995; Abedi and Zachary 1997; Karkkainen and Petrova 2000; Veikkola et al. 2000; Stoletov et al. 2001). The activation of endothelial cells results in vasorelaxation, increased vascular permeability, endothelial cell migration, proliferation and survival (Carmeliet and Collen 2000; Karkkainen and Petrova 2000; Veikkola et al. 2000). New blood vessels originating from surrounding, pre-existing normal vessels generate a tumor neovasculature that allows further tumor growth, tumor progression and development of metastasis.

14.3
Anti-VEGF Strategies

Based on increasing insight into the molecular mechanisms underlying the biological effects of the VEGFs and their receptors, various rationally designed strategies to inhibit VEGF-dependent angiogenesis were developed (Table 14.1). The best investigated approaches include antibodies against VEGF or VEGFR and VEGF receptor tyrosine kinase inhibitors (RTKI).

Neutralizing antibodies against VEGF or VEGFR2 can reduce the growth rate of tumors and metastases in experimental animals (Kim et al. 1993; Asano et al. 1995; Borgström et al. 1996; Presta et al. 1997; Gorski et al. 1999; Prewett et al. 1999; Bruns et al. 2000; Lee et al. 2000; Kozin et al. 2001; Gupta et al. 2002). However, considerable intertumoral heterogeneity in response to anti-VEGF or anti-VEGFR antibodies was observed. In some tumors treated with anti-VEGF antibodies, a nearly complete inhibition of angiogenesis, a decline in vessel permeability and a decrease in vascular density compared with control tumors has been demonstrated by intravital

Table 14.1. Strategies to inhibit angiogenesis by the VEGF/VEGFR -pathway

Target	Mechanism	References
Ligand	Neutralizing monoclonal antibodies	Kim et al. 1993; Asano et al. 1995; Borgström et al. 1996; Presta et al. 1997
	Neutralizing chimeric proteins	Aiello et al. 1995
	Soluble VEGFR-1	Lin et al. 1998; Goldman et al. 1998; Davidoff et al. 2001
	Antisense oligonucleotides	Bell et al. 1999; Im et al. 1999
Receptor	Neutralizing monoclonal antibodies	Prewett et al. 1999
	Mutant VEGF receptor 2 (VEGFR-2)	Machein et al. 1999
	Ribozyme targeted to mRNA	Parry et al. 1999
	Antisense oligonucleotides	Rockwell et al. 1997
	Tyrosine kinase inhibitors	Fong et al. 1999; Laird et al. 2000; Wood et al. 2000; Wedge et al. 2000

microscopy and histology (BORGSTRÖM et al. 1996; YUAN et al. 1996). To generate VEGF antibodies suitable for clinical trials, mouse monoclonal antibodies were humanized in order to combine high affinity to human VEGF with little or no immunogenicity (PRESTA et al. 1997; FERRARA and ALITALO 1999). In a phase I clinical trial including 25 patients with advanced solid tumors, no dose-limiting toxicity up to the highest dose of recombinant human anti-VEGF monoclonal antibody (rhumab, 10 mg/kg body weight) was observed (GORDON et al. 2001). However, in this trial three episodes of tumor bleeding were noted. In two additional patients with known pulmonary metastasis, minor hemoptysis occurred. It was not possible to discriminate whether these bleedings were caused by the treatment or by the underlying disease. In combination with chemotherapy rhumabVEGF (3 mg/kg body weight) was safely administered without hemorrhagic complications (MARGOLIN et al. 2001). In a multicenter trial, 99 patients with advanced non-small cell lung cancer were randomized to standard chemotherapy or standard chemotherapy plus rhumabVEGF (DEVORE et al. 2000). Response rate and time to progression were increased after combined treatment. In six patients, four of them with a central tumor location, severe tumor bleeding occurred, which was fatal in four patients. According to the NCI-trial list (www.cancer.gov, last up-date 08/02/02) 15 phase II and 5 phase III clinical trials are now ongoing, testing VEGF-antibodies in combination with cytotoxic drugs in the treatment of different malignant diseases.

VEGF-dependent angiogenesis can also be suppressed by receptor tyrosine kinase inhibitors (RTKIs). Agents such as SU5416, SU6668, ZD4190, and PTK787/ZK222584 competitively inhibit ATP-dependent phosphorylation of tyrosine residues of the VEGF receptor, resulting in a decrease in proliferation and survival of endothelial cells in vitro, angiogenesis in vivo, and growth rate of tumor and metastasis (FONG et al. 1999; SHAHEEN et al. 1999; DREVS et al. 2000; LAIRD et al. 2000; MENDEL et al. 2000; WEDGE et al. 2000; WOOD et al. 2000). Although these compounds were designed to inhibit VEGFR-2, some of them show also activity against other receptors involved in angiogenesis (LAIRD et al. 2000). In a clinical phase I study on single-agent SU5416 treatment in patients with advanced malignant disease, the dose-limiting toxicity was vomiting, nausea, and severe headache (CROPP et al. 1999; ROSEN et al. 1999; STOPECK 2000). In a subsequent phase I clinical trial investigating SU5416 combined with cisplatin and gemcitabine in a total of 19 patients with solid tumors, an unexpectedly high rate of thromboembolic events was observed (KUENEN et al. 2002). These discouraging results may be a consequence of the specific regimen of chemotherapy applied. This illustrates the importance of further, detailed investigations of interactions and optimal scheduling of administration (MARX et al. 2002). Of special importance in this context are preclinical investigations into normal tissue effects of combined approaches, exploiting suitable animal models.

14.4
Combination of Anti-VEGF Strategies with Radiotherapy

14.4.1
Anti-VEGF Strategies and Irradiation of Experimental Tumors

Experimental and clinical data indicate that anti-VEGF compounds have little effect on the growth of established, macroscopic tumors. Whether anti-VEGF strategies can be used to improve tumor response when combined with irradiation was studied in a number of experimental investigations (Table 14.2). In these studies human and murine tumors, grown in experimental animals, of different histology were treated with various anti-VEGF compounds combined with single-dose or fractionated irradiation. Although VEGF inhibition alone had only a modest or no significant impact on tumor growth, the combination with irradiation consistently resulted in improved outcome. For example, in the study published by GORSKI et al. (1999) anti-$VEGF_{165}$ antibody alone did not reduce the tumor growth rate in U87 human glioblastoma xenografts, while the combination of 40 Gy given in eight fractions with anti-$VEGF_{165}$ antibody 3 h before each irradiation increased tumor growth delay compared with irradiation alone. In another study performed by KOZIN and colleagues (2001), two different human xenograft tumors were treated with an anti-VEGFR2 antibody combined with fractionated irradiation. In both tumor models, the combined treatment resulted in a statistically significant decrease in the dose necessary for permanent local tumor control compared to tumors that were only irradiated. This result demonstrates that anti-VEGFR antibody treatment increases the inactivation of clonogenic tumor cells and supports the hypothesis that anti-VEGF strategies

Table 14.2. Preclinical in vivo studies testing anti-VEGF strategies in combination with radiotherapy

Compound	Mechanism of VEGF-inhibition	Tumor	Treatment schedule	Endpoint	Result	Reference
SU5416	RTKI[a]	Murine SCC[b] VII	5×2 Gy plus concomitant SU5416	Growth delay	+[c]	Ning et al. 2002
SU6668	RTKI	Murine SCC VII	5×2 Gy plus concomitant SU6668	Growth delay	+	Ning et al. 2002
SU6668	RTKI	Human mammary carcinoma SCK, human fibrosarcoma FSIIa, human pancreatic carcinoma CFPAC	2 administrations of SU6668 prior to irradiation with a single dose of 15 Gy	Growth delay	+	Griffin et al. 2002
SU5416	RTKI	Murine malignant glioma GL261	6 fractions of 3 Gy with concomitant SU5416	Growth delay	+	Geng et al. 2001
ZK 222584/ PTK 787	RTKI	Human SW480 colon carcinoma	12 Gy in 4 fractions with concomitant ZK222584/ PTK787	Growth delay	+	Hess et al. 2001
A.4.6.1	Anti-VEGF antibody	Human glioblastoma U87, human colon adenocarcinoma LS174T	Single dose under normoxic or hypoxic conditions after antibody treatment	Growth delay	+	Lee et al. 2000
DC101	Anti-VEGFR2 antibody	Human small cell lung cancer 54A, human glioblastoma U87	5 fractions in 5 days with 6 administrations of DC101 every 3rd day	Growth delay, tumor control rate	+	Kozin et al. 2001
Anti-VEGF$_{165}$	Anti-human VEGF$_{165}$ antibody	Human SCC SQ20B, Seg-1 human adenocarcinoma, human glioblastoma U87	Anti-VEGF$_{165}$ prior to irradiation with 4 or 8 fractions	Growth delay	+	Gorski et al. 1999
Anti-VEGF$_{165}$	Anti-murine	Murine Lewis lung carcinoma	40 Gy in 2 fractions with anti-VEGF$_{165}$ prior to irradiation	Growth delay	+	Gorski et al. 1999
Anti-VEGF$_{165}$	Anti-human VEGF$_{165}$ antibody	Seg-1 human adenocarcinoma, human glioblastoma U87	Anti-VEGF$_{165}$ plus 20 Gy in 5 fractions (Seg-1) or 40 Gy in 8 fractions (U87)	Growth delay	+	Gupta et al. 2002

[a] RTKI receptor tyrosine kinase inhibitor. [b] Squamous cell carcinoma. [c] + Denotes better outcome with combined treatment compared to control tumors.

may improve the outcome of curative radiotherapy. However, in the majority of the experiments listed in Table 14.2, tumor growth delay was the experimental endpoint. Therefore, further experiments studying tumor control are necessary to corroborate the findings of Kozin and colleagues (2001). Importantly, total dose, dose per fraction, overall treatment time and the sequence of the modalities in combined treatment may impact on the outcome of combination treatment. Hence, further preclinical studies in relevant animal models addressing these parameters need to be conducted to investigate whether the benefit of the combined therapy holds true for clinically relevant irradiation schedules.

14.4.2
Mechanisms Underlying the Enhanced Effect of Anti-VEGF Agents When Combined withI rradiation

The observation that anti-VEGF compounds given alone only modestly impact the tumor growth rate while in combination with irradiation anti-VEGF agents consistently improve the response of tumors suggests a radiosensitizing effect. This might be restricted to endothelial cells because VEGF-receptors are almost exclusively expressed on this cell type (Jakeman et al. 1992; Ning et al. 2002). This notion is supported by the fact that neither unirradiated nor irradiated tumor cells were affected by anti-VEGF compounds (GORSKI et al. 1999; HESS et al. 2001; GUPTA et al. 2002). VEGFs are potent mitogens and survival factors for endothelial cells (see Chap. 10.2). Irradiation of endothelial cells in vitro results in decreased proliferation and decreased clonogenic survival (DE GOWIN et al. 1974; HEI et al. 1987; HAIMOWITZ-FRIEDMAN et al. 1991; FUKS et al. 1994; GORSKI et al. 1999; HESS et al. 2001; KERMANI et al. 2001; GUPTA et al. 2002). When VEGF is added to culture media, the effects of irradiation on proliferation and survival of endothelial cells were attenuated (GORSKI et al. 1999; HESS et al. 2001; KERMANI et al. 2001; GUPTA et al. 2002). Vice versa, VEGF-inhibitors reduce these effects of VEGF on irradiated endothelial cells (GORSKI et al. 1999; HESS et al. 2001; GUPTA et al. 2002). However, complete cell survival curves for endothelial cells irradiated in the presence or absence of VEGF are currently not available. In studies using another angiogenic growth factor, bFGF, increased clonogenic survival of irradiated bovine aortic endothelial cells was observed (HAIMOWITZ-FRIEDMAN et al. 1991; FUKS et al. 1994). In these studies, the slope of the dose–survival curves was not significantly different between endothelial cells incubated with or without bFGF. However, the shoulder region of the dose effect curve was almost completely eliminated when no bFGF was added to culture media. An interesting hypothesis of the mechanism of anti-VEGF combined with irradiation was proposed by GORSKI and colleagues based on the fact that many cell types, including tumor cells, respond to irradiation with an increased release of growth factors (1999, Fig. 14.1). These growth factors such as VEGF or bFGF may, in an autocrine and/or paracrine manner, increase endothelial cell survival after irradiation (WITTE et al. 1989; HAIMOVITZ-FRIEDMAN et al. 1991; GORSKI et al. 1999; GUPTA et al. 2002). The authors hypothesized that the inhibition of VEGF can abrogate the effects of radiation-induced VEGF on irradiated endothelial cells in tumors. This may result in increased radiation-induced endothelial cell kill, which eventually leads to impaired tumor vascularization. As a result, the tumor cell production rate

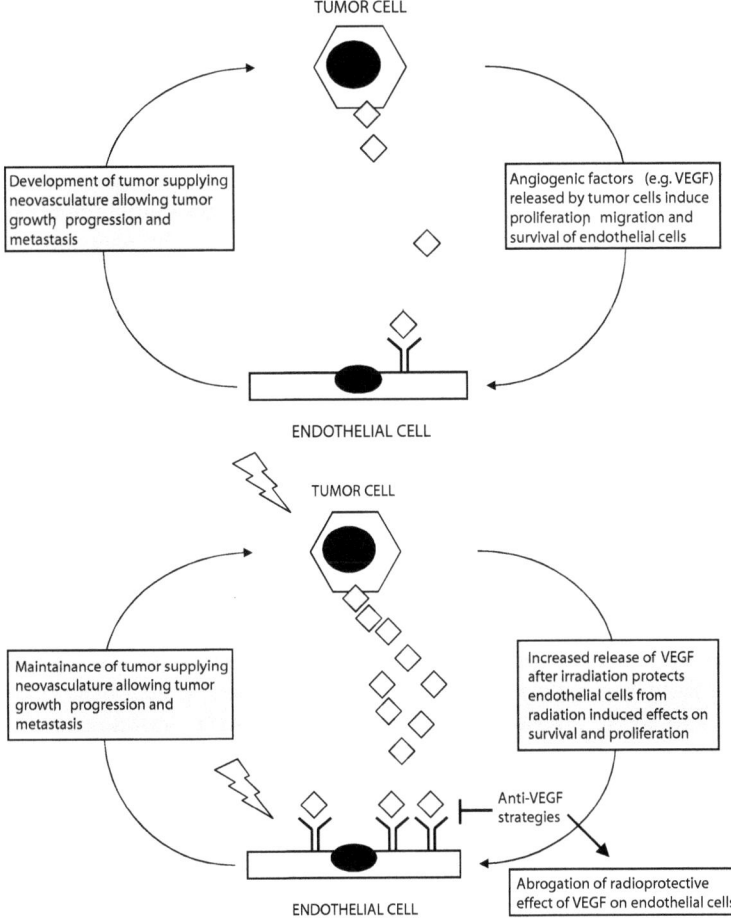

Fig. 14.1A, B. Interaction of the tumor and endothelial cells in tumors. Angiogenic factors released by tumor cells induce neoangiogenesis that allows further tumor growth, progression and metastasis (A). Possible mechanisms underlying the effectiveness of anti-VEGF agents combined with irradiation (B) include the abrogation of the radioprotective effect of VEGF on endothelial cells and the sensitization of endothelial cells against anti-VEGF agents by irradiation (see Sect. 14.4.2)

decreases and/or the tumor cell loss increases, which may result in improved tumor response after irradiation. Further experimental studies are required to elucidate the interaction of the endothelial cell and the tumor cell compartment after a combination of anti-VEGF compounds with irradiation.

14.4.3
Impact of Anti-VEGF Strategies on Radiobiological Hypoxia

A major concern of the combination of anti-angiogenic approaches with irradiation is that tumor hypoxia might increase. Anoxic cells are less sensitive to irradiation compared to normoxic cells by a factor of about 3 (GRAY et al. 1953; WRIGHT and HOWARD-FLANDERS 1957). Thus, inhibitors of angiogenesis, by decreasing vessel density or vessel function, might increase the proportion of poorly oxygenated clonogenic tumor cells and thereby decrease the efficacy of irradiation. A negative effect of anti-angiogenic agents on the results of irradiation was observed in an experiment by MURATA and colleagues (1997). The authors investigated the effect of TNP-470 on local tumor control after single-dose and fractionated irradiation of murine mammary carcinoma in C3H/He mice. The radiobiological hypoxic fraction of clonogenic tumor cells, as determined from the tumor control data after single-dose irradiation, was not affected significantly by TNP-470. However, for fractionated irradiation under normal blood flow conditions, tumors treated with TNP-470 were more resistant compared with control tumors. In contrast, no differences were observed for fractionated irradiation under clamp hypoxia. The authors concluded that inhibition of angiogenesis by TNP-470 impairs reoxygenation during fractionated irradiation and thus increases the radioresistance of tumors. In a study on human colon carcinoma growing in nude mice, another anti-angiogenic compound, suramin, was also found to increase radiobiological hypoxia (LEITH et al. 1992). Yet both TNP-470 (ZHANG et al. 2000) and suramin do not specifically inhibit VEGF or VEGF receptors but decrease angiogenesis, at least in part by other mechanisms. Whether anti-VEGF drugs similarly increase radiobiological hypoxia was addressed in two experimental studies using anti-VEGF and anti-VEGF-receptor antibodies (LEE et al. 2000; KOZIN et al. 2001). Tumor growth delay after graded single radiation doses given under normal blood flow conditions was compared with tumor growth delay after irradiations administered under clamp hypoxia. In both studies, anti-VEGF and anti-VEGF-receptor antibodies increased tumor growth delay compared with control tumors, irrespective of the tumor oxygenation status at the time of irradiation. These results suggest that VEGF inhibition does not increase the radiobiological hypoxic cell fraction in tumors. The contradiction that VEGF inhibitors reduce vessel density but apparently do not increase radiobiological hypoxia may be attributed to an impact on the quality of vascular organization by selective ablation of immature tumor blood vessels, a decrease in the number of oxygen-consuming cells and a decrease in vessel permeability (BENJAMIN et al. 1999; LEE et al. 2000).

14.4.4
Sequencing of Anti-VEGF Strategies Combined with Radiotherapy

VEGF-inhibitors can be administrated before (neoadjuvant), during (simultaneous) and/or after (adjuvant) a course of fractionated radiotherapy. No conclusion on the optimal sequence can be drawn from the studies listed in Table 14.2. Current data indicate that VEGF inhibitors have only a minor effect on tumor volume when given alone. Neoadjuvant application should have only a small effect on the number of clonogenic tumor cells that need to be killed by irradiation. Thus, a substantial improvement of the results of radiotherapy by neoadjuvant VEGF inhibition can not be expected, although these substances may possibly be useful to bridge waiting times before radiotherapy or unscheduled treatment gaps. Table 14.2 shows that simultaneous application of VEGF-inhibitors with fractionated irradiation improved the radiation response of several tumor models. As discussed under 14.4.2, these results might be caused by abrogation of the radioprotective effects of radiation-induced VEGF on endothelial cells. So far the experimental results do not support the idea that neoadjuvant or simultaneous application of VEGF inhibitors increase tumor hypoxia. However, it should be recognized that the data base still is relatively weak. To circumvent the possibility of increased hypoxia, anti-angiogenic agents may be applied after the end of fractionated irradiation. In a study by MURATA and colleagues (1997), TNP-470 administered after a course of ten fractions in 2 weeks significantly increased tumor growth delay compared to irradiation alone. In our own experiments, different combination schedules of a VEGFR tyrosine kinase inhibitor with fractionated irradiation of human squamous cell carcinomas in nude mice were compared. Short-term neoadjuvant and simultaneous administration showed no effect on tumor growth delay, while long-term adjuvant treatment resulted in prolonged tumor growth delay (ZIPS et al. 2001). Several reasons might explain the efficacy of adjuvant administration of VEGF inhibitors. Firstly, tumors may shrink after irradiation and smaller tumors are more likely to respond to anti-angiogenic compounds than larger tumors (GRIFFIN et al. 2002). Secondly, a negative impact of increased radiobiological hypoxia can be avoided. Thirdly, irradiated vessels appear to be more sensitive to VEGF inhibition, which is supported by the observation that in vitro irradiated endothelial cells show an increased VEGFR2 expression (KERMANI et al. 2001). An obvious disadvantage of the adjuvant sequence is that the radioprotective effect of VEGF on endothelial cells will not be counteracted. Further studies to determine the optimal sequence of VEGF inhibition in combination with fractionated irradiation are needed.

14.4.5
Side Effects of Anti-VEGF Compounds Combined with Radiotherapy

In most of the studies listed in Table 14.2, the combination of anti-VEGF with irradiation was well tolerated. Skin reactions after irradiation of the subcutaneously growing experimental tumors on the hind leg or flank of the animals were not increased. However, after whole body irradiation in combination with anti-VEGFR2 antibody DC101, 40% of 54A tumor-bearing mice developed ascites and half of them died (KOZIN et al. 2001). Histology revealed focal segmental glomerulonecrosis associated with increased expression of VEGFR2 on the surface of glomerular endothelial cells in the kidneys (KOZIN et al. 2002). This indicates that although angiogenesis in adult organisms is almost exclusively confined to tumor tissue, inhibition of VEGF-dependent processes may result in increased normal tissue reactions after irradiation. This might be explained by the fact that VEGF does not only stimulate angiogenesis but is also important for survival and maintenance of normal function of endothelial cells. This is supported by the observation of apoptosis in alveolar septal cells of the lung and emphysema in rats chronically treated with VEGF receptor inhibitor SU5416 (KASAHARA et al. 2000). Such results underline the importance of further studies into normal tissue reactions, particularly those dominated by a vascular component, after combined anti-VEGF strategies with radiotherapy.

14.4.6
Conclusions

Preclinical experiments in a variety of tumor models indicate that inhibition of VEGF or VEGF receptor in combination with irradiation is a promising concept for the improvement of the radiation response of tumors. The mechanisms underlying this approach, however, are not fully understood. Both radiosensitization of endothelial cells by VEGF inhibition as well as sensitization of endothelial cells against anti-angiogenic agents by irradiation appear to play an important role. Future research must include investigations into the efficacy of VEGF inhibition in combination with irradiation regarding dose-fractionation parameters, optimization of the sequence, identification of predictive factors for response, and studies on normal tissue toxicity of anti-VEGF strategies in combination with radiotherapy, not only in vitro but in relevant experimental animal tumor and normal tissue models.

References

Abedi H, Zachary I (1997) Vascular endothelial growth factor stimulates tyrosine phosphorylation and recruitment to new focal adhesions of focal adhesion kinase and paxillin in endothelial cells. J Biol Chem 272:15442–15451

Aiello LP, Pierce EA, Foley ED, Takagi H, Chen H, Riddle L, Ferrara N, King GL, Smith LE (1995) Suppression of retinal neovascularization in vivo by inhibition of vascular endothelial growth factor (VEGF) using soluble VEGF-receptor chimeric proteins. Proc Natl Acad Sci U S A 92: 10457–10461

Asano M, Yukita A, Matsumoto T, Kondo S, Suzuki H (1995) Inhibition of tumor growth and metastasis by an immunoneutralizing monoclonal antibody to human vascular endothelial growth factor/vascular permeability factor 121. Cancer Res 55:5296–5301

Ausprunk DH, Folkman J (1977) Migration and proliferation of endothelial cells in preformed and newly formed blood vessels during tumor angiogenesis. Microvasc Res 14:53–65

Bell C, Lynam E, Landfair DJ, Janjic N, Wiles ME (1999) Oligonucleotide NX1838 inhibits VEGF165-mediated cellular responses in vitro. In Vitro Cell Dev Biol Anim 35: 533–542

Benjamin LE, Golijanin D, Itin A, Pode D, Keshet E (1999) Selective ablation of immature blood vessels in established human tumors follows vascular endothelial growth factor withdrawal. J Clin Invest 103:159-165

Borgström P, Hillan KJ, Sriramarao P, Ferrara N (1996) Complete inhibition of angiogenesis and growth of microtumors by anti-vascular endothelial growth factor neutralizing antibody: novel concepts of angiostatic therapy from intravital videomicroscopy. Cancer Res 56:4032-4039

Bruns CJ, Liu W, Davis DW, Shaheen RM, McConkey DJ, Wilson MR, Bucana CD, Hicklin DJ, Ellis LM (2000) Vascular endothelial growth factor is an in vivo survival factor for tumor endothelium in a murine model of colorectal carcinoma liver metastases. Cancer 89:488-499

Carmeliet P (2000) Mechanisms of angiogenesis and arteriogenesis. Nat Med 6:389-395

Carmeliet P, Collen D (2000) Molecular basis of angiogenesis. Role of VEGF and VE-cadherin. Ann N Y Acad Sci 902:249-262

Carmeliet P, Jain RK (2000) Angiogenesis in cancer and other diseases. Nature 407:249-257

Cropp G, Rosen L, Mulay M et al (1999) Pharmacokinetics and pharmacodynamics of SU5416 in a phase I, dose-escalating trial in patients with advanced malignancies (abstract 619). Proc Am Soc Clin Oncol 18:161a

Davidoff AM, Leary MA, Ng CY, Vanin EF (2001) Gene therapy-mediated expression by tumor cells of the angiogenesis inhibitor flk-1 results in inhibition of neuroblastoma growth in vivo. J Pediatr Surg 36:30-36

De Gowin RL, Lewis LJ, Hoak JC, Mueller AL, Gibson DP (1974) Radiosensitivity of human endothelial cells in culture. J Lab Clin Med 84:42-48

Denekamp J (1993) Review article: angiogenesis, neovascular proliferation and vascular pathophysiology as targets for cancer therapy. Br J Radiol 66:181-196

DeVore RF, Fehrenbacher L, Herbst RS et al. (2000) A randomized phase II trial comparing Rhumab VEGF (recombinant humanized monoclonal antibody to vascular endothelial growth factor) plus carboplatin/paclitaxel (CP) to CP alone in patients with stage IIIB/IV NSCLC (abstract 1896). Proc Am Soc Clin Oncol 19:454a

Drevs J, Hofmann I, Hugenschmidt H, Wittig C, Madjar H, Muller M, Wood J, Martiny-Baron G, Unger C, Marme D (2000) Effects of PTK787/ZK 222584, a specific inhibitor of vascular endothelial growth factor receptor tyrosine kinases, on primary tumor, metastasis, vessel density, and blood flow in a murine renal cell carcinoma model. Cancer Res 60:4819-4824

Dvorak HF, Brown LF, Detmar M, Dvorak AM (1995) Vascular permeability factor/vascular endothelial growth factor, microvascular hyperpermeability, and angiogenesis. Am J Pathol 146:1029-1039

Endrich B, Vaupel P (1998) The role of the microcirculation in the treatment of malignant tumors: facts and fiction. In: Molls M, Vaupel P (eds) Blood perfusion and microenvironment of human tumors. Springer, Berlin Heidelberg, pp 19-39

Ferrara N (1999) Molecular and biological properties of vascular endothelial growth factor. J Mol Med 77:527-543

Ferrara N, Alitalo K (1999) Clinical applications of angiogenic growth factors and their inhibitors. Nat Med 5:1359-1364

Folkman J (1971) Tumor angiogenesis: therapeutic implications. N Engl J Med 285:1182-1186

Folkman J (1986) How is blood vessel growth regulated in normal and neoplastic tissue? G.H.A. Clowes Memorial Award lecture. Cancer Res 46:467-473

Folkman J (1995) Angiogenesis in cancer, vascular, rheumatoid and other disease. Nat Med 1:27-31

Fong TA, Shawver LK, Sun L, Tang C, App H, Powell TJ, Kim YH, Schreck R, Wang X, Risau W, Ullrich A, Hirth KP, McMahon G (1999) SU5416 is a potent and selective inhibitor of the vascular endothelial growth factor receptor (Flk-1/KDR) that inhibits tyrosine kinase catalysis, tumor vascularization, and growth of multiple tumor types. Cancer Res 59:99-106

Fuks Z, Persaud RS, Alfieri A, McLoughlin M, Ehleiter D, Schwartz JL, Seddon AP, Cordon-Cardo C, Haimovitz-Friedman A (1994) Basic fibroblast growth factor protects endothelial cells against radiation-induced programmed cell death in vitro and in vivo. Cancer Res 54:2582-2590

Geng L, Donnelly E, McMahon G, Lin PC, Sierra-Rivera E, Oshinka H, Hallahan DE (2001) Inhibition of vascular endothelial growth factor receptor signaling leads to reversal of tumor resistance to radiotherapy. Cancer Res 61:2413-2419

Goldman CK, Kendall RL, Cabrera G, Soroceanu L, Heike Y, Gillespie GY, Siegal GP, Mao X, Bett AJ, Huckle WR, Thomas KA, Curiel DT (1998) Paracrine expression of a native soluble vascular endothelial growth factor receptor inhibits tumor growth, metastasis, and mortality rate. Proc Natl Acad Sci U S A 95:8795-8800

Gordon MS, Margolin K, Talpaz M, Sledge GW Jr, Holmgren E, Benjamin R, Stalter S, Shak S, Adelman D (2001) Phase I safety and pharmacokinetic study of recombinant human anti-vascular endothelial growth factor in patients with advanced cancer. J Clin Oncol 19:843-850

Gorski DH, Beckett MA, Jaskowiak NT, Calvin DP, Mauceri HJ, Salloum RM, Seetharam S, Koons A, Hari DM, Kufe DW, Weichselbaum RR (1999) Blockage of the vascular endothelial growth factor stress response increases the antitumor effects of ionizing radiation. Cancer Res 59:3374-3378

Gray LH, Conger AD, Ebert M et al (1953) The concentration of oxygen dissolved in tissues at the time of irradiation as a factor in radiotherapy. Br J Radiol 26: 638-648

Griffin RJ, Williams BW, Wild R, Cherrington JM, Park H, Song CW (2002) Simultaneous inhibition of the receptor kinase activity of vascular endothelial, fibroblast, and platelet-derived growth factors suppresses tumor growth and enhances tumor radiation response. Cancer Res 62:1702-1706

Guo D, Jia Q, Song HY, Warren RS, Donner DB (1995) Vascular endothelial cell growth factor promotes tyrosine phosphorylation of mediators of signal transduction that contain SH2 domains. Association with endothelial cell proliferation. J Biol Chem 270:6729-6733

Gupta VK, Jaskowiak NT, Beckett MA, Mauceri HJ, Grunstein J, Johnson RS, Calvin DA, Nodzenski E, Pejovic M, Kufe DW, Posner MC, Weichselbaum RR (2002) Vascular endothelial growth factor enhances endothelial cell survival and tumor radioresistance. Cancer J 8:47-54

Haimovitz-Friedman A, Vlodavsky I, Chaudhuri A, Witte L, Fuks Z (1991) Autocrine effects of fibroblast growth factor in repair of radiation damage in endothelial cells. Cancer Res 51:2552-2558

Hei TK, Marchese MJ, Hall EJ (1987) Radiosensitivity and sublethal damage repair in human umbilical cord vein endothelial cells. Int J Radiat Oncol Biol Phys 13:879-884

Hess C, Vuong V, Hegyi I, Riesterer O, Wood J, Fabbro D, Glanzmann C, Bodis S, Pruschy M (2001) Effect of VEGF receptor inhibitor PTK787/ZK222584 [correction of ZK222548] combined with ionizing radiation on endothelial cells and tumour growth. Br J Cancer 85:2010–2016

Im SA, Gomez-Manzano C, Fueyo J, Liu TJ, Ke LD, Kim JS, Lee HY, Steck PA, Kyritsis AP, Yung WK (1999) Antiangiogenesis treatment for gliomas: transfer of antisense-vascular endothelial growth factor inhibits tumor growth in vivo. Cancer Res 59:895–900

Jakeman LB, Winer J, Bennett GL, Altar CA, Ferrara N (1992) Binding sites for vascular endothelial growth factor are localized on endothelial cells in adult rat tissues. J Clin Invest 89:244–253

Karkkainen MJ, Petrova TV (2000) Vascular endothelial growth factor receptors in the regulation of angiogenesis and lymphangiogenesis. Oncogene 19:5598–5605

Kasahara Y, Tuder RM, Taraseviciene-Stewart L, Le Cras TD, Abman S, Hirth PK, Waltenberger J, Voelkel NF (2000) Inhibition of VEGF receptors causes lung cell apoptosis and emphysema. J Clin Invest 106:1311–1319

Kerbel RS (2000) Tumor angiogenesis: past, present and the near future. Carcinogenesis 21:505–515

Kerbel RS, Viloria-Petit A, Okada F, Rak J (1998) Establishing a link between oncogenes and tumor angiogenesis. J Mol Med 4:286–295

Kermani P, Leclerc G, Martel R, Fareh J (2001) Effect of ionizing radiation on thymidine uptake, differentiation, and VEGFR2 receptor expression in endothelial cells: the role of VEGF(165). Int J Radiat Oncol Biol Phys 50:213–220

Kim KJ, Li B, Winer J, Armanini M, Gillett N, Phillips HS, Ferrara N (1993) Inhibition of vascular endothelial growth factor-induced angiogenesis suppresses tumour growth in vivo. Nature 362:841–844

Koukourakis MI (2001) Tumour angiogenesis and response to radiotherapy. Anticancer Res 21:4285–4300

Kozin SV, Boucher Y, Hicklin DJ, Bohlen P, Jain RK, Suit HD (2001) Vascular endothelial growth factor receptor-2-blocking antibody potentiates radiation-induced long-term control of human tumor xenografts. Cancer Res 6:39–44

Kozin SV, Boucher Y, di Tomaso E, Padera TP, Xavier R, Hicklin DJ, Bohlen P, Jain RK (2002) Glomerulopathy in mice treated with whole-body irradiation and VEGFR2-blocking antibody (abstract). 49th Annual Meeting of the Radiation Research Society, Reno, Nevada, p 65

Kuenen BC, Rosen L, Smit EF, Parson MR, Levi M, Ruijter R, Huisman H, Kedde MA, Noordhuis P, van der Vijgh WJ, Peters GJ, Cropp GF, Scigalla P, Hoekman K, Pinedo HM, Giaccone G (2002) Dose-finding and pharmacokinetic study of cisplatin, gemcitabine, and SU5416 in patients with solid tumors. J Clin Oncol 20:1657–1667

Laird AD, Vajkoczy P, Shawver LK, Thurnher A, Liang C, Mohammadi M, Schlessinger J, Ullrich A, Hubbard SR, Blake RA, Fong TA, Strawn LM, Sun L, Tang C, Hawtin R, Tang F, Shenoy N, Hirth KP, McMahon G, Cherrington JF (2000) SU6668 is a potent antiangiogenic and antitumor agent that induces regression of established tumors. Cancer Res 60:4152–4160

Lee CG, Heijn M, di Tomaso E, Griffon-Etienne G, Ancukiewicz M, Koike C, Park KR, Ferrara N, Jain RK, Suit HD, Boucher Y (2000) Anti-vascular endothelial growth factor treatment augments tumor radiation response under normoxic or hypoxic conditions. Cancer Res 60:5565–5570

Leith JT, Papa G, Quaranto L, Michelson S (1992) Modification of the volumetric growth responses and steady-state hypoxic fractions of xenografted DLD-2 human colon carcinomas by administration of basic fibroblast growth factor or suramin. Br J Cancer 66:345–348

Lin P, Sankar S, Shan S, Dewhirst MW, Polverini PJ, Quinn TQ, Peters KG (1998) Inhibition of tumor growth by targeting tumor endothelium using a soluble vascular endothelial growth factor receptor. Cell Growth Differ 9:49–58

Machein MR, Risau W, Plate KH (1999) Antiangiogenic gene therapy in a rat glioma model using a dominant-negative vascular endothelial growth factor receptor 2. Hum Gene Ther 10:1117–1128

Margolin K, Gordon MS, Holmgren E, Gaudreault J, Novotny W, Fyfe G, Adelman D, Stalter S, Breed J (2001) Phase Ib trial of intravenous recombinant humanized monoclonal antibody to vascular endothelial growth factor in combination with chemotherapy in patients with advanced cancer: pharmacologic and long-term safety data. J Clin Oncol 19:851–856

Marx GM, Steer CB, Harper P, Pavlakis N, Rixe O, Khayat D (2002) Unexpected serious toxicity with chemotherapy and antiangiogenic combinations: time to take stock! J Clin Oncol 20:1446–1448

Mendel DB, Schreck RE, West DC, Li G, Strawn LM, Tanciongco SS, Vasile S, Shawver LK, Cherrington JM (2000) The angiogenesis inhibitor SU5416 has long-lasting effects on vascular endothelial growth factor receptor phosphorylation and function. Clin Cancer Res 6:4848–4858

Murata R, Nishimura Y, Hiraoka M (1997) An antiangiogenic agent (TNP-470) inhibited reoxygenation during fractionated radiotherapy of murine mammary carcinoma. Int J Radiat Oncol Biol Phys 37:1107–1113

Ning S, Laird D, Cherrington JM, Knox SJ (2002) The antiangiogenic agents SU5416 and SU6668 increase the antitumor effects of fractionated irradiation. Radiat Res 157:45–51

Okada F, Rak JW, Croix BS, Lieubeau B, Kaya M, Roncari L, Shirasawa S, Sasazuki T, Kerbel RS (1998) Impact of oncogenes in tumor angiogenesis: mutant K-ras up-regulation of vascular endothelial growth factor/vascular permeability factor is necessary, but not sufficient for tumorigenicity of human colorectal carcinoma cells. Proc Natl Acad Sci U S A 95:3609–3614

O'Reilly MS, Holmgren L, Chen C, Folkman J (1996) Angiostatin induces and sustains dormancy of human primary tumors in mice. Nat Med 2:689–692

O'Reilly MS, Boehm T, Shing Y, Fukai N, Vasios G, Lane WS, Flynn E, Birkhead JR, Olsen BR, Folkman J (1997) Endostatin: an endogenous inhibitor of angiogenesis and tumor growth. Cell 88:277–285

Parry TJ, Cushman C, Gallegos AM, Agrawal AB, Richardson M, Andrews LE, Maloney L, Mokler VR, Wincott FE, Pavco PA (1999) Bioactivity of anti-angiogenic ribozymes targeting Flt-1 and KDR mRNA. Nucleic Acids Res 27:2569–2577

Presta LG, Chen H, O'Connor SJ, Chisholm V, Meng YG, Krummen L, Winkler M, Ferrara N (1997) Humanization of an anti-vascular endothelial growth factor monoclonal antibody for the therapy of solid tumors and other disorders. Cancer Res 57:4593–4599

Prewett M, Huber J, Li Y, Santiago A, O'Connor W, King K, Overholser J, Hooper A, Pytowski B, Witte L, Bohlen P, Hicklin DJ (1999) Antivascular endothelial growth factor receptor (fetal liver kinase 1) monoclonal antibody inhibits tumor angiogenesis and growth of several mouse and human tumors. Cancer Res 59:5209–5218

Ramakrishnan S, Olson TA, Bautch VL, Mohanraj D (1996) Vascular endothelial growth factor-toxin conjugate specifically inhibits KDR/flk-1-positive endothelial cell proliferation in vitro and angiogenesis in vivo. Cancer Res 56:1324–1330

Rockwell P, O'Connor WJ, King K, Goldstein NI, Zhang LM, Stein CA (1997) Cell-surface perturbations of the epidermal growth factor and vascular endothelial growth factor receptors by phosphorothioate oligodeoxynucleotides. Proc Natl Acad Sci U S A 94:6523–6528

Rosen LS (2002) Clinical experience with angiogenesis signaling inhibitors: focus on vascular endothelial growth factor (VEGF) blockers. Cancer Control 9 [Suppl 2]:36–44

Rosen L, Mulay M, Mayers A et al (1999) Phase I dose-escalating trial of SU5416, a novel angiogenesis inhibitor in patients with advanced malignancies (abstract 618). Proc Am Soc Clin Oncol 18:161a

Shaheen RM, Davis DW, Liu W, Zebrowski BK, Wilson MR, Bucana CD, McConkey DJ, McMahon G, Ellis LM (1999) Antiangiogenic therapy targeting the tyrosine kinase receptor for vascular endothelial growth factor receptor inhibits the growth of colon cancer liver metastasis and induces tumor and endothelial cell apoptosis. Cancer Res 59:5412–5416

Siemann DW, Warrington KH, Horsman MR (2000) Targeting tumor blood vessels: an adjuvant strategy for radiation therapy. Radiother Oncol 57:5–12

Stoletov KV, Ratcliffe KE, Spring SC, Terman BI (2001) NCK and PAK participate in the signaling pathway by which vascular endothelial growth factor stimulates the assembly of focal adhesions. J Biol Chem 276:22748–22755

Stopeck A (2000) Results of a phase I dose-escalating study of the antiangiogenic agent, SU5416, in patients with advanced malignancies. Proc Am Soc Clin Oncol 19:206a (abstract 802)

Tao Q, Backer MV, Backer JM, Terman BI (2001) Kinase insert domain receptor (KDR) extracellular immunoglobulin-like domains 4–7 contain structural features that block receptor dimerization and vascular endothelial growth factor-induced signaling. J Biol Chem 276:21916–21923

Teicher BA, Sotomayor EA, Huang ZD (1992) Antiangiogenic agents potentiate cytotoxic cancer therapies against primary and metastatic disease. Cancer Res 52:6702–6704

Veikkola T, Karkkainen M, Claesson-Welsh L, Alitalo K (2000) Regulation of angiogenesis via vascular endothelial growth factor receptors. Cancer Res 60:203–212

Wedge SR, Ogilvie DJ, Dukes M, Kendrew J, Curwen JO, Hennequin LF, Thomas AP, Stokes ES, Curry B, Richmond GH, Wadsworth PF (2000) ZD4190: an orally active inhibitor of vascular endothelial growth factor signaling with broad-spectrum antitumor efficacy. Cancer Res 60:970–975

Witte L, Fuks Z, Haimovitz-Friedman A, Vlodavsky I, Goodman DS, Eldor A (1989) Effects of irradiation on the release of growth factors from cultured bovine, porcine, and human endothelial cells. Cancer Res 49:5066–5072

Wood JM, Bold G, Buchdunger E, Cozens R, Ferrari S, Frei J, Hofmann F, Mestan J, Mett H, O'Reilly T, Persohn E, Rosel J, Schnell C, Stover D, Theuer A, Towbin H, Wenger F, Woods-Cook K, Menrad A, Siemeister G, Schirner M, Thierauch KH, Schneider MR, Drevs J, Martiny-Baron G, Totzke F (2000) PTK787/ZK 222584, a novel and potent inhibitor of vascular endothelial growth factor receptor tyrosine kinases impairs vascular endothelial growth factor-induced responses and tumor growth after oral administration. Cancer Res 60:2178–2189

Wright EA, Howard-Flanders P (1957) The influence of oxygen on the radiosensitivity of mammalian tissues. Acta Radiol 48:26–32

Yancopoulos GD, Davis S, Gale NW, Rudge JS, Wiegand SJ, Holash J (2000) Vascular-specific growth factors and blood vessel formation. Nature 407:242–248

Yuan F, Chen Y, Dellian M, Safabakhsh N, Ferrara N, Jain RK (1996) Time-dependent vascular regression and permeability changes in established human tumor xenografts induced by an anti-vascular endothelial growth factor/vascular permeability factor antibody. Proc Natl Acad Sci U S A 93:14765–14770

Zhang Y, Griffith EC, Sage J, Jacks T, Liu JO (2000) Cell cycle inhibition by the anti-angiogenic agent TNP-470 is mediated by p53 and p21WAF1/CIP1. Proc Natl Acad Sci U S A 97:6427–6432

Zips D, Krause M, Westphal J, Brüchner K, Eicheler W, Dörfler A, Hoinkis C, Grenman R, Petersen C, Baumann M (2001) Combination of VEGF receptor tyrosine kinase inhibition by ZK 222584/ PTK 787 (ZK) with fractionated radiotherapy (RT) in human squamous cell carcinoma (hSCC) in nude mice: first results. Radiother Oncol 60 [Suppl 2]: S19

15 Role of Epidermal Growth Factor Receptor and Its Inhibition in Radiotherapy

L. Milas, Z. Fan, K. A. Mason, and K. K. Ang

CONTENTS

15.1 Introduction 189
15.2 Epidermal Growth Factor Receptor and Cancer 190
15.2.1 Molecular Structure of Epidermal Growth Factor Receptor 190
15.2.2 Substrates of Epidermal Growth Factor Receptor Tyrosine Kinase and Signal Transduction 190
15.2.3 Biological Functions of Epidermal Growth Factor Receptor in Tumorigenesis and Tumor Growth 191
15.3 Role of Epidermal Growth Factor Receptor in Radiotherapy 192
15.3.1 Epidermal Growth Factor Receptor Expression and Tumor Radioresponse 192
15.3.2 Effects of Epidermal Growth Factor Receptor and Its Ligands on In Vitro Cell Radioresponse 193
15.3.3 Activation of Epidermal Growth Factor Receptor Signaling by Radiation 194
15.3.4 Epidermal Growth Factor Receptor and Cellular Changes in Tumors Undergoing Radiotherapy 195
15.4 Inhibition of Epidermal Growth Factor Receptor for Cancer Therapy 197
15.4.1 Combining Anti-Epidermal Growth Factor Receptor Agents with Radiation: Preclinical Findings 197
15.4.2 Mechanisms of Enhancement of Tumor Radioresponse 198
15.4.3 Clinical Trials 200
15.5 Conclusions 200
References 201

L. Milas, MD, PhD; K. A. Mason, MD
The University of Texas M.D. Anderson Cancer Center, Department of Experimental Radiation Oncology, 1515 Holcombe Boulevard, Houston, TX 77030-4009, USA
Z. Fan, MD
The University of Texas M.D. Anderson Cancer Center, Department of Experimental Therapeutics, 1515 Holcombe Boulevard, Houston, TX 77030-4009, USA
K. K. Ang, MD, PhD
The University of Texas M.D. Anderson Cancer Center, Department of Radiation Oncology, 1515 Holcombe Boulevard, Houston, TX 77030-4009, USA

15.1 Introduction

Growth factors are substances that regulate cell growth and proliferation, and maintain architectural and functional homeostasis in normal tissues. They bind to specific cell membrane receptors setting in motion a highly regulated network of cellular events, signal transduction, gene activation, transcription, etc., which then regulate cell cycle checkpoints. Growth factors act locally by autocrine or paracrine functions or on distant tissues via endocrine activities. Over a hundred different growth factors have been identified, many of which interact with each other rendering complimentary or opposing effects on cell growth. Compared to normal tissues, growth factor signaling pathways in tumors are commonly subverted to result in inordinate division and function of cells. Tumors, which are composed of both malignant cells and many types of normal cells that infiltrate tumors, including endothelial cells, fibroblasts and lymphoid cells, secrete a variety of growth factors, which regulate tumor growth and dissemination. Comparable to their action in normal tissues, these factors can be autocrine, paracrine or affect cells at a distance from their production site and may have complementary or opposing effects on tumor cell growth.

The growth factor receptor-mediated signal transduction plays important roles not only in the biological process of cancer cell proliferation, mobility, invasion and metastasis, but also in conferring resistance of cancer cells to various treatments, including radiation. It has been shown that growth factors play a critical role in pathogenesis of radiation injury, both in normal tissues and tumors (Milas et al. 1998; Ruifrok and McBride 1999). Radiation induces the expression of new factors and alters both the magnitude and dynamics of existing ones. Through their action on cell and tissue proliferation, as well as cell loss, mediated via regulation of cell cycle check points, growth factors can influence major determinants of cell and tissue (both normal and tumor) radioresponse. The determinants include total number of clonogenic cells, cell cycle redistribution, cell repopulation, cellular repair mechanisms and tissue microenvironment such as tumor hypoxia and acidity. Cells respond to radiation and other external signals using the same receptors and signal transduction pathways as they use for self-regulation. In recent years it has become clear that radiation can induce alterations in production of growth factors and their receptors. Although our knowledge on biology of growth factors has greatly increased recently, research on the interaction of these factors with radiation has been limited. Hence, this interaction is still poorly understood.

Much of our knowledge on the regulation of radiosensitivity of cancer cells and tumor radioresponse by growth factors comes from the studies of the expression of epidermal growth factor receptor (EGFR) in cancer cells and the signals that are regulated by EGFR-mediated signal transduction pathways. This chapter will overview our current understanding of the effects of epidermal growth factor (EGF) and its receptor in cell and tumor response to radiation and their implications to tumor radiotherapy.

15.2
Epidermal Growth Factor Receptor and Cancer

15.2.1
Molecular Structure of Epidermal Growth Factor Receptor

The human EGFR is a 170-kDa transmembrane glycoprotein, which is composed of 1186 amino acids and stretched into an extracellular ligand-binding domain, a transmembrane segment, and an intracellular portion. The intracellular portion includes a tyrosine kinase domain [also referred as to *Src*-homology-1 (SH1) domain] that mediates the signals produced by growth factors into growth and survival regulatory signals, and an important regulatory region that serves as the docking site for the receptor downstream substrate to anchor and to be phosphorylated (Fig. 15.1).

EGFR is the founding member of a family of structurally related receptors, known as the *erbB* receptor family. The *erbB* receptor family derives its name from the avian erythroblastosis retroviral oncogenes (*v-erbB*) due to sequence homology to *v-erbB*. The gene products are also frequently referred to as HERs, based on their homology to the human EGF receptor. There are four members in this family, including EGFR/HER1 (*c-erbB1*), HER-2 (*c-erbB2*, referred to as the *neu* gene in the rat), HER-3 (*c-erbB3*), and HER-4 (*c-erbB4*). The *erbB* family is also often referred to as the type I growth receptor family, when compared with other structurally different receptor protein tyrosine kinase families such as the insulin-like growth factor (IGF) receptor (type II), the platelet-derived growth factor (PDGF) receptor (type III), and the fibroblast growth factor (FGF) receptor (type IV). These HER receptors have been shown to differ in their ligand-binding and substrate specificity. They function principally as heterodimers when more than one receptor type is present in cells. EGF binds with higher affinity to heterodimers of the EGF receptor and HER2 receptor than to homodimers of the EGF receptor; and similarly, neural differentiation factor (NDF), a ligand for HER3 and HER4, binds with much higher affinity to heterodimers of HER3 and HER2 than to homodimers of HER3 (SLIWKOWSKI et al. 1994). Binding of the appropriate growth factor is accompanied by receptor dimerization and autophosphorylation on tyrosine residues (ULLRICH and SCHLESINGER 1990).

EGFR (*c-erbB1*/HER1) was initially purified from the squamous carcinoma cell line A431 cells in which it is overexpressed (WRANN and FOX 1979) and some years later its cDNA sequence (3633 bp) (DOWNWARD et al. 1984; LIN et al. 1984; ULLRICH et al. 1984; XU et al. 1984), chromosome localization (*7p12-p22*) (DAVIES et al. 1980; CARLIN and KNOWLES 1982) and genomic structure (HALEY et al. 1987) were determined.

In addition to EGF, several other homologous molecules have been identified to bind to EGFR. These ligands include transforming growth factor-α (TGF-α) (DERYNCK 1988), amphiregulin (AR) (SHOYAB et al. 1988, 1989), heparin-binding EGF-like growth factor (HB-EGF) (HIGASHIYAMA et al. 1991), *cripto* (CICCODICOLA et al. 1989; CIARDIELLO et al. 1991), vaccinia virus growth factor (VVGF) (REISNER 1985; CHANG et al. 1987), betacellulin (BTC) (SHING et al. 1993; WATANABE et al. 1994; RIESE et al. 1996; BEERLI and HYNES 1996) and epiregulin (TOYODA et al. 1995). The most widely expressed ligands for EGFRs are EGF and TGF-α.

15.2.2
Substrates of Epidermal Growth Factor Receptor Tyrosine Kinase and Signal Transduction

The regulatory tail at the carboxyl terminus of EGFR (shown in Fig. 15.1) contains all currently known tyrosine autophosphorylation sites that are critical for the transduction of the signals following EGFR

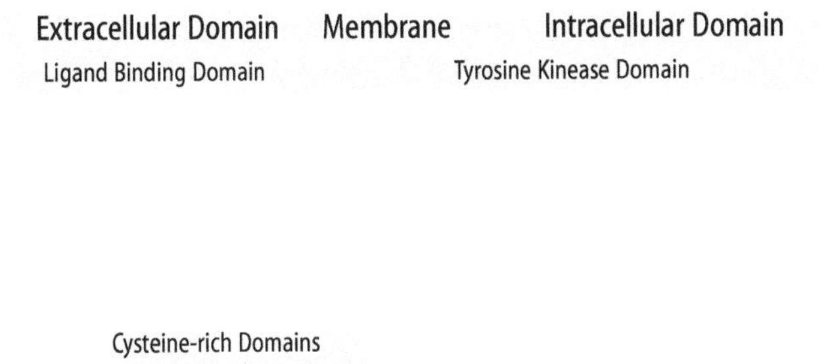

Extracellular Domain   Membrane   Intracellular Domain
Ligand Binding Domain   Tyrosine Kinease Domain

Cysteine-rich Domains

Fig. 15.1. Schematic structure of the human EGF receptor. The extracellular region of the receptor is divided into four domains: domain I (amino acids 1–165), cysteine-rich domain II (166–309), domain III (310–481), and cysteine-rich domain IV (482–621). Domain III is believed to be the major ligand-binding domain. The intracellular region is mainly composed of the protein tyrosine kinase domain (683–958), and the carboxyl-terminus tail (959–1186). Five currently known EGFR autophosphorylation sites are listed. K721 is the ATP-binding site on the receptor. ● stands for Asn-linked glycosylation sites

tyrosine kinase activation. An essential function of these sites is to allow intracellular substrates to bind to the receptors via the SH2 domains (a conserved motif of approximately 100 residues that bind to tyrosine-phosphorylated amino acid stretches) of EGF receptor downstream substrates and therefore to stimulate their activities (ANDERSON et al. 1990).

Substrate binding to the receptor via SH2 domain of the substrate is followed by phosphorylation of substrate molecules on tyrosine residues and transmission of the signals from the cell surface to the nucleus (a cascade of biochemical reactions that is collectively referred to as signal transduction pathways) through a series of protein–protein interactions via their SH2 and SH3 domains, and protein–lipid interactions via their pleckstrin homology (PH) domain (PAWSON et al. 2001; PAWSON 1995; MAYER et al. 1993; HASLAM et al. 1993). SH3 domains are conserved motifs of 50–75 residues that are involved in the protein–protein interaction. SH3-binding sites consist of proline-rich peptides of approximately 10 amino acids. SH3 domain links the signals transmitted from the cell surface by protein tyrosine kinase to downstream effector proteins during the signal transduction. The PH domain consists of approximately 100 amino acids and may tether signaling proteins to membrane, thus mediating protein–lipid interactions (HARLAN et al. 1994).

Several downstream pathways have been well-demonstrated following EGFR dimerization and activation. In addition to the major Grb/SOS/Ras/Raf/MEK/MAPK mitogenic pathway, there are the phosphotidylinositol-3 kinase/Akt pathway, the phospholipase-g/protein kinase C pathway, and the Janus kinase (JAK)/signal transducers and activators of transcription (STATs) pathways that activate a set of differential gene expressions, collectively leading to increased cell adhesion and mobility potential, enhanced cell cycle traversal, and inhibition of cell death. These biological effects are considered to be important contributing factors for tumor cell survival, proliferation, invasiveness and metastasis.

15.2.3
Biological Functions of Epidermal Growth Factor Receptor in Tumorigenesis and Tumor Growth

EGFR plays an important role both in development and growth of malignant tumors. Overexpression of EGFR results in ligand (EGF or TGF-α)-dependent cell transformation (VELU et al. 1987; DIFIORE et al. 1987; DI MARCO et al. 1989). Overexpression of a 140-kDa extracellular binding domain truncated form of EGFR mutant (EGFRvIII) (HUMPHREY et al. 1990) can transform NIH3T3 cells via a ligand-independent mechanism, as a result of constitutive activation of the receptor kinase (MOSCATELLO et al. 1996).

Many types of epithelial malignancies display increased EGFR on their cell surface membranes. Examples include cancers of the lung, breast, prostate, head and neck, colon, bladder, pancreas, cervix, vulva, and glioblastoma. Gene amplification is not a frequent finding in these tumors, with the exception of the glioblastoma. In several types of cancers, the EGF receptor status has been shown to be an important prognostic indicator (GULLICK 1991). Increased receptor expression often is associated with increased production of TGF-α by the same tumor cells. This establishes conditions conducive to receptor activation by an autocrine stimulatory pathway.

The mechanisms by which EGFR contributes to tumorigenesis are multiple and may include stimulation of cell cycle progression leading to increased cell proliferation, activation of cytoskeletal molecules leading to increased cell mobility, invasion, and enhanced angiogenesis. Expression of D-cyclins is stimulated by EGFR stimulation, suggesting a role for D-type cyclins as one of the sensors that link EGFR stimulation with the cell cycle machinery (SHERR and ROBERTS 1995; SHERR 1996). Experimental elevation of D-type cyclin level shortens duration of the G1 cell cycle phase, reduces the requirement for exogenous growth factors, and prevents terminal cell differentiation (SHERR and ROBERTS 1995). Genetic aberrations affecting D-type cyclin, their dependent kinases CDK4/6 and their inhibitors such as p21 and p27, and the substrate Rb are frequent events occurring in human cancer.

Recent research has shown that exposure of cells to growth factors causes cytoskeleton reorganization, formation of lamellipodia and membrane ruffling and altered cell morphology, implicating the roles of growth factors in stimulating cell migration and invasion, which constitute the basis for cancer metastasis.

15.3
Role of Epidermal Growth Factor Receptor in Radiotherapy

15.3.1
Epidermal Growth Factor Receptor Expression and Tumor Radioresponse

Although many studies reported positive association between overexpression of EGFR and adverse patient survival, including poor response to various anticancer therapies (MENDELSOHN 1997, 2000; MENDELSOHN and FAN 1997; WOODBURN 1999), information on the relevance of EGFR expression on tumor response to radiotherapy is still limited. However, the available information from both preclinical research and clinical studies implicates the role of EGFR in tumor resistance to radiotherapy. Our group explored the relationship between EGFR expression and radioresponse of mouse carcinomas that display a broad range in radioresponse, measured by TCD_{50} (radiation dose yielding 50% local tumor control) (AKIMOTO et al. 1999a). EGFR protein levels were analyzed by Western blotting in nine tumors of different histological type and were shown to vary by more than 20-fold among these tumors. As shown in Fig. 15.2, there was a highly significant ($r=0.8$, $P<0.01$) positive correlation between the level of EGFR and TCD_{50} value (AKIMOTO et al. 1999a). Thus, tumors with higher EGFR protein levels were less responsive to radiation. In a subsequent study (MILAS et al. 2002), using the same cohort of nine murine tumors, we investigated whether a relationship exists between the extent of expression of cyclin D1, which is a downstream sensor of EGFR signaling, and tumor radiocurability. Cyclin D1 expression, determined by Western blotting, varied by 40-fold among these tumors and its magnitude positively correlated with poorer tumor radioresponse (higher TCD_{50} values). The level of cyclin D1 expression paralleled that of EGFR.

These findings suggest that EGFR and its sensor cyclin D1 may be important determinants of tumor radioresponse in vivo. The clinical implications of these findings are that the pretreatment assessment of EGFR expression may serve as a useful predictor of radiotherapy outcome and may assist in selecting an effective treatment modality. Our preclinical investigations were followed by a clinical study to determine whether the expression of EGFR in head and neck cancer is correlated with treatment outcome to radiotherapy. It has already been shown that the vast majority of head and neck carcinomas have elevated levels of EGFR and its ligand, TGF-α. For example, GRANDIS and TWEARDY (1993) reported that the EGFR mRNA and TGF-α mRNA were elevated by a mean of 69- and 5-fold, respectively, in a cohort of 24 tumors compared to corresponding mRNA levels in control normal mucosa. In a subsequent immunohistochemical (IHC) study of 91 head and neck carcinomas of various stages (T1–4, N0–1) treated

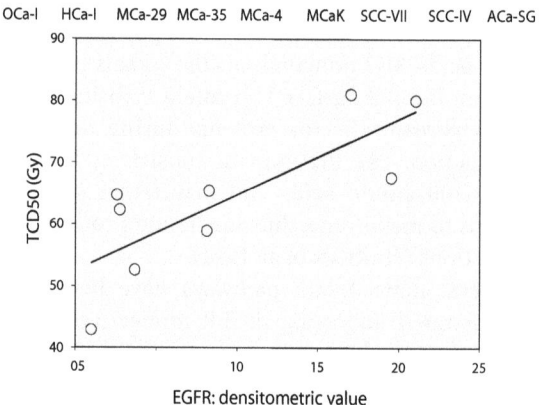

Fig. 15.2. Expression of epidermal growth factor receptor (EGFR) protein in nine murine carcinomas determined by Western blotting (*top panel*). Relationship between EGFR expression and radiocurability (TCD_{50} = radiation dose yielding 50% tumor cure) of these nine carcinomas (*lower panel*). (From AKIMOTO et al. 1999a, with permission)

with surgical resection with or without radiotherapy/chemotherapy, GRANDIS et al. (1998) correlated the expression of EGFR and TGF-α proteins with treatment outcome. Perhaps due to the relatively small sample size, this study did not address the effects of protein expression on the pattern of failure.

Our own study analyzed the immunohistochemical expression of EGFR in a series of 155 representative head and neck cancer patients enrolled into a prospective clinical trial treated with a consistent radiation regimen (unpublished). Tumors of advanced stage, mainly III–IV, displayed a wide range of EGFR expression (Fig. 15.3), which did not correlate with the tumor or nodal stage, other established prognostic stage groupings (AJCC or RTOG-RPA), or patient performance status. Correlative analysis showed that EGFR expression was a strong, independent prognostic determinant of overall and disease-free survival ($P=0.0006$ and $P=0.0016$, respectively). Analysis of the patterns of relapse in this series revealed a new, clinically relevant finding that EGFR expression was a robust predictor for local-regional relapse ($P=0.0031$) but not for distant metastasis ($P=0.96$). We thus showed that EGFR expression is a strong predictor of tumor resistance to radiotherapy in a relatively homogeneous group of patients in terms of disease stage and therapy received.

That the level of EGFR expression can influence tumor cell radiosensitivity was recently shown by SHERIDAN et al. (1997). These investigators determined sensitivity to 2-Gy single-dose radiation of primary cultures derived from 14 head and neck carcinoma patients, and found that cell cultures expressing high levels of EGFR were more radioresistant than those expressing low levels of EGFR. Resistance was measured by the extent of radiation-induced cell growth inhibition.

15.3.2
Effects of Epidermal Growth Factor Receptor and Its Ligands on In Vitro Cell Radioresponse

Our knowledge on the effect of EGFR or its ligands on tumor cell response to radiation or other cytotoxic agents comes mainly from in vitro studies performed within the last decade. Although some studies showed that EGF can enhance the cytotoxic effect of ionizing radiation, more evidence implicates EGF as having radioprotective effects. KWOK and SUTHERLAND (1991, 1992) observed that EGF increased radioresponse of squamous cell carcinoma cell lines that had high-affinity cell surface receptors to EGF. The radioenhancement was most significant in G_1-phase cells and was associated mainly with a reduction of the shoulder region of the dose-survival curve. Another study showed that radioenhancement induced by EGF depended on the intrinsic sensitivity of tumor cells to radiation, with the effect being greater in more radiosensitive cells (BONNER et al. 1994). A number of studies, however, showed that EGF can provide protection to cells against radiation damage (WOLLMAN et al. 1994; BALABAN et al. 1996). Addition of EGF to cultures of hormone-deprived MCF-7 cells before irradiation resulted in increased radioresistance of these cells, and this radioprotective effect was abrogated by a specific antibody to the EGF receptor (WOLLMAN et al. 1994). The induced resistance was associated with an increase in the number of cells in the radioresistant S-phase of the cell cycle, and in a rise in the level of intracellular glutathione that acts radioprotectively. In a similar study, BALABAN et al. (1996) showed that the presence of EGF during and after irradiation resulted in a decreased radiosensitivity of A431 carcinoma cells. In contrast, treatment of cells with monoclonal antibodies to the EGFR sensitized cells to radiation by enhancing radiation-induced apoptosis. They suggested that radiation activates EGFR and hence initiates downstream signaling processes resulting in increased cellular radioresistance. A causal relationship between EGFR and increased resistance of cells to cytotoxic agents was provided by transfection experiments. DICKSTEIN et al. (1995) were the first to report that transfection of EGFR into human breast cancer cells increased the resistance of these cells to cytotoxic drugs. In a gene transfection experi-

Fig. 15.3. Immunohistochemistry of human head and neck squamous cell carcinoma showing high EGFR positivity (stained brown). Unstained portion is stromal tissue within the tumor ment, we recently addressed the causal relationship between EGFR overexpression and radiation sensitivity using a low EGFR expressing an ovarian adenocarcinoma cell line (OCA-I). The *EGFR*-gene transfection, but not transfer of the control vector, induced EGFR overexpression in OCA-I cells, which rendered these cells more resistant to radiation compared to the original nontransfected cell line. When these EGFR transfected cells were treated with anti-EGFR antibody, their original radiosensitivity was restored (unpublished).

15.3.3
Activation of Epidermal Growth Factor Receptor Signaling by Radiation

A number of in vitro and in vivo studies showed that ionizing radiation can mimic the action of ligand-receptor binding and on its own activate transduction processes involved in EGFR signaling (BALABAN et al. 1996; GOLDKORN et al. 1997; SCHMIDT-ULLRICH et al. 1996, 1997; AKIMOTO et al. 1999a; MILAS et al. 2002). BALABAN et al. (1996) showed that radiation affects multiple signaling pathways in A431 carcinoma cells, but that induction of radioresistance was predominantly associated with the activation of EGFR. SCHMIDT-ULLRICH et al. (1996, 1997) reported that irradiation of human mammary and squamous carcinoma cell lines induces EGFR phosphorylation followed by activation of transduction pathways, including Raf-1 and MAPK. Blockade of EGFR phosphorylation by the specific inhibitor tyrphostin AG1478 abolished the transduction signal (SCHMIDT-ULLRICH et al. 1997). These investigators postulated that activation of EGFR-mediated signals stimulates cell proliferation, which may underlie acceleration of tumor clonogen repopulation during the course of fractionated radiotherapy.

Our studies showed that radiation induces activation of EGFR signaling pathways in tumors growing in vivo (AKIMOTO et al. 1999a; MILAS et al. 2002). AKIMOTO et al. (1999a) reported that tumor irradiation with 15-Gy single-dose γ-rays induced EGFR phosphorylation within 30 min of irradiation and that the phosphorylation persisted for the observation period of 2 h. (Fig. 15.4). However, the induced phosphorylation depended on the basal level of EGFR expression and occurred in SCC-VII, a high-EGFR-expressing tumor, but not in OCA-I, a low-EGFR-expressing tumor. Tumor irradiation also induced an increase in protein tyrosine kinase (PTK) activity. Similar to EGFR phosphorylation, the increase in PTK activity

Fig. 15.4. Effect of ionizing radiation (15 Gy) on EGFR autophosphorylation of SCC-VII and OCA-1 tumors. 0 h, nonirradiated. The immunoprecipitates were subjected to Western blotting with an antiphosphotyrosine (PY-20; **a** and **c**) or a polyclonal EGFR antibody (**b** and **d**). Note that intensities of EGFR (**b** and **d**) are almost the same for all samples that were taken before and after irradiation. (From AKIMOTO et al. 1999a, with permission)

occurred in tumors with higher basal PTK activity (SCC-VII and HCA-I tumors). In contrast, in tumors with low basal PTK activity, irradiation either had no effect (MCA-29 tumor) or reduced PTK activity (MCA-4 tumor). Basal PTK activity was about twice as high in tumors with high EGFR levels than in tumors with low EGFR levels.

The downstream EGFR-mediated signaling molecules are also affected by radiation, including cyclin D1 and p27, the latter being an inhibitory protein that regulates downstream transfer of molecular signals mediated by the G1-cell cycle phase cyclins and their associated cdks. Namely, upon receiving afferent signals, cyclin D1 binds to its corresponding cdk, and the complex then interacts with the Rb/E2F complex. This interaction can be constrained by a number of cdk inhibitors, including p27, and if constrained the cells become arrested in G1 or may undergo apoptosis. The effect of tumor irradiation on the expression of cyclin D1 and p27 proteins was determined in the radiosensitive OCA-I and in the radioresistant SCC-VII tumors (MILAS et al. 2002). The results of this study, shown in Fig. 15.5, showed that the expression of both cyclin D1 and p27 was

15.3.4
Epidermal Growth Factor Receptor and Cellular Changes in Tumors Undergoing Radiotherapy

Taken together the findings of in vivo studies described above (AKIMOTO et al. 1999a; MILAS et al. 2002) imply that radiation initiates EGFR signaling in radioresistant tumors and facilitates the transfer of signals through cyclin D1. On the other hand, in radiosensitive tumors, radiation is ineffective in inducing and propagating EGFR-mediated cell proliferation signals. In fact, radiation blocked signal transfer at the level of cyclin D1 and p27. We provided some evidence that these alterations in EGFR-mediated signaling molecules were associated with cellular changes in tumors exposed to radiation, including changes in cell proliferation and apoptotic response to radiation. PCNA labeling, used for assessing cell proliferation, showed no significant change in the radioresistant SCC-VII tumors within 2 days of 15 Gy, which is consistent with the general view that radioresistant tumors are relatively insensitive to radiation-induced disruption of cell proliferation. In contrast, in the radiosensitive OCA-I tumors, cell proliferation was greatly reduced by irradiation. Decline in PCNA positivity was visible within several hours of irradiation and its magnitude continued to decline within the observation period of 2 days following irradiation. The inability of radiation to reduce the percentage of PCNA-positive SCC-VII cells may be attributed to high intrinsic cell radioresistance, possibly linked to the involvement of PCNA in repairing DNA damage after radiation (KELMAN 1997). This repair would be expected to result in increased survival of clonogenic tumor cells.

Differences in susceptibility of cells to radiation-induced apoptosis are also a factor involved in the radioresponse of radioresistant vs radiosensitive tumors, including the SCC-VII and OCA-I tumors studied by MILAS et al. (2002). While SCC-VII is highly resistant, OCA-I is sensitive to induction of apoptosis by radiation (MEYN et al. 1993). The loss of PCNA positive cells in OCA-I tumor can be largely attributed to induced apoptosis, as the loss of PCNA staining was associated with significant increase in apoptotic cells (MILAS et al. 2002). This loss of cells by apoptosis is accompanied by molecular changes in terms of high up-regulation

Fig. 15.5. Effect of ionizing radiation (15 Gy) on (*A*) cyclin D1 protein expression and (*B*) p27 protein expression in radioresistant SCC-VII and radiosensitive OCA-I tumors. Both Western blots and calculated densitometric values of protein expression as a function of time after irradiation are shown. The densitometric value of protein expression in nonirradiated tumors was taken as 1.0. (From MILAS et al. 2002, with permission)

influenced by ionizing radiation, but the effect in radioresistant tumors was different from that in radiosensitive tumors. In radioresistant tumors, the expression of cyclin D1 was unaffected by radiation, whereas the expression of p27 was reduced. This suggests that in radioresistant tumors the cell cycle progression signals received by cyclin D1 are further transmitted uninhibited. Moreover, transmission of these signals might even be facilitated, as suggested by the radiation-induced reduction in p27 expression. In contrast, radiation reduced the level of cyclin D1 in radiosensitive tumors, which could mean that less of it is available to receive the afferent signals. In addition, radiation up-regulated the expression of p27, which is suggestive of increased inhibition of the transfer of the received signals to the Rb/E2F complex.

of p21 (AKIMOTO et al. 1999b), as well as of p27 (Fig. 15.5B) proteins that inhibit progression of cells through the G1 cell cycle phase. A number of recent reports show that p27 in addition to being involved in cell cycle arrest has pro-apoptotic activity (KATAYOSE et al. 1997; WANG et al. 1997; SCHREIBER et al. 1999).

As already mentioned, SCHMIDT-ULLRICH et al. (1996, 1997) found that activation of EGFR-mediated signals stimulates tumor cell proliferation in vitro, and they suggested that this may underlie acceleration of tumor clonogen repopulation during the course of fractionated radiotherapy. It has long been recognized that the time of onset and the extent of regeneration of tumor clonogens during radiotherapy play an important role in tumor control (WITHERS et al. 1988). In an in vivo study, we addressed the question of whether the onset of regeneration of tumor cells that survive irradiation is different in tumors that have high levels of EGFR and cyclin D1 from those that have low levels of these proteins. Our study (THAMES et al. 1996) showed that the regeneration of tumor cell clonogens in the radiosensitive, low-EGFR- and low-cyclin D1-expressing OCA-I tumor was negligible within 10 days of tumor irradiation, after which the regeneration began and assumed an accelerated mode. Similar dynamics of postradiation tumor cell repopulation was exhibited by another low-EGFR- and cyclin D1-expressing tumor, designated MCA-4, where clonogen regeneration began approximately 8 days after radiation delivery (MILAS et al. 1991). Figure 15.6 shows that cell repopulation in the radioresistant, high-EGFR- and high-cyclin D1-expressing tumor began much earlier than in either OCA-I or MCA-4; it began between 1 and 4 days after irradiation. In fact, the extent of cell repopulation present at 4 days after irradiation was high enough to result in a significant inhibition of tumor response to the second dose of radiation compared to that when the second dose of radiation was given 1 day after the priming dose. The details of this experiment are described in the legend of Fig. 15.6. Therefore, rapid repopulation of tumor cell clonogens after irradiation is another characteristic of tumors with high levels of EGFR and cyclin D1, which contributes to poor tumor radioresponse. Rapid repopulation of tumor cell clonogens would result in earlier onset of postirradiation recurrences and would have a strong negative impact on tumor curability after fractionated radiotherapy.

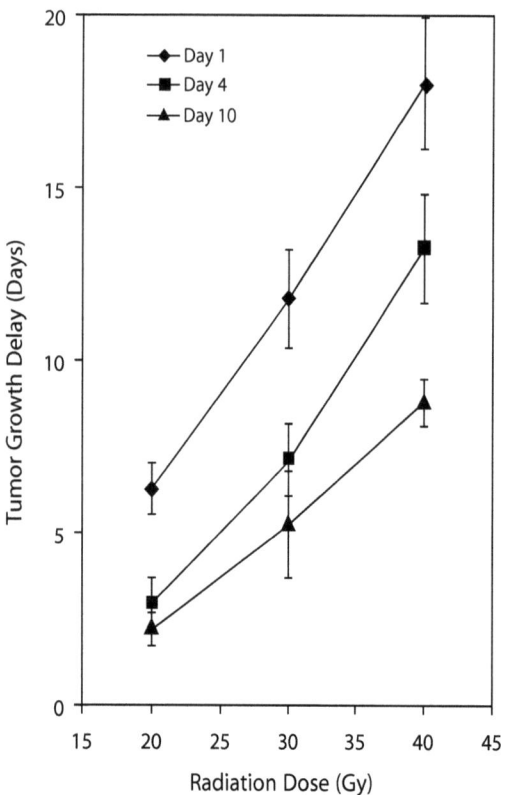

Fig. 15.6. Cell repopulation in SCC-VII tumors after irradiation. Tumors were exposed to 45-Gy single-dose irradiation (priming dose) when 6.5 mm in diameter, and 1, 4 or 10 days later they were reirradiated under hypoxic conditions with 20 Gy, 30 Gy, or 40 Gy. Reirradiation was performed under hypoxic conditions to exclude the influence of reoxygenation that might have taken place after the priming dose. The plot of tumor growth delay in days produced by the second radiation dose shows that the second dose given 1 day after the priming dose was the most effective, and tumor growth was delayed more as the dose of radiation was increased. The second doses of radiation were less effective when given 4 days after the priming dose, and even less effective when given 10 days after the priming dose. This reduction in efficacy can be attributed to the regeneration of tumor cell clonogens that survived the priming dose of radiation. The magnitude of repopulation was estimated by dividing the radiation dose given 10 days after the priming dose with that given 1 day after the priming dose that produced the same tumor growth delay. For example, a tumor growth delay of 8.5 days required a 40-Gy dose when radiation was given 10 days after and only 24 Gy when radiation was given 1 day after the priming dose. Thus, tumor repopulation offset the efficacy of radiation by 16 Gy in 9 days or 1.78 Gy per day

15.4
Inhibition of Epidermal Growth Factor Receptor for Cancer Therapy

Targeting EGFR as a potential therapy for cancer has attracted extensive interest over the past decade. Currently, two major pharmacological approaches are being explored for inhibiting EGF receptor function in cancer cells. One approach uses monoclonal antibodies (mAb) such as C225 and ABX-EGF, which are directed to the extracellular domain of EGF receptor and block natural ligand for receptor binding, thereby preventing receptor activation (Fig. 15.7). The other approach uses a class of small molecule ATP analogues (such as Iressa [ZD-1839], Tarceva [OSI774]) that are highly selective to the ATP binding site on the intracytoplasmic portion of EGFR. These small molecules inhibit tyrosine kinase and prevent further downstream transduction of the EGFR initiated signals. C225 is a human mouse chimeric anti-EGFR monoclonal antibody. It is in clinical phase II and III trials in combination with chemotherapy or radiation therapy for a number of human cancers including head and neck, colorectal, pancreatic, and lung cancers. Many small molecules that target intracellular domain of EGFR are already available and have entered clinical testing. Of these, the most commonly used is Iressa, an ATP-binding competitor. Other tyrosine kinase inhibitors such as Tarceva are also in clinical trial. There are a number of newer inhibitors including CI-1033 and PKI-166, which are still in relatively early stages of development. Clinical application of EGFR inhibitors will be discussed later in Sec. 15.4.3, Clinical Trials.

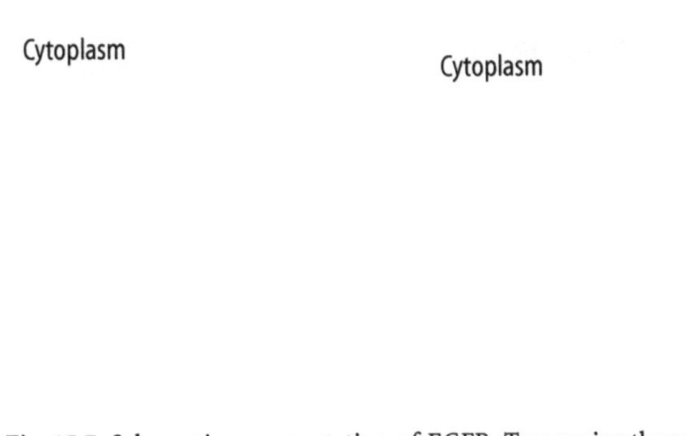

15.4.1
Combining Anti-Epidermal Growth Factor Receptor Agents with Radiation: Preclinical Findings

Increasing evidence from preclinical studies shows that interference with EGFR signaling pathways has therapeutic potential (MENDELSOHN 1997, 2000; WOODBURN 1999). This is particularly evident when anti-EGFR substances are combined with cytotoxic agents, including radiation (BASELGA et al. 1993; FAN et al. 1993; MENDELSOHN 1997, 2000; WOODBURN 1999; HUANG et al. 1999; HUANG and HARARI 2000; BIANCO et al. 2000; MILAS et al. 2000; NASU et al. 2001). As most studies thus far have been performed using the combination of C225 with radiation, we briefly describe their findings. HUANG et al. (1999) reported that in vitro exposure of SCC-13Y head and neck squamous cell carcinoma cells to C225-anti-EGFR monoclonal antibody either for 3 days prior to, or during and after irradiation enhanced cell radiosensitivity. The major mechanism for enhanced radioresponse was attributed to the ability of the antibody to enhance susceptibility of tumor cells to radiation-induced apoptosis. There have been a number of in vivo studies by others (BIANCO et al. 2000; HUANG and HARARI 2000) and our team (MILAS et al. 2000; NASU et al. 2001) showing that treatment of mice bearing human tumor xenografts with C225 potentiates the antitumor efficacy of radiation. This was observed using A431 squamous cell carcinoma (MILAS et al. 2000; NASU et al. 2001), SCC-1 and SCC-6 head and neck squamous cell carcinomas (HUANG and HARARI 2000) and GEO colon carcinoma (BIANCO et al. 2000) xenografts. Potentiation of tumor radioresponse was significant in all studies. The treatment endpoints were tumor growth delay (BIANCO et al. 2000; HUANG and HARARI 2000; MILAS et al. 2000), tumor cure rate (NASU et al. 2001), onset of postradiation tumor recurrences (NASU et al. 2001), and mouse survival (BIANCO et al. 2000). All treatment endpoints showed that the combined treatment effect was more than the additive effects of individual treatments. In our own study, where tumor growth delay was the treatment endpoint, tumor radioresponse was enhanced by a factor of 1.59 when C225 was given once 6 h before single-dose local tumor irradiation and by a factor of 3.62 when two additional doses of C225 were

Fig. 15.7. Schematic representation of EGFR. Two major therapeutic approaches to inhibit EGFR are being tested. One is to block the extracellular domain of the receptor by anti-EGFR antibodies (such as C225) to prevent EGFR binding to its ligands (EGF, TGF-α). The other approach uses chemical agents that inhibit PTK phosphorylation given 3 and 6 days after irradiation (MILAS et al. 2000; Fig. 15.8). The same treatment schedules augmented tumor radiocurability, assessed by the TCD_{50} assay 120 days after treatment, and delayed the onset of tumor recurrence (NASU et al. 2001; Fig. 15.9). Tumor radiocurability was enhanced by a factor of 1.18 by a single dose and by a factor of 1.92 by three doses of C225. Likewise, the appearance of tumor recurrences was delayed by a factor of 1.37 by a single dose and by a factor of 2.13 by three doses of C225.

15.4.2
Mechanisms of Enhancement of Tumor Radioresponse

The mechanisms by which EGFR inhibitors augment tumor response to radiation and other cytotoxic agents are multiple, involving direct and indirect interaction with tumor cells. The following consideration of possible mechanisms is based mainly on studies with C225. This antibody on its own can be cytotoxic or inhibit proliferation of tumor cells (MENDELSOHN 1997; FAN et al. 1993, 1994; BASELGA et al. 1993; PREWETT et al. 1996; WU et al. 1995). Cytotoxic action of C225 is commonly attributed to the ability of the antibody to induce apoptotic cell death, and therefore a possibility that C225 increases susceptibility of tumor cells to radiation-induced apoptosis will be the first mechanism considered (MENDELSOHN 1997; WU et al. 1995). A number of studies demonstrated the ability of anti-EGFR antibodies to enhance in vitro response of tumor cells to cytotoxic drugs (MENDELSOHN 1997; FAN et al. 1993; BASELGA et al. 1993; MENDELSOHN and FAN 1997) or ionizing irradiation (BALABAN et al. 1996; HUANG et al. 1999), and the enhancement was attributed to augmentation of drug- or radiation-induced apoptosis. Information on the apoptotic effect of C225 when combined with radiation in treating tumors in vivo is very limited. Our findings do not support induction of apoptosis as the major underlying mechanism of antitumor action of C225 combined with irradiation (MILAS et al. 2000). In this particular tumor (A431), neither C225 nor radiation, nor the combination of the two agents caused significant apoptosis. Instead, C225 combined with radiation produced significant tumor necrosis. In some tumors, necrosis was very extensive, occupying the whole tumor except for a tiny peripheral rim (illustrated in Fig. 15.10). Cell death by necrosis in treated tumors could have resulted from direct damage to tumor cells, indirectly through the damage of tumor vascularization, or more likely both. The involvement of the vascular effect was supported by histological features that included intravascular thrombosis, tumor hemorrhage, and massive necrosis positioned centrally within the tumor. Regarding apoptosis, it might be that there are differences in induction or detection of C225-induced apoptosis between in vitro and in

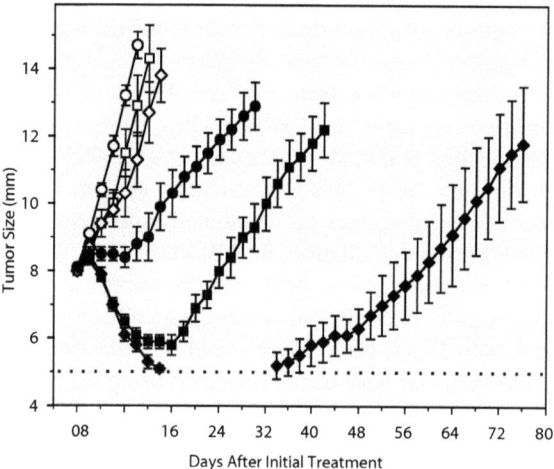

Fig. 15.8. Effect of C225 antibody on radioresponse of A431 tumor xenograft: ○, no treatment; □, treated with a single injection of C225; ◇, treated with three injections of C225; ●, 18 Gy of local tumor irradiation; ■, single dose of C225 plus 18 Gy of local tumor irradiation; ◆, three doses of C225 plus 18 Gy. (From MILAS et al. 2000, with permission)

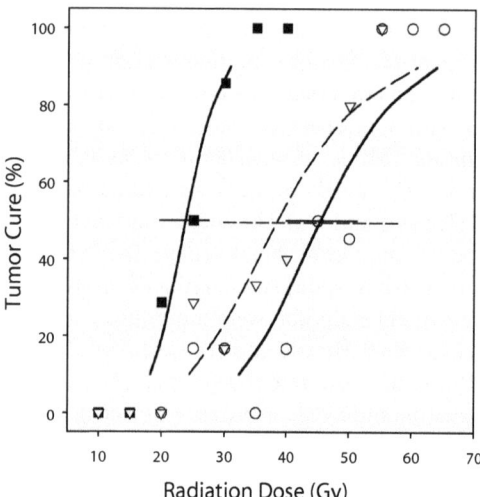

Fig. 15.9. Radiocurability of 8-mm A431 tumor xenografts in nude mice. Radiation dose-response curves were generated for local tumor control at 120 days after treatment with radiation alone (○), a single dose of C225 plus radiation (▽), or three doses of C225 plus radiation (■). (From NASU et al. 2001, with permission)

Fig. 15.10. Histological appearance of A431 xenografts, untreated or 7 days after treatment with C225 and 18 Gy. The treated xenograft shows central necrosis. (From MILAS et al. 2000, with permission)

vivo settings, or that massive necrosis induced by radiation masked the apoptotic response.

Interference of C225 with cellular repair mechanisms is likely another mechanism underlying the direct radiosensitizing effect of this antibody. BANDYOPADHYAY et al. (1998) showed that EGFR physically interacts with DNA-dependent protein kinase (DNA-PK) and that inhibition of EGFR signaling by anti-EGFR antibody is accompanied by a reduction in the level of the DNA-PK and its activity in the nuclear fraction. HUANG and HARARI (2000) subsequently reported that EGFR blockade leads to redistribution of DNA-PK from the nucleus to the cytosol, resulting in reduced radiation-induced DNA damage repair detectable through the classic split-dose experiment.

Interference with tumor neovascularization is an additional mechanism for increased tumor radioresponse by C225. EGFR ligands, EGF, and TGF-α were reported to play a role in tumor angiogenesis, directly (SCHRIEBER et al. 1986) or indirectly by interaction with VEGF (GILLE et al. 1997). Our own study (MILAS et al. 2000) demonstrated that C225 significantly inhibited formation of new vessels at the site of A431 tumor cell inoculation, which was also associated with significant delay in tumor growth. This delay could have resulted either from a direct effect of C225 on tumor angiogenesis or from inhibition of tumor cell proliferation, thus indirectly inhibiting angiogenesis. The direct inhibitory effect of C225 is supported by a recent study showing that the antibody inhibited mRNA and protein production of the VEGF, IL-8, and bFGF angiogenic factors in cultured bladder cancer cells as well as in xenografts derived from these cells (PERROTTE et al. 1999). C225 caused significant endothelial cell apoptosis in treated tumors. Inhibition of tumor angiogenesis as a mechanism of C225-induced enhancement of tumor radioresponse is suggested by a number of reports showing that treatment with antiangiogenic agents such as angiostatin and TNP-470 increases tumor radioresponse (GORSKI et al. 1998, 1999; MAUCERI et al. 1998; TEICHER et al. 1995; KAKEJI and TEICHER 1997). The effect was attributed primarily to the damage of endothelial cells. Some angiogenic agents may act radioprotectively for tumor or endothelial cells. For example, GORSKI et al. (1999) reported that VEGF protects endothelial cells from radiation and that the radioprotection can be abolished by treatment with an anti-VEGF antibody. Since C225 inhibits VEGF production (PETIT et al. 1997; PERROTTE et al. 1999), it is possible that it enhances tumor radioresponse by eliminating the protective effect of VEGF.

We observed some characteristic histological features associated with C225 treatment, primarily tumor infiltration with granulocytes and an increase in terminal cell differentiation (MILAS et al. 2000). The infiltrating cells were present throughout tumor tissue but were particularly pronounced in the perivascular region. Most likely the granulocytic response was related to clearing dead tumor cells, but a possibility exists that these infiltrating cells were involved in tumor cell kill on their own. STOCKMEYER et al. (1997) reported that granulocytes primed with the granulocyte colony-stimulating factor were cytolytic to a number of breast cancer cell lines expressing HER-2/neu in the presence of anti-HER-2/neu monoclonal antibodies. Also, it is possible that perivascular infiltration with granulocytes could damage vascular walls and indirectly contribute to tumor cell kill and development of the severe necrosis discussed above in this section.

Treatment with C225 was associated with increased terminal cell differentiation in tumors and was especially pronounced when the antibody was combined with irradiation. Terminal cell differentiation was also found in cultured tumor cells exposed to anti-EGFR antibodies (ICR63 or ICR80) or tyrosine kinase inhibitors (MODJTAHEDI et al. 1998). It is also possible that C225, through its antiproliferative effect, delayed the onset of cell repopulation in irradiated tumors. This repopulation-inhibitory effect could account for the dramatic retardation in tumor growth when C225 was administered both before and after radiation treatment (see Fig. 15.8).

Overall, it seems that multiple mechanisms underlie the enhancement of cell and tumor response to radiation by EGFR inhibitors, including induction of apoptosis, inhibition of repair from radiation damage, inhibition of tumor angiogenesis, vascular damage, tumor infiltration with polymorphonuclear cells and an increase in cell differentiation.

15.4.3
Clinical Trials

As mentioned in Sec. 15.4, "Inhibition of Epidermal Growth Factor Receptor for Cancer Therapy", the number of agents that interfere with EGFR and its signaling pathways is rapidly increasing, and some of them have been moved from preclinical investigations to clinical trials. Most of these agents are in their early clinical testing. A series of Phase I and I/II clinical trials using C225 antibody have been performed showing dose-dependent EGFR saturable pharmacokinetics and the lack of significant antibody response against C225 (PEREZ-SOLER et al. 1994, 1998; MODJTAHEDI et al. 1996). The recommended dose of C225 for clinical trials consists of a 400 mg/m^2 loading dose, followed by a weekly maintenance dose of 250 mg/m^2 (BASELGA et al. 2000a). Related to radiotherapy, a Phase I/II trial was performed in patients with advanced head and neck cancer where weekly administration of C225 was combined with a 60-Gy total radiation dose to the tumor given by standard fractionation regimen of 2 Gy per day (EZEKIEL et al. 1998). The response rate was 100%, with 13 of 15 patients having complete remission. One year after treatment completion, more than 50% of patients remained in complete remission (BONNER et al. 2000). These encouraging findings have led to a multi-institutional Phase III trial in head and neck patients. The treatment is well tolerated and the major associated toxicity is acneiform skin rash occurring in about 10% of patients. Clinical trials that combined C225 with chemotherapy have also provided encouraging results (MENDELSOHN et al. 1999).

A number of clinical trials have investigated the efficacy of agents that inhibit tyrosine kinase. Recently, the results of a Phase I study of oral administration of Iressa, administered daily for 14 consecutive days every 28-day cycle, in patients with different tumor types were reported (RANSON et al. 2002). The treatment was well tolerated; the major side effects were acneiform-like rash and diarrhea. In Phase II trials, tumor response rate after Iressa treatment is between 10% and 20% (BASELGA et al. 2000b, 2001). No clinical study that combined Iressa with radiotherapy has thus far been reported. An overview of ongoing clinical studies of EGFR inhibitors, both anti-EGFR antibodies and tyrosine kinase inhibitors, can be found in recent reports by BASELGA (2002) and KIM et al. (2002).

15.5
Conclusions

There is compelling evidence that overexpression or mutation in EGFR plays a critical role in the growth of many tumors. About one-third of all epithelial cancers in humans have elevated EGFR, which is also commonly associated with production of TGF-α, an EGFR ligand, by these tumors. Overexpression of EGFR and high levels of its ligands have two major clinical implications: to serve as a prognostic tool of treatment outcome and to be a target for therapy, including radiotherapy. Elevated EGFR is associated with more aggressive tumors, poor response to standard treatment modalities, and poor patient survival. Our own preclinical studies using murine epithelial tumors provided clear evidence showing that an inverse correlation exists between EGFR expression and tumor radiocurability. Also, our recent clinical study revealed that high levels of EGFR in head and neck cancer were associated with local-regional relapse after radiotherapy. Thus, quantitation of EGFR and its ligands may be a useful tool for identifying subgroups of patients with high-risk adverse treatment outcome, and enable the use of the most rational individualized therapeutic strategy.

Another crucial implication of dysregulated EGFR and its signaling pathways is that they may serve as targets for cancer therapy. It is possible to interfere with EGFR binding or with individual steps in downstream processes. Antibodies are being developed to prevent binding of ligands to EGFR. One of these antibodies, C225, was shown in preclinical tumor models to suppress tumor growth and potentiate antitumor efficacy of chemotherapeutic agents and radiation. Therapeutic efficacy of C225 is currently undergoing clinical trials when combined with radiotherapy or chemotherapy and the initial results are encouraging.

Many chemical agents, such as Iressa and Tarceva, that inhibit tyrosine kinase phosphorylation and thus block downstream propagation of EGFR-initiated signals have recently been developed. They have also entered initial clinical testing that has already exhibited encouraging therapeutic effects. Therefore, interference with EGFR binding or EGFR-mediated intracellular signal transduction pathways has high therapeutic potential, particularly when combined with standard treatment modalities including tumor radiotherapy.

Acknowledgements. This work was supported in part by National Institutes of Health research grants CA-06294, CA-42060, CA-84415 and CA-16672, and Texas Tobacco Settlements Funds.

References

Akimoto T, Hunter NR, Buchmiller L et al (1999a) Inverse relationship between epidermal growth factor receptor expression and radiocurability of murine carcinomas. Clin Cancer res 5:2884–2890

Akimoto T, Seong J, Hunter NR, Buchmiller L, Mason K, Milross CG, Milas L (1999b) Association of increased radiocurability of murine carcinomas with low constitutive expression of P21$^{WAF1/CIP1}$ protein. Int J Radiat Oncol Biol Phys 44:413–419

Anderson D, Koch CA, Grey L et al (1990) Binding of SH2 domains of phospholipase C gamma 1, GAP, and Src to activated growth factor receptors. Science 250:979–982

Balaban N, Moni J, Shannon M, Dang L, Murphy E, Goldkorn T (1996) The effect of ionizing radiation on signal transduction: antibodies to EGF receptor sensitize A431 cells to radiation. Biochim Biophys Acta 1314:147–156

Bandyopadhyay D, Mandal M, Adam L et al (1998) Physical interaction between epidermal growth factor receptor and DNA-dependent protein kinase in mammalian cells. J Biol Chem 273:1568–1573

Baselga J (2002) Targeting the epidermal growth factor receptor with tyrosine kinase inhibitors: small molecules, big hopes. J Clin Oncol 20:2217–2219

Baselga J, Norton L, Masui H et al (1993) Antitumor effects of doxorubicin in combination with anti-epidermal growth factor receptor monoclonal antibodies. J Natl Cancer Inst 85:1327–1333

Baselga J, Pfister D, Cooper MR et al (2000a) Phase I studies of anti-epidermal growth factor receptor chimeric antibody C225 alone and in combination with cisplatin. J Clin Oncol 18:904–914

Baselga J, Herbst R, LoRusso P et al (2000b) Continuous administration of AD1839, a novel oral epidermal growth factor receptor tyrosine kinase inhibitors (EGFR-TKI), in patients with five selected tumor types: evidence of activity and good tolerability (abstract 686). Proc Am Soc Clin Oncol 19:177a

Baselga J, Rano S, Giaccone G et al (2001) Initial results from a phase II trial of AD1839 ('Iressa') as second- and third-line monotherapy for patients with advanced non-small-cell lung cancer (IDEAL 1) (abstract 630). Proc AACR-NCI-EORTC, Miami Beach, FL, p 128

Beerli RR, Hynes NE (1996) Epidermal growth factor-related peptides activate distinct subsets of ErbB receptors and differ in their biological activities. J Biol Chem 271:6071–6076

Bianco C, Bianco R, Tortora G et al (2000) Antitumor activity of combined treatment of human cancer cells with ionizing radiation and anti-epidermal growth factor receptor monoclonal antibody C225 plus type I protein kinase A antisense oligonucleotide. Clin Cancer Res 6:4343–4350

Bonner JA, Maible NJ, Folven BR, Christianson TJH, Spain K (1994) The interaction of epidermal growth factor and radiation in human head and neck squamous cell carcinoma cell lines with vastly different radiosensitivities. Int J Radiat Oncol Biol Phys 29:243–247

Bonner JA, Ezekial MP, Robert F et al (2000) Combined response following treatment with IMC-C225, an EGFr MoAb, combined with RT in advanced head and neck malignancies. Proc Am Soc Clin Oncol 19:A5F, 4a

Carlin CR, Knowles BB (1982) Identity of human epidermal growth factor (EGF) receptor with glycoprotein SA-7: evidence for differential phosphorylation of the two components of the EGF receptor from A431 cells. Proc Natl Acad Sci U S A 79:5026–5030

Chang W, Upton C, Hu SL et al (1987) The genome of Shope fibroma virus, a tumorigenic poxvirus, contains a growth factor gene with sequence similarity to those encoding epidermal growth factor and transforming growth factor alpha. Mol Cell Biol 7:535–540

Ciardiello F, Dono R, Kim N et al (1991) Expression of cripto, a novel gene of the epidermal growth factor gene family, leads to in vitro transformation of a normal mouse mammary epithelial cell line. Cancer Res 51:1051–1054

Ciccodicola A, Dono R, Obici S et al (1989) Molecular characterization of a gene of the 'EGF family' expressed in undifferentiated human NTERA2 teratocarcinoma cells. EMBO J 8:1987–1991

Davies Rl, Grosse VA, Kucherlapati R, Bothwell M (1980) Genetic analysis of epidermal growth factor action: assignment of human epidermal growth factor receptor gene to chromosome 7. Proc Natl Acad Sci U S A 77:4188–4192

Derynck R (1988) Transforming growth factor alpha. Cell 54:593–595

Di Fiore PP, Pierce JH, Fleming TP et al (1987) Overexpression of the human EGF receptor confers an EGF-dependent transformed phenotype to NIH 3T3 cells. Cell 51:1063–1070

Di Marco E, Pierce JH, Fleming TP et al (1989) Autocrine interaction between TGF alpha and the EGF-receptor: quantitative requirements for induction of the malignant phenotype. Oncogene 4:831–838

Dickstein BN, Wosikowski K, Bates S (1995) Increased resistance to cytotoxic agents in ZR75B human breast cancer cells transfected with epidermal growth factor receptor. Mol Cell Endocrinol 110:205–211

Downward J, Yarden Y, Mayes E et al (1984) Close similarity of epidermal growth factor receptor and v-erb-B oncogene protein sequences. Nature 307:521–527

Ezekial MP, Robert F, Meredith RF et al (1998) Phase I study of anti-epidermal growth factor receptor (EGFR) antibody C225 in combination with irradiation in patients with advanced squamous cell carcinoma of the head and neck (SCCHN). Proc Am Soc Clin Oncol 17:A1522, 395a

Fan Z, Baselga J, Masui H et al (1993) Antitumor effect of anti-epidermal growth factor receptor monoclonal antibodies plus cis-diaminedichloroplatinum on well-established A431 cell xenografts. Cancer Res 53:4637–4642

Fan Z, Lu Y, Wu X, Mendelsohn J (1994) Antibody-induced epidermal growth factor receptor dimerization mediates inhibition of autocrine proliferation of A431 squamous carcinoma cells. J Biol Chem 269:27595–27602

Gille J, Swerlick RA, Caughman SW (1997) Transforming growth factor-alpha-induced transcriptional activation of the vascular permeability factor (VPF/VEGF) gene requires AP-2 dependent DNA binding and transactivation. EMBO J 16:750–759

Goldkorn T, Balaban N, Shannon M, Matsukuma K (1997) EGF receptor phosphorylation is affected by ionizing radiation. Biochim Biophys Acta 1358:289–299

Gorski DH, Mauceri HJ, Salloum RM et al (1998) Potentiation of the antitumor effect of ionizing radiation by brief concomitant exposures to angiostatin. Cancer Res 58:5686–5689

Gorski DH, Beckett MA, Jaskowiak NT et al (1999) Blockage of the vascular endothelial growth factor stress response increases the antitumor effects of ionizing radiation. Cancer Res 59:3374–3378

Grandis J, Tweardy D (1993) Elevated levels of transforming growth factor-α and epidermal growth factor receptor messenger RNA are early markers of carcinogenesis in head and neck cancer. Cancer Res 53:3579–3584

Grandis J, Melhem M, Gooding W et al (1998) Levels of TGF-α and EGFR protein in head and neck squamous cell carcinoma and patient survival. J Natl Cancer Inst 90:824–832

Gullick WJ (1991) Prevalence of aberrant expression of the epidermal growth factor receptor in human cancers. Br Med Bull 47:87–98

Haley J, Whittle N, Bennet P et al (1987) The human EGF receptor gene: structure of the 110-kb locus and identification of sequences regulating its transcription. Oncogene Res 1:375–396

Haslam RJ, Koide HB, Hemmings BA (1993) Pleckstrin domain homology. Nature 363:309–310

Harlan JE, Hajduk PJ, Yoon HS et al (1994) Pleckstrin homology domains bind to phosphatidylinositol-4,5- bisphosphate. Nature 371:168–170

Higashiyama S, Abraham JA, Miller J et al (1991) A heparin-binding growth factor secreted by macrophage-like cells that is related to EGF. Science 251:936–939

Huang S-M, Harari PM (2000) Modulation of radiation response after epidermal growth factor receptor blockade in squamous cell carcinomas: inhibition of damage repair, cell cycle kinetics, and tumor angiogenesis. Clin Cancer Res 6:2166–2174

Huang S-M, Bock JM, Harari PM (1999) Epidermal growth factor receptor blockade with C225 modulates proliferation, apoptosis, and radiosensitivity in squamous cell carcinomas of the head and neck. Cancer Res 59:1935–1940

Humphrey PA, Wong AJ, Vogelstein B et al (1990) Anti-synthetic peptide antibody reacting at the fusion junction of deletion-mutant epidermal growth factor receptors in human glioblastoma. Proc Natl Acad Sci U S A 87:4207–4211

Kakeji Y, Teicher BA (1997) Preclinical studies of the combination of angiogenic inhibitors with cytotoxic agents. Invest New Drugs 15:39–48

Katayose Y, Kim M, Rakkar ANS et al (1997) Promoting apoptosis: a novel activity associated with the cyclin-dependent kinase inhibitor p27. Cancer Res 57:5441–5445

Kelman Z (1997) PCNA: structure, functions and interactions. Oncogene 4:629–640

Kim ES, Kies M, Herbst R (2002) Novel therapeutics for head and neck cancer. Curr Opin Oncol 14:334–342

Kwok TT, Sutherland RM (1991) Differences in EGF-related radiosensitization of human squamous carcinoma cells with high and low numbers of EGF receptors. Br J Cancer 64:251–254

Kwok TT, Sutherland RM (1992) Cell cycle dependence of epidermal growth factor induced radiosensitization. Int J Radiat Oncol Biol Phys 22:525–527

Lin CR, Chen WS, Kruiger W et al (1984) Expression cloning of human EGF receptor complementary DNA: gene amplification and three related messenger RNA products in A431 cells. Science 224:843–848

Mauceri HJ, Hanna NN, Beckett MA et al (1998) Combined effects of angiostatin and ionizing radiation in antitumour therapy. Nature 394:287–291

Mayer BJ, Ren R, Clark KL et al (1993) A putative modular domain present in diverse signaling proteins. Cell 73:629–630

Mendelsohn J (1997) Epidermal growth factor receptor inhibition by a monoclonal antibody as anticancer therapy. Clin Cancer Res 3:2703–2707

Mendelsohn J (2000) Blockade of receptors for growth factors: an anticancer therapy – the Fourth Annual Joseph H. Burchenal American Association for Cancer Research Clinical Research Award Lecture. Clin Cancer Res 6:747–753

Mendelsohn J, Fan Z (1997) Epidermal growth factor receptor family and chemosensitization. J Natl Cancer Inst 89:341–343

Mendelsohn J, Shin DM, Donato N et al (1999) A phase I study of chimerized anti-epidermal growth factor receptor (EGFr) monoclonal antibody, C225, in combination with cisplatin (CDDP) in patients (pts) with recurrent head and neck squamous cell carcinoma (SCC). Proc Am Soc Clin Oncol 18:A1502, 389a

Meyn RE, Stephens LC, Ang K et al (1993) Heterogeneity in the development of apoptosis in irradiated murine tumours of different histologies. Int J Radiat Biol 64:583–591

Milas L, Yamada S, Hunter N et al (1991) Changes in TCD50 as a measure of clonogen doubling time in irradiated and unirradiated tumors. Int J Radiat Oncol Biol Phys 21:1195–1202

Milas L, Ang KK, McBride W (1998) Growth factors and cytokines: implications for radiotherapy. In: Kogelnik HD and Sedlmayer F (eds) Proceedings of the 6th International Meeting on Progress in radio-oncology VI, Monduzzi Editori, Salzburg, Austria, pp 15–23

Milas L, Mason K, Hunter N et al (2000) In vivo enhancement of tumor radioresponse by C225 antiepidermal growth factor receptor antibody. Clin Cancer Res 6:701–708

Milas L, Akimoto T, Hunter NR et al (2002) Relationship between cyclin D1 expression and poor radioresponse of murine carcinomas. Int J Radiat Oncol Biol Phys 52:514–521

Modjtahedi H, Hickish T, Nicolson M et al (1996) Phase I trial and tumour localization of the anti-EGFR monoclonal antibody ICR62 in head and neck or lung cancer. Br J Cancer 73:228–235

Modjtahedi H, Affleck K, Stubberfield C, Dean C (1998) EGFR blockade by tyrosine kinase inhibitor or monoclonal antibody inhibits growth, directs terminal differentiation and induced apoptosis in the human squamous cell carcinoma HN5. Int J Oncol 13:335–342

Moscatello DK, Montgomery RB, Sundareshan P et al (1996) Transformational and altered signal transduction by a naturally occurring mutant EGF receptor. Oncogene 13: 85–96

Nasu S, Ang KK, Fan Z et al (2001) C225 antiepidermal growth factor receptor antibody enhances tumor radiocurability. Int J Radiat Oncol Biol Phys 51:474–477

Pawson T (1995) Protein modules and signalling networks. Nature 373:573–580

Pawson T, Gish GD, Nash P (2001) SH2 domains, interaction modules and cellular wiring. Trends Cell Biol 11:504–511

Perez-Soler R, Donato NJ, Shin DM et al (1994) Tumor epidermal growth factor receptor studies in patients with non-small cell lung cancer or head and neck cancer treated with monoclonal antibody. J Clin Oncol 12:730–739

Perez-Soler R, Shim DM, Donato N et al (1998) Tumor studies in patients with head and neck cancer treated with humanized anti-epidermal growth factor (EGFR) monoclonal antibody C225 in combination with cisplatin. Proc Am Soc Clin Oncol 17:1514, 393a

Perrotte P, Matsumoto T, Inoue K, Kuniyasu H, Eve BY, Hicklin DJ, Radinsky R, Dinney CP (1999) Anti-epidermal growth factor receptor antibody C225 inhibits angiogenesis in human transitional cell carcinoma growing orthotopically in nude mice. Clin Cancer Res 5:257–265

Petit AM, Rak J, Hung MC, Rockwell P, Goldstein N, Fendly B, Kerbel RS (1997) Neutralizing antibodies against epidermal growth factor and ErB-2/neu receptor tyrosine kinases down-regulate vascular endothelial growth factor production by tumor cells in vitro and in vivo: angiogenic implications for signal transduction therapy of solid tumors. Am J Pathol 151:1523–1530

Prewett M, Rockwell P, Rockwell RF, Giorgio NA, Mendelsohn J, Scher HI, Goldstein NI (1996) The biologic effects of C225, a chimeric monoclonal antibody to the EGFR, on human prostate carcinoma. J Immunother Emphasis Tumor Immunol 19:419–427

Ranson M, Hammond LA, Ferry D et al (2002) ZD1839, a selective oral epidermal growth factor receptor-tyrosine kinase inhibitor, is well tolerated and active in patients with solid, malignant tumors: results of a phase I trial. J Clin Oncol 20:2240–2250

Reisner AH (1985) Similarity between the vaccinia virus 19K early protein and epidermal growth factor. Nature 313: 801–803

Riese DJ Jr, Bermingham Y, van Raaij TM et al (1996) Betacellulin activates the epidermal growth factor receptor and erbB-4, and induces cellular response patterns distinct from those stimulated by epidermal growth factor or neuregulin-beta. Oncogene 12:345–353

Ruifrok A, McBride W (1999) Growth factors: biological and clinical aspects. Int J Radiat Oncol Biol Phys 43:877–881

Schmidt-Ullrich RK, Valerie K, Fogleman PB, Walters J (1996) Radiation-induced autophosphorylation of epidermal growth factor receptor in human malignant mammary and squamous epithelial cells. Radiat Res 145:81–85

Schmidt-Ullrich RK, Mikkelsen RB, Dent P et al (1997) Radiation-induced proliferation of the human A431 squamous carcinoma cells is dependent on EGFR tyrosine phosphorylation. Oncogene 15:1191–1197

Schreiber M, Muller WJ, Singh G et al (1999) Comparison of the effectiveness of adenovirus vectors expressing cyclin kinase inhibitors $p16^{INK4C}$, $P19^{INK4D}$, $p21^{WAFI/CIPI}$ and $p27^{KIP1}$ in inducting cell cycle arrest, apoptosis and inhibition of tumorigenicity. Oncogene 18:1663–1676

Schrieber AB, Winkler ME, Derynck R (1986) Transforming growth factor-alpha: a more potent angiogenic mediator than epidermal growth factor. Science 232:1250–1253

Sheridan MT, O'Dwyer T, Seymour CB, Mothersill CE (1997) Potential indicators of radiosensitivity in squamous cell carcinoma of the head and neck. Radiat Oncol Invest 5: 180–186

Sherr CJ (1996) Cancer cell cycles. Science 274:1672–1677

Sherr CJ, Roberts JM (1995) Inhibitors of mammalian G1 cyclin-dependent kinases. Genes Dev 9:1149–1163

Shoyab M, McDonald VL, Bradley JG et al (1988) Amphiregulin: a bifunctional growth-modulating glycoprotein produced by the phorbol 12-myristate 13-acetate-treated human breast adenocarcinoma cell line MCF-7. Proc Natl Acad Sci U S A 85:6528–6532

Shoyab M, Plowman GD, McDonald VL et al (1989) Structure and function of human amphiregulin: a member of the epidermal growth factor family. Science 243:1074–1076

Shing Y, Christofori G, Hanahan D et al (1993) Betacellulin: a mitogen from pancreatic beta cell tumors. Science 259: 1604–1607

Sliwkowski MX, Schaefer G, Akita RW et al (1994) Coexpression of erbB2 and erbB3 proteins reconstitutes a high affinity receptor for heregulin. J Biol Chem 269: 14661–14665

Stockmeyer B, Valerius T, Repp R et al (1997) Preclinical studies with Fc(gamma)R bispecific antibodies and granulocyte colony-stimulating factor-primed neutrophils as effector cells against HER-2/neu overexpressing breast cancer. Cancer Res 57:696–701

Teicher BA, Holden SA, Dupuis NP, Kakeji Y, Ikebe M, Emi Y, Goff D (1995) Potentiation of cytotoxic therapies by TNP-470 and minocycline in mice bearing EMT-6 mammary carcinoma. Breast Cancer Res Treat 36:227–236

Thames H Jr, Rulfrok ACC, Milas L et al (1996) Accelerated repopulation during fractionated irradiation of a murine ovarian carcinoma: downregulation of apoptosis as a possible mechanism. Int J Radiat Oncol Biol Phys 35:951–962

Toyoda H, Komurasaki T, Uchida D et al (1995) Epiregulin. A novel epidermal growth factor with mitogenic activity for rat primary hepatocytes. J Biol Chem 270:7495–7500

Ullrich A, Schlessinger J (1990) Signal transduction by receptors with tyrosine kinase activity. Cell 61:203–212

Ullrich A, Coussens L, Hayflick JS et al (1984) Human epidermal growth factor receptor cDNA sequence and aberrant expression of the amplified gene in A431 epidermoid carcinoma cells. Nature 309:418–425

Velu TJ, Beguinot L, Vass WC et al (1987) Epidermal-growth-factor-dependent transformation by a human EGF receptor proto-oncogene. Science 238:1408–1410

Wang X, Gorospe M, Huang Y et al (1997) $p27^{Kip1}$ overexpression causes apoptotic death of mammalian cells. Oncogene 15:2991–2997

Watanabe T, Shintani A, Nakata M et al (1994) Recombinant human betacellulin. Molecular structure, biological activities, and receptor interaction. J Biol Chem 269: 9966-9973

Withers HR, Taylor JMG, Maciejewski B (1988) The hazard of accelerated tumor clonogen repopulation during radiotherapy. Acta Oncol 27:131-145

Wollman R, Yahalom J, Maxy R, Pinto J, Fuks Z (1994) Effect of epidermal growth factor on the growth and radiation sensitivity of human breast cancer cells in vitro. Int J Radiat Oncol Biol Phys 30:91-98

Woodburn JR (1999) The epidermal growth factor receptor and its inhibition in cancer treatment. Pharmacol Ther 82:241-250

Wrann MM, Fox CF (1979) Identification of epidermal growth factor receptors in a hyperproducing human epidermoid carcinoma cell line. J Biol Chem 254:8083-8086

Wu X, Fan Z, Masui H, Rosen N, Mendelsohn J (1995) Apoptosis induced by an anti-epidermal growth factor receptor monoclonal antibody in a human colorectal carcinoma cell line and its delay by insulin. J Clin Invest 95:1897-1905

Xu YH, Ishii S, Clark AJ et al (1984) Human epidermal growth factor receptor cDNA is homologous to a variety of RNAs overproduced in A431 carcinoma cells. Nature 309:806-810

16 Enhancement of the Radiation Response with Interleukins and Interferons

F. Lohr, C. Herskind, J. Lohr, F. Wenz, and C.-Y. Li

CONTENTS

16.1 Introduction 205
16.2 Aspects of the Cytotoxic Immune Response 206
16.2.1 General Aspects 206
16.2.2 The Th1/Th2 Paradigm 208
16.3 Cytokines and the Effector Network 208
16.3.1 Interleukins 209
16.3.2 Interferons 209
16.4 Why Do Tumor Cells Escape Detection by the Immune System? 210
16.5 Immunological Effects of Ionizing Radiation 211
16.5.1 Effects of Ionizing Radiation on the Immune System 211
16.5.2 Immunogenic Effects of Ionizing Radiation on Tumor Cells 211
16.6 Antitumoral Effects of Cytokines and Enhancement of the Radiation Response 212
16.6.1 IL-1, IL-3, IL-6 212
16.6.2 IL-2 212
16.6.2.1 Antitumoral Effects 212
16.6.2.2 Enhancement of the Radiation Response 213
16.6.3 IL-4 213
16.6.4 IL-12 214
16.6.4.1 Antitumoral Effects 214
16.6.4.2 Enhancement of the Radiation Response 215
16.6.5 IFN-α, -β 215
16.6.5.1 Antitumoral Effects 215
16.6.5.2 Enhancement of the Radiation Response 216
16.6.6 IFN-γ 217
16.6.6.1 Antitumoral Effects and Enhancement of the Radiation Response 217
16.6.7 Toxicity of Interferon Combined with Radiotherapy 218
16.7 Conclusions and Future Prospects 218
References 219

F. Lohr, MD; F. Wenz, MD
Institut für Klinische Radiologie, Sektion Strahlentherapie, Theodor-Kutzer-Ufer 1–3, 68167 Mannheim, Germany
C. Herskind, PhD
Department of Experimental Clinical Oncology, Aarhus University Hospital, Nørrebrogade 44, Building 5, 8000 Aarhus C, Denmark
J. Lohr, MD
Department of Pathology, University of California San Francisco School of Medicine, Parnassus Ave., San Francisco, CA 94143, USA
C.-Y. Li, PhD
Department of Radiation Oncology, Duke University Medical Center, 201B MSRB, Box 3455, Durham, NC, 27710, USA

16.1 Introduction

Physical and technical developments and refinements of the last decade in radiation oncology have been impressive. Particle therapy is on the rise again, and photon therapy has received a major boost from intensity modulation, making delivery of tumor-conformal radiation treatment easier than ever before. Intensity-modulated particle therapy, regarded by some as the holy grail of radiotherapy, is on the horizon, combining highly conformal dose distributions with low integral doses. However, while any desired dose distribution can be created now or in a not too distant future, this does not solve the problem of normal tissue present within the irradiated target volumes due to infiltration by the tumor. Therefore, further progress can only be expected from efforts directed at widening the therapeutic window between tumors and normal tissue through specific modulation of their responses to radiotherapy.

One of several approaches currently pursued is to unlock synergies between radiotherapy and natural antitumoral systems of the body such as the immune system. Cytokines provide a means to modulate the immune system. Although much progress has been made, the broad range of their functions has not been fully elucidated and, therefore, the optimal mode of their use still needs to be explored. However, it has become clear that cytokines do not only play an important role in the regulation of the immune system but some can have other features such as antiangiogenic properties providing them with additional antitumoral leverage.

This chapter will concentrate on the mode of action of different cytokines, mainly within the confines of the immune system, although it has become clear that the nonimmunological component of the mode of action of cytokines is larger than initially thought, especially when combined with radio- or chemotherapy. We will discuss the theoretical basis of the potentially beneficial effects of a combined treatment with radiotherapy and cytokines. Finally, preclinical and clinical data obtained with such combination treatments will be reviewed.

16.2 Aspects of the Cytotoxic Immune Response

16.2.1 General Aspects

The immune system is a complex network which – for a simplified operational approach – can be divided into two effector elements, a *humoral system* and a *cellular system*. The humoral system is the main line of defense against extracellular pathogens. Its effector cells are the B lymphocytes which act through production of specific antibodies (Fig. 16.1). The cellular system is directed mainly against intracellular pathogens such as viruses, and its effector cells are cytotoxic T lymphocytes (CTL), natural killer (NK) cells and phagocytes. B and T lymphocytes belong to the adaptive immune system which is clonal and has evolved in vertebrates (HUGHES and YEAGER 1997). It is capable of creating and memorizing responses to specific antigens not previously encountered by the individual organism and forms the basis for immunization through vaccination. The innate immune system, on the other hand, is nonclonal and is directed against a broad spectrum of non-self antigens, providing a defense mechanism against pathogens which is conserved throughout invertebrate and vertebrate species (MUSHEGIAN and MEDZHITOV 2001). Phagocytes and granulocytes (neutrophils, eosinophils and basophils) are part of the mammalian innate immune system. NK cells are effectors of the innate immune response but participate also in adaptive responses. Thus the adaptive and the innate immune systems do not act isolated from each other but interact via a network of cytokines and other signals.

Prerequisite for an effective immune reaction against a pathogen is an appropriate *presentation* of the antigens to stimulate effector cells (Fig. 16.2). T cells react only to antigens presented to them in conjunction with major histocompatibility complex (MHC) antigens whereas B cells can detect antigen directly through their membrane-bound immunoglobulins (Ig). NK cells have intermediate properties since they can detect non-MHC-bound antigen through Ig-like receptors. The two main T cell subsets, T4 and T8 in humans, are characterized by the CD4 and CD8 antigens, respectively. Although the functional distinction between T4 and T8 cells is

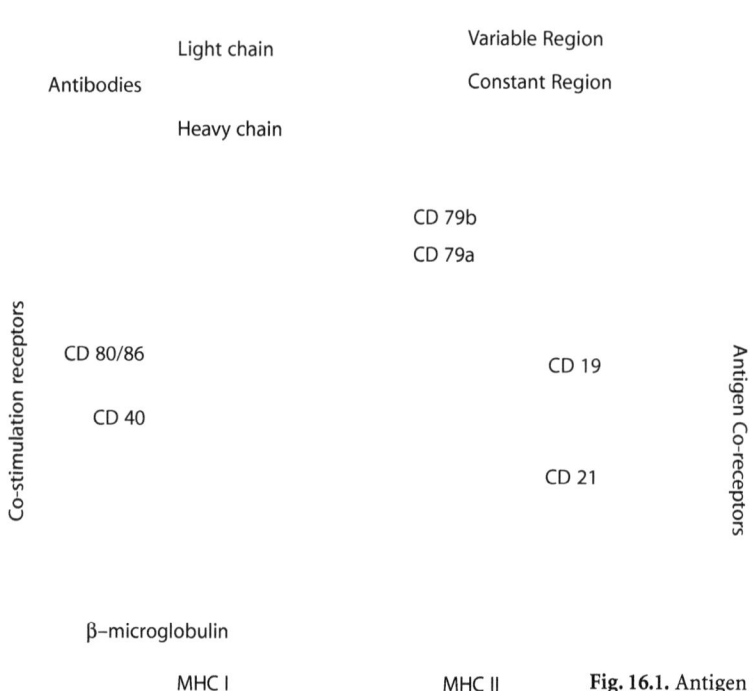

Fig. 16.1. Antigen receptors, antigen co-receptors, co-stimulation receptors, and presentation molecules of B-lymphocytes. (From RADBRUCH 2001, with permission)

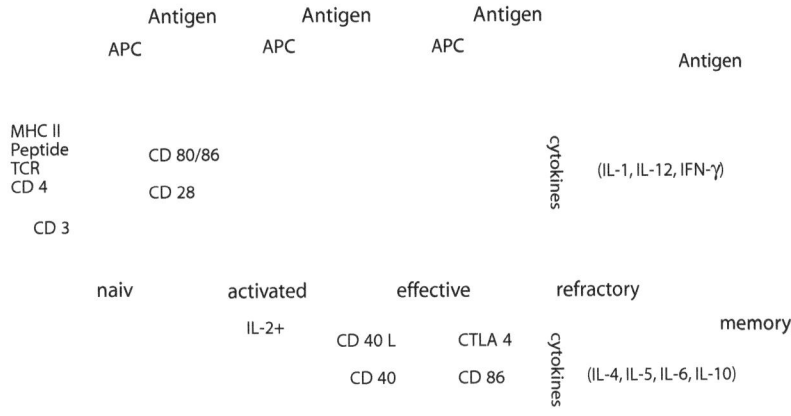

Fig. 16.2. Activation of T-lymphocytes and their interaction with antigen-presenting cells and B-lymphocytes. (From RADBRUCH 2001, with permission)

not strict, most T4 cells are MHC class II restricted helper cells, which modulate the immune response through various cytokines (PARDOLL and TOPALIAN 1998) whereas most T8 lymphocytes are killer T cells (CTL) having mainly cytotoxic functions.

More effective responses are elicited when antigens are acquired by so-called professional antigen presenting cells (APC) such as monocytes, macrophages and – most importantly – dendritic cells (DC), e.g., by incorporation of fragments of necrotic cells (BENDELAC and MEDZHITOV 2002; MEDZHITOV and JANEWAY 1997). The antigen is then processed intracellularly and presented on these cells conjugated to both MHC I and MHC II antigens (so-called cross-priming) together with surface molecules that further modulate the immune response. Such co-stimulatory molecules are essential for creating immunity in most situations, and presentation of antigen without co-stimulation may result in peripheral T cell tolerance (TOWNSEND and ALLISON 1993). In contrast to MHC I, MHC II is only found on professional APC. Thus the following elements are involved in the process of antigen presentation between APC and effector or regulatory cells:

1. The T cell receptor is a heterodimer that primarily interacts with the MHC-coupled antigen on APC. It is associated with the CD3 complex on the surface of all T cells.
2. The CD4 and CD8 surface antigens interact with both the T cell receptor and MHC molecules. CD4 reacts only with MHC II, and CD8 with MHC I, which causes the MHC I – or MHC II – restriction of CD8+ and CD4+ T cells.
3. Co-stimulatory signals are important for an efficient immune response by T cells and include B7.1 (CD80), B7.2 (CD86), CD2 and CD137w on APC as well as CD40 on B lymphocytes. Antigen recognition in the absence of these molecules may lead to the induction of tolerance.

Although CD8+ lymphocytes mediating the CTL response were previously considered the main effector elements of the cellular system, similar functions of other cells emerge. While T lymphocytes are MHC-restricted, NK cells have the potential to directly lyse MHC I-negative cells, a process that also seems to be facilitated by co-stimulatory molecules (GELDHOF et al. 1998). The relative importance of these different elements in a response to tumor cells, therefore, seems to depend on tumor immune phenotype, which can even change during the course of the disease, e.g., by shedding of MHC I (CHEN et al. 1994; COULIE et al. 1999). As a general pattern, the NK-axis is the major early component of the immune reaction, which is important for effective initial reduction of tumor load whereas the CD4+/CD8+ lymphocyte system seems to be a prerequisite for a durable and protective immunity upon re-challenge (KAWAKITA et al. 1997; PHAM-NGUYEN et al. 1999). In this context, the importance of heat shock proteins (HSP) currently emerges. Recent data point out the important role of these molecules as general danger signals and facilitators of antigen presentation by virtue of being chaperones for intracellular antigens both for direct presentation on a somatic cell surface and for acquisition by APC in the process of cross-priming (SRIV-

ASTAVA 2002; SUTO and SRIVASTAVA 1995; TAMURA et al. 1997; TODRYK et al. 1999).

For CD4+/CD8+ lymphocytes as well as for NK cells, the eventual elimination of target cells is in part mediated by the perforin/granzyme system inducing the apoptotic cascade in the target cell (SHRESTA et al. 1998). CD4+ lymphocytes can also initiate this cascade through activation of Fas/Apo-1 through Fas-ligand. However, other systems of the execution of antitumoral effects seem to exist (KODAMA et al. 1999).

16.2.2
The Th1/Th2 Paradigm

Based on studies in murine model systems, CD4+ T lymphocytes can be divided into two subsets, Th1 and Th2, characterized by their cytokine expression profiles (ABBAS et al. 1996; MOSMANN et al. 1986). Th1 cells express interleukin (IL)-2, interferon (IFN)-γ and tumor necrosis factor (TNF)-β, and have been associated with a phagocyte-dependent response whereas Th2 cells are characterized by IL-4 and frequently express IL-5, IL-6, and IL-13, and are associated with the humoral immune response (ABBAS et al. 1996). IL-10 was initially considered to be a product of Th2 but can also be secreted by Th1 (SORNASSE et al. 1996). The process of cells developing production of either IFN-γ or IL-4 is termed polarization. An important feature of this process is the auto-stimulatory effects of IFN-γ on Th1 cells and of IL-4 on Th2 cells, and the negative cross-regulation of Th2 cells by IFN-γ and of Th1 cells by IL-4. A third subclass of T4 lymphocytes, Th0, expresses IFN-γ as well as IL-4 and may be viewed as a partially differentiated state. This basic classification has recently been complicated by the discovery of various subtypes of regulatory CD4+ T cells, which have been shown to negatively regulate immune responses. Tolerance induction by these cells may be dependent on cytokines, e.g., IL-10 and TGF-β (Tr1, Th3) (AKBARI et al. 2001) or on cell-to-cell contact (CD4+CD25+ regulatory T cells) (DIECKMANN et al. 2001; LEVINGS et al. 2001; TAYLOR et al. 2001). The mechanisms of induction and the exact classification of lineages in humans and mice are subject to current investigations.

It has been shown that cytotoxic T cells (CD8+) can also be divided into two subclasses, Tc1 and Tc2, displaying Th1 and Th2 cytokine profiles, respectively (SAD et al. 1995). In humans, the segregation of the cytokine profiles is less strict than in the murine systems. Furthermore, some degree of switching between classes is possible. For these reasons, it appears more appropriate to put the emphasis on the functional effects rather than on the actual type of cells producing the polarized cytokine response. Thus the Type 1 (Th1-like) response promotes cell-mediated immunity whereas the Type 2 (Th2-like) response promotes humoral-mediated immunity (ABBAS et al. 1996; CLERICI et al. 1998; LAPPIN and CAMPBELL 2000; LUCEY 1999). Nevertheless, the Th1/Th2 paradigm provides a useful framework for understanding the function of the adaptive immune system.

16.3
Cytokines and the Effector Network

Cytokines are secreted polypeptides acting as intercellular messengers, thus providing a means for communication between the cellular elements of the immune system to create an effector network. Cytokines can act in a proinflammatory or immunosuppressive fashion but a strict distinction based on these properties is not possible since the same cytokine can act in either way depending on the context (O'SHEA et al. 2002). Cytokines are produced by many different cells including cell types not belonging to the immune system, such as fibroblasts and endothelial cells. Historically they have been given different names but although new cytokines are assigned an IL number for systematic purposes, "cytokine" is the appropriate generic term.

Some general features are common for most cytokines (ABBAS et al. 2001). Secretion of cytokines is usually a brief and self-limiting event, and the effects of the individual cytokine are often pleiotropic and sometimes even sequentially counteractive. Because of the tightly woven interactive network of the immune system, secretion of one cytokine often leads to the secretion of multiple other cytokines. Cytokines usually act locally in an autocrine or paracrine fashion but some can also act systemically in an endocrine fashion, which is the therapeutic pathway commonly used, although it is frequently fraught with side effects.

The effects of cytokines are mediated through specific receptors on target cells which themselves can be up- or down-regulated. Most cytokines act through Type I or II cytokine receptors whose extracellular domain contains two conserved pairs of cysteine residues. Downstream of the Type I and II cytokine receptors, the signal transduction pathway commonly involves so-called Janus kinases (JAK) attached to the intracellular domain of the cytokine receptors. Upon receptor activation, STAT proteins (signal transduction and activation of transcription) are recruited to the receptor complex by JAK, become phosphorylated, dimerize and translocate to the nucleus where the STAT dimer binds to the promoter region of cytokine-responsive genes. The specificity of this signaling pathway depends on the combination of JAKs and STATs that is activated for a particular cytokine. Thus the array of cellular and physiological responses for each cytokine is vast and for most cytokines probably only partially known.

16.3.1
Interleukins

- IL-1 is a mediator of local inflammation and is produced by mononuclear phagocytes and other cell types after induction by lipopolysaccharide (LPSs) or cytokines. IL-1 exists in two structurally distinct but functionally similar forms, IL-1α, which is the predominant form in serum, and IL-1b, which has a shorter half-life and is the main form synthesized by activated macrophages. IL-1 is important in attracting lymphocytes and helps activating T helper cells (CD4+) during the acute-phase response. Together with colony stimulating factor (CSF) it helps stimulate proliferation of hematopoietic stem cells (HESTDAL et al. 1992).
- IL-2 is the primary cytokine produced by Th1 cells upon antigen recognition. It is, in an autocrine or paracrine way, responsible for expansion of the specific effector T cell clones. It also stimulates other immunologically active cells such as NK cells, thus generating lymphokine-activated killer cells (LAK), and activates tumor-infiltrating lymphocytes (TIL). Termination of a specific response, at least partly through induction of apoptotic death of antigen-activated T cells, is a further function of this important cytokine, hence mice deficient in IL-2 production or IL-2 receptor expression (CD25–/–) show symptoms of aggressive autoimmune disease (O'SHEA et al. 2002).
- IL-3 is produced by Th2 cells and stimulates the proliferation of pluripotent stem cells as well as of several types of committed progenitor cells.
- IL-4 both promotes Th2 differentiation and is then also produced by Th2 cells. It is therefore defining the Type-2 cytokine response. The cellular source of the initially secreted IL-4 is unclear. IL-4 activates B cells to proliferate and become mature clonal plasma cells secreting an immunoglobulin against a specific antigen. Upon binding of the antigen, this is internalized and presented in MHC II to the T cells, which binds via the T cell receptor. IL-4 together with IL-10 also acts as an immunosuppressor in Th1 cells following a successful Type-1 cytokine response.
- IL-5 is synthesized by Th2 cells and stimulates proliferation of B cells.
- IL-6 is produced by macrophages and by Th2 cells. It stimulates the synthesis of acute-phase proteins and is a differentiation factor for B cells to become mature Ig-secreting plasma cells. Furthermore, IL-6 helps activate T cells.
- IL-10 is a predominantly anti-inflammatory regulatory cytokine produced mainly by Th2 but also by Th1. It inhibits macrophage function as a negative feedback regulator by down-regulating co-stimulatory and class II MHC molecules on macrophages as well as by inhibiting production of IL-12 and TNF-α by activated macrophages (BOGDAN et al. 1992). Furthermore IL-10 blocks secretion of IFN-γ by NK cells and Th1 cells. IL-10 has been demonstrated to contain immune responses in various systems (MOORE et al. 2001).
- IL-12 is produced only by antigen-presenting cells (APC) such as activated monocytes/macrophages, dendritic cells and B lymphocytes. It was initially described as an activator of NK cell cytolytic function. However, its most obvious effect is the induction of IFN-γ (through transcriptional and posttranscriptional control [HODGE et al. 2002]) in T lymphocytes and NK cells, which in turn activates macrophages.
- IL-15 and IL-18. These cytokines contribute to the acute-phase response. IL-15 and IL-18, though acting through different pathways and receptors, share some of the functional features of IL-2 and IL-12. They act synergistically with these cytokines, in part through antiangiogenic properties (COUGHLIN et al. 1998) or through effects on the Type-1 response. In particular, the expression of IL-18 can be precisely modulated by IL-12 through induction of IL-18 binding protein expression, an IFN-γ dependent process (VEENSTRA et al. 2002).

16.3.2
Interferons

- Type I Interferons (IFN-α and -β) are early mediators of the immune response to viral infections. IFN-α is mainly produced by mononuclear phagocytes although most cell types can produce it. IFN-α comprises several subtypes of structurally similar proteins encoded by separate genes. IFN-β is produced by a number of cells, including fibroblasts. Type I interferons inhibit viral replication and increase expression of class I MHC molecules, thereby enhancing the recognition of class I-associated antigens by cytotoxic T lymphocytes. They inhibit the proliferation of hematopoietic cells and help stimulate the differentiation of Th0 to Th1 lymphocytes. The anti-inflammatory properties of IFN-β are used clinically in the treatment of multiple sclerosis, a putative Th1 disease. Moreover, type I IFN can up-regulate IL-18 mRNA in T and NK cells, thereby facilitating IL-18-mediated activation of these cells in the acute phase (SARENEVA et al. 2000).

- Type II Interferon (IFN-γ) is the only interferon binding to the type II receptor and is the main activator of macrophage function, initiated by T lymphocytes and NK cells. It stimulates the expression of MHC II and, similar to type I interferons, of MHC I on a number of cells (RESTIFO et al. 1993). It is, therefore, a major enhancer of MHC-associated antigen presentation. It promotes phagocytosis by increasing production of reactive oxygen molecules and up-regulation of Fcg receptors. IL-12 stimulates the production of IFN-γ in Th1 cells where INF-γ induces – and finally defines – the differentiation of Th0 to Th1 cells. Furthermore, it exerts effects on B cells and potentiates the cytotoxic effects of TNF on endothelial cells, possibly through induction of nitric oxide production (YAMAOKA et al. 2002).

16.4
Why Do Tumor Cells Escape Detection by the Immune System?

In the recent past, numerous tumor associated antigens (TAA) were discovered, rendering the hypothesis invalid that lack of specific antigens is responsible for the inability of the immune system to recognize tumor cells (e.g., OSTRAND-ROSENBERG et al. 1999). These TAA can be classified as
a) Non-mutated molecules such as the MAGE and MART group, RAGE and MUC, whose expression is normal and which therefore do not elicit an immune response
b) Tissue-specific (but not tumor-specific) antigens such as PSA, CEA, tyrosinase and gp100, which are also expressed in normal tissues
c) Tumor-specific mutated proteins such as CASP-8
d) Inappropriately expressed oncogenes, such as Her-2/neu

The tolerance of the immune system towards tumor cells therefore seems to be caused by escape mechanisms rendering a tumor invisible despite its specific antigens (OSTRAND-ROSENBERG et al. 1999). This is corroborated by the fact that active immunization with isolated peptides or lethally irradiated tumor cells has not met with much success (VELDERS et al. 1998). Only when high-dose IL-2 was applied simultaneously, or when mutated peptides with enhanced MHC I-activity were used, could immunity be generated. This suggests that – in addition to some general immune suppression induced by malignancy (LEVEY and SRIVASTAVA 1995) – tumor cells manage to escape the immune system by behaving as "immunologically privileged tissue" (OCHSENBEIN et al. 2001). This idea is further supported by the fact that for many murine tumor models there is a window for comparatively easy induction of immunity against a transplanted tumor within the first 10 days after implantation when there is still an inflammatory, immunostimulatory environment. After this time window has elapsed, immunotherapeutic intervention succeeds less often, in part because peripheral T cell tolerance may develop in the absence of the stimulating environment (STAVELEY-O'CARROLL et al. 1998; VAN ELSAS et al. 1999). Evidence from animal models shows that while necrotic cell death leads to an immune response via cross-priming, apoptotic cell death may – depending on the targeted DC-subset (HUANG et al. 2000) – rather lead to cross-tolerization, demonstrating that products released by stress and damaged tissues can act as adjuvants, even though stimulatory effects were initially described (ALBERT et al. 1998). Recognition of these substances is mediated by a family of pattern recognition receptors called toll receptors (BENDELAC and MEDZHITOV 2002; MEDZHITOV and JANEWAY 1997). Understanding the regulation of these molecules will be instrumental for alteration of tumor immunogenicity.

Although a humoral response against tumor cells is possible (anti-p53 autoantibodies have been observed in tumor patients (e.g., SCANLAN et al. 1998) the immunological response is mainly directed against external epitopes. The more relevant system for eliminating tumor cells, therefore, is likely to be the cellular system and its effector cells (ROTH et al. 1994).

Various mechanisms may contribute to suppressing an immune response to tumor antigens. Thus, the expression of MHC I is frequently down-regulated in tumor cells, e.g., through Ras-induced intratumoral TGF-β expression (SELIGER et al. 1998). Furthermore, solid tumors in general lack co-stimulatory molecules (O'CONNELL et al. 1999), resulting in incomplete antigen presentation and potential tolerance. This tolerance may even persist against tumor cells that are manipulated in such a way as to present co-stimulatory molecules (SCHWARTZ 1990), suggesting that more than one pathway of co-stimulation may be essential. Another possible, albeit still controversial, pathway of reduced effector cell efficiency might be the expression of Fas-ligand on tumor cells, which would lead to apoptosis of activated lymphocytes expressing Fas. So far, however, data have been contradictory (CHAPPELL et al. 1999; HAHNE et al. 1996), since Fas-ligand transfected tumor cells were more immunogenic in a preclinical model, probably secondary to enhanced neutrophil influx (ARAI et al. 1997; KANG et al. 1997). Another controversial issue is the occasionally observed down-regulation of the T cell receptor's zeta-chain (VELDERS et al. 1998), potentially diminishing T cell function.

Antigen presentation by APCs such as dendritic cells also seems to be impaired in tumor-bearing hosts (GABRILOVICH et al. 1996). This impairment is, in part, a consequence of the down-regulation of NF-κB mediated by vascular endothelial growth factor (VEGF), which is produced by a wide array of human tumors (OYAMA et al. 1998). IL-10, also prevalent in human tumors, results in impaired DC maturation, which then leads to antigen presentation in a tolerogenic rather than immunogenic fashion (STEINBRINK et al. 1999).

This line of thought leads to the conclusion that tumor-specific antigens exist, but that tumor cells and even APCs lack effective ways to present these antigens to effector cells. Successful immunization, therefore, requires breaking certain escape mechanisms, for example by creating an inflammatory environment in the tumor. Cytokines may help to create such an inflammatory and thus immunogenic environment.

16.5
Immunological Effects of Ionizing Radiation

16.5.1
Effects of Ionizing Radiation on the Immune System

Radiation has several direct and indirect immunological effects, ranging from complete immunosuppression after high total body doses to local changes in the immune phenotype of tumor cells after irradiation.

Total-body irradiation (TBI), either administered as a single dose of 7 Gy or as fractionated treatment with a total dose of 12–16 Gy, is used for complete depletion of hematopoietic cells. Extended loco-regional radiation of head and neck or abdomen influences systemic immunity (BELKA et al. 1999; TISCH et al. 1998). Although the effects depend on the target volume, CD4+ cells seem to be more susceptible to radiation than CD8+ cells, and naive T cells generally seem to be more susceptible than memory T cells. Normal titers are sometimes reached only months after radiation. By contrast, NK cells seem to be comparatively radioresistant, reverting to normal values a few weeks after the end of radiotherapy (BELKA et al. 1999; OLKOWSKI 1999).

Antigen presenting DC, unfortunately, represent an extremely radiosensitive cell subset (EVERSON et al. 1989; ROBERTS et al. 1990). However, recruitment of DCs into irradiated tissue occurs shortly after irradiation (COLE et al. 1984; KAWASE et al. 1990) and the number of DCs around untreated tumors may be a general prognostic indicator for the course of the disease (IKEGUCHI et al. 1998).

Several cytokines can be induced by radiation, the most prominent among them being IL-1, IL-6 and TNF-α, which are under the control of NFk B (HONG et al. 1999; RAJU et al. 1999), as well as IL-10 (MIZUTANI et al. 2002).

16.5.2
Immunogenic Effects of Ionizing Radiation on Tumor Cells

Low-dose TBI (total dose of 1.5–2 Gy in fractions of 0.1–0.25 Gy/fraction) has been used frequently and is still used occasionally as a treatment for lymphocytic leukemia and low-grade non-Hodgkin's lymphoma. Its antitumor effect seems to be partly mediated by the immune system, possibly through induction of cytokines such as IL-2, IFN-γ and TNF-α, thereby activating NK and T cells (HASHIMOTO et al. 1999; SAFWAT 2000).

Radiation-induced apoptosis is one of the mechanisms that may contribute to killing tumor cells. Apoptosis as a consequence of radiation may, among other mechanisms, be induced by activation of Fas. Baseline and probably also radiation-induced differential expression of Fas and Fas ligand differs from tumor to tumor. Frequently, Fas has been found to be down- and Fas ligand to be up-regulated in tumors (GRATAS et al. 1998; KONTNY et al. 1998). However, this controversial issue has been the focus of discussion (CHAPPELL et al. 1999; HAHNE et al. 1996; TAKAGI et al. 1998). While radiation induces both Fas and Fas-ligand in lymphocytes (FARIS et al. 1998; OGAWA et al. 1998) the situation is less clear for solid tumors where some, such as melanoma, require high single doses (>15 Gy) (LOHR et al. 2000a) while others, such as nasopharyngeal carcinoma (NPC) cells, seem to express Fas ligand already in response to 2 Gy (ABDULKARIM et al. 2000). Thus Fas ligand seemed to be inducible in vitro in B16 cells, but this could not be reproduced in vivo.

Tumor cells that were irradiated in vitro seem to be more immunogenic than their untreated counterparts (DRANOFF et al. 1993). Thus the growth of unirradiated tumor cells could be slowed by the injection of irradiated tumor cells into the same animal (YOUNES et al. 1995b). Furthermore, increased peritumoral infiltration with T lymphocytes (mainly of the CD4+ subset) after local tumor radiotherapy has been described in clinical specimens (OBOSHI et al. 1967; YAMASHITA et al. 1987). In some tumor model systems such as the KMT 17 fibrosarcoma, radiotherapy can revert the down-regulation of tumor-associated antigens (SHIBATA et al. 1998). On the same note, molecules involved in antigen presentation, e.g., ICAM-1, MHC I, B7.1 and gp96 are induced by radiation, either directly or indirectly through induction of TNF-α (HAREYAMA et al. 1998; MOREL et al. 1998; RÜBE et al. 1997; SANTIN et al. 1998). However, neither for MHC I nor for B7.1 could we demonstrate induction in B16 melanoma and in 4T1 breast cancer at doses of up to 18 Gy (LOHR et al. 2000a).

cell vaccines were more efficient than the parental cell vaccines in delaying tumor growth after irradiation (CHIANG et al. 2000). This response was specific against each particular tumor and depended on the ability of the host to produce TNF-α.

Some studies suggest that the effect of interleukins may depend on the tumor system. Thus, IL-6 caused radiosensitization of B-leukemia cells (WADDICK et al. 1995) whereas in experimental pancreas tumors, radiation-induced apoptosis was inhibited by IL-6 (MIYAMOTO et al. 2001). Furthermore, transduction of basal cell carcinoma cells with an IL-6 expression vector resulted in increased anti-apoptotic activity and induction of angiogenic factors, as well as potentiating tumor formation in athymic (nude) mice (JEE et al. 2001). Obviously, a proper understanding of the effects of these interleukins in different tumors is required when clinical application is considered.

IL-1 protects mice against whole-body irradiation (BARBERA et al. 1993; ZUCALI et al. 1994) although this might not be the case in tumor-bearing subjects (KOVACS et al. 1991). It acts as a radioprotector of hematopoietic cells in vivo where stem cell factor was required for the recovery of bone marrow cells (NETA et al. 1994). A similar radioprotective effect of IL-3 on hematopoietic cells has been reported in baboons (DOWN et al. 2000). Furthermore, accelerated recovery of hematopoietic stem cells after irradiation has been reported as an effect of IL-6 (PATCHEN et al. 1991). Although, potentially, a therapeutic benefit might be achievable for tumors responding to these interleukins plus irradiation, this approach does not seem to have been pursued further.

16.6
Antitumoral Effects of Cytokines and Enhancement of the Radiation Response

16.6.1
IL-1, IL-3, IL-6

In RIF-1 tumors, Dorie and co-workers reported enhancement of cytotoxic effects of cyclophosphamide and radiotherapy by IL-1, which was observed only under very specific circumstances (combination of agents, timing of the sequence, etc. (DORIE et al. 1989, 1991). However, other authors observed the induction of radioresistance by IL-1, which was presumably secondary to IL-1-induced hypoxia (BRAUNSCHWEIGER et al. 1996).

An immunogenic approach in a murine system showed that IL-3 gene-transduced fibrosarcoma

16.6.2
IL-2

16.6.2.1
Antitumoral Effects

IL-2 is one of the cytokines that have been successfully applied clinically, albeit with problems due to its short half-life and high toxicity. These problems, however, may be overcome with new gene therapy-based delivery techniques (ADDISON et al. 1998; KIMURA et al. 1999). Initial studies reported objective responses with high doses of IL-2 in one-third of patients suffering from metastatic malignant melanoma, and durable complete remissions in a very small fraction of patients (ROSENBERG et al. 1994). However, in combination with chemotherapy, which itself did not succeed in prolonging survival for patients with metastatic disease, IL-2 and IFN-α did not improve the outcome but resulted in increased toxicity (ATZPODIEN et al. 2002; KEILHOLZ et al. 1997; ROSENBERG et al. 1999).

16.6.2.2
Enhancement of the Radiation Response

Studies of the interaction between IL-2 and radiation have been performed in vitro and with experimental tumor systems. Preirradiation in combination with 5-FU or cisplatinum treatment of a squamous cell carcinoma cell line enhanced their susceptibility to apoptosis by IL-2-activated lymphocytes (LAK) (YAMAMOTO et al. 2000). Improved tumor response after radiotherapy combined with subcutaneous IL-2 and histamine was observed in an androgen-sensitive subline of the transplantable Dunning R3327 rat prostate tumor in Copenhagen rats, a syngeneic tumor model particularly pertinent to prostate cancer (JOHANSSON et al. 1998). IL-2 also seemed to synergize with photon and even neutron radiation in a mouse prostate tumor (HILLMAN et al. 2001).

Syngeneic SL2 lymphomas and M8013 mammary carcinomas were used to study the effect of peritumoral IL-2 injection on radiotherapy. When tumors were inoculated in both flanks of the murine host, radioimmunotherapy of only one tumor also caused the untreated tumor to regress, indicating a systemic antitumoral effect (JURGENLIEMK-SCHULZ et al. 1997). In the murine renal adenocarcinoma (Renca) model, unilateral irradiation of pulmonary metastases followed by systemic IL-2 treatment slowed the growth of unirradiated tumor cells in the contralateral lung, suggesting that the systemic effect of the immunostimulatory action is enhanced by irradiation (YOUNES et al. 1995a). In the same system, tumor cell vaccines that were genetically engineered to produce IL-2 seemed to synergize with local irradiation of lung metastases (NISHISAKA et al. 1999). The effect was also observed in nude mice, suggesting that the antitumoral immune response is mediated by NK cells, which can be activated by IL-2 to become LAK. A synergism between radiotherapy, IL-2 and tumor-infiltrating lymphocytes (TIL) has also been reported (CAMERON et al. 1990).

IL-2 transfected murine EMT6 mammary tumors were more sensitive to radiation than parental tumors (LEE et al. 2000). This effect, however, was ascribed to a decreased hypoxic tumor cell fraction resulting from the increased vascularity of transfected tumors.

In most of the studies conducted with IL-2, increased tumor infiltration with inflammatory cells was reported but no functional experiments elucidating the mechanism of action of the reported synergism were performed. Experimental therapy combining IL-2 and radiotherapy in murine models underlined that lung metastases and subcutaneous tumors just after inoculation were easily treated by combined therapy whereas for larger primary tumors no synergy was observed (HUNTER et al. 1992). In none of the animal studies with local injection of IL-2 was excessive toxicity observed. One should keep in mind, however, that due to the different composition of subcutaneous tissues, most murine tissues may not be adequate models of human normal tissues.

The outcome of the studies with murine kidney tumors mentioned above (YOUNES et al. 1995a,b) led to a clinical phase I/II trial at the same institution, combining radiotherapy (8 Gy) and IL-2 injections in patients with metastatic renal cell cancer. In a first report, the results were comparable to high-dose IL-2 and no unexpected toxicity was observed (REDMAN et al. 1998). Whereas a study including just 12 patients with metastatic renal cell cancer claimed a synergistic effect of combined radio- and chemoimmunotherapy (BRINKMANN et al. 1999), an earlier report from ROSENBERG's group on the combination of IL-2, TIL and a rapid fractionation regimen such as radiotherapy did not find a significant synergy in 28 patients (LANGE et al. 1992).

For non-small cell lung cancer, a randomized trial claimed a significant advantage of adjuvant therapy on local tumor control by combining tumor-infiltrating lymphocytes and IL-2 in the postoperative setting whereas the incidence of distant metastases was not reduced (RATTO et al. 1996).

16.6.3
IL-4

Systemic treatment with IL-4 on day 5–9 after inoculation of tumor cells resulted in regression of pulmonary metastasis in the murine Renca tumor model (HILLMAN et al. 1995). Tumor regression was abrogated by depletion of CD8+ cells or asiolo(as)GM1+ cells (mainly NK) but not CD4+ cells, suggesting the involvement of CD8+ cells and NK cells. On the other hand, growth of Renca tumors in the kidney was suppressed by injection of anti-IL-4 mAb at the time of tumor implantation (TAKEUCHI et al. 1997). The anti-IL-4 mAb-induced growth suppression was abrogated by antibodies against CD4+ and CD8+ T cells and was not observed in nude mice, strongly implicating both types of T cells. It appeared that high levels of IL-4 may be required for tumor regression or rejection by non-T mechanisms whereas low levels of IL-4 produced by the tumor cells favor Type 2 polarization, thus suppressing the Type 1 cell-mediated immune response (TAKEUCHI et al. 1997). Furthermore, although IL-4 inhibits growth of several cancer cell lines in vitro, it has been found to stimulate the growth of head and neck SCC cell lines (MYERS et al. 1996). Thus, the conditions of application, including cytokine level and timing, as well as the type of tumor, may be critical for clinical application of IL-4 and other cytokines such as IL-1 and IL-6.

The antitumoral effects of modulating the Type-1 vs Type-2 cytokine responses by IL-4 does not appear to have been investigated in combination with radiation. However, IL-4 has been shown to restore the radiation-induced inhibition of the ability of Th2 clones to induce IgE synthesis in primed B cells (DEKRUYFF et al. 1995). Furthermore, IL-4 enhanced the survival of lethally irradiated mice but, in contrast with the protective effects of IL-1 and IL-3, this was not associated with any hematopoietic activity of IL-4 (MEEREN et al. 1999). In a subsequent study by the same group, IL-4 was found to be able to down-regulate radiation-induced mediators of the inflammatory response, and it was suggested that this down-regulation might be involved in enhancing survival (VAN DER MEEREN et al. 2001).

16.6.4
IL-12

16.6.4.1
Antitumoral Effects

Stimulation of the cellular (Type 1) immune response via induction of IFN-γ is the rationale for the considerable interest in IL-12 as an immune modulator in cancer therapy. Thus, antitumoral effects of IL-12 in experimental mouse tumors were reported early by BRUNDA and co-workers although it did not inhibit tumor cell proliferation in vitro (BRUNDA et al. 1993).

Intraperitoneal daily injections of IL-12, initiated between day 1 and up to day 28 after tumor inoculation efficiently delayed the growth of primary tumor and metastases of B16 melanoma and Renca renal cell carcinoma but tumor cures were not observed (BRUNDA et al. 1993). The effect was identical in NK-deficient beige mice or mice depleted of NK cell activity by anti-asGM1 mAb when IL-12 treatment was initiated on day 14. By contrast, the efficacy of IL-12 was strongly reduced in Balb/c nude mice compared with immunocompetent animals. CD8+ depletion decreased the antitumoral effect whereas CD4+ depletion did not, implicating CD8+ T cells rather than NK- or CD4+ cells as the critical cell type.

Similar antitumoral effects with actual tumor cure and a tumor-specific cytotoxic T lymphocyte (CTL) reaction in cured animals were reported in MC38 adenocarcinoma and MCA205 fibrosarcoma when IL-12-producing adenovirus was injected within the first 7 days after tumor inoculation (GAMBOTTO et al. 1999). However, a CTL response in tumor-bearing animals is a rare event (FERNANDEZ et al. 1999) and the function of CD8+ cells has been found to be suppressed early after IL-12 injection (KURZAWA et al. 1998). This notion has been supported by a lack of tumor cure and CTL activity in IL-12-injected animals (LOHR et al. 2000a).

The time window for immunological manipulation after tumor inoculation appeared to be short and confined to early times after inoculation (NORTH and BURSUKER 1984; VAN ELSAS et al. 1999). This may also explain why so-called prophylactic use of IL-12 combining allogeneic tumor cell vaccination and systemic interleukin 12 was successful in preventing mammary carcinogenesis in HER-2/neu transgenic mice (NANNI et al. 1998).

The exact role of NK cells in mediating IL-12 effects is still unclear. Although a connection between NK cells and generation of a CTL response is postulated (Kos and ENGLEMAN 1996; KUROSAWA et al. 1995), and NK cells seem to be necessary for elimination of metastasis in murine tumors, their actual importance for IL-12 effects on the primary tumor is controversial and ranges from negligible (KODAMA et al. 1999; NASU et al. 1999; WANG et al. 1999) to moderately relevant (BRUNDA et al. 1993; LOHR et al. 2000a; VAN ELSAS et al. 1999).

IFN-γ is a secondary messenger for IL-12 and the production of IFN-γ seems to be a necessary event in the antitumoral activity of IL-12 (DIGHE et al. 1994), which would explain the requirement of T cells despite the lack of a specific CTL response. IFN-γ itself has antitumoral effects for some tumors but is without effects in most tumor models (BRUNDA et al. 1993; FERNANDEZ et al. 1999; PUISIEUX et al. 1998). This is also corroborated by the fact that the antitumoral effects of IL-12 in nude mice are usually weaker than in immunocompetent mice although up to fivefold higher IFN-γ levels can be induced in nude mice (BRUNDA et al. 1993).

IL-12 induces the expression of MHC I, MHC II and ICAM-1 in melanoma cells and APCs either directly or via stimulation of IFN-γ production by NK and T cells (YUE et al. 1999). An approach using dendritic cells (DC) that are genetically engineered to produce IL-12 has met with great success in preclinical tests (MELERO et al. 1999; NISHIOKA et al. 1999).

As a nonimmunological feature, the antiangiogenic effects of IL-12 have been described (COUGHLIN et al. 1998; LEE et al. 2002; STRASLY et al. 2001; VOEST et al. 1995). Delivery of IL-12 targeted to neovasculature seems to further enhance its antitumor efficacy (HALIN et al. 2002). The preclinical data, therefore, imply that the antitumoral effect of IL-12 very much depends on the tumor model, the immune phenotype, the mode of application (single dose vs repeated), the time schedule of its application, etc. However, the early antitumoral effects of IL-12 may well be due to nonspecific mechanisms (macrophages, antiangiogenicity, etc.), and long-lasting specific immunity has been the exception.

Clinically, IL-12 was first administered intravenously in 1994 (ATKINS et al. 1997), but due to excessive toxicity, the mode of application was soon changed (LEONARD et al. 1997). Subcutaneous delivery was less problematic and is still in clinical trials (MOTZER et al. 2001). Responses in metastatic renal cell cancer, however, have been disappointing so far, despite the expected increase in IFN-γ levels and NK activity, both of which seem to be of importance in metastatic disease. The same is the case for treatment with IL-12 gene-modified autologous melanoma cell vaccines (SUN et al. 1998, 1999).

16.6.4.2
Enhancement of the Radiation Response

Early preclinical studies showed synergy between systemic IL-12 application and radiotherapy for Lewis lung carcinoma for different application schedules of IL-12 (TEICHER et al. 1998). More recent data on the combination of adenovirus-mediated IL-12 gene therapy and local radiotherapy in a murine fibrosarcoma suggested antiangiogenic properties of IL-12 as the main mode of action in conjunction with radiotherapy (SEETHARAM et al. 1999). This conclusion, however, was only based on the observation of rarified vessels in the tumor after combined treatment. No studies with regard to the contribution of different cellular elements of the immune system to the immediate tumor regression were performed. Nevertheless, immunity against tumors was observed in cured animals upon re-challenge and this immunity could be abrogated by depletion of CD8+ cells.

Our own data on combined fractionated local radiotherapy of the 4T1 mouse mammary carcinoma and B16 mouse melanoma with intratumoral injections of IL-12/B7.1 encoding adenovirus also showed an enhanced effect of the combined-modality therapy over each single modality that was clearly supra-additive for B16 melanoma, in particular when the vector was injected after radiotherapy (LOHR et al. 2000a). We could show that both T and NK cells contribute to the overall effect, although they are not the sole contributors. Nonspecific mechanisms such as macrophage activity or the antiangiogenic properties of IL-12 probably account for some of the effects since there was an effect of IL-12 even in NK-depleted nude mice.

16.6.5
IFN-α,-β

16.6.5.1
Antitumoral Effects

Interferons have been used to treat various malignancies, with varying success. The antitumor effects of IFN-α and IFN-β seem to be the consequence of immunostimulatory features and direct antiproliferative effects. Among the hematological malignancies effectively treated with IFN-α are hairy cell leukemia, chronic myelogenous leukemia (CML) and follicular lymphoma. However, this treatment seems to delay the course of the disease rather than improve eradication (JONASCH and HALUSKA 2001).

Experience with solid tumors has been mixed. In metastatic renal cell carcinoma (RCC), mean response rates of 15% seem realistic, apparently translating into a modest survival benefit (MOTZER et al. 1998; MRC/RCC 1999). Combinations with IL-2 were not convincing, unless also combined with 5-FU (ATZPODIEN et al. 1993). Confirmatory trials, however, did not succeed in reproducing the high response rates initially reported with this regimen (TOURANI et al. 1998; VAN HERPEN et al. 2000).

In metastatic melanoma, response rates were around 20%, but the hopes for prolonged survival, both for single-modality therapy as well as chemoimmunotherapy, were not fulfilled despite initial euphoria based on phase II trials (LEGHA et al. 1996). Several recently published large randomized multicenter trials showed no benefit whatsoever for chemotherapy combined with IL-2/IFN-α over chemotherapy alone (ATZPODIEN et al. 2002; KEILHOLZ et al. 1997; ROSENBERG et al. 1999). Nevertheless, for lymph node-positive disease, there seems to be a measurable benefit of adjuvant IFN therapy, as suggested by ECOG 1684 (KIRKWOOD et al. 1996), which led to FDA approval of adjuvant IFN-α in high-risk (node-positive and deep primary) malignant melanoma although a recent meta-analysis shed doubt on this (LENS and DAWES 2002). Initial positive reports about treatment of nasopharyngeal cancer were based mainly on studies with comparatively few patients (CONNORS et al. 1985; TREUNER et al. 1980) and only rarely involved larger trials (MERTENS et al. 1997). So far, no randomized data are available.

A phase III trial of modulation of cisplatinum/fluorouracil by IFN-α in patients with recurrent or metastatic head and neck cancer of the Head and Neck Interferon Cooperative Study Group (SCHRIJVERS et al. 1998) did not show any advantage of adding IFN-α to chemotherapy. In metastatic or unresectable bladder cancer, a phase III trial showed that a combination of IFN-α and chemotherapy with fluorouracil and cisplatinum was inferior when compared with M-VAC chemotherapy (SIEFKER-RADTKE et al. 2002).

16.6.5.2
Enhancement of the Radiation Response

The rationale for using interferons in combination with radiotherapy was initially based on their virus-clearing properties. Thus IFN may be of particular interest in diseases with a presumed viral component, such as Epstein-Barr virus (EBV) in nasopharyngeal cancer (NPC) or human papilloma virus (HPV) in cancer of the uterine cervix.

The interest in combining interferons with radiotherapy for the treatment of nasopharyngeal cancer (NPC) is the result of an early observation by CONNORS and co-workers, who saw measurable tumor regression in advanced NPC (CONNORS et al. 1985). IFN-α, -β and -γ have been used in combination with radiotherapy on a case-by-case basis (without any success for IFN-γ but suggesting some efficacy for IFN-α and -β), and systematically in a pediatric trial though only in a nonrandomized fashion (MERTENS et al. 1997). To our knowledge, no randomized data exist for this disease. Initially promising data in head and neck cancer (VOKES 1994) have not been substantiated by phase III results, either.

In early studies, it was found that IFN-α or -β increases the radiosensitivity of various human cancer cell lines in vitro, including squamous cell carcinomas of the head and neck and of cervix origin, lung and renal cell cancer in vitro (CHANG and KENG 1987; GOULD et al. 1984; HOLSTI et al. 1987; SCHMIDBERGER et al. 1999). One of the mechanisms contributing to radiosensitization is probably the accumulation of cells in G2-M-phase (CHANG and KENG 1987), although this did not seem to be the main mode of action in skin cancer, where increased apoptosis seemed to play a role (SHIN et al. 2002). IFN-β may also impair radiation damage repair (SCHMIDBERGER et al. 1999). Interestingly, nontransformed MRC-5 fibroblasts were not sensitized by IFN-β (SCHMIDBERGER et al. 1999).

IFN-α in combination with retinoids has shown a synergistic radiosensitizing effect in several in vitro studies with cervical and head-and-neck squamous cell carcinoma (SCC) cell lines (ANGIOLI et al. 1992, 1993; DELANEY et al. 1996; HOFFMANN et al. 1997). In general, squamous cell cancer of the cervix and skin seemed to be more responsive than head-and-neck SCC (HOFFMANN et al. 1997). However, effective radiosensitization of tumor cells appeared to depend mainly on low basal expression levels of cytoplasmatic retinoic acid (RA) binding protein I (CRABP I), which is responsible for degradation of RA (HOFFMANN et al. 1999). In murine colon epithelium, pretreatment with a combination of IFN-α and 13-cis RA was moderately radioprotective whereas, clinically, proctitis had been observed in patients (MASON and TOFILON 1994). Possibly, differences in timing and administration of the treatment may influence the reaction of normal tissue and thus determine whether a therapeutic benefit is obtained.

The promising preclinical results for the combination of IFN and RA prompted combination therapy trials in tumors that pose a significant local problem, such as non-small-cell lung cancer and cancer of the cervix (ANGIOLI et al. 1992, 1993; TOMA et al. 1994). Consequently, several phase I/II trials were begun in lung cancer, most of these with limited success (MAASILTA et al. 1992; TORRISI et al. 1986) and some resulting in excessive toxicity. Neurological toxicity and recall effects have been reported (THOMAS and STEA 2002). From these initial trials with interferons and radiotherapy in lung cancer, the phase I/II trial by MCDONALD et al. combining radiotherapy and IFN-β stood out (MCDONALD et al. 1993). The response rate of 81% compared very favorably with a historical 35%, and 5-year survival seemed to be improved. Unfortunately, an intended follow-up phase III trial has not been published to date. By contrast, a recent randomized phase III trial (RTOG 93-04) on locally advanced non-small cell lung cancer showed no difference in survival rates or survival time between patients receiving IFN-β plus radiotherapy and patients receiving only radiotherapy (BRADLEY et al. 2002). However, patients receiving IFN-β showed more severe acute and late lung toxicities.

The picture for cancer of the uterine cervix, a tumor, where viral infection also plays an eminent role, is very similar. A large body of promising phase I/II data exists (MURAD et al. 1994; PARK et al. 1998; TOMA et al. 1994; VERASTEGUI-AVILES et al. 1999), especially in conjunction with RA (HOFFMANN et al. 1997; LIPPMAN et al. 1993). However, a randomized phase II trial on recurrent cervical cancer did not show a benefit of IFN-α combined with 13-cis RA or all-trans RA and radiotherapy although the treatment was well tolerated (WEISS et al. 1998).

In brain cancer, IFN-α was tested in a limited number of patients, either with inconclusive (DILLMAN et al. 1995) or outright disappointing results (PACKER et al. 1996). An in vitro study has shown a radiosensitizing effect of IFN-α in combination with 13-cis-RA on glioma cells (MALONE et al. 1999). However, a non-randomized study of high-grade glioma patients treated with IFN-α and 13-cis-RA plus radiotherapy showed no evidence of improved survival compared with a previous study of patients receiving concurrent IFN-α and radiotherapy or only radiotherapy in other studies (DILLMAN et al. 2001). A phase III trial comparing adjuvant chemotherapy (BCNU) with BCNU + IFN-α after surgery and radiotherapy also did not show any advantage of adjuvant cytokine treatment (BUCKNER et al. 2001).

A potential advantageous effect of IFN-α/RA may be the improved oxygenation of cervix tumors undergoing radiotherapy, thereby decreasing the fraction of radioresistant hypoxic cells (DUNST et al. 1999). A randomized trial has recently been completed (DUNST and HAENSGEN, in preparation), which confirms the oxygenation data but does not demonstrate superiority for the combination of IFN-α/RA with radiotherapy (DUNST and HAENSGEN, personal communication).

The development of novel combinations of therapy modalities may hold some promise for improved outcome. A recent nonrandomized retrospective study of pancreatic cancer compared GITSG-type radiochemotherapy in the adjuvant setting with radiochemotherapy and additional IFN-α. The 2-year survival (84%) was higher than in the GITSG-group (54%) data and actuarial survival curves significantly favored IFN-α treatment in spite of a more advanced tumor stage in this group (NUKUI et al. 2000). These data represent the highest survival rate after IFN treatment published to date and strongly encourage randomized trials to evaluate this promising approach further.

A preclinical immunogenic approach using the murine Renca lung metastasis model takes advantage of the ability of IFN-α to activate NK cells. It was shown that subcutaneous vaccination with IFN-α-secreting Renca tumor cells combined with unilateral lung irradiation reduced the number of tumors and total tumor volume in both lungs (NISHISAKA et al. 2000). This indicates the potential for eliciting an immunogenic response against tumors by exploiting the actions of cytokines on immune cells.

16.6.6
IFN-γ

16.6.6.1
Antitumoral Effects and Enhancement of the Radiation Response

The use of IFN-γ in the clinical setting has not been met with overwhelming success. IFN-γ was ineffective in nasopharyngeal cancer (MAHJOUBI et al. 1993). In a phase III trial in complete responders with small-cell lung cancer after conventional radiotherapy/chemotherapy, median time to progression was increased by IFN-γ therapy, although not significantly (JETT et al. 1994). A phase I study on NSCLC with concomitant IFN-γ and accelerated hyperfractionated radiotherapy (60 Gy in 1.5-Gy twice daily fractions) showed unacceptably severe pneumonitis, which was partly fatal, as well as cases of severe esophagitis (SHAW et al. 1995). In a large randomized phase I/II trial on metastatic melanoma, IFN-γ showed little effect. A tumor response was observed only in 4 out of 81 patients and involved different dose levels (SCHILLER et al. 1996). A randomized study on treatment of newly diagnosed glioblastoma with adjuvant IFN-γ and radiotherapy showed no difference in tumor progression or survival (FARKKILA et al. 1994).

A synergistic radiosensitizing effect of IFN-γ in combination with 9-cis-RA was observed in breast cancer cell lines (WINDBICHLER et al. 1996). Like some other cytokines, IFN-γ has been reported to protect hematopoietic stem cells from radiation damage (GARDNER 1998). This has, however, not led to any clinical use so far.

The inconsistent antitumoral effects of IFN-γ (BRUNDA et al. 1993; DIGHE et al. 1994; FERNANDEZ et al. 1999; PUISIEUX et al. 1998) have led to the conclusion that IFN-γ needs to be provided by specific cellular elements to be effective. This has formed the basis for developing strategies based on stimulating IFN-γ secretion by IL-12 (see Sec. 16.3.1, "Interleukins").

In the immunological approach using the murine Renca lung metastasis model described in Sec. 16.6.4, "IL-12" injection of IFN-γ-secreting tumor cells resulted in s.c. tumors in only 1 of 8 immunocompetent mice but in 8 of 8 Balb/c nude mice (Nishisaka et al. 1999). Since NK cells were implicated as the cytotoxic mediator (based on the efficacy of IL-2 in nude mice described in Sec. 16.6.4, "IL-12"), IFN-γ did not seem to activate NK cells in the absence of T cells. Multiple vaccinations with IFN-γ-producing cells into Balb/c mice plus lung irradiation with a single dose of 3 Gy had significant antitumoral effect on lung metastases (Nishisaka et al. 1999).

16.6.7
Toxicity of Interferon Combined with Radiotherapy

Although most reports describe only mild and manageable toxicity of combined cytokine/radiotherapy regimens, some toxicity patterns seem to be reproducible (Mollman 1992). The side effects of cytokines fall into four major groups: constitutional (fever, chills, rigors, anorexia, fatigue), neuropsychiatric (somnolence, confusion, neuropathy, depression), hematologic and hepatic.

Special caution seems to be warranted when large lung volumes are treated with IFN-α, IFN-β (Bradley et al. 2002; Hoffmann et al. 1997) or INF-γ (Shaw et al. 1995), although in the latter case the accelerated hyperfractionation scheme may have contributed to the severe toxicity observed. Rectal toxicity was dose limiting in combined treatments of advanced cervical cancer (Lippman et al. 1993; Verastegui-Aviles et al. 1999). Combinations with other compounds, especially with membrane destabilizing agents, may be even more detrimental. In a recent letter, a higher rate of neurological toxicity than expected for each single agent was reported when IFN-α was combined with thalidomide in metastatic renal cell cancer (Nathan et al. 2002). Radiation recall has been observed both with IFN-γ (pneumonitis) (Shaw et al. 1995) and as skin recall with IFN-α (Thomas and Stea 2002).

The biggest concern with combination therapy is neurotoxicity, which is already a problem with cytokine therapy as a single modality (Meriggioli and Rowin 2000). The combination with radiotherapy can be extremely dangerous when large volumes of nerve tissue are within the irradiated volume. Such problems have been reported, especially with IFN-α (Hazard et al. 2002).

16.7
Conclusions and Future Prospects

Clinical application of cytokines in cancer therapy so far has focused on the interferons -α, -β and -γ, IL-2 and IL-12. In combination with radiotherapy, the cytokines have mostly been applied systemically. Although preclinical studies have been encouraging and some success has been reported in smaller clinical studies, subsequent randomized phase III trials have, with few exceptions, not confirmed an enhancing effect and have frequently been associated with considerable toxicity. Thus a therapeutic benefit of systemic application appears doubtful. On the other hand, preclinical studies have indicated some potential for radioimmunotherapy with tumor cell vaccines in combination with cytokines injected locally or expressed locally using gene-transfer techniques, although long-lasting immunity may not have been achieved.

With recent improvements in distributions of radiation dose, a further widening of the therapeutic window in radiotherapy is likely to result from the combination with other modalities such as chemotherapy, which has proved successful in rectal cancer, cancer of the cervix and esophageal cancer. Similarly, biological response modifiers are candidates for such combination therapies.

New ways of delivering immunostimulating cytokines are necessary and the methods of gene transfer offer viable alternatives. Although such methods may pose their own toxicity problems (Lohr et al. 2001), these may be overcome by novel (e.g., gene-based) approaches (Lohr et al. 2000b). Since some cytokines may actually stimulate growth of certain tumors, preclinical studies, preferably in syngeneic tumor model systems, are important to test the applicability of each cytokine in particular types of tumors.

Another path worth pursuing is the combination of cytokines and key elements of the immune system such as dendritic cells. In using such systems, optimal timing of the application of conventional methods such as radio- and chemotherapy and the immunostimulatory approaches is of paramount importance. It may also be prudent to apply different agents in different locations (primary tumor vs lymph nodes), depending on where they exert the greatest effect. Further insight into the mechanisms causing tolerance against tumors and the ways it can be broken should lead to a new generation of combined treatments entering clinical trials. It is the hope that this approach may eventually be successful in improving the therapy of such cancers that presently have a poor prognosis.

Acknowledgements. CH was supported by an EDRO Research Fellowship from ESTRO under an ESQUIRE contract with the EU.

References

Abbas AK, Murphy KM, Sher A (1996) Functional diversity of helper T lymphocytes. Nature 383:787–793

Abbas AK, Lichtman AH, Pober JS (2001) Cellular and molecular immunology. Saunders, Philadelphia

Abdulkarim B, Sabri S, Deutsch E, Vaganay S, Marangoni E, Vainchenker W, Bongrand P, Busson P, Bourhis J (2000) Radiation-induced expression of functional Fas ligand in EBV-positive human nasopharyngeal carcinoma cells. Int J Cancer 86:229–237

Addison CL, Bramson JL, Hitt MM, Muller WJ, Gauldie J, Graham FL (1998) Intratumoral coinjection of adenoviral vectors expressing IL-2 and IL-12 results in enhanced frequency of regression of injected and untreated distal tumors. Gene Ther 5:1400–1409

Akbari O, DeKruyff RH, Umetsu DT (2001) Pulmonary dendritic cells producing IL-10 mediate tolerance induced by respiratory exposure to antigen. Nat Immunol 2:725–731

Albert ML, Sauter B, Bhardwaj N (1998) Dendritic cells acquire antigen from apoptotic cells and induce class I-restricted CTLs. Nature 392:86–89

Angioli R, Sevin BU, Perras JP, Untch M, Hightower RD, Nguyen HN, Steren A, Villani C, Averette HE (1992) Rationale of combining radiation and interferon for the treatment of cervical cancer. Oncology 49:445–449

Angioli R, Sevin BU, Perras JP, Untch M, Koechli OR, Nguyen HN, Steren A, Schwade JG, Villani C, Averette HE (1993) In vitro potentiation of radiation cytotoxicity by recombinant interferons in cervical cancer cell lines. Cancer 71:3717–3725

Arai H, Gordon D, Nabel EG, Nabel GJ (1997) Gene transfer of Fas ligand induces tumor regression in vivo. Proc Natl Acad Sci U S A 94:13862–13867

Atkins MB, Robertson MJ, Gordon M, Lotze MT, DeCoste M, DuBois JS, Ritz J, Sandler AB, Edington HD, Garzone PD, Mier JW, Canning CM, Battiato L, Tahara H, Sherman ML (1997) Phase I evaluation of intravenous recombinant human interleukin 12 in patients with advanced malignancies. Clin Cancer Res 3:409–417

Atzpodien J, Kirchner H, Hanninen EL, Deckert M, Fenner M, Poliwoda H (1993) Interleukin-2 in combination with interferon-alpha and 5-fluorouracil for metastatic renal cell cancer. Eur J Cancer 29A [Suppl 5]:S6–S8

Atzpodien J, Neuber K, Kamanabrou D, Fluck M, Brocker EB, Neumann C, Runger TM, Schuler G, von den Driesch P, Muller I, Paul E, Patzelt T, Reitz M (2002) Combination chemotherapy with or without s.c. IL-2 and IFN-alpha: results of a prospectively randomized trial of the Cooperative Advanced Malignant Melanoma Chemoimmunotherapy Group (ACIMM). Br J Cancer 86:179–184

Barbera N, Palmucci T, Chiarenza A, Bartoloni G, Cordaro S, Greco S, Scapagnini U, Bernardini R (1993) Radioprotective effects of the association thymopentin-interleukin-1 alpha in the C57BL/6 mouse. Pharmacol Toxicol 72:256–261

Belka C, Ottinger H, Kreuzfelder E, Weinmann M, Lindemann M, Lepple-Wienhues A, Budach W, Grosse-Wilde H, Bamberg M (1999) Impact of localized radiotherapy on blood immune cell counts and function in humans. Radiother Oncol 50:199–204

Bendelac A, Medzhitov R (2002) Adjuvants of immunity: harnessing innate immunity to promote adaptive immunity. J Exp Med 195:F19–F23

Bogdan C, Paik J, Vodovotz Y, Nathan C (1992) Contrasting mechanisms for suppression of macrophage cytokine release by transforming growth factor-beta and interleukin-10. J Biol Chem 267:23301–23308

Bradley JD, Scott CB, Paris KJ, Demas WF, Machtay M, Komaki R, Movsas B, Rubin P, Sause WT (2002) A phase III comparison of radiation therapy with or without recombinant beta-interferon for poor-risk patients with locally advanced non-small-cell lung cancer (RTOG 93-04). Int J Radiat Oncol Biol Phys 52:1173–1179

Braunschweiger PG, Basrur V, Santos O, Adessa A, Houdek P, Markoe AM (1996) Radioresistance in murine solid tumors induced by interleukin-1. Radiat Res 145:150–156

Brinkmann OA, Bruns F, Prott FJ, Hertle L (1999) Possible synergy of radiotherapy and chemo-immunotherapy in metastatic renal cell carcinoma (RCC). Anticancer Res 19:1583–1587

Brunda MJ, Luistro L, Warrier RR, Wright RB, Hubbard BR, Murphy M, Wolf SF, Gately MK (1993) Antitumor and antimetastatic activity of interleukin 12 against murine tumors. J Exp Med 178:1223–1230

Buckner JC, Schomberg PJ, McGinnis WL, Cascino TL, Scheithauer BW, O'Fallon JR, Morton RF, Kuross SA, Mailliard JA, Hatfield AK, Cole JT, Steen PD, Bernath AM (2001) A phase III study of radiation therapy plus carmustine with or without recombinant interferon-alpha in the treatment of patients with newly diagnosed high-grade glioma. Cancer 92:420–433

Cameron RB, Spiess PJ, Rosenberg SA (1990) Synergistic antitumor activity of tumor-infiltrating lymphocytes, interleukin 2, and local tumor irradiation. Studies on the mechanism of action. J Exp Med 171:249–263

Chang AY, Keng PC (1987) Potentiation of radiation cytotoxicity by recombinant interferons, a phenomenon associated with increased blockage at the G2-M phase of the cell cycle. Cancer Res 47:4338–4341

Chappell DB, Zaks TZ, Rosenberg SA, Restifo NP (1999) Human melanoma cells do not express Fas (Apo-1/CD95) ligand. Cancer Res 59:59–62

Chen L, McGowan P, Ashe S, Johnston J, Li Y, Hellstrom I, Hellstrom KE (1994) Tumor immunogenicity determines the effect of B7 costimulation on T cell-mediated tumor immunity. J Exp Med 179:523–532

Chiang CS, Hong JH, Wu YC, McBride WH, Dougherty GJ (2000) Combining radiation therapy with interleukin-3 gene immunotherapy. Cancer Gene Ther 7:1172–1178

Clerici M, Shearer GM, Clerici E (1998) Cytokine dysregulation in invasive cervical carcinoma and other human neoplasias: time to consider the TH1/TH2 paradigm. J Natl Cancer Inst 90:261–263

Cole S, Lewkowicz SJ, Townsend KM (1984) Langerhans cell number and morphology in mouse footpad epidermis after X irradiation. Radiat Res 100:594–606

Connors JM, Andiman WA, Howarth CB, Liu E, Merigan TC, Savage ME, Jacobs C (1985) Treatment of nasopharyngeal carcinoma with human leukocyte interferon. J Clin Oncol 3:813–817

Coughlin CM, Salhany KE, Wysocka M, Aruga E, Kurzawa H, Chang AE, Hunter CA, Fox JC, Trinchieri G, Lee WMF (1998) Interleukin-12 and interleukin-18 synergistically induce murine tumor regression which involves inhibition of angiogenesis. J Clin Invest 101:1441–1452

Coulie PG, Ikeda H, Baurain JF, Chiari R (1999) Antitumor immunity at work in a melanoma patient. Adv Cancer Res 76:213–242

DeKruyff RH, Fang Y, Umetsu DT (1995) IL-4-based helper activity of CD4+ T cells is radiation sensitive. Cell Immunol 160:248–256

DeLaney TF, Afridi N, Taghian AG, Sanders DA, Fuleihan NS, Faller DV, Nogueira CP (1996) 13-cis-retinoic acid with alpha-2a-interferon enhances radiation cytotoxicity in head and neck squamous cell carcinoma in vitro. Cancer Res 56:2277–2280

Dieckmann D, Plottner H, Berchtold S, Berger T, Schuler G (2001) Ex vivo isolation and characterization of CD4(+)CD25(+) T cells with regulatory properties from human blood. J Exp Med 193:1303–1310

Dighe AS, Richards E, Old LJ, Schreiber RD (1994) Enhanced in vivo growth and resistance to rejection of tumor cells expressing dominant negative IFN gamma receptors. Immunity 1:447–456

Dillman RO, Wiemann M, Oldham RK, Soori G, Bury M, Hafer R, Church C, DePriest C (1995) Interferon alpha-2a and external beam radiotherapy in the initial management of patients with glioma: a pilot study of the National Biotherapy Study Group. Cancer Biother 10:265–271

Dillman RO, Shea WM, Tai DF, Mahdavi K, Barth NM, Kharkar BR, Poor MM, Church CK, DePriest C (2001) Interferon-alpha2a and 13-cis-retinoic acid with radiation treatment for high-grade glioma. Neurooncology 3:35–41

Dorie MJ, Allison AC, Zaghloul MS, Kallman RF (1989) Interleukin 1 protects against the lethal effects of irradiation of mice but has no effect on tumors in the same animals. Proc Soc Exp Biol Med 191:23–29

Dorie MJ, Kallman RF, Cebulska-Wasilewska A (1991) Interleukin-1 modification of the effects of cyclophosphamide and fractionated irradiation. Int J Radiat Oncol Biol Phys 20:311–314

Down JD, Awwad M, Kurilla-Mahon B, Moran K, Ericsson T, Oldmixon B, Lachance A, Watts A, Treter S, Nash K, Gojo S, Sachs DH, White-Scharf ME, Cooper DK (2000) Increases in autologous hematopoietic progenitors in the blood of baboons following irradiation and treatment with porcine stem cell factor and interleukin-3. Transplant Proc 32:1045–1046

Dranoff G, Jaffee E, Lazenby A, Golumbek P, Levitsky H, Brose K, Jackson V, Hamada H, Pardoll D, Mulligan RC (1993) Vaccination with irradiated tumor cells engineered to secrete murine granulocyte-macrophage colony-stimulating factor stimulates potent, specific, and long-lasting antitumor immunity. Proc Natl Acad Sci U S A 90:3539–3543

Dunst J, Hansgen G, Lautenschlager C, Fuchsel G, Becker A (1999) Oxygenation of cervical cancers during radiotherapy and radiotherapy + cis-retinoic acid/interferon. Int J Radiat Oncol Biol Phys 43:367–373

Everson MP, Spalding DM, Koopman WJ (1989) Exquisite sensitivity of dendritic cells to ultraviolet radiation and temperature changes. Transplantation 48:666–671

Faris M, Latinis KM, Kempiak SJ, Koretzky GA, Nel A (1998) Stress-induced Fas ligand expression in T cells is mediated through a MEK kinase 1-regulated response element in the Fas ligand promoter. Mol Cell Biol 18:5414–5424

Farkkila M, Jaaskelainen J, Kallio M, Blomstedt G, Raininko R, Virkkunen P, Paetau A, Sarelin H, Mantyla M (1994) Randomised, controlled study of intratumoral recombinant gamma-interferon treatment in newly diagnosed glioblastoma. Br J Cancer 70:138–141

Fernandez NC, Levraud JP, Haddada H, Perricaudet M, Kourilsky P (1999) High frequency of specific CD8+ T cells in the tumor and blood is associated with efficient local IL-12 gene therapy of cancer. J Immunol 162:609–617

Gabrilovich DI, Ciernik IF, Carbone DP (1996) Dendritic cells in antitumor immune responses. I. Defective antigen presentation in tumor-bearing hosts. Cell Immunol 170:101–110

Gambotto A, Tuting T, McVey DL, Kovesdi I, Tahara H, Lotze MT, Robbins PD (1999) Induction of antitumor immunity by direct intratumoral injection of a recombinant adenovirus vector expressing interleukin-12. Cancer Gene Ther 6:45–53

Gardner RV (1998) Interferon-gamma (IFN-gamma) as a potential radio- and chemo-protectant. Am J Hematol 58:218–223

Geldhof AB, Moser M, Lespagnard L, Thielemans K, De Baetselier P (1998) Interleukin-12-activated natural killer cells recognize B7 costimulatory molecules on tumor cells and autologous dendritic cells. Blood 91:196–206

Gould MN, Kakria RC, Olson S, Borden EC (1984) Radiosensitization of human bronchogenic carcinoma cells by interferon beta. J Interferon Res 4:123–128

Gratas C, Tohma Y, Barnas C, Taniere P, Hainaut P, Ohgaki H (1998) Up-regulation of Fas (APO-1/CD95) ligand and down-regulation of Fas expression in human esophageal cancer. Cancer Res 58:2057–2062

Hahne M, Rimoldi D, Schroter M, Romero P, Schreier M, French LE, Schneider P, Bornand T, Fontana A, Lienard D, Cerottini J, Tschopp J (1996) Melanoma cell expression of Fas(Apo-1/CD95) ligand: implications for tumor immune escape. Science 274:1363–1366

Halin C, Rondini S, Nilsson F, Berndt A, Kosmehl H, Zardi L, Neri D (2002) Enhancement of the antitumor activity of interleukin-12 by targeted delivery to neovasculature. Nat Biotechnol 20:264–269

Hareyama M, Imai K, Oouchi A, Takahashi H, Hinoda Y, Tsujisaki M, Adachi M, Shonai T, Sakata K, Morita K (1998) The effect of radiation on the expression of intercellular adhesion molecule-1 of human adenocarcinoma cells. Int J Radiat Oncol Biol Phys 40:691–696

Hashimoto S, Shirato H, Hosokawa M, Nishioka T, Kuramitsu Y, Matsushita K, Kobayashi M, Miyasaka K (1999) The suppression of metastases and the change in host immune response after low-dose total-body irradiation in tumor-bearing rats. Radiat Res 151:717–724

Hazard LJ, Sause WT, Noyes RD (2002) Combined adjuvant radiation and interferon-alpha 2B therapy in high-risk melanoma patients: the potential for increased radiation toxicity. Int J Radiat Oncol Biol Phys 52:796–800

Hestdal K, Jacobsen SE, Ruscetti FW, Dubois CM, Longo DL, Chizzonite R, Oppenheim JJ, Keller JR (1992) In vivo effect of interleukin-1 alpha on hematopoiesis: role of colony-stimulating factor receptor modulation. Blood 80:2486–2494

Hillman GG, Younes E, Visscher D, Ali E, Lam JS, Montecillo E, Pontes JE, Haas GP, Puri RK (1995) Systemic treatment with interleukin-4 induces regression of pulmonary metastases in a murine renal cell carcinoma model. Cell Immunol 160: 257–263

Hillman GG, Maughan RL, Grignon DJ, Yudelev M, Rubio J, Tekyi-Mensah S, Layer A, Che M, Forman JD (2001) Neutron or photon irradiation for prostate tumors: enhancement of cytokine therapy in a metastatic tumor model. Clin Cancer Res 7:136–144

Hodge DL, Martinez A, Julias JG, Taylor LS, Young HA (2002) Regulation of nuclear gamma interferon gene expression by interleukin 12 (IL-12) and IL-2 represents a novel form of posttranscriptional control. Mol Cell Biol 22:1742–1753

Hoffmann W, Schiebe M, Hirnle P, Souchon R, Clemens M, Adamietz I, Bamberg M (1997) 13-cis retinoic acid and interferon-alpha +/- irradiation in the treatment of squamous-cell carcinomas. Int J Cancer 70:475–477

Hoffmann W, Blase MA, Santo-Hoeltje L, Herskind C, Bamberg M, Rodemann HP (1999) Radiation sensitivity of human squamous cell carcinoma cells in vitro is modulated by all-trans and 13-cis-retinoic acid in combination with interferon-alpha. Int J Radiat Oncol Biol Phys 45:991–998

Holsti LR, Mattson K, Niiranen A, Standertskiold-Nordenstam CG, Stenman S, Sovijarvi A, Cantell K (1987) Enhancement of radiation effects by alpha interferon in the treatment of small cell carcinoma of the lung. Int J Radiat Oncol Biol Phys 13:1161–1166

Hong JH, Chiang CS, Tsao CY, Lin PY, McBride WH, Wu CJ (1999) Rapid induction of cytokine gene expression in the lung after single and fractionated doses of radiation. Int J Radiat Biol 75:1421–1427

Huang FP, Platt N, Wykes M, Major JR, Powell TJ, Jenkins CD, MacPherson GG (2000) A discrete subpopulation of dendritic cells transports apoptotic intestinal epithelial cells to T cell areas of mesenteric lymph nodes. J Exp Med 191:435–444

Hughes AL, Yeager M (1997) Molecular evolution of the vertebrate immune system. Bioessays 19:777–786

Hunter N, Nakayama T, Ito H, Woo S, Milas L (1992) Combination of interleukin-2 and irradiation in therapy of murine tumors. Clin Exp Metastasis 10:431–436

Ikeguchi M, Ikeda M, Tatebe S, Maeta M, Kaibara N (1998) Clinical significance of dendritic cell infiltration in esophageal squamous cell carcinoma. Oncol Rep 5:1185–1189

Jee SH, Shen SC, Chiu HC, Tsai WL, Kuo ML (2001) Overexpression of interleukin-6 in human basal cell carcinoma cell lines increases anti-apoptotic activity and tumorigenic potency. Oncogene 20:198–208

Jett JR, Maksymiuk AW, Su JQ, Mailliard JA, Krook JE, Tschetter LK, Kardinal CG, Twito DI, Levitt R, Gerstner JB (1994) Phase III trial of recombinant interferon gamma in complete responders with small-cell lung cancer. J Clin Oncol 12:2321–2326

Johansson S, Landstrom M, Hellstrand K, Henriksson R (1998) The response of Dunning R3327 prostatic adenocarcinoma to IL-2, histamine and radiation. Br J Cancer 77:1213–1219

Jonasch E, Haluska FG (2001) Interferon in oncological practice: review of interferon biology, clinical applications, and toxicities. Oncologist 6:34–55

Jurgenliemk-Schulz IM, Renes IB, Rutgers DH, Everse LA, Bernsen MR, Den Otter W, Battermann JJ (1997) Antitumor effects of local irradiation in combination with peritumoral administration of low doses of recombinant interleukin-2 (rIL-2). Radiat Oncol Invest 5:54–61

Kang SM, Schneider DB, Lin Z, Hanahan D, Dichek DA, Stock PG, Baekkeskov S (1997) Fas ligand expression in islets of Langerhans does not confer immune privilege and instead targets them for rapid destruction. Nat Med 3: 738–743

Kawakita M, Rao GS, Ritchey JK, Ornstein DK, Hudson MA, Tartaglia J, Paoletti E, Humphrey PA, Harmon TJ, Ratliff TL (1997) Effect of canarypox virus (ALVAC)-mediated cytokine expression on murine prostate tumor growth. J Natl Cancer Inst 89:428–436

Kawase Y, Naito S, Ito M, Sekine I, Fujii H (1990) The effect of ionizing radiation on epidermal Langerhans cells – a quantitative analysis of autopsy cases with radiation therapy. J Radiat Res (Tokyo) 31:246–255

Keilholz U, Goey SH, Punt CJ, Proebstle TM, Salzmann R, Scheibenbogen C, Schadendorf D, Lienard D, Enk A, Dummer R, Hantich B, Geueke AM, Eggermont AM (1997) Interferon alfa-2a and interleukin-2 with or without cisplatin in metastatic melanoma: a randomized trial of the European Organization for Research and Treatment of Cancer Melanoma Cooperative Group. J Clin Oncol 15: 2579–2588

Kimura M, Yoshida Y, Narita M, Takenaga K, Takenouchi T, Yamaguchi T, Saisho H, Sakiyama S, Tagawa M (1999) Acquired immunity in nude mice induced by expression of the IL-2 or IL-4 gene in human pancreatic carcinoma cells and anti-tumor effect generated by in vivo gene transfer using retrovirus. Int J Cancer 82:549–555

Kirkwood JM, Strawderman MH, Ernstoff MS, Smith TJ, Borden EC, Blum RH (1996) Interferon alfa-2b adjuvant therapy of high-risk resected cutaneous melanoma: the Eastern Cooperative Oncology Group Trial EST 1684. J Clin Oncol 14:7–17

Kodama T, Takeda K, Shimozato O, Hayakawa Y, Atsuta M, Kobayashi K, Ito M, Yagita H, Okumura K (1999) Perforindependent NK cell cytotoxicity is sufficient for anti-metastatic effect of IL-12. Eur J Immunol 29:1390–1396

Kontny HU, Lehrnbecher TM, Chanock SJ, Mackall CL (1998) Simultaneous expression of Fas and nonfunctional Fas ligand in Ewing's sarcoma. Cancer Res 58:5842–5849

Kos FJ, Engleman EG (1996) Immune regulation: a critical link between NK cells and CTLs. Immunol Today 17: 174–176

Kovacs CJ, Gooya JM, Harrell JP, McGowan KM, Evans MJ (1991) Altered radioprotective properties of interleukin I alpha (IL-1) in non-hematologic tumor-bearing animals. Int J Radiat Oncol Biol Phys 20:307–310

Kurosawa S, Harada M, Matsuzaki G, Shinomiya Y, Terao H, Kobayashi N, Nomoto K (1995) Early-appearing tumour-infiltrating natural killer cells play a crucial role in the generation of anti-tumour T lymphocytes. Immunology 85:338–346

Kurzawa H, Wysocka M, Aruga E, Chang AE, Trinchieri G, Lee WM (1998) Recombinant interleukin 12 enhances cellular immune responses to vaccination only after a period of suppression. Cancer Res 58:491–499

Lange JR, Raubitschek AA, Pockaj BA, Spencer WF, Lotze MT, Topalian SL, Yang JC, Rosenberg SA (1992) A pilot study of the combination of interleukin-2-based immunotherapy and radiation therapy. J Immunother 12:265–271

Lappin MB, Campbell JD (2000) The Th1-Th2 classification of cellular immune responses: concepts, current thinking and applications in haematological malignancy. Blood Rev 14:228–239

Lee J, Moran JP, Fenton BM, Koch CJ, Frelinger JG, Keng PC, Lord EM (2000) Alteration of tumour response to radiation by interleukin-2 gene transfer. Br J Cancer 82:937–944

Lee S, Zheng M, Deshpande S, Eo SK, Hamilton TA, Rouse BT (2002) IL-12 suppresses the expression of ocular immunoinflammatory lesions by effects on angiogenesis. J Leukoc Biol 71:469–476

Legha SS, Ring S, Bedikian A, Plager C, Eton O, Buzaid AC, Papadopoulos N (1996) Treatment of metastatic melanoma with combined chemotherapy containing cisplatin, vinblastine and dacarbazine (CVD) and biotherapy using interleukin-2 and interferon-alpha. Ann Oncol 7:827–835

Lens MB, Dawes M (2002) Interferon alfa therapy for malignant melanoma: a systematic review of randomized controlled trials. J Clin Oncol 20:1818–1825

Leonard JP, Sherman ML, Fisher GL, Buchanan LJ, Larsen G, Atkins MB, Sosman JA, Dutcher JP, Vogelzang NJ, Ryan JL (1997) Effects of single-dose interleukin-12 exposure on interleukin-12-associated toxicity and interferon-gamma production. Blood 90:2541–2548

Levey DL, Srivastava PK (1995) T cells from late tumor-bearing mice express normal levels of p56lck, p59fyn, ZAP-70, and CD3 zeta despite suppressed cytolytic activity. J Exp Med 182:1029–1036

Levings MK, Sangregorio R, Roncarolo MG (2001) Human cd25(+)cd4(+) t regulatory cells suppress naive and memory T cell proliferation and can be expanded in vitro without loss of function. J Exp Med 193:1295–1302

Lippman SM, Kavanagh JJ, Paredes-Espinoza M, Delgadillo-Madrueno F, Paredes-Casillas P, Hong WK, Massimini G, Holdener EE, Krakoff IH (1993) 13-cis-retinoic acid plus interferon-alpha 2a in locally advanced squamous cell carcinoma of the cervix. J Natl Cancer Inst 85:499–500

Lohr F, Hu K, Haroon Z, Samulski TV, Huang Q, Beaty J, Dewhirst MW, Li CY (2000a) Combination treatment of murine tumors by adenovirus-mediated local B7/IL12 immunotherapy and radiotherapy. Mol Ther 2:195–203

Lohr F, Hu K, Huang Q, Zhang L, Samulski TV, Dewhirst MW, Li CY (2000b) Enhancement of radiotherapy by hyperthermia-regulated gene therapy. Int J Radiat Oncol Biol Phys 48:1513–1518

Lohr F, Huang Q, Hu K, Dewhirst MW, Li CY (2001) Systemic vector leakage and transgene expression by intratumorally injected recombinant adenovirus vectors. Clin Cancer Res 7:3625–3628

Lucey DR (1999) Evolution of the type-1 (Th1)-type-2 (Th2) cytokine paradigm. Infect Dis Clin North Am 13:1–9

Maasilta P, Holsti LR, Halme M, Kivisaari L, Cantell K, Mattson K (1992) Natural alpha-interferon in combination with hyperfractionated radiotherapy in the treatment of non-small cell lung cancer. Int J Radiat Oncol Biol Phys 23:863–868

Mahjoubi R, Bachouchi M, Munck JN, Busson P, Gasmi J, Azli N, Brandely M, Trusz T, Cvitkovic E, Armand JP (1993) Phase II trial of recombinant interferon gamma in refractory undifferentiated carcinoma of the nasopharynx. Head Neck 15:115–118

Malone C, Schiltz PM, Nayak SK, Shea MW, Dillman RO (1999) Combination interferon-alpha2a and 13-cis-retinoic acid enhances radiosensitization of human malignant glioma cells in vitro. Clin Cancer Res 5:417–423

Mason KA, Tofilon PJ (1994) Unexpected radiation protection with 13-cis-retinoic acid plus interferon alpha-2a. Cancer Chemother Pharmacol 33:435–437

McDonald S, Chang AY, Rubin P, Wallenberg J, Kim IS, Sobel S, Smith J, Keng P, Muhs A (1993) Combined Betaseron R (recombinant human interferon beta) and radiation for inoperable non-small cell lung cancer. Int J Radiat Oncol Biol Phys 27:613–619

Medzhitov R, Janeway CA Jr (1997) Innate immunity: the virtues of a nonclonal system of recognition. Cell 91:295–298

Meeren AV, Gaugler MH, Mouthon MA, Squiban C, Gourmelon P (1999) Interleukin 4 promotes survival of lethally irradiated mice in the absence of hematopoietic efficacy. Radiat Res 152:629–636

Melero I, Duarte M, Ruiz J, Sangro B, Galofre J, Mazzolini G, Bustos M, Qian C, Prieto J (1999) Intratumoral injection of bone-marrow-derived dendritic cells engineered to produce interleukin-12 induces complete regression of established murine transplantable colon adenocarcinomas. Gene Ther 6:1779–1784

Meriggioli MN, Rowin J (2000) Chronic inflammatory demyelinating polyneuropathy after treatment with interferon-alpha. Muscle Nerve 23:433–435

Mertens R, Granzen B, Lassay L, Gademann G, Hess CF, Heimann G (1997) Nasopharyngeal carcinoma in childhood and adolescence: concept and preliminary results of the cooperative GPOH study NPC-91. Gesellschaft für Padiatrische Onkologie und Hamatologie. Cancer 80:951–959

Miyamoto Y, Hosotani R, Doi R, Wada M, Ida J, Tsuji S, Kawaguchi M, Nakajima S, Kobayashi H, Masui T, Imamura M (2001) Interleukin-6 inhibits radiation-induced apoptosis in pancreatic cancer cells. Anticancer Res 21:2449–2456

Mizutani N, Fujikura Y, Wang YH, Tamechika M, Tokuda N, Sawada T, Fukumoto T (2002) Inflammatory and anti-inflammatory cytokines regulate the recovery from sublethal X irradiation in rat thymus. Radiat Res 157:281–289

Mollman JE (1992) Neuromuscular toxicity of therapy. Curr Opin Oncol 4:540–546

Moore KW, de Waal Malefyt R, Coffman RL, O'Garra A (2001) Interleukin-10 and the interleukin-10 receptor. Annu Rev Immunol 19:683–765

Morel A, Fernandez N, de La Coste A, Haddada H, Viguier M, Polla BS, Antoine B, Kahn A (1998) Gamma-ray irradiation induces B7.1 costimulatory molecule neoexpression in various murine tumor cells. Cancer Immunol Immunother 46:277–282

Mosmann TR, Cherwinski H, Bond MW, Giedlin MA, Coffman RL (1986) Two types of murine helper T cell clone. I. Definition according to profiles of lymphokine activities and secreted proteins. J Immunol 136:2348–2357

Motzer RJ, Rakhit A, Schwartz LH, Olencki T, Malone TM, Sandstrom K, Nadeau R, Parmar H, Bukowski R (1998) Phase I trial of subcutaneous recombinant human interleukin-12 in patients with advanced renal cell carcinoma. Clin Cancer Res 4:1183–1191

Motzer RJ, Rakhit A, Thompson JA, Nemunaitis J, Murphy BA, Ellerhorst J, Schwartz LH, Berg WJ, Bukowski RM (2001) Randomized multicenter phase II trial of subcutaneous recombinant human interleukin-12 versus interferon-alpha 2a for patients with advanced renal cell carcinoma. J Interferon Cytokine Res 21:257–263

MRC/RCC (1999) Interferon-alpha and survival in metastatic renal carcinoma: early results of a randomised controlled trial. Medical Research Council Renal Cancer Collaborators. Lancet 353:14–17

Murad AM, Oliveira M, Saldanha TM (1994) Phase II trial of isotretinoin and interferon alpha-2a in the treatment of advanced recurrent cervical carcinoma. Int J Gynecol Cancer 4:414–418

Mushegian A, Medzhitov R (2001) Evolutionary perspective on innate immune recognition. J Cell Biol 155:705–710

Myers JN, Yasumura S, Suminami Y, Hirabayashi H, Lin W, Johnson JT, Lotze MT, Whiteside TL (1996) Growth stimulation of human head and neck squamous cell carcinoma cell lines by interleukin 4. Clin Cancer Res 2:127–135

Nanni P, Rossi I, De Giovanni C, Landuzzi L, Nicoletti G, Stoppacciaro A, Parenza M, Colombo MP, Lollini PL (1998) Interleukin 12 gene therapy of MHC-negative murine melanoma metastases. Cancer Res 58:1225–1230

Nasu Y, Bangma CH, Hull GW, Lee HM, Hu J, Wang J, McCurdy MA, Shimura S, Yang G, Timme TL, Thompson TC (1999) Adenovirus-mediated interleukin-12 gene therapy for prostate cancer: suppression of orthotopic tumor growth and pre-established lung metastases in an orthotopic model. Gene Ther 6:338–349

Nathan PD, Gore ME, Eisen TG (2002) Unexpected toxicity of combination thalidomide and interferon alpha-2a treatment in metastatic renal cell carcinoma. J Clin Oncol 20:1429–1430

Neta R, Oppenheim JJ, Wang JM, Snapper CM, Moorman MA, Dubois CM (1994) Synergy of IL-1 and stem cell factor in radioprotection of mice is associated with IL-1 up-regulation of mRNA and protein expression for c-kit on bone marrow cells. J Immunol 153:1536–1543

Nishioka Y, Hirao M, Robbins PD, Lotze MT, Tahara H (1999) Induction of systemic and therapeutic antitumor immunity using intratumoral injection of dendritic cells genetically modified to express interleukin 12. Cancer Res 59:4035–4041

Nishisaka N, Maini A, Kinoshita Y, Yasumoto R, Kishimoto T, Jones RF, Morse P, Hillman GG, Wang CY, Haas GP (1999) Immunotherapy for lung metastases of murine renal cell carcinoma: synergy between radiation and cytokine-producing tumor vaccines. J Immunother 22:308–314

Nishisaka N, Jones RF, Morse P, Kuratsukuri K, Romanowski R, Wang CY, Haas GP (2000) Inhibition of lung metastases of murine renal cell carcinoma by the combination of radiation and interferon-alpha-producing tumor cell vaccine. Cytokines Cell Mol Ther 6:199–206

North RJ, Bursuker I (1984) T cell-mediated suppression of the concomitant antitumor immune response as an example of transplantation tolerance. Transplant Proc 16:463–469

Nukui Y, Picozzi VJ, Traverso LW (2000) Interferon-based adjuvant chemoradiation therapy improves survival after pancreaticoduodenectomy for pancreatic adenocarcinoma. Am J Surg 179:367–371

Oboshi S, Shimosato Y, Itakura K, Umegaky S (1967) Radiation pathology for cancer II: the immunological significance of the infiltration of lymphocytes surrounding the tumor tissue during irradiation. Igakunoyumi 61:725–730

Ochsenbein AF, Sierro S, Odermatt B, Pericin M, Karrer U, Hermans J, Hemmi S, Hengartner H, Zinkernagel RM (2001) Roles of tumour localization, second signals and cross priming in cytotoxic T-cell induction. Nature 411:1058–1064

O'Connell J, Bennett MW, O'Sullivan GC, Collins JK, Shanahan F (1999) Fas counter-attack – the best form of tumor defense? Nat Med 5:267–268

Ogawa Y, Nishioka A, Kubonishi II, Inomata T, Yoshida S, Kataoka S (1998) Cytotoxicity of Fas ligand against lymphoma cells with radiation-induced Fas antigen. Int J Mol Med 2:435–436

Olkowski ZL (1999) Functional response of human natural killer (NK) cells to ionizing radiation. Int J Radiat Oncol Biol Phys 45:282–283

O'Shea JJ, Ma A, Lipsky P (2002) Cytokines and autoimmunity. Nat Rev Immunol 2:37–45

Ostrand-Rosenberg S, Gunther V, Armstrong T, Pulaski B, Pipeling M, Clements V, Namouse-Smith N (1999) Immunologic targets for the gene therapy of cancer. In: Lattime EC, Gerson SL (eds) Gene therapy of cancer. Academic Press, New York

Oyama T, Ran S, Ishida T, Nadaf S, Kerr L, Carbone DP, Gabrilovich DI (1998) Vascular endothelial growth factor affects dendritic cell maturation through the inhibition of nuclear factor-kappa B activation in hemopoietic progenitor cells. J Immunol 160:1224–1232

Packer RJ, Prados M, Phillips P, Nicholson HS, Boyett JM, Goldwein J, Rorke LB, Needle MN, Sutton L, Zimmerman RA, Fitz CR, Vezina LG, Etcubanas E, Wallenberg JC, Reaman G, Wara W (1996) Treatment of children with newly diagnosed brain stem gliomas with intravenous recombinant beta-interferon and hyperfractionated radiation therapy: a children's cancer group phase I/II study. Cancer 77:2150–2156

Pardoll DM, Topalian SL (1998) The role of CD4+ T cell responses in antitumor immunity. Curr Opin Immunol 10:588–594

Park TK, Lee JP, Kim SN, Choi SM, Kudelka AP, Kavanagh JJ (1998) Interferon-alpha 2a, 13-cis-retinoic acid and radiotherapy for locally advanced carcinoma of the cervix: a pilot study. Eur J Gynaecol Oncol 19:35–38

Patchen ML, MacVittie TJ, Williams JL, Schwartz GN, Souza LM (1991) Administration of interleukin-6 stimulates multilineage hematopoiesis and accelerates recovery from radiation-induced hematopoietic depression. Blood 77:472–480

Pham-Nguyen KB, Yang W, Saxena R, Thung SN, Woo SL, Chen SH (1999) Role of NK and T cells in IL-12-induced anti-tumor response against hepatic colon carcinoma. Int J Cancer 81:813–819

Puisieux I, Odin L, Poujol D, Moingeon P, Tartaglia J, Cox W, Favrot M (1998) Canarypox virus-mediated interleukin 12 gene transfer into murine mammary adenocarcinoma induces tumor suppression and long-term antitumoral immunity. Hum Gene Ther 9:2481–2492

Radbruch A (2001) Immunsystem und Immunität (German). In: Zeidler H, Zacher J, Hiepe F (eds) Interdisziplinäre klinische Rheumatologie. Springer, Berlin Heidelberg New York, pp 4–25

Raju U, Gumin GJ, Tofilon PJ (1999) NF kappa B activity and target gene expression in the rat brain after one and two exposures to ionizing radiation. Radiat Oncol Invest 7:145–152

Ratto GB, Zino P, Mirabelli S, Minuti P, Aquilina R, Fantino G, Spessa E, Ponte M, Bruzzi P, Melioli G (1996) A randomized trial of adoptive immunotherapy with tumor-infiltrating lymphocytes and interleukin-2 versus standard therapy in the postoperative treatment of resected nonsmall cell lung carcinoma. Cancer 78:244–251

Redman BG, Hillman GG, Flaherty L, Forman J, Dezso B, Haas GP (1998) Phase II trial of sequential radiation and interleukin 2 in the treatment of patients with metastatic renal cell carcinoma. Clin Cancer Res 4:283–286

Restifo N, Kawakami Y, Marincola F et al (1993) Molecular mechanisms used by tumors to escape immune recognition: immunotherapy and the cell biology of major histocompatibility complex I. J Immunother 14:182–190

Roberts JL, Sharrow SO, Singer A (1990) Clonal deletion and clonal anergy in the thymus induced by cellular elements with different radiation sensitivities. J Exp Med 171:935–940

Rosenberg SA, Yannelli JR, Yang JC, Topalian SL, Schwartzentruber DJ, Weber JS, Parkinson DR, Seipp CA, Einhorn JH, White DE (1994) Treatment of patients with metastatic melanoma with autologous tumor-infiltrating lymphocytes and interleukin 2. J Natl Cancer Inst 86:1159–1166

Rosenberg SA, Yang JC, Schwartzentruber DJ, Hwu P, Marincola FM, Topalian SL, Seipp CA, Einhorn JH, White DE, Steinberg SM (1999) Prospective randomized trial of the treatment of patients with metastatic melanoma using chemotherapy with cisplatin, dacarbazine, and tamoxifen alone or in combination with interleukin-2 and interferon alfa-2b. J Clin Oncol 17:968–975

Roth C, Rochlitz C, Kourilsky P (1994) Immune response against tumors. Adv Immunol 57:281–351

Rübe C, Finke C, van Valen F, Schafer KL, Dockhorn-Dworniczak B, Willich N (1997) The demonstration of the radiation-induced production of tumor necrosis factor-alpha in Ewing's sarcoma RM 82 in vitro and in vivo. Strahlenther Onkol 173:407–414

Sad S, Marcotte R, Mosmann TR (1995) Cytokine-induced differentiation of precursor mouse CD8+ T cells into cytotoxic CD8+ T cells secreting Th1 or Th2 cytokines. Immunity 2:271–279

Safwat A (2000) The immunobiology of low-dose total-body irradiation: more questions than answers. Radiat Res 153:599–604

Santin A, Hermonat P, Ravaggi A, Chiriva-Internati M, Hiserodt J, Batchus R, Barclay D, Pecorelli S, Parham G (1998) The effects of irradiation on the expression of a tumor rejection antigen (heat shock protein gp96) in human cervical cancer. Int J Radiat Biol 73:699–704

Sareneva T, Julkunen I, Matikainen S (2000) IFN-alpha and IL-12 induce IL-18 receptor gene expression in human NK and T cells. J Immunol 165:1933–1938

Scanlan MJ, Chen YT, Williamson B, Gure AO, Stockert E, Gordan JD, Tureci O, Sahin U, Pfreundschuh M, Old LJ (1998) Characterization of human colon cancer antigens recognized by autologous antibodies. Int J Cancer 76:652–658

Schiller JH, Pugh M, Kirkwood JM, Karp D, Larson M, Borden E (1996) Eastern cooperative group trial of interferon gamma in metastatic melanoma: an innovative study design. Clin Cancer Res 2:29–36

Schmidberger H, Rave-Frank M, Lehmann J, Schweinfurth S, Rehring E, Henckel K, Hess CF (1999) The combined effect of interferon beta and radiation on five human tumor cell lines and embryonal lung fibroblasts. Int J Radiat Oncol Biol Phys 43:405–412

Schrijvers D, Johnson J, Jiminez U, Gore M, Kosmidis P, Szpirglas H, Robbins K, Oliveira J, Lewensohn R, Schuller J, Riviere A, Arvay C, Langecker P, Jacob H, Cvitkovic E, Vokes E (1998) Phase III trial of modulation of cisplatin/fluorouracil chemotherapy by interferon alfa-2b in patients with recurrent or metastatic head and neck cancer. Head and Neck Interferon Cooperative Study Group. J Clin Oncol 16:1054–1059

Schwartz RH (1990) A cell culture model for T lymphocyte clonal anergy. Science 248:1349–1356

Seetharam S, Staba MJ, Schumm LP, Schreiber K, Schreiber H, Kufe DW, Weichselbaum RR (1999) Enhanced eradication of local and distant tumors by genetically produced interleukin-12 and radiation. Int J Oncol 15:769–773

Seliger B, Harders C, Lohmann S, Momburg F, Urlinger S, Tampe R, Huber C (1998) Down-regulation of the MHC class I antigen-processing machinery after oncogenic transformation of murine fibroblasts. Eur J Immunol 28:122–133

Shaw EG, Deming RL, Creagan ET, Nair S, Su JQ, Levitt R, Steen PD, Wiesenfeld M, Mailliard JA (1995) Pilot study of human recombinant interferon gamma and accelerated hyperfractionated thoracic radiation therapy in patients with unresectable stage IIIA/B nonsmall cell lung cancer. Int J Radiat Oncol Biol Phys 31:827–831

Shibata T, Akiyama N, Noda M, Sasai K, Hiraoka M (1998) Enhancement of gene expression under hypoxic conditions using fragments of the human vascular endothelial growth factor and the erythropoietin genes. Int J Radiat Oncol Biol Phys 42:913–916

Shin DM, Glisson BS, Khuri FR, Clifford JL, Clayman G, Benner SE, Forastiere AA, Ginsberg L, Liu D, Lee JJ, Myers J, Goepfert H, Lotan R, Hong WK, Lippman SM (2002) Phase II and biologic study of interferon alfa, retinoic acid, and cisplatin in advanced squamous skin cancer. J Clin Oncol 20:364–370

Shresta S, Pham CT, Thomas DA, Graubert TA, Ley TJ (1998) How do cytotoxic lymphocytes kill their targets? Curr Opin Immunol 10:581–587

Siefker-Radtke AO, Millikan RE, Tu SM, Moore DF Jr, Smith TL, Williams D, Logothetis CJ (2002) Phase III trial of fluorouracil, interferon alpha-2b, and cisplatin versus methotrexate, vinblastine, doxorubicin, and cisplatin in metastatic or unresectable urothelial cancer. J Clin Oncol 20:1361–1367

Sornasse T, Larenas PV, Davis KA, de Vries JE, Yssel H (1996) Differentiation and stability of T helper 1 and 2 cells derived from naive human neonatal CD4+ T cells, analyzed at the single-cell level. J Exp Med 184:473–483

Srivastava P (2002) Roles of heat-shock proteins in innate and adaptive immunity. Nat Rev Immunol 2:185–194

Staveley-O'Carroll K, Sotomayor E, Montgomery J, Borrello I, Hwang L, Fein S, Pardoll D, Levitsky H (1998) Induction of antigen-specific T cell anergy: an early event in the course of tumor progression. Proc Natl Acad Sci U S A 95:1178–1183

Steinbrink K, Jonuleit H, Muller G, Schuler G, Knop J, Enk AH (1999) Interleukin-10-treated human dendritic cells induce a melanoma-antigen-specific anergy in CD8(+) T cells resulting in a failure to lyse tumor cells. Blood 93:1634–1642

Strasly M, Cavallo F, Geuna M, Mitola S, Colombo MP, Forni G, Bussolino F (2001) IL-12 inhibition of endothelial cell functions and angiogenesis depends on lymphocyte-endothelial cell cross-talk. J Immunol 166:3890–3899

Sun Y, Jurgovsky K, Moller P, Alijagic S, Dorbic T, Georgieva J, Wittig B, Schadendorf D (1998) Vaccination with IL-12 gene-modified autologous melanoma cells: preclinical results and a first clinical phase I study. Gene Ther 5:481–490

Sun Y, Paschen A, Schadendorf D (1999) Cell-based vaccination against melanoma – background, preliminary results, and perspective. J Mol Med 77:593–608

Suto R, Srivastava PK (1995) A mechanism for the specific immunogenicity of heat shock protein-chaperoned peptides. Science 269:1585–1588

Takagi A, Imai A, Horibe S, Ohno T, Tamaya T (1998) Lack of evidence for expression of Fas ligand in Fas-bearing tumors. Oncol Rep 5:377–380

Takeuchi T, Ueki T, Sasaki Y, Kajiwara T, Li B, Moriyama N, Kawabe K (1997) Th2-like response and antitumor effect of anti-interleukin-4 mAb in mice bearing renal cell carcinoma. Cancer Immunol Immunother 43:375–381

Tamura Y, Peng P, Liu K, Daou M, Srivastava PK (1997) Immunotherapy of tumors with autologous tumor-derived heat shock protein preparations. Science 278:117–120

Taylor PA, Noelle RJ, Blazar BR (2001) CD4(+)CD25(+) immune regulatory cells are required for induction of tolerance to alloantigen via costimulatory blockade. J Exp Med 193:1311–1318

Teicher BA, Ara G, Buxton D, Leonard J, Schaub RG (1998) Optimal scheduling of interleukin-12 and fractionated radiation therapy in the murine Lewis lung carcinoma. Radiat Oncol Invest 6:71–80

Thomas R, Stea B (2002) Radiation recall dermatitis from high-dose interferon alfa-2b. J Clin Oncol 20:355–357

Tisch M, Heimlich F, Daniel V, Opelz G, Maier H (1998) Cellular immune defect caused by postsurgical radiation therapy in patients with head and neck cancer. Otolaryngol Head Neck Surg 119:412–417

Todryk S, Melcher AA, Hardwick N, Linardakis E, Bateman A, Colombo MP, Stoppacciaro A, Vile RG (1999) Heat shock protein 70 induced during tumor cell killing induces Th1 cytokines and targets immature dendritic cell precursors to enhance antigen uptake. J Immunol 163:1398–1408

Toma S, Palumbo R, Vincenti M, Aitini E, Paganini G, Pronzato P, Grimaldi A, Rosso R (1994) Efficacy of recombinant alpha-interferon 2a and 13-cis-retinoic acid in the treatment of squamous cell carcinoma. Ann Oncol 5:463–465

Torrisi J, Berg C, Harter K, Lvovsky E, Yeung K, Woolley P, Bonnem E, Dritschilo A (1986) Phase I combined modality clinical trial of alpha-2-interferon and radiotherapy. Int J Radiat Oncol Biol Phys 12:1453–1456

Tourani JM, Pfister C, Berdah JF, Benhammouda A, Salze P, Monnier A, Paule B, Guillet P, Chretien Y, Brewer Y, Di Palma M, Untereiner M, Malaurie E, Tadrist Z, Pavlovitch JM, Hauteville D, Mejean A, Azagury M, Mayeur D, Lucas V, Krakowski I, Larregain-Fournier D, Abourachid H, Andrieu JM, Chastang C (1998) Outpatient treatment with subcutaneous interleukin-2 and interferon alfa administration in combination with fluorouracil in patients with metastatic renal cell carcinoma: results of a sequential nonrandomized phase II study. Subcutaneous Administration Proleukin Program Cooperative Group. J Clin Oncol 16:2505–2513

Townsend SE, Allison JP (1993) Tumor rejection after direct costimulation of CD8+ T cells by B7- transfected melanoma cells. Science 259:368–370

Treuner J, Niethammer D, Dannecker G, Hagmann R, Neef V, Hofschneider PH (1980) Successful treatment of nasopharyngeal carcinoma with interferon. Lancet 1:817–818

Van der Meeren A, Monti P, Lebaron-Jacobs L, Marquette C, Gourmelon P (2001) Characterization of the acute inflammatory response after irradiation in mice and its regulation by interleukin 4 (Il4). Radiat Res 155:858–865

Van Elsas A, Hurwitz AA, Allison JP (1999) Combination immunotherapy of B16 melanoma using anti-cytotoxic T lymphocyte-associated antigen 4 (CTLA-4) and granulocyte/macrophage colony-stimulating factor (GM-CSF)-producing vaccines induces rejection of subcutaneous and metastatic tumors accompanied by autoimmune depigmentation. J Exp Med 190:355–366

Van Herpen CM, Jansen RL, Kruit WH, Hoekman K, Groenewegen G, Osanto S, De Mulder PH (2000) Immunochemotherapy with interleukin-2, interferon-alpha and 5-fluorouracil for progressive metastatic renal cell carcinoma: a multicenter phase II study. Dutch Immunotherapy Working Party. Br J Cancer 82:772–776

Veenstra KG, Jonak ZL, Trulli S, Gollob JA (2002) IL-12 induces monocyte IL-18 binding protein expression via IFN-gamma. J Immunol 168:2282–2287

Velders MP, Schreiber H, Kast WM (1998) Active immunization against cancer cells: impediments and advances. Semin Oncol 25:697–706

Verastegui-Aviles E, Mohar A, Mota A, Guadarrama A, De La Garza-Salazar J (1999) Combination of radiation therapy and interferon alpha-2b in patients with advanced cervical carcinoma: a pilot study. Int J Gynecol Cancer 9:401–405

Voest EE, Kenyon BM, O'Reilly MS, Truitt G, D'Amato RJ, Folkman J (1995) Inhibition of angiogenesis in vivo by interleukin 12. J Natl Cancer Inst 87:581–586

Vokes EE (1994) The promise of biochemical modulation in combined modality therapy. Semin Oncol 21:29–33

Waddick KG, Finnegan DM, Chelstrom LM, Uckun FM (1995) In vivo radiosensitizing effects of recombinant interleukin 6 on radiation resistant BCL-1 B-lineage leukemia cells in a murine syngeneic bone marrow transplant model system. Leuk Lymph 19:121–128

Wang C, Quevedo ME, Lannutti BJ, Gordon KB, Guo D, Sun W, Paller AS (1999) In vivo gene therapy with interleukin-12 inhibits primary vascular tumor growth and induces apoptosis in a mouse model. J Invest Dermatol 112:775–781

Weiss GR, Liu PY, Alberts DS, Peng YM, Fisher E, Xu MJ, Scudder SA, Baker LH Jr, Moore DF, Lippman SM (1998) 13-cis-retinoic acid or all-trans-retinoic acid plus interferon-alpha in recurrent cervical cancer: a Southwest Oncology Group phase II randomized trial. Gynecol Oncol 71:386–390

Windbichler GH, Hensler E, Widschwendter M, Posch A, Daxenbichler G, Fritsch E, Marth C (1996) Increased radiosensitivity by a combination of 9-cis-retinoic acid and interferon-y in breast cancer cells. Gynecol Oncol 61:387–394

Yamamoto T, Yoneda K, Ueta E, Doi S, Osaki T (2000) Enhanced apoptosis of squamous cell carcinoma cells by interleukin-2-activated cytotoxic lymphocytes combined with radiation and anticancer drugs. Eur J Cancer 36:2007–2017

Yamaoka J, Kabashima K, Kawanishi M, Toda K, Miyachi Y (2002) Cytotoxicity of IFN-gamma and TNF-alpha for vascular endothelial cell is mediated by nitric oxide. Biochem Biophys Res Commun 291:780–786

Yamashita T, Mizukoshi T, Tomita K, Kobayashi H (1987) Antitumor immunity and tumor metastases as influenced by the radiation dosage in local radiotherapy. Gan No Rinsho 33:1205–1210

Younes E, Haas GP, Dezso B, Ali E, Maughan RL, Kukuruga MA, Montecillo E, Pontes JE, Hillman GG (1995a) Local tumor irradiation augments the response to IL-2 therapy in a murine renal adenocarcinoma. Cell Immunol 165: 243–251

Younes E, Haas GP, Dezso B, Ali E, Maughan RL, Montecillo E, Pontes JE, Hillman GG (1995b) Radiation-induced effects on murine kidney tumor cells: role in the interaction of local irradiation and immunotherapy. J Urol 153: 2029–2033

Yue FY, Geertsen R, Hemmi S, Burg G, Pavlovic J, Laine E, Dummer R (1999) IL-12 directly up-regulates the expression of HLA class I, HLA class II and ICAM-1 on human melanoma cells: a mechanism for its antitumor activity? Eur J Immunol 29:1762–1773

Zucali JR, Moreb J, Gibbons W, Alderman J, Suresh A, Zhang Y, Shelby B (1994) Radioprotection of hematopoietic stem cells by interleukin-1. Exp Hematol 22:130–135

17 Enhancement of Radiation Response with TNF/TRAIL

A. MUNSHI and R. E. MEYN

CONTENTS

17.1 Introduction 227
17.2 Death Receptors and Their Ligands 228
17.2.1 Members of the TNF Family 228
17.2.2 Death Receptor Signaling 230
17.3 TNF and Radiation 232
17.4 TRAIL and Radiation 234
References 238

17.1 Introduction

Radiotherapy continues to play an important role in the treatment of cancer and, currently, about one-half of all cancer patients receive radiotherapy as part of the overall management of their disease. Radiotherapy is especially useful in controlling local-regional cancer and notable improvements have been made in recent years that involve combinations with chemotherapy, altered fractionation schemes, and conformal radiation delivery. However, despite these important innovations, an unacceptable proportion of patients still die of local-regional disease progression and additional improvements are sorely needed. One explanation for these failures is that some tumors appear to be resistant to doses of radiation as high as 75–80 Gy. Even with conformal therapy, it may be difficult to escalate the dose much beyond these levels without increasing the probability of late normal tissue complications. Thus, strategies for sensitizing tumor cells to radiation must be considered. Advances in our understanding of the molecular and cellular biology of cancer offer a broad range of possible radiosensitizing approaches. One approach that has been examined over the last several years has been to restore the mode of cell death known as apoptosis in irradiated tumors.

Apoptosis is a genetically programmed and physiological mode of cell death that results in the elimination of unwanted cells (WYLLIE et al. 1980). It is characterized by a number of unique features that include cell shrinkage, chromatin condensation and fragmentation of the cell into apoptotic bodies (KERR et al. 1972). In addition to its central role during development and in maintenance of homeostasis in adult tissues, apoptosis occurs following exposure to genotoxic agents such as chemotherapeutic agents and radiation (THOMPSON 1995). Apoptosis is also a critically important pathway for physiologically regulating the presence of certain cells in the immune system (KRAMMER 2000). Here, one of the principal mechanisms for mediating apoptosis is through interaction of "death receptors" on the cell surface with their respective and specific "death ligands" (ASHKENAZI and DIXIT 1998). The death ligands belong to the tumor necrosis factor (TNF) family of proteins. Once the death receptor on the cell surface is activated by its ligand, apoptosis is mediated through intracellular processes that are at least partially shared by chemotherapy agent- or radiation-induced apoptosis (EL-DEIRY 2001).

In the case of radiation-induced apoptosis, the initial lesion produced in the cell by the radiation that triggers apoptosis has not been clearly defined. However, reactive oxygen species that damage cellular components such as the plasma membrane or DNA have been implicated (HAIMOVITZ-FRIEDMAN et al. 1994; WARD 1988). The importance of apoptosis in tumor response to radiotherapy has been debated. Some reports have suggested that apoptosis is not a major pathway in tumor response (STEEL 2001) whereas other studies have correlated the radioresponsiveness of tumors with the respective levels of apoptosis following the treatment (MEYN et al. 1993). Regardless, it has been noted that most tumors do not display a robust apoptotic response to radiation

A. MUNSHI, MD
Instructor, The University of Texas M.D. Anderson Cancer Center, 1515 Holcombe Blvd., Box 66, Houston, TX 77030, USA
R. E. MEYN, PhD
Kathryn O'Connor Research Professor, The University of Texas M.D. Anderson Cancer Center, 1515 Holcombe Blvd., Box 66, Houston, TX 77030, USA

and, thus, strategies for enhancing radiation-induced apoptosis through genetic manipulation or gene therapy have been tested. Many of these studies have demonstrated that enhancing the apoptotic response leads to an enhanced tumor response to radiotherapy (RUPNOW et al. 1998; SPITZ et al. 1996). In a similar context, several laboratories have investigated whether the combination of apoptosis-inducing death ligands of the TNF family would synergize with radiation to enhance the apoptotic response leading to an enhanced tumor response. The purpose of this chapter is to review the status of these efforts.

17.2
Death Receptors and Their Ligands

17.2.1
Members of the TNF Family

The TNF family of genes continues to grow as new members are identified but comprises a series of death ligands and their associated death receptors (SINGH et al. 1998). The receptors are type I transmembrane proteins that share sequence homology in the cysteine-rich, extracellular domain and contain in their cytoplasmic domain a region termed the "death domain" (Fig. 17.1). The ligands trimerize and induce receptor trimerization upon binding. Once activated, the receptors recruit death-domain-containing adaptor molecules that interact with the death domain of the receptor (ASHKENAZI and DIXIT 1998). These adaptor proteins then engage the downstream effectors of the apoptosis pathway. Although there are several known TNF family members, this review will focus on the three that have been studied in detail. These are TNFα, Fas ligand (FasL), and tumor necrosis factor-related apoptosis-inducing ligand (TRAIL).

TNF-α, the prototypic member of this family, was identified many years ago on the basis of its antitumor activity (CARSWELL et al. 1975). It is now known to have a number of important activities in addition to inducing apoptosis. It mediates the inflammatory response, regulates certain aspects of immune function, and has antiviral activity. Aberrant TNF-α production has been associated with cachexia, respiratory distress syndrome, certain autoimmune diseases and septic shock (BEUTLER and CERAMI 1988). TNF-α is primarily produced by activated macrophages and interacts with its target cell through two specific cell surface receptors, TNF-R1 and TNF-R2. Most of TNF-α's biological effects appear to be mediated through the TNF-R1 receptor (CHEN and GOEDDEL 2002). Following engagement of the receptor, the intracellular death domain of TNF-R1 interacts with its associated death-domain-containing adapter protein, TNF receptor-associated death domain (TRADD) (ASHKENAZI and DIXIT 1998). Though TNF-α is cytotoxic to a number of tumor cell lines in vitro, several lines are resistant to the apoptotic effects of TNF-α. This resistance can, however, be overcome by the addition of protein synthesis inhibitors, suggesting the existence of some cellular proteins that may act to suppress the apoptotic signaling induced by this death ligand (SHEIKH and FORNACE 2000; WONG et al. 1989).

The cell surface death receptor Fas (also known as APO-1 and CD95) was simultaneously discovered in two independent laboratories in 1989 (TRAUTH et al. 1989; YONEHARA et al. 1989). Apoptosis is triggered through engagement of Fas receptor by its specific ligand FasL (CD95L) (SUDA et al. 1993). Similar to TNF-α, the intracellular domain of Fas then recruits its appropriate adapter protein called Fas-associ-

Fig. 17.1. TNF family members: death receptors and death ligands ated death domain (FADD) (ASHKENAZI and DIXIT 1998; WALCZAK and KRAMMER 2000). Fas receptor is expressed by a wide variety of normal cells in addition to many types of tumor cell lines. FasL is naturally expressed on the surface of activated cytotoxic T lymphocytes and natural killer (NK) cells (ASHKENAZI and DIXIT 1998; FRIESEN et al. 1999). Cell stress induces Fas expression leading to apoptosis, suggesting that one physiological role for this death-receptor–ligand interaction is the elimination of damaged cells. The Fas–FasL system is also involved in the deletion of unwanted T and B cells and mutations in the genes for Fas or FasL can lead to serious autoimmune syndromes (FISHER et al. 1995). In the liver, it participates in maintaining liver homeostasis and, therefore, FasL can not be administered systemically as a cancer therapeutic in vivo because it is extremely hepatotoxic (NAGATA 1997; WALCZAK and KRAMMER 2000). Some tumors may avoid immune surveillance by triggering apoptosis of tumor-reactive immune cells through the constitutive expression of FasL on their surface. In this regard, it is interesting to note that several laboratories have reported the up-regulation of Fas and FasL in tumor cells following treatment with ionizing radiation, suggesting that activation of the Fas–FasL system may participate in the killing of tumor cells by radiation (BELKA et al. 1998; FULDA et al. 1998; REAP et al. 1997). Although this may occur in irradiated tumors, it is difficult to envision a strategy for taking advantage of this effect to enhance tumor radiation response in vivo based on the profound liver toxicity of FasL. Thus, the Fas–FasL system will not be discussed further in this article in the context of its therapeutic implications.

TRAIL, also referred to as APO-2L, is the most recently discovered member of the TNF family and was identified independently by two groups based on its sequence homology to other members of the TNF family (PITTI et al. 1996; WILEY et al. 1995). Similar to TNF-α and FasL, TRAIL is expressed in a variety of cell types, including cells of the hematopoietic system (FIUMARA and YOUNES 2001). TRAIL forms a soluble ligand when its extracellular domain is cleaved from the membrane by metalloproteases (HELD and SCHULZE-OSTHOFF 2001). It is now well established that both membrane-bound and soluble forms of TRAIL can signal apoptosis. The normal role of TRAIL is not understood. Some reports suggest that TRAIL is involved in T-cell-mediated cytotoxicity (FIUMARA and YOUNES 2001; HELD and SCHULZE-OSTHOFF 2001). However, in contrast to TNF-α and FasL, TRAIL has a high degree of specificity for transformed cells over normal cells (FRENCH and TSCHOPP 1999). Indeed, recombinant TRAIL protein has been tested as a therapeutic in SCID mice bearing xenograft tumors derived from human tumor cell lines (ASHKENAZI et al. 1999; WALCZAK et al. 1999). The tumors regressed following IP injection of TRAIL but no toxicity of normal tissues was observed. The initial hypothesis to explain this finding was based on possible differences in expression of TRAIL receptors. There are five known receptors for TRAIL: these are known as DR4 (TRAIL-R1), DR5 (TRAIL-R2), DcR1 (TRAIL-R3), DcR2 (TRAIL-R4), and osteoprotegerin (OPG) (FIUMARA and YOUNES 2001). DR4 and DR5 are fully functional, having complete death domains in their intracellular portions. DcR1 and DcR2 lack or have an incomplete death domain, respectively (Fig. 17.2), and are referred to as decoy receptors (ASHKENAZI and DIXIT 1998; HELD and SCHULZE-OSTHOFF 2001). The OPG receptor is shared with another ligand known as RANK (FIUMARA and YOUNES 2001). Initially, it was thought that normal cells may either lack the expression of DR4 and/or DR5 or, alternatively, would express high levels of the decoy receptors when compared to tumor cells, and this might act to prevent engagement of TRAIL with the active receptors. This idea has not held up on further examination of receptor expression across many different tumor and normal cells and it is now believed that cells that are resistant to the apoptosis-inducing effects of TRAIL have blocks to TRAIL signaling downstream of receptor engagement (FIUMARA and YOUNES 2001). The specificity of TRAIL for transformed cells was recently questioned in a report demonstrating toxicity of TRAIL for human liver cells (JO et al. 2000). However, it appears that the toxicity of recombinant TRAIL for liver cells is highly dependent on the technique used to produce trimerization and formulations designed for clinical use are not hepatotoxic (LAWRENCE et al. 2001). TRAIL is very similar to TNF-α and FasL with regard to the intracellular signaling pathway stimulated upon receptor engagement. In fact, it appears to use the same adapter protein, FADD, as is used by Fas. The role of FADD as the adaptor molecule used by TRAIL has been controversial in the past; however, the consensus now is that FADD serves this purpose. The existence of other adaptor proteins that may be used by TRAIL upon receptor engagement have not been rued out (PETER 2000). Thus, of the three death receptor–ligand systems discussed above, TRAIL appears to be the most promising as a single agent for cancer therapy due to its differential cytotoxicity for transformed cells compared to normal cells (NAGANE et al. 2001). This promise must ultimately be proven in clinical trials.

Fig. 17.2. Scheme of TRAIL-activated apoptosis signaling. *TRAIL*, tumor necrosis factor-related apoptosis-inducing ligand; *c-FLIP*, FLICE-like inhibitory protein; *FADD*, Fas-associated death domain

17.2.2
Death Receptor Signaling

All three death receptor–ligand systems introduced in the preceding section signal apoptosis in a very similar if not identical manner. In order to ascertain how death receptor–ligand interactions may act to enhance radiation response, it is important to understand the signaling pathway through which these ligands stimulate apoptosis and how that pathway intersects with the apoptotic pathway stimulated by ionizing radiation. Independent of the specific stimulus, apoptosis, once signaled, is universally mediated intracellularly by a cascade of proteolytic events (HENGARTNER 2000). A series of cysteine proteases called caspases carry out these steps. At least 14 different caspases have been identified in mammalian cells thus far (THORNBERRY and LAZEBNIK 1998). Prior to the induction of apoptosis, these caspases exist in the cell as inactive proenzymes and, upon apoptotic stimulus, they are proteolytically cleaved into active units. Two different subunits are formed from the proenzyme and they associate to create a heterodimeric complex that is the active form of the enzyme (HENGARTNER 2000). The caspases are divided into two groups depending on whether they are involved in the initiation of apoptosis, whereby they are called initiator caspases, or are activated by the initiator caspases to carry out downstream degradation of other cellular proteins, which, when cleaved, produce the morphological features of apoptosis (THORNBERRY and LAZEBNIK 1998). These latter caspases are known as effector caspases. Caspase 3 is the prototypic member of the family of caspases since it was one of the first to be shown to have a role in apoptosis. As it happens, caspase 3 actually plays a very central role in apoptosis and it is generally considered that, once caspase 3 is activated by processing of its pro-caspase form, apoptosis is irreversible after that point in time.

Caspase 3 is an effector caspase that can be activated by two different initiator caspases, caspases 8 and 9 (BUDIHARDJO et al. 1999). Caspases 8 and 9 reside in two ostensibly different apoptotic pathways referred to as the receptor-mediated (or extrinsic) and the mitochondrial-mediated (or intrinsic) pathways, respectively (Fig. 17.3). As the names imply, apoptosis is initiated in these pathways either at the level of a cell surface receptor, namely one of the three described in Sec. 17.2.1, "Members of the TNF Family" or through signals generated in the cell's mitochondria (BUDIHARDJO et al. 1999). These two pathways will be described separately. The receptor-mediated pathway is activated when, following engagement of

Fig. 17.3. Pathways of receptor-mediated and mitochondrial-mediated apoptosis

the receptor with its specific ligand, the death domain of the intracellular portion of the receptor molecule associates with its appropriate death-domain-containing adapter protein. In the case of Fas and the active TRAIL receptors, FADD is the adapter protein (Ashkenazi and Dixit 1998; Daniel 2000; Walczak and Krammer 2000). In the case of TNF-R1, the primary adapter protein is TRADD; however, FADD in turn associates with TRADD and becomes a secondary adapter protein for this receptor as well (Ashkenazi and Dixit 1998). In addition to its death domain, FADD also contains a death effector domain that is similar to a domain found in the proenzyme form of caspase 8. Thus, pro-caspase 8 is recruited to this complex of the receptor and FADD causing caspase 8 oligomerization and activation by self-cleavage (Daniel 2000). This complex with pro-caspase 8 is referred to as a death-inducing signaling complex or DISC (Kischkel et al. 1995). Caspase 8, once activated at the DISC, in turn activates caspase 3 by cleaving pro-caspase 3. This entire process has been defined in more detail than is mentioned here and several additional proteins are involved in this process. Some of these activate other signal transduction pathways such as NF-kB, whereas others may negatively regulate DISC function (Ashkenazi and Dixit 1998). One of these latter proteins is especially critical in this regard, namely cellular FLICE-like inhibitory protein (c-FLIP) (Irmler et al. 1997). It has been shown that c-FLIP has potent inhibitory effects and its expression or the expression of other similar molecules may explain why different types of cells have different sensitivities to death-receptor-mediated apoptosis (Irisarri et al. 2000; Walczak and Krammer 2000).

In the mitochondria-mediated or intrinsic pathway of apoptosis, caspase activation occurs as a direct result of severe perturbations in mitochondrial metabolism (Green and Reed 1998). This appears to be initiated through damage to or alterations of the mitochondrial membranes. In irradiated cells, these alterations may be produced by reactive oxygen species or triggered by signals originating from the nucleus in response to the DNA damage induced by radiation (Coultas and Strasser 2000; Rich et al. 2000). It seems highly probable that the p53 tumor suppressor gene participates in this latter mechanism (El-Deiry 2001; Sheikh and Fornace 2000). Alternatively, radiation may directly damage the plasma membrane resulting in the release of ceramide (Haimovitz-Friedman et al. 1994). Ceramide, once released into the cytoplasm, is able to directly damage mitochondrial membranes to stimulate the initiation of apoptosis (Loeffler and

Kroemer 2000; Zhivotovsky et al. 1999). Once the signal for apoptosis is perceived at the level of the mitochondrial membranes, mitochondrial metabolism is disrupted and a number of critical events take place that involve loss of the mitochondrial transmembrane potential and the release of proteins from the mitochondria (Loeffler and Kroemer 2000). One of these proteins that is critically involved with mediating downstream events is cytochrome c (Liu et al. 1996). Cytochrome c, once released from the mitochondria, then interacts with a protein complex comprised of pro-caspase 9 and its cofactor called Apaf-1 (Green and Reed 1998). This interaction leads to the activation of caspase 9 via a conformational change in the protein (Hengartner 2000). Pro-caspase 3 is a substrate for caspase 9 and, thus, mitochondrial-mediated apoptosis and receptor-mediated apoptosis both converge at activation of caspase 3 as their common downstream step.

The mitochondrial-mediated apoptotic pathway is tightly regulated by members of the Bcl-2 family of proteins (Adams and Cory 1998). A complete discussion of this family of proteins is beyond the scope of this chapter but basically it is comprised of pro-apoptotic members such as Bax and Bak and anti-apoptotic members such as Bcl-2 and Bcl-XL (Antonsson and Martinou 2000). These proteins apparently function at the level of the mitochondrial membranes. For example, Bax interacts with these membranes to facilitate the alterations required to initiate cytochrome c release whereas the presence of Bcl-2 blocks this process, presumably through binding to Bax and abrogating its function. Thus, the ratio of expression of these pro- and anti-apoptotic proteins governs the propensity for the cell to undergo the intrinsic pathway of apoptosis. The Bcl-2 family also has some ability to govern receptor-mediated apoptosis through its participation in a cross-talk mechanism that exists between these two apoptosis pathways (Daniel 2000). This cross-talk is mediated by another member of the Bcl-2 family called Bid. Bid, a pro-apoptotic protein somewhat similar to Bax, exists in the cell in an inactive form until activated by proteolytic cleavage (Antonsson and Martinou 2000). However, Bid is a substrate for caspase 8 and, once activated by caspase 8, the truncated Bid translocates to the mitochondrial membrane where it facilitates mitochondrial-mediated apoptosis (Fulda et al. 2001). Apoptosis is, therefore, enhanced in the receptor-mediated pathway when this mechanism is activated in cells that express Bid. Note that the anti-apoptotic members of the Bcl-2 family are still fully able to block this enhancement. There is also a mechanism for enhancing the mitochondrial-mediated pathway in Bid-expressing cells. It is now understood that pro-caspase 8 is a substrate for caspase 3 (Slee et al. 1999). Therefore, even in the absence of death receptor engagement, caspase 8 can be activated by caspase 3 during mitochondrial-mediated apoptosis and cleave Bid, resulting in a further amplification of the overall apoptotic signaling cascade (Wieder et al. 2001).

These cross-talk and amplification mechanisms may provide a basis for enhancing tumor response when death cytokines such as TNF-α or TRAIL are combined with radiotherapy. Two major possibilities are evident. First, it is well-established that the expression of a number of pro-apoptotic proteins is enhanced following irradiation and therefore, if radiation is delivered prior to cytokine treatment, these factors may sensitize the cells to the cytokine (El-Deiry 2001; Rich et al. 2000). Bax is one good example; however, this list also includes certain death receptors such as Fas, DR4 and DR5 (Coultas and Strasser 2000). Thus, tumor cells may be more responsive to death cytokines following irradiation. Second, if radiation is delivered after death cytokine treatment, the initiation of receptor-mediated apoptosis may lower the threshold for radiation-induced, mitochondrial-mediated apoptosis due to the cross-talk between these two pathways mentioned above in this paragraph resulting in a radiosensitizing effect. Both TNF-α and TRAIL have been combined with radiation in a number of studies with the goal of enhancing tumor cell response to treatment. The remainder of this chapter will be devoted to a review of the results of these investigations.

17.3
TNF and Radiation

The interaction of TNF and radiation has been investigated since the late 1980s (Table 17.1). The earliest paper examined the effects of recombinant human TNF alone or in combination with radiation in two murine tumor models treated in vivo (Sersa et al. 1988). Both agents produced a significant delay in tumor growth when used alone. However, the combination produced an effect that was greater than the additive effect of the individual treatments. For the combination treatments, TNF was administered IV for 7 consecutive days commencing 3 h after irradiation. In addition, TNF was found to enhance radiocurability when tumor control was assessed as the endpoint. These initial studies were followed up in a

Table 17.1. TNF and radiation

Reference	Model system
SERSA et al. (1988)	Murine mammary carcinoma transplantable tumor
LEONARD et al. (1992)	Murine neuroblastoma transplantable tumor
HALLAHAN et al. (1990)	Human tumor cell lines in vitro
NISHIGUCHI et al. (1990)	Murine mammary carcinoma transplantable tumor
GRIDLEY et al. (1994)	Human colon adenocarcinoma xenograft tumor
GRIDLEY et al. (1996)	Human lung adenocarcinoma xenograft tumor
GRIDLEY et al. (1997)	Rat glioma xenograft tumor
HUANG et al. (1995)	Human glioblastoma xenograft tumor
HALLAHAN et al. (1995b)	Human squamous cell carcinoma xenograft tumor
WEICHSELBAUM et al. (1994)	Human squamous cell carcinoma xenograft tumor
SEUNG et al. (1995)	Murine fibrosarcoma transplantable tumor
HALLAHAN et al. (1995a)	Phase I clinical trial
MAUCERI et al. (1996)	Human squamous cell carcinoma xenograft tumor
CHUNG et al. (1998)	Human prostate cancer xenograft tumor
BAHER et al. (1999)	Rat glioma xenograft tumor
STABA et al. (1998)	Human malignant glioma xenograft tumor
GRIDLEY et al. (2000)	Rat glioma xenograft tumor
GUPTA et al. (2002)	Human esophageal adenocarcinoma xenograft tumor
KIM et al. (2001a)	Human colon xenograft tumor

subsequent study by the same group where TNF as an adjunct to fractionated radiotherapy was examined in the same murine tumor models (NISHIGUCHI et al. 1990). Again, the combination of TNF and radiation produced a greater than additive effect on tumor growth delay compared to the effect of the individual treatments. In this case, TNF was given IV 3 h after each daily dose of radiation for 10 days. These early reports stimulated other investigators to examine this combination in other tumor cell models and LEONARD et al. (1992) reported that TNF enhanced the radiosensitivity of a murine neuroblastoma when treated in vivo with TNF delivered in two IP injections 12 and 36 h after irradiation.

HALLAHAN et al. (1990) measured the radiosensitizing properties of TNF in 13 different human tumor cell lines using colony forming assays. They included in this analysis a determination of the optimal sequence and timing of TNF administration relative to the delivery of ionizing irradiation. Their results indicated that synergistic or additive cell killing was produced by the combination in 7 of 10 cell lines while independent cell killing by each agent occurred in two lines. The best synergistic effect was observed when TNF was given 4–10 h prior to irradiation and this interaction was absent when the TNF was given after irradiation. This latter finding contrasts with the in vivo studies described above in this section with regard to the optimum schedule of administration of TNF and radiation, suggesting that the mechanisms of this interaction may differ between the in vitro and in vivo situations.

Xenograft tumors growing in nude mice have also been used as a model system to test the interaction of TNF and radiation. Gridley et al. have published three reports describing the results of investigations using three different xenograft tumor models; human colon adenocarcinoma (GRIDLEY et al. 1994), human lung adenocarcinoma (GRIDLEY et al. 1996), and a rat glioma (GRIDLEY et al. 1997). A similar treatment protocol was used in all three studies; a series of fractionated doses of radiation were given over a time period of several days and TNF was delivered as IV injections starting prior to commencement of irradiation and on the intervening days during the radiation treatments. TNF enhanced the antitumor effect of radiation in all three tumor models as assessed by tumor growth delay. In one of these studies, apoptosis was measured on the basis of its characteristic morphological features seen in histological sections taken from the treated tumors (GRIDLEY et al. 1994). Apoptosis levels appeared to be enhanced in the tumors that received TNF plus radiation compared to controls.

With regard to its examination in the clinical treatment of human cancers, TNF was initially tested as a single agent based on promising preclinical studies demonstrating its selective toxicity for malignant cells (SPRIGGS et al. 1987, 1988). However, when given systemically, TNF was found to be very toxic in humans, producing dose-limiting toxicities that included shock-like syndromes, fever, and hypotension (FREI and SPRIGGS 1989). The further use of TNF as a cancer therapeutic was stimulated by the laboratory findings reviewed above in this section that indicated a synergistic interaction between TNF and radiation and a phase I clinical trial testing this combination was initiated in the early 1990s. The results of that phase I trial were published in 1995 (HALLAHAN et al. 1995b). In that trial, a total of 31 patients were treated with the combination of TNF and radiotherapy in a dose-escalation study. Recombinant human TNF-α was given IV 4 h prior to radiation treatment and the doses of TNF ranged from 10–150 µg/m². Although complete tumor regression was seen in a subset of patients, significant toxicities similar to those reported in the earlier trials of TNF alone prevented continued use of systemically administered TNF. The authors concluded that a therapeutic benefit might be achieved in the absence of systemic toxicity if TNF-α could be delivered locally.

One strategy for delivering TNF locally would be using gene therapy and several such strategies have been tested in preclinical models. One such strategy takes advantage of the fact that radiation activates the transcription of certain immediate early genes that encode transcription factors. These include the early growth response gene *Egr-1*. WEICHSELBAUM et al. (1994) linked DNA sequences from the *Egr-1* promoter region to a sequence that encodes for human TNF-α. This Egr-TNF construct was used to transfect a human leukemic cell line HL525. HL525 cells that express this Egr-TNF construct were then injected into established xenograft tumors produced using the human squamous cell carcinoma cell line SQ-20B and the tumor was given a dose of 20 Gy followed 1 day later with another dose of 20 Gy. The animals that received HL525 cells plus radiation displayed a higher rate of tumor cure compared to control animals treated with either agent alone. No increase in local or systemic toxicity was observed. These results suggested that delivering TNF-α using a radiation-inducible gene therapy approach enhanced tumor cure without increasing toxicity.

Weichselbaum's group has subsequently tested further variations of this approach. A similar Egr-TNF construct was encapsulated into cationic liposomes and murine fibrosarcomas growing in vivo were injected with this liposome preparation prior to irradiation (SEUNG et al. 1995). Analysis of the tumors indicated that radiation-induced, TNF-protein levels were 29 times control levels. Moreover, mean tumor volumes in the group of animals receiving the combination treatment were significantly reduced compared to control groups that received either agent alone. This group of investigators also tested the efficacy of adenoviral-mediated expression of the Egr-TNF construct, Ad.Egr-TNF (HALLAHAN et al. 1995a). They used this vector in combination with radiation to treat human xenograft tumors made using SQ-20B cells (MAUCERI et al. 1996) and observed very positive results. Examination of the tumors receiving the combination treatment indicated extensive intratumoral vascular thrombosis and tumor necrosis that was not observed in the controls. No vascular thrombosis was observed in the normal tissues. Thus, they concluded that the combination of Ad.Egr-TNF plus radiation selectively produced occlusion of tumor vessels. Additional tests of the combination of Ad.Egr-TNF and radiation were conducted by this group in human malignant glioma and human prostate cancer xenograft models with similar success (CHUNG et al. 1998; STABA et al. 1998). Recently, this group has produced a clinical grade version of this same vector that is referred to as Ad.Egr-TNF.11D and preclinical tests of this vector in combination with radiation in Seg-1 human esophageal adenocarcinoma xenografts were also successful (GUPTA et al. 2002). This new vector is currently in phase I clinical trials (SHARMA et al. 2001).

Another group of investigators, GRIDLEY et al. (2000) constructed a plasmid-based TNF-α expression vector that they have shown to have potent antitumor effects on rat glioma xenograft tumors treated in vivo in combination with radiation. In another of their studies, the vector was combined with a cationic polyamine just prior to injection, which facilitated tumor cell uptake of the plasmid (BAHER et al. 1999). Expression of TNF in the transfected tumor cells in these approaches is constitutive rather than radiation-induced. More recently, this same group has published a report demonstrating that liposome-encapsulation of TNF-α protein enhances the effects of radiation in human colon tumor xenografts treated in vivo (KIM et al. 2001a). In this protocol, the animals are treated with the liposome formulation by IV injection prior to irradiation. Collectively, these systems developed by the Gridley and Weichselbaum groups for local delivery of TNF-α to tumors appear to be promising approaches in combination with radiation for the local control of tumors, without increasing systemic toxicity.

17.4
TRAIL and Radiation

Compared to TNF-α, less has been done with TRAIL in combination with radiation due to the fact that

TRAIL was only discovered in 1995 and many of its activities at the biochemical and molecular level have only recently been elucidated. However, of the two, TRAIL may hold more promise as a cancer therapeutic because of its lack of toxicity to normal tissues. As with other such agents, TRAIL will most likely be used in the clinic in combination with other cancer therapeutic modalities and not used alone. Therefore, a number of investigators have undertaken preclinical, laboratory studies directed at determining if TRAIL synergizes with conventional chemotherapy drugs or radiotherapy. TRAIL appears to synergize with radiation and this has been demonstrated in several reports that have been published over the last 3 years (Table 17.2). CHINNAIYAN et al. (2000) examined TRAIL in combination with radiation in a breast cancer model. Several human breast cancer cell lines were tested for an enhanced apoptotic response. Two cell lines that had wild-type p53 status displayed a synergistic apoptotic response when TRAIL and radiation were combined whereas 3 lines with mutant p53 status did not. This effect also correlated with an up-regulation of the TRAIL receptor, DR5, in the lines with wild-type p53. Further experiments conducted using a breast cancer xenograft model treated in vivo showed an enhanced tumor growth delay when the combination was used compared to when either treatment was used alone. Enhanced apoptosis was also observed in histological sections taken from these tumors following the combination treatment. No toxicity was observed in the mice that received systemic treatments of TRAIL.

GONG and ALMASAN tested the efficacy of the combination of TRAIL and radiation in human leukemia/lymphoma cell lines treated in vitro (GONG and ALMASAN 2000). Both the Molt-4 and Jurkat cell lines expressed higher levels of TRAIL mRNA following exposure to radiation. In addition, the Molt-4 line, which has wild-type p53, but not the Jurkat line, which has mutant p53, expressed higher levels of DR5 mRNA after irradiation. However, the combination of radiation and recombinant TRAIL protein had a synergistic effect on the loss of clonogenic survival in both cell lines. In the paper by BELKA et al. (2001), the Jurkat cell line was also used as a model system; however, these authors also examined a Bcl-2 overexpressing Jurkat line. Interestingly, whereas apoptosis induction appeared to be only additive in the control Jurkat line, a synergistic effect was observed in the line overexpressing Bcl-2 with the combination of TRAIL and radiation. A strong effect of TRAIL plus radiation on loss of clonogenic survival was also found in this study. In a third paper where the Jurkat cell system was used, KIM et al. (2001b) showed that a TRAIL-resistant Jurkat line could be sensitized to TRAIL by radiation. Apoptosis following the combination treatment associated with activation of caspases 8, 9, and 3 and cleavage of Bid protein. No changes in DR4 or DR5 expression were observed following irradiation in this line.

DI PIETRO et al. (2001) investigated the effects of TRAIL in combination with radiation in three different erythroleukemic cell lines compared to normal erythroblasts. When TRAIL and radiation were combined, an additive effect was observed in the erythroleukemic cell lines when the radiation was given 3–6 h prior to the addition of TRAIL. This additive effect correlated with an up-regulation of DR4. This additive effect on apoptosis induction was not observed when normal erythroblasts were treated with the combination. Radiation did not induce the up-regulation of DR4 in the erythroblasts but up-regulated the expression of the TRAIL decoy receptor DcR1 instead. Finally, RAVI and BEDI (2002) have shown that TRAIL sensitizes human colon adenocarcinoma cell lines to radiation. They compared the responses of the HCT116 line that contains wild-type p53 and has one intact Bax allele with isogenic p53-deficient (p53–/–) or Bax-deficient (Bax–/–) derivatives of HCT116 cells generated by targeted disruption of the *p53* or *Bax* genes. TRAIL sensitized HCT116 cells to radiation independently of their p53 status. However, the Bax-deficient line was insensitive to either TRAIL or radiation or their combination. Thus, the combination of TRAIL and radiation may be a useful treatment strategy for colorectal cancer but perhaps not in Bax-deficient tumors.

Table 17.2. TRAIL and radiation

Reference	Model system
CHINNAIYAN et al. (2000)	Human breast carcinoma xenograft tumor
GONG and ALMASAN (2000)	Human leukemic cell lines
BELKA et al. (2001)	Human lymphoma cell line
KIM et al. (2001b)	Human lymphoma cell line
DI PIETRO et al. (2001)	Murine and human leukemic cell lines
RAVI and BEDI (2002)	Human colon adenocarcinoma cell lines

In addition to these investigations of TRAIL in combination with radiation, a number of studies have been conducted examining TRAIL in combination with chemotherapy drugs (Table 17.3). KEANE et al. (1999) examined human breast cancer lines and observed that incubation of the cells with either doxorubicin or 5-fluorouracil augmented TRAIL-induced apoptosis in a synergistic manner. This enhancement correlated with caspase 3 activation. Similar findings for breast cancer cell lines treated with TRAIL plus etoposide were reported by GIBSON et al. (2000). GLINIAK and LE tested TRAIL in combination with CPT-11, a water-soluble analogue of camptothecin, in models of colon carcinoma (GLINIAK and LE 1999). Mice bearing xenograft tumors were treated with CPT-11 plus TRAIL. This combination produced a significant inhibition of tumor growth. LACOUR et al. (2001) also show that colon cancer cells could by sensitized to TRAIL by cisplatin and doxorubicin. This effect correlated with enhanced activation of caspase 8 and cleavage of Bid. TRAIL in combination with topotecan was examined in renal carcinoma cell lines by DEJOSEZ et al. (2000). A synergistic effect on suppression of cell proliferation was observed. WEN et al. (2000) tested antileukemic drugs in combination with TRAIL in HL-60 cells. They observed that etoposide, Ara-c, and doxorubicin up-regulated DR5 expression and sensitized HL-60 cells to TRAIL in a p53-independent manner. Human hepatocellular carcinoma cell lines were studied by YAMANAKA et al. (2000). Doxorubicin and camptothecin augmented TRAIL-induced cytotoxicity in these lines. TRAIL in combination with a variety of chemotherapy agents has also shown efficacy in laboratory investigations of other types of cancer including gliomas (NAGANE et al. 2000), bladder (MIZUTANI et al. 2001), ovarian (CUELLO et al. 2001), mesothelioma (LIU et al. 2001), prostate (NIMMANAPALLI et al. 2001), pancreatic (MATSUZAKI et al. 2001), and multiple myeloma (JAZIREHI et al. 2001). A more complete review of this topic can be found in the recent article by HELD and SCHULZE-OSTHOFF (2001).

Our interest in TRAIL started a few years ago and we have examined its effect in combination with both chemotherapeutic agents and ionizing radiation. In the first study, we determined if TRAIL-induced apoptosis would be suppressed by Bcl-2 in human prostate tumor cells (MUNSHI et al. 2001). Thus, pairs of isogenic cell lines that expressed or did not express Bcl-2 were exposed to recombinant human TRAIL. Three lines were examined, PC3, DU145 and LNCaP and apoptosis was the endpoint. All three lines were resistant to low doses of TRAIL but could be sensitized by the addition of a protein synthesis inhibitor, cycloheximide (CHX). The three variant lines that expressed Bcl-2 were resistant to TRAIL plus CHX. Both caspases 8 and 3 were activated in the PC3 cell line that lacked Bcl-2 expression but activation of these caspases was blocked in the Bcl-2-overexpressing PC3 cell line. Based on the kinetics of these events and the fact that Bid was cleaved and cytochrome c was released into the cytosol, we concluded that TRAIL-induced apoptosis in these cells was facilitated through the mitochondria-mediated pathway and that Bcl-2 suppressed apoptosis at this level.

In our second study, we tested whether chemotherapeutic agents would enhance TRAIL-induced apoptosis in prostate cancer cells (MUNSHI et al. 2002). Thus, the PC3 and LNCaP human prostate cancer cell lines were treated with TRAIL alone, drug alone, or the combination and cytotoxicity was determined by apoptosis and clonogenic survival.

Table 17.3. TRAIL and chemotherapy drugs

Reference	Model system	Drug
KEANE et al. (1999)	Human breast cancer cell lines	Doxorubicin, 5-FU
GIBSON et al. (2000)	Human breast cancer cell lines	Etoposide
GLINIAK and LE (1999)	Human colon carcinoma xenograft tumors	CPT-11
LACOUR et al. (2001)	Human colon carcinoma cell lines	Cisplatin, doxorubicin
DEJOSEZ et al. (2000)	Human renal cell carcinoma cell lines	Topotecan
WEN et al. (2000)	Human leukemic cell lines	Etoposide, doxorubicin, Ara-C
YAMANAKA et al. (2000)	Human hepatocellular carcinoma cell lines	Doxorubicin, camptothecin
NAGANE et al. (2000)	Human glioblastoma xenograft tumors	Cisplatin, etoposide
MIZUTANI et al. (2001)	Human bladder cell line	5-FU, mitomycin C, cisplatin
CUELLO et al. (2001)	Human ovarian carcinoma cell lines	Cisplatin, doxorubicin, paclitaxel
LIU et al. (2001)	Human mesothelioma cell lines	Doxorubicin, cisplatin, etoposide
NIMMANAPALLI et al. (2001)	Human prostate cancer cell lines	Paclitaxel
MATSUZAKI et al. (2001)	Human pancreatic cancer cell lines	actinomycin D
JAZIREHI et al. (2001)	Human multiple myeloma cell lines	Doxorubicin, etoposide
MUNSHI et al. (2002)	Human prostate cancer cell lines	Doxorubicin, etoposide, cisplatin

Three drugs were used: etoposide, doxorubicin, and cisplatin. The results indicated that these three drugs all enhanced TRAIL-induced apoptosis in both cell lines. This effect was partially abrogated in the Bcl-2-overexpressing versions of these lines. Similar effects were observed when clonogenic survival was used as the endpoint. When the chemotherapeutic drugs or TRAIL were used alone, only a weak activation of either caspase 8 or caspase 3 could be detected. However, activation of caspase 8 and caspase 3 became significant when these agents were used in combination. We concluded that the drugs overcome the cellular resistance to TRAIL by enhancing this activation of caspases.

More recently, we have begun to examine the effects of the combination of TRAIL and radiation in models of non-small cell lung cancer (NSCLC) and colorectal cancer. The SW620 human colorectal cancer cell line was examined for DR4 expression following a single dose of 6 Gy of radiation. The results shown in Fig. 17.4 indicate that DR4 expression is enhanced by irradiation beginning 3 h after exposure to radiation and this enhancement lasts for up to 48 h. To see if TRAIL and radiation can synergize for cell killing, we treated SW620 cells with different doses of radiation and waited for 48 h before treating the cells with TRAIL for 6 h. Following TRAIL treatment, the cells were plated for clonogenic survival. The results, shown in Fig. 17.5, show a small but significant sensitizing effect when TRAIL and radiation were used in combination. Optimization of the dose of TRAIL and schedule of these treatments could lead to an even greater enhancement of synergy in this cell system. Our results shown here are consistent with the recent report by Ravi and Bedi (2002), reviewed above in this section, who observed enhanced apoptosis in human colorectal cancer cells treated with the combination of TRAIL and radiation. In a similar approach, we have also begun to examine the NSCLC line A549. A549 cells were treated with a dose of 4 Gy and tested for DR4 expression. Similar to the SW620 cells, DR4 expression was up-regulated quickly after irradiation in the A549 cell line and this enhanced expression was maintained for up to 48 h (Fig. 17.4). Although these preliminary findings will have to be followed up in expanded studies, the results to date suggest that

Fig. 17.4. Immunoblot analysis of DR4 expression following irradiation in SW620 and A549 cells

Fig. 17.5. Clonogenic survival curves for SW620 cells exposed to different doses of radiation with or without the addition of TRAIL the combination of the TRAIL and radiation may be efficacious in the treatment of NSCLC.

In conclusion, we have reviewed the current status of research being conducted on combining death cytokines with radiotherapy for the treatment of cancer. Although there are several death cytokines that have now been recognized, only three – FasL, TNF-α and TRAIL – have been studied in any great detail. FasL may not have any clinical utility because of its systemic toxicity. Although TNF-α also has systemic toxicity, its local and/or targeted delivery through the use of gene therapy strategies appears to be promising. TRAIL is perhaps the most promising of the three based on its apparent lack of toxicity to normal tissues when administered systemically. At the present time, this needs to be confirmed in phase I clinical trials. If TRAIL's selective toxicity to transformed cells is validated in patients, combinations of TRAIL therapy and radiotherapy or chemotherapy would appear to be potentially efficacious based on the preclinical studies referenced here. These investigations have clearly established that TRAIL can synergize with radiation and several different anticancer drugs in laboratory models of a wide variety of human cancers using clinically relevant endpoints of tumor response.

References

Adams JM, Cory S (1998) The Bcl-2 protein family: arbiters of cell survival. Science 281:1322–1326

Antonsson B, Martinou JC (2000) The Bcl-2 protein family. Exp Cell Res 256:50–57

Ashkenazi A, Dixit VM (1998) Death receptors: signaling and modulation. Science 281:1305–1308

Ashkenazi A, Pai RC, Fong S et al (1999) Safety and antitumor activity of recombinant soluble Apo2 ligand. J Clin Invest 104:155–162

Baher AG, Andres ML, Folz-Holbeck J et al (1999) A model using radiation and plasmid-mediated tumor necrosis factor-alpha gene therapy for treatment of glioblastomas. Anticancer Res 19:2917–2924

Belka C, Marini P, Budach W et al (1998) Radiation-induced apoptosis in human lymphocytes and lymphoma cells critically relies on the up-regulation of CD95/Fas/APO-1 ligand. Radiat Res 149:588–595

Belka C, Schmid B, Marini P et al (2001) Sensitization of resistant lymphoma cells to irradiation-induced apoptosis by the death ligand TRAIL. Oncogene 20:2190–2196

Beutler B, Cerami A (1988) Tumor necrosis, cachexia, shock, and inflammation: a common mediator. Annu Rev Biochem 57:505–518

Budihardjo I, Oliver H, Lutter M et al (1999) Biochemical pathways of caspase activation during apoptosis. Annu Rev Cell Dev Biol 15:269–290

Carswell EA, Old LJ, Kassel RL et al (1975) An endotoxin-induced serum factor that causes necrosis of tumors. Proc Natl Acad Sci U S A 72:3666–3670

Chen G, Goeddel DV (2002) TNF-R1 signaling: a beautiful pathway. Science 296:1634–1635

Chinnaiyan AM, Prasad U, Shankar S et al (2000) Combined effect of tumor necrosis factor-related apoptosis-inducing ligand and ionizing radiation in breast cancer therapy. Proc Natl Acad Sci U S A 97:1754–1759

Chung TD, Mauceri HJ, Hallahan DE et al (1998) Tumor necrosis factor-alpha-based gene therapy enhances radiation cytotoxicity in human prostate cancer. Cancer Gene Ther 5:344–349

Coultas L, Strasser A (2000) The molecular control of DNA damage-induced cell death. Apoptosis 5:491–507

Cuello M, Ettenberg SA, Nau MM et al (2001) Synergistic induction of apoptosis by the combination of trail and chemotherapy in chemoresistant ovarian cancer cells. Gynecol Oncol 81:380–390

Daniel PT (2000) Dissecting the pathways to death. Leukemia 14:2035–2044

Dejosez M, Ramp U, Mahotka C et al (2000) Sensitivity to TRAIL/APO-2L-mediated apoptosis in human renal cell carcinomas and its enhancement by topotecan. Cell Death Differ 7:1127–1136

Di Pietro R, Secchiero P, Rana R et al (2001) Ionizing radiation sensitizes erythroleukemic cells but not normal erythroblasts to tumor necrosis factor-related apoptosis-inducing ligand (TRAIL) – mediated cytotoxicity by selective up-regulation of TRAIL-R1. Blood 97:2596–2603

El-Deiry WS (2001) Insights into cancer therapeutic design based on p53 and TRAIL receptor signaling. Cell Death Differ 8:1066–1075

Fisher GH, Rosenberg FJ, Straus SE et al (1995) Dominant interfering Fas gene mutations impair apoptosis in a human autoimmune lymphoproliferative syndrome. Cell 81:935–946

Fiumara P, Younes A (2001) CD40 ligand (CD154) and tumour necrosis factor-related apoptosis inducing ligand (Apo-2L) in haematological malignancies. Br J Haematol 113:265–274

Frei E III, Spriggs D (1989) Tumor necrosis factor: still a promising agent. J Clin Oncol 7:291–294

French LE, Tschopp J (1999) The TRAIL to selective tumor death. Nat Med 5:146–147

Friesen C, Fulda S, Debatin KM (1999) Cytotoxic drugs and the CD95 pathway. Leukemia 13:1854–1858

Fulda S, Scaffidi C, Pietsch T et al (1998) Activation of the CD95 (APO-1/Fas) pathway in drug- and gamma-irradiation-induced apoptosis of brain tumor cells. Cell Death Differ 5:884–893

Fulda S, Meyer E, Friesen C et al (2001) Cell type specific involvement of death receptor and mitochondrial pathways in drug-induced apoptosis. Oncogene 20:1063–1075

Gibson SB, Oyer R, Spalding AC et al (2000) Increased expression of death receptors 4 and 5 synergizes the apoptosis response to combined treatment with etoposide and TRAIL. Mol Cell Biol 20:205–212

Gliniak B, Le T (1999) Tumor necrosis factor-related apoptosis-inducing ligand's antitumor activity in vivo is enhanced by the chemotherapeutic agent CPT-11. Cancer Res 59:6153–6158

Gong B, Almasan A (2000) Apo2 ligand/TNF-related apoptosis-inducing ligand and death receptor 5 mediate the apoptotic signaling induced by ionizing radiation in leukemic cells. Cancer Res 60:5754–5760

Green DR, Reed JC (1998) Mitochondria and apoptosis. Science 281:1309–1312

Gridley DS, Hammond SN, Liwnicz BH (1994) Tumor necrosis factor-alpha augments radiation effects against human colon tumor xenografts. Anticancer Res 14:1107–1112

Gridley DS, Andres ML, Garner C et al (1996) Evaluation of TNF-alpha effects on radiation efficacy in a human lung adenocarcinoma model. Oncol Res 8:485–495

Gridley DS, Archambeau JO, Andres MA et al (1997) Tumor necrosis factor-alpha enhances antitumor effects of radiation against glioma xenografts. Oncol Res 9:217–227

Gridley DS, Li J, Kajioka EH et al (2000) Combination of pGL1-TNF-alpha gene and radiation (proton and gamma-ray) therapy against brain tumor. Anticancer Res 20:4195–4203

Gupta VK, Park JO, Jaskowiak NT et al (2002) Combined gene therapy and ionizing radiation is a novel approach to treat human esophageal adenocarcinoma. Ann Surg Oncol 9:500–504

Haimovitz-Friedman A, Kan CC, Ehleiter D et al (1994) Ionizing radiation acts on cellular membranes to generate ceramide and initiate apoptosis. J Exp Med 180:525–535

Hallahan DE, Beckett MA, Kufe D et al (1990) The interaction between recombinant human tumor necrosis factor and radiation in 13 human tumor cell lines. Int J Radiat Oncol Biol Phys 19:69–74

Hallahan DE, Mauceri HJ, Seung LP et al (1995a) Spatial and temporal control of gene therapy using ionizing radiation. Nat Med 1:786–791

Hallahan DE, Vokes EE, Rubin SJ et al (1995b) Phase I dose-escalation study of tumor necrosis factor-alpha and concomitant radiation therapy. Cancer J Sci Am 1:204–209

Held J, Schulze-Osthoff K (2001) Potential and caveats of TRAIL in cancer therapy. Drug Resist Updat 4:243–252

Hengartner MO (2000) The biochemistry of apoptosis. Nature 407:770–776

Huang P, Allam A, Perez LA, Taghian A, Freeman J, Suit HD (1995) The effect of combining recombinant human tumor necrosis factor-alpha with local radiation on tumor control probability of a human glioblastoma multiforme xenograft in nude mice. Int J Radiat Oncol biol Phys 32:93–98

Irisarri M, Plumas J, Bonnefoix T et al (2000) Resistance to CD95-mediated apoptosis through constitutive c-FLIP expression in a non-Hodgkin's lymphoma B cell line. Leukemia 14:2149–2158

Irmler M, Thome M, Hahne M et al (1997) Inhibition of death receptor signals by cellular FLIP. Nature 388:190–195

Jazirehi AR, Ng CP, Gan XH et al (2001) Adriamycin sensitizes the adriamycin-resistant 8226/Dox40 human multiple myeloma cells to Apo2L/tumor necrosis factor-related apoptosis-inducing ligand-mediated (TRAIL) apoptosis. Clin Cancer Res 7:3874–3883

Jo M, Kim TH, Seol DW et al (2000) Apoptosis induced in normal human hepatocytes by tumor necrosis factor-related apoptosis-inducing ligand. Nat Med 6:564–567

Keane MM, Ettenberg SA, Nau MM et al (1999) Chemotherapy augments TRAIL-induced apoptosis in breast cell lines. Cancer Res 59:734–741

Kerr JF, Wyllie AH, Currie AR (1972) Apoptosis: a basic biological phenomenon with wide-ranging implications in tissue kinetics. Br J Cancer 26:239–257

Kim DW, Andres ML, Li J et al (2001a) Liposome-encapsulated tumor necrosis factor-alpha enhances the effects of radiation against human colon tumor xenografts. J Interferon Cytokine Res 21:885–897

Kim MR, Lee JY, Park MT et al (2001b) Ionizing radiation can overcome resistance to TRAIL in TRAIL-resistant cancer cells. FEBS Lett 505:179–184

Kischkel FC, Hellbardt S, Behrmann I et al (1995) Cytotoxicity-dependent APO-1 (Fas/CD95)-associated proteins form a death-inducing signaling complex (DISC) with the receptor. EMBO J 14:5579–5588

Krammer PH (2000) CD95's deadly mission in the immune system. Nature 407:789–795

Lacour S, Hammann A, Wotawa A et al (2001) Anticancer agents sensitize tumor cells to tumor necrosis factor-related apoptosis-inducing ligand-mediated caspase-8 activation and apoptosis. Cancer Res 61:1645–1651

Lawrence D, Shahrokh Z, Marsters S et al (2001) Differential hepatocyte toxicity of recombinant Apo2L/TRAIL versions. Nat Med 7:383–385

Leonard MP, Jeffs RD, Gearhart JP et al (1992) Recombinant human tumor necrosis factor enhances radiosensitivity and improves animal survival in murine neuroblastoma. J Urol 148:743–746

Liu W, Bodle E, Chen JY et al (2001) Tumor necrosis factor-related apoptosis-inducing ligand and chemotherapy cooperate to induce apoptosis in mesothelioma cell lines. Am J Respir Cell Mol Biol 25:111–118

Liu X, Kim CN, Yang J et al (1996) Induction of apoptotic program in cell-free extracts: requirement for dATP and cytochrome c. Cell 86:147–157

Loeffler M, Kroemer G (2000) The mitochondrion in cell death control: certainties and incognita. Exp Cell Res 256:19–26

Matsuzaki H, Schmied BM, Ulrich A et al (2001) Combination of tumor necrosis factor-related apoptosis-inducing ligand (TRAIL) and actinomycin D induces apoptosis even in TRAIL-resistant human pancreatic cancer cells. Clin Cancer Res 7:407–414

Mauceri HJ, Hanna NN, Wayne JD et al (1996) Tumor necrosis factor alpha (TNF-alpha) gene therapy targeted by ionizing radiation selectively damages tumor vasculature. Cancer Res 56:4311–4314

Meyn RE, Stephens LC, Ang KK et al (1993) Heterogeneity in the development of apoptosis in irradiated murine tumours of different histologies. Int J Radiat Biol 64:583–591

Mizutani Y, Nakao M, Ogawa O et al (2001) Enhanced sensitivity of bladder cancer cells to tumor necrosis factor-related apoptosis inducing ligand-mediated apoptosis by cisplatin and carboplatin. J Urol 165:263–270

Munshi A, Pappas G, Honda T et al (2001) TRAIL (APO-2L) induces apoptosis in human prostate cancer cells that is inhibitable by Bcl-2. Oncogene 20:3757–3765

Munshi A, McDonnell TJ, Meyn RE (2002) Chemotherapeutic agents enhance TRAIL-induced apoptosis in prostate cancer cells. Cancer Chemother Pharmacol 50:46–52

Nagane M, Pan G, Weddle JJ et al (2000) Increased death receptor 5 expression by chemotherapeutic agents in human gliomas causes synergistic cytotoxicity with tumor necrosis factor-related apoptosis-inducing ligand in vitro and in vivo. Cancer Res 60:847–853

Nagane M, Huang HJ, Cavenee WK (2001) The potential of TRAIL for cancer chemotherapy. Apoptosis 6:191–197

Nagata S (1997) Apoptosis by death factor. Cell 88:355–365

Nimmanapalli R, Perkins CL, Orlando M et al (2001) Pretreatment with paclitaxel enhances apo-2 ligand/tumor necrosis factor-related apoptosis-inducing ligand-induced apoptosis of prostate cancer cells by inducing death receptors 4 and 5 protein levels. Cancer Res 61:759–763

Nishiguchi I, Willingham V, Milas L (1990) Tumor necrosis factor as an adjunct to fractionated radiotherapy in the treatment of murine tumors. Int J Radiat Oncol Biol Phys 18:555–558

Peter ME (2000) The TRAIL DISCussion: it is FADD and caspase-8! Cell Death Differ 7:759–760

Pitti RM, Marsters SA, Ruppert S et al (1996) Induction of apoptosis by Apo-2 ligand, a new member of the tumor necrosis factor cytokine family. J Biol Chem 271:12687–12690

Ravi R, Bedi A (2002) Requirement of BAX for TRAIL/Apo2L-induced apoptosis of colorectal cancers: synergism with sulindac-mediated inhibition of Bcl-x(L). Cancer Res 62: 1583–1587

Reap EA, Roof K, Maynor K et al (1997) Radiation and stress-induced apoptosis: a role for Fas/Fas ligand interactions. Proc Natl Acad Sci U S A 94:5750–5755

Rich T, Allen RL, Wyllie AH (2000) Defying death after DNA damage. Nature 407:777–783

Rupnow BA, Murtha AD, Alarcon RM et al (1998) Direct evidence that apoptosis enhances tumor responses to fractionated radiotherapy. Cancer Res 58:1779–1784

Sersa G, Willingham V, Milas L (1988) Anti-tumor effects of tumor necrosis factor alone or combined with radiotherapy. Int J Cancer 42:129–134

Seung LP, Mauceri HJ, Beckett MA et al (1995) Genetic radiotherapy overcomes tumor resistance to cytotoxic agents. Cancer Res 55:5561–5565

Sharma A, Mani S, Hanna N et al (2001) Clinical protocol. An open-label, phase I, dose-escalation study of tumor necrosis factor-alpha (TNFerade Biologic) gene transfer with radiation therapy for locally advanced, recurrent, or metastatic solid tumors. Hum Gene Ther 12:1109–1131

Sheikh MS, Fornace AJ Jr (2000) Death and decoy receptors and p53-mediated apoptosis. Leukemia 14:1509–1513

Singh A, Ni J, Aggarwal BB (1998) Death domain receptors and their role in cell demise. J Interferon Cytokine Res 18:439–450

Slee EA, Harte MT, Kluck RM et al (1999) Ordering the cytochrome c-initiated caspase cascade: hierarchical activation of caspases-2, -3, -6, -7, -8, and -10 in a caspase-9-dependent manner. J Cell Biol 144:281–292

Spitz FR, Nguyen D, Skibber JM et al (1996) Adenoviral-mediated wild-type p53 gene expression sensitizes colorectal cancer cells to ionizing radiation. Clin Cancer Res 2:1665–1671

Spriggs DR, Sherman ML, Frei E III et al (1987) Clinical studies with tumour necrosis factor. Ciba Found Symp 131: 206–227

Spriggs DR, Sherman ML, Michie H et al (1988) Recombinant human tumor necrosis factor administered as a 24-hour intravenous infusion. A phase I and pharmacologic study. J Natl Cancer Inst 80:1039–1044

Staba MJ, Mauceri HJ, Kufe DW et al (1998) Adenoviral TNF-alpha gene therapy and radiation damage tumor vasculature in a human malignant glioma xenograft. Gene Ther 5:293–300

Steel GG (2001) The case against apoptosis. Acta Oncol 40: 968–975

Suda T, Takahashi T, Golstein P et al (1993) Molecular cloning and expression of the Fas ligand, a novel member of the tumor necrosis factor family. Cell 75:1169–1178

Thompson CB (1995) Apoptosis in the pathogenesis and treatment of disease. Science 267:1456–1462

Thornberry NA, Lazebnik Y (1998) Caspases: enemies within. Science 281:1312–1316

Trauth BC, Klas C, Peters AM et al (1989) Monoclonal antibody-mediated tumor regression by induction of apoptosis. Science 245:301–305

Walczak H, Krammer PH (2000) The CD95 (APO-1/Fas) and the TRAIL (APO-2L) apoptosis systems. Exp Cell Res 256: 58–66

Walczak H, Miller RE, Ariail K et al (1999) Tumoricidal activity of tumor necrosis factor-related apoptosis-inducing ligand in vivo. Nat Med 5:157–163

Ward JF (1988) DNA damage produced by ionizing radiation in mammalian cells: identities, mechanisms of formation, and reparability. Prog Nucleic Acid Res Mol Biol 35: 95–125

Weichselbaum RR, Hallahan DE, Beckett MA et al (1994) Gene therapy targeted by radiation preferentially radiosensitizes tumor cells. Cancer Res 54:4266–4269

Wen J, Ramadevi N, Nguyen D et al (2000) Antileukemic drugs increase death receptor 5 levels and enhance Apo-2L-induced apoptosis of human acute leukemia cells. Blood 96:3900–3906

Wieder T, Essmann F, Prokop A et al (2001) Activation of caspase-8 in drug-induced apoptosis of B-lymphoid cells is independent of CD95/Fas receptor-ligand interaction and occurs downstream of caspase-3. Blood 97:1378–1387

Wiley SR, Schooley K, Smolak PJ et al (1995) Identification and characterization of a new member of the TNF family that induces apoptosis. Immunity 3:673–682

Wong GH, Elwell JH, Oberley LW et al (1989) Manganous superoxide dismutase is essential for cellular resistance to cytotoxicity of tumor necrosis factor. Cell 58:923–931

Wyllie AH, Kerr JF, Currie AR (1980) Cell death: the significance of apoptosis. Int Rev Cytol 68:251–306

Yamanaka T, Shiraki K, Sugimoto K et al (2000) Chemotherapeutic agents augment TRAIL-induced apoptosis in human hepatocellular carcinoma cell lines. Hepatology 32: 482–490

Yonehara S, Ishii A, Yonehara M (1989) A cell-killing monoclonal antibody (anti-Fas) to a cell surface antigen co-downregulated with the receptor of tumor necrosis factor. J Exp Med 169:1747–1756

Zhivotovsky B, Joseph B, Orrenius S (1999) Tumor radiosensitivity and apoptosis. Exp Cell Res 248:10–17

18 Role of Cyclooxygenase-2 (COX-2) and Its Inhibition in Tumor Biology and Radiotherapy

L. Milas, K. Mason, Z. Liao, U. Raju, M. Milas, A. Husain, K. K. Ang

CONTENTS

18.1 Introduction 241
18.2 COX-2, Prostanoids and COX-2 Inhibitors 242
18.2.1 Cyclooxygenase Enzymes 242
18.2.2 Prostanoids 242
18.2.3 Cyclooxygenase Inhibitors 243
18.3 Tumorigenesis, Tumor Growth and Metastasis 244
18.3.1 Tumorigenesis 244
18.3.2 Established Tumors 245
18.3.3 Metastasis 246
18.3.4 Mechanisms of COX-2 and Its Inhibitors in Tumorigenesis, Tumor Growth and Metastasis 247
18.4 Interactions with Ionizing Radiation 249
18.4.1 Radioprotective Effects of PGs 249
18.4.2 Effect of COX-2 Inhibitors on Tumor Radioresponse 249
18.4.3 Effect of COX-2 Inhibitors on Normal Tissue Radioresponse 251
18.4.4 Clinical Trials Related to Radiotherapy 252
18.4.5 Mechanisms of Increased Tumor Radioresponse 252
18.5 Conclusions 254
References 255

18.1 Introduction

In recent years our understanding of the fundamental biology of cancer has greatly increased. It has become clear that many molecular processes and signaling pathways that normally regulate growth, survival and function of cells become dysregulated in cancer cells, contributing to the more aggressive behavior of malignant tumors. In parallel, the knowledge of molecular, biochemical and cellular effects of ionizing radiation in both tumors and normal tissues has broadened, allowing design and implementation of more effective therapy. Increasing evidence shows that dysregulation in epidermal growth factor receptor (EGFR) signaling, presence of cyclooxygenase-2 (COX-2) enzyme, mutated *ras*, and secretion of proangiogenic molecules by tumor cells are associated with tumor resistance to cytotoxic therapies, including radiotherapy. Targeting these molecules or their signaling pathways has increasingly been explored as a therapeutic strategy, and newly developed agents directed against these molecules are already reaching the clinic. In preclinical studies, many of these novel agents have been particularly effective when combined with chemotherapeutic drugs or radiation, where they rendered tumor cells more susceptible to the cytotoxic action of chemotherapy and radiation. Targeting dysregulated molecular processes should, in theory, affect only malignant cells and thus is unlikely to sensitize normal tissues to injury by cytotoxic drugs or radiation.

Our laboratory has been actively exploring a number of molecular targeting strategies, and has been instrumental in introducing targeting COX-2 in combination with radiation (Milas et al. 1999; Kishi et al. 2000). The COX-2 enzyme mediates production of prostanoids in various pathological states, primarily in inflammatory tissues and tumors. Either via prostanoids or by other signaling pathways, COX-2 plays an important role in carcinogenesis, tumor growth and response of tumors and normal tissues to radiation, and consequently represents a potential target for tumor therapy. In this review, we describe the involvement of COX-2 in the biology of cancer and discuss the therapeutic potential of targeting homeostatic pathways mediated by COX-2 and prostanoids through the use of selective COX-2 inhibitors in combination with radiotherapy.

L. Milas, MD, PhD; K. Mason; U. Raju, PhD;
A. Husain, MD
Department of Experimental Radiation Oncology, The University of Texas M.D. Anderson Cancer Center, 1515 Holcombe Blvd., Box 66, Houston, TX 77030, USA
Z. Liao, MD
Department of Radiation Oncology, The University of Texas M.D. Anderson Cancer Center, 1515 Holcombe Blvd., Box 97, Houston, TX 77030, USA
M. Milas, MD
Department of General Surgery, The Cleveland Clinic Foundation, 9500 Euclid Avenue A80, Cleveland, Ohio 44195, USA
K.K. Ang, MD, PhD
Department of Radiation Oncology, The University of Texas M.D. Anderson Cancer Center, 1515 Holcombe Blvd., Box 66, Houston, TX 77030, USA

18.2
COX-2, Prostanoids and COX-2 Inhibitors

18.2.1
Cyclooxygenase Enzymes

Cyclooxygenase (COX), also known as prostaglandin endoperoxide synthase, is the key enzyme involved in synthesis of prostanoids, a collective term for prostaglandins (PGs) and thromboxanes (TXs). Slightly over a decade ago, it was discovered that COX enzyme consists of two isoforms, COX-1 and COX-2 (Fu et al. 1990). COX-1, a ubiquitous enzyme expressed constitutively in virtually all tissues, is responsible for production of the prostanoids that regulate normal homeostatic physiological functions. In contrast, COX-2 is normally absent from most cells and tissues, although it is constitutively expressed in some tissues such as brain and kidney (Fosslien 2000). COX-2, however, appears rapidly in pathological states, such as in inflamed tissues and tumors in which it mediates prostanoid production (Williams and DuBois 1996; O'Banion 1999). COX-2 is an inducible enzyme, induced by a variety of substances including pro-inflammatory cytokines (i.e., TNF-α, IL-1β, platelet activity factors), growth factors (i.e., EGF, PDGF, bFGF, TGF-β), mitogenic substances, oncogenes, etc.

As isoenzymes, COX-1 and COX-2 are genetically independent proteins with different properties and are encoded by genes located on different chromosomes. The *COX-1* gene is located on chromosome 9 (*9q32-q33.3*), has a size of 22 kb, which is composed of 11 exons producing a 2.7-kb mRNA message. The *COX-2* gene is located on chromosome 1 (*1q25.2-q25.3*), has a size of 8.3 kb, which is much smaller than that of COX-1, and includes 10 exons generating a 4.3- to 4.5-kb message. While the intron/exon structures of these genes are nearly identical and the encoded proteins are 75% homologous, the regulatory elements within the genes are quite different. The greater size of the COX-2 mRNA is due to a larger 3'-untranslated region (Kujubu et al. 1991; Xie et al. 1991). Unlike COX-1, COX-2 is an immediate, early response gene whose expression is regulated by transcriptional activation sites as well as motifs controlling message stability. The COX-2 promoter contains a TATA box absent from COX-1 and cis-acting elements responsive to factors up-regulated during inflammation, specifically NF-kB, NF-IL-6, and adenosine 3', 5'-cyclic monophosphate. In addition, the first exon of COX-2 contains a TPA-response element. The 3' untranslated region contains 17 copies of the Shaw-Kamen motif (AUUUnA) that controls message stability and three polyadenylation signals. There is some evidence for alternative splicing of the COX-2 message that would further regulate COX-2 expression.

Both COX-1 and COX-2 are membrane-bound enzymes in the endoplasmic reticulum. In addition, COX-2 localizes to the perinuclear envelope. The molecular weight of COX-1 protein is 67 kDa and that of COX-2 72 kDa (Garavito 1996). Each protein has three structural domains: an epidermal growth factor domain, a membrane-binding domain and a large catalytic domain that is structurally similar to the mammalian peroxidase. Both the cyclooxygenase and peroxidase regions are conserved between the two enzyme isoforms, but the amino acid sequence of COX-2 is truncated at its amino terminus and contains an additional block of 18 amino acids at the carboxy terminus. Major characteristics of COX-1 and COX-2 are listed in Table 18.1. Additional details regarding the biochemistry and molecular biology of these enzymes are described in recent reviews (Marnett 2000; O'Banion 1999; Bakhle 2001; Dannhardt and Kiefer 2001).

18.2.2
Prostanoids

In response to physiological signals, stress or injury, cells produce prostanoids, a family of diverse, highly biologically active lipids derived from enzymatic metabolism of arachidonic acid by COX enzymes. Arachidonic acid is a polyunsaturated fatty acid bound as an ester to cell membrane phospholipids. The initial step in synthesis of prostanoids is the liberation of arachidonic acid from the membrane phospholipids by phospholipase A2. The liberated acid is then catalyzed by COX enzymes, which by the cyclooxygenase activity insert molecular oxygen into the acid to generate prostaglandin (PG) G2. This prostaglandin is unstable and undergoes rapid conversion to PGH2 by the peroxidase activity of COX. The cyclooxygenase and peroxidase sites are located on opposite sides of the catalytic domain of COX. Because COX catalyzes two sequential enzymatic reactions, it is also called prostaglandin peroxide synthase, PGH synthase, or PGG/H synthase. Once generated, PGH2 undergoes further metabolism to PGs and TXA2 through the action of specific isomerases that exert a wide range of biological actions specific to an individual prostanoid. There are several PGs, including PGE_2, $PGF_{2\alpha}$, PGD_2 and PGI_2 (prostacyclin).

Table 18.1. Major characteristics of COX-1 and COX-2

	COX-1	COX-2
Regulation	Constitutive	Inducible
Molecular weight	67 kDa	72 kDa
Gene size	22 kb	8.3 kb
Human chromosome	Chromosome 9	Chromosome 1
mRNA size	2.7 kb	4.3–4.5 kb
Localization	Endoplasmic reticulum	Endoplasmic reticulum, perinuclear envelope
Tissue expression	Ubiquitous	Mainly pathological states
TATA motif (5¢-end)	No	Yes
Promoter	Unknown	NF-κB, NF-IL6, CRE; TCF

Prostanoids regulate many physiological homeostatic functions, including vasomotility (constriction and dilation), platelet aggregation, maintenance of the integrity of gastrointestinal mucosa, immunomodulation, and regulation of cell growth and differentiation. Different PGs may have agonistic or antagonistic effects; the following are only some of the major activities of individual PGs. PGE_2 is a potent vasodilator and an immunosuppressive substance. PGI_2, produced primarily by endothelial cells, is both a vasodilator and an inhibitor of platelet aggregation. $PGF_{2\alpha}$ is a potent vasoconstrictor. PGD_2, produced mainly by plasma cells, inhibits platelet aggregation and causes bronchoconstriction. TXA2, the major arachidonic acid metabolite produced by platelets, induces platelet aggregation and vasoconstriction. It should be noted that although some prostanoids are produced predominantly by certain specific types of cells, most cells produce more than one prostanoid with complementary or antagonistic activities. Therefore, the final biological effect on tissues depends on the balance of similar and opposing actions of the prostanoids involved.

Prostanoids also play a role in the pathogenesis of various pathological states, including inflammation, rheumatoid states, autoimmune diseases, and cancer, where PGE_2 is the major prostaglandin involved. PGE_2, produced in abundance by proinflammatory mononuclear cells such as macrophages, mediates the typical symptoms of inflammation due to its vasodilatory action. This augments edema formation caused by substances that increase vascular permeability such as histamine. PGE_2 is also involved in the development of erythema and heat at the site of inflammation and it potentiates pain. In tumors, although many different prostanoids are formed, PGE_2 production by both neoplastic and tumor infiltrating normal cells predominates.

Prostanoids are short-lived locally acting substances (autocoids) released from cells immediately after being synthesized. By binding to high-affinity membrane receptors they may act on cells that produce them (autocrine activity) or on neighboring cells (paracrine activity). Each prostanoid has a single receptor with the exception of PGE_2 that has four separate receptors. The receptors are designated DP receptors for PGD_2, FP receptors for $PGF_{2\alpha}$, IP receptors for PGI_2, TP receptors for thromboxane, and EP receptors for PGE_2. The four PGE_2 receptors are designated EP_1, EP_2, EP_3 and EP_4. Each receptor binds to its own ligand; however, most prostanoids cross-bind to receptors other than their own. The prostanoid receptors are coupled to G (guanine nucleotide)-binding proteins and generate second messengers, primarily cAMP, Ca^{2+}, and inositol triphosphate (GILMAN 1987; SMITH 1989). A number of protein kinases are activated, including protein kinases C and A and likely protein tyrosine kinase.

There is recent evidence indicating that prostanoids can initiate signaling not only via binding to membrane receptors but also through nuclear hormone receptors, notably the peroxisome proliferator-activated receptors (PPARs). There are three distinct PPAR isoforms, designated PPARα, PPARδ and PPARγ (LEMBERGER et al. 1996), which bind to sequence-specific DNA response elements as heterodimers with the retinoic acid receptor RXR (KLIEWER et al. 1994). The identity of natural ligands for PPARs is still unknown, but it seems that prostanoids, particularly the PGJ_2 metabolite of PGD_2 and PGI_2, can serve as activating ligands (FORMAN et al. 1995, 1997; LIM et al. 1999).

A schematic diagram of prostanoid synthesis and the involvement of COX-1 and COX-2 enzymes is shown in Fig. 18.1.

18.2.3
Cyclooxygenase Inhibitors

As discussed in the preceding section, prostanoids play important roles in both normal physiological

- ubiquitous
- normal tissue
- various physiological functions:
  - GI integrity
  - Vasodilation, vasoconstriction
  - Platelet aggregation
  - Kidney function

- inducible
- inflammatory states
- cancer

Fig. 18.1. A flow diagram of prostanoid synthesis from arachidonic acid, and the involvement of COX-1 and COX-2. Phospholipase A_2 generates free arachidonic acid from membrane phospholipids. Cyclooxygenase-1 or -2 (COX-1, COX-2) convert arachidonic acid to prostaglandin (PG) G_2 via a cyclooxygenase activity followed by conversion to PGH_2 into other prostaglandin isoforms or thromboxane (TX) A_2. Nonsteroidal anti-inflammatory drugs (NSAIDs) inhibit both COX-1 and COX-2 whereas specific COX-2 inhibitors inhibit COX-2 only

regulation and in pathogenesis of various disease states. Aspirin and other nonsteroidal anti-inflammatory drugs (NSAIDs) have for many decades been used for treatment of different inflammatory states. Three decades ago, VANE (1971) proposed that the cyclooxygenase enzyme was the molecular target. Because these agents block both COX-1 and COX-2, their use is associated with significant toxicity, primarily gastrointestinal due to inhibition of protective PGs whose production is mediated by COX-1. The discovery of COX-2 enzyme, shown to be responsible for pathogenesis of inflammatory diseases, thus offered an opportunity for development of agents that would selectively target COX-2 and consequently avoid toxicity associated with the use of standard NSAIDs.

The mechanism of selective COX-2 inhibition is based on structural differences between COX-1 and COX-2. The basic three-dimensional structure of these membrane-associated enzymes consists of a long narrow channel with the opening through which arachidonic acid passes to reach the catalytic site of the enzyme. Only COX-2 enzyme has a side pocket in the channel wall created by a single aminoacid difference between the two enzymes. At position 523, COX-2 contains a smaller valine molecule instead of a larger isoleucine molecule. This difference in size is essentially the cause of the side pocket in COX-2 enzyme regarded to be the binding site of many selective inhibitors. A detailed description of structural differences between the two enzymes and strategies for constructing selective COX-2 inhibitors is reviewed elsewhere (HAWKEY 1999; DANNHARDT and KIEFER 2001; MARNETT and DuBOIS 2002).

18.3
Tumorigenesis, Tumor Growth and Metastasis

18.3.1
Tumorigenesis

Tumorigenesis is a multistep process in which multiple genetic and epigenetic factors are involved. That PGs play a role in this process has long been recognized, leading to the investigations of aspirin and other NSAIDs as possible chemopreventive agents. Ample data from experimental, epidemiological and clinical studies have been accumulated showing that these agents are potent inhibitors of tumorigenesis, particularly colon carcinoma. Regular intake of these drugs for an extended period of time can reduce development of colorectal cancer in humans by 40%–50%. Some NSAIDs such as sulindac were also effective in decreasing the number and size of existing colonic polyps. Development of tumors other than colon carcinoma has also been affected by exposure to NSAIDs, including esophageal, breast and bladder carcinomas. A large body of available information on the effect of aspirin and other NSAIDs on development of cancer was recently reviewed by TAKETO (1998a,b), JANNE and MAYER (2000) and THUN et al. (2002).

Though these studies with NSAIDs implicate cyclooxygenase enzymes as having a role in pathogenesis of tumor development, they could not provide evidence that COX-2 is the principal enzyme responsible. That COX-2 plays a major role in colon carcinogenesis is suggested by findings that COX-2 is present in a high percentage of premalignant lesions and established tumors. The enzyme is detected in about 40%–50% of malignant adenomas and in more than 80% of adenocarcinomas (EBERHART et al. 1994; KOKI et al. 1999). However, the most compelling evidence of a causal relationship between COX-2 and colon carcinogenesis is provided by genetic studies in Min (multiple intestinal neoplasms) mice that have mutations in the *APC* (adenopolyposis coli) gene (OSHIMA et al. 1996). The Min mouse is a good animal model for human familial adenomatous polyposis (FAP). Using these mice that spontaneously develop numerous intestinal polyps, OSHIMA et al. (1996) investigated whether deletions of the *COX-2* gene influenced development of polyps. The APC$^{\Delta 716}$ mice were produced, which were homozygous (+/+), or heterozygous (+/-) for *COX-2*, or were lacking both copies of the gene (-/-). Dramatic differences in polyp formation depending on the presence of the *COX-2* gene were observed. At 10 weeks of age, the homozygous mice developed an average of 652 polyps, whereas mice lacking both copies of *COX-2* developed only 93 polyps, a reduction of 86%. When a single copy of the *COX-2* gene was deleted, polyp development was reduced by 66%. This study provided definitive genetic evidence that COX-2 plays a crucial role in an early event in colon carcinogenesis. Further research showed that treatment of the Min mice with selective COX-2 inhibitors was highly effective in preventing polyp development (OSHIMA et al. 1996; JACOBY et al. 2000). In a study by JACOBY et al. (2000), celecoxib, a selective COX-2 inhibitor, reduced the formation of polyps by 83%. In addition, the size of polyps that formed after treatment with celecoxib was significantly smaller than that of polyps in untreated mice. Piroxicam, a standard NSAID, was also effective in preventing polyp development. However, in contrast to celecoxib, its administration was associated with significant toxicity that included formation of ulcers and perforation and bleeding in the gastrointestinal tract. Selective COX-2 inhibitors were also effective in suppressing development of chemically induced colon cancer (KAWAMORI et al. 1998; KOKI et al. 1999).

Selective COX-2 inhibitors have already entered clinical trials of chemoprevention. STEINBACH et al. (2000) reported a study that assessed the effect of celecoxib on colorectal polyps in patients with familial adenomatous polyposis. These patients have a nearly 100% risk for developing colorectal cancer. The patients were given 100 mg or 400 mg celecoxib twice daily for 6 months, at which time the number and size of polyps was determined by endoscopy and compared to the same polyp parameters at the beginning of the study. Celecoxib was effective in reducing both the number and size of polyps; the drug dose of 400 mg reduced the number of polyps by 28% and the size of polyps by 31%.

18.3.2
Established Tumors

COX-2 and its products play a role in tumor growth and metastases. It has been known for some time that malignant tumors, both experimental and human, often produce excessive amounts of PGs (BENNETT et al. 1979; FURUTA et al. 1988a; RIGAS et al. 1993). Although both the amount and the type of PGs produced vary among tumors, PGE_2 is most commonly produced. Both tumor cells and tumor infiltrating cells including macrophages, lymphocytes, fibroblasts, and endothelial cells produce PGs. As discussed earlier in the chapter the final biological effect of prostanoids depends on the type and quantity of prostanoids produced. With respect to tumors, however, ample evidence suggests that tumor-produced prostanoids stimulate tumor growth and its metastatic spread (FURUTA et al. 1988a; TANG and HONN 1994; KOKI et al. 1999).

Recently, there has been a flare of clinical studies assessing the expression of COX-2 in tumors and its relevance to tumor growth behavior, patient prognosis, and response to conventional treatments. Most studies used immunohistochemistry to detect COX-2, and they showed that COX-2 is present in a broad range of human cancers including colon, esophagus, lung, pancreas and head and neck cancers (reviewed in KOKI et al. 1999). Results of several investigations will be mentioned here. Colorectal carcinomas were found to display high levels of COX-2 expression, whereas the expression of this enzyme in normal intestinal mucosa was either absent or detectable only at low levels (SANO et al. 1995; KARGMAN et al. 1995; SHEEHAN et al. 1999). SHEEHAN et al. (1999) demonstrated a positive relationship between the extent of COX-2 expression and more aggressive tumor behavior. High expression of COX-2 was related to advanced Dukes staging, lymph node metastasis, and poorer long-term outcome for colorectal cancer patients.

ZIMMERMANN et al. (1999) reported that COX-2 was expressed in a high percentage of esophageal tumors: 78% of adenocarcinomas and 91% of squamous cell carcinomas. They also measured COX-2 expression in two esophageal cancer cell lines to evaluate the functional relevance of COX-2-derived PGs and found that PGE_2 synthesis was 600 times higher in the cell line that expressed COX-2. Selective COX-2 inhibitors suppressed PGE_2 synthesis in this cell line, which resulted in inhibition of cell proliferation and induction of apoptosis. This study, therefore, suggested that COX-2-derived PGs play an important role in the regulation of cell proliferation and cell death in esophageal cancer and that the inhibition of COX-2 may be useful in the therapy and prevention of this cancer. Another study (WILSON et al. 1998) measured the expression of the genes encoding inducible nitric oxide synthase and COX-2, both of which are mediators of inflammation and regulators of epithelial cell growth, in patients with Barrett's metaplasia and esophageal adenocarcinomas. The mRNA for the nitric oxide gene was elevated in 76% and the *COX-2* gene in 80% of patients with Barrett's metaplasia, and in 80% and 100%, respectively, of patients with esophageal carcinomas.

COX-2 is frequently overexpressed in premalignant lesions as well as established carcinomas in the lung (HIDA et al. 1998; WOLFF et al. 1998; ACHIWA et al. 1999; KHURI et al. 2001). For example, using immunohistochemical analysis, HIDA et al. (1998) detected COX-2 expression in about one-third of cases of atypical adenomatous hyperplasia and carcinomas in situ and in 70% of cases of invasive adenocarcinomas. The percentage of COX-2-positive cells in adenocarcinomas was greater in lymph node metastases than in the primary tumors. Another lung study (WOLFF et al. 1998) reported COX-2 positivity in 90% of the adenocarcinomas and in 100% of the squamous cell carcinomas, but the intensity of COX-2 positivity varied widely. COX-2 was not detected in normal lung tissue and only rarely in hyperplastic bronchiolar epithelium. There appears to be a positive relationship between COX-2 overexpression and the poor survival of patients with lung carcinoma (ACHIWA et al. 1999; KHURI et al. 2001). Using in situ hybridization with a digoxigenin-labeled COX-2 antisense riboprobe, KHURI et al. (2001) analyzed COX-2 status in 185 patients with stage I non-small cell lung carcinoma (NSCLC) treated with surgical resection and found an inverse correlation between the level of COX-2 positivity and 5-year survival. The level of COX-2 expression was an independent prognostic factor for survival in the multivariate analysis.

Using quantitative reverse transcription-polymerase chain reaction, immunoblotting, and immunohistochemistry, TUCKER et al. (1999) assessed the expression of COX-2 in pancreatic cancer and normal pancreatic tissue. There was a more then 60-fold greater expression of COX-2 mRNA in pancreatic cancer than in adjacent non-tumorous tissue. COX-2 protein was present in 9 of 10 adenocarcinomas of the pancreas but was undetectable in non-tumorous pancreatic tissue. Immunohistochemical analysis showed that *COX-2* was expressed in malignant epithelial cells. The exact same methods revealed overexpression of COX-2 in squamous cell carcinomas of the head and neck, compared with normal mucosa from healthy volunteers (CHAN et al. 1999). In our ongoing study (unpublished) of head and neck carcinomas, we observed that COX-2 is present in more than 85% of analyzed tumors. The extent of expression, determined by both the percentage of tumor cells positive and the intensity of staining, broadly varied. Figure 18.2 shows COX-2 positivity in head and neck tumors.

Taken together, the evidence is compelling that many cancers in humans do possess COX-2 enzyme, but there exists broad variability both in the percentage of tumors that contain it and also in the level of the enzyme among COX-2-positive tumors. Also, increasing evidence shows that tumors that express COX-2 show more malignant behavior and adversely impact patient prognosis.

18.3.3
Metastasis

Metastasis, migration of tumor cells beyond tissue compartment and spread to distant organs, is a complex, multistep event in the progression of malignant tumors that is influenced by many systemic and local factors as well as the properties of the tumor cell.

Fig. 18.2. COX-2 expression in a head and neck squamous cell carcinoma. Brown stain shows cells positive for COX-2. COX-2 negative stroma is stained blue

Levels of *COX-2* expression were found to correlate with in vitro motility and invasion and the in vivo metastasis of a highly metastatic human lung cancer cell line (LNM35) (KOZAKI et al. 2001). KOZAKI et al. (2001) and DOHADWALA et al. (2001) suggested that the invasion of NSCLC occurred through a COX-2-mediated and CD44-dependent pathway. Cell surface CD44 is a cell surface transmembrane receptor of hyaluronate that mediates cellular adhesion to extracellular matrix, an important step in tumor cell migration. A direct link between COX-2 and enhanced adhesion of carcinoma cells to endothelial cells, and enhanced liver metastasis potential has been reported (KAKIUCHI et al. 2002). In addition, clinical data has demonstrated frequent co-expression of COX-2 and Laminin-5, another extracellular matrix protein that plays a key role in cell migration and tumor invasion, at the invasive front of early-stage adenocarcinoma of the lung (NIKI et al. 2002). *COX-2* expression enhances lymphatic invasion and metastasis in human gastrointestinal tract cancers (MURATA et al. 1999; SHEEHAN et al. 1999).

On the other hand, nonsteroidal anti-inflammatory drugs (NSAIDs) and selective COX-2 inhibitors have been reported to inhibit COX-2 activity and the proliferation of malignant cells in vitro (HIDA et al. 1998; TSUBOUCHI et al. 2000) to retard tumor progression and to reduce metastasis in vivo (FULTON 1987; MASFERRER et al. 2000; KOKI et al. 1999). Treatment with celecoxib, a selective COX-2 inhibitor, showed a dose-dependent inhibitory effect on both tumor growth and the number of lung metastases that developed in tumor-bearing mice. This effect was attributed at least partly to the antiangiogenic effect of celecoxib, since the drug caused a substantial reduction in the number and length of sprouting capillaries in a rat corneal model (MASFERRER et al. 2000).

18.3.4
Mechanisms of COX-2 and Its Inhibitors in Tumorigenesis, Tumor Growth and Metastasis

COX-2 contributes to tumorigenesis and the growth and metastases of already-established tumors by multiple mechanisms; the major mechanisms are discussed in the following sections.

Production of Mutagens and Carcinogens. COX-2 is a bifunctional enzyme, having both cyclooxygenase and peroxidase activities. The latter activity can break down PGH2 to a mutagen, malondialdehyde, which forms adducts with DNA. The peroxidase reaction is important in xenobiotic metabolism, generating different mutagens and carcinogens. This is particularly relevant to the gastrointestinal and upper aerodigestive tracts where cells are constantly exposed to a variety of xenobiotics (MARNETT 1994; ELING and CURTIS 1992; PRESCOTT and WHITE 1996). As an example, many chemicals present in tobacco smoke are converted by the peroxidase action of COX-2 into carcinogens that bind to DNA (WIESE et al. 2001). Logically then, it can be expected that the inhibition of COX-2 would suppress formation of mutagens and carcinogens, thus reducing carcinogenesis.

Cell Growth Dysregulation and Induction of Apoptosis. Dysregulation of cell division and growth as well as the propensity of cells to undergo apoptosis are characteristic features not only of tumorigenesis but also of the growth of established tumors and tumors' propensity to metastasize. Ample experimental data show that COX-2 or its products can cause these imbalances in cell growth and death. Most PGs stimulate cell growth by autocrine or paracrine signaling involving the G-protein family of receptors and cell proliferation. In contrast, inhibitors of COX-2 inhibit cell growth. COX-2 can cause dysregulation of cell growth on its own or in cooperation with other tumor cell growth factors or signaling pathways, such as through the involvement of epidermal growth factor receptor (EGFR). Inhibition of these so-called cooperative signals can inhibit cell growth and carcinogenesis. Recently, TORRANCE et al. (2000) reported that development of intestinal neoplasms in mice was reduced by EK1-568, an inhibitor of EGFR kinase, although to a lesser extent than by the NSAID sulindac. When the two drugs were combined, the inhibition of intestinal tumorigenesis was synergistic. The inhibitory effect of sulindac on polyp formation in Min mice was partially prevented by administering PGE_2 to mice, which demonstrates the role of COX-2 products in induction of colon tumorigenesis (HANSEN-PETRIK et al. 2002).

COX-2 is involved in resistance of cells to undergo apoptotic cell death, and via this mechanism may exert its pro-carcinogenic effect and its stimulatory actions on tumor growth. There is a positive correlation between COX-2 expression and resistance to apoptosis (WATSON 1998; SMITH et al. 2000). More direct evidence for the apoptosis-inhibitory role of COX-2 was provided by transfection-type experiments. For example, when intestinal epithelial cells were transfected with COX-2, they became resistant to butyrate-induced apoptosis (TSUJII and DUBOIS 1995). The transfected cells exhibited an increased adhesion to extracellular matrix and showed elevated expression of Bcl2 protein, an apoptosis-inhibitory molecule. These effects of COX-2 transfection were reversed by treatment of cells with the NSAID sulindac sulfide. The inhibitory role of COX-2 or PGs on apoptosis and reversal of that by NSAIDs or selective COX-2 inhibitors is not limited to colorectal cancer cells but is observed in many other tumor cell types; for more details see KOKI et al. (1999) and DEMPKE et al. (2001). Collectively, these findings demonstrate that COX-2 can increase tumorigenic potential by inducing various phenotypic changes in cells conducive to their survival and by reducing cell loss through apoptosis. COX-2 would thus prolong the survival of cells, likely including cells that had already accumulated sufficient sequential genetic changes to result in malignant transformation. Likewise, reduced cell loss in established tumors results in more rapid tumor growth.

At the molecular level, various downstream molecules in signaling pathways have been identified that are modulated by the COX-2 inhibitors, which can lead to apoptotic cell death. ZHANG and DUBOIS (2000) showed that NS-398 increased a prostate apoptosis-response gene, *Par-4*, in human colon carcinoma cells (HCA-7), suggesting that COX-2 inhibition induced apoptosis via Par-4 induction. Accumulation of arachidonic acid after COX inhibition led to the increased formation of ceramide from sphingomyelin that resulted in increased apoptosis in colorectal cancer cells (CHAN et al. 1998). Cytochrome-c pathway has been implicated in the NS-398-induced apoptosis, where treatment with the inhibitor induced cytochrome c release from mitochondria, followed by activation of caspase-9 and caspase-3 which in turn induced PARP cleavage leading to apoptosis in esophageal cancer cells (LI et al. 2001). In LNCaP cells, NS-398 induced apoptosis by down-regulating bcl-2 expression. Also, inhibition of NFkB activity by COX-2 inhibitors and NSAIDs has been reported in several cell types in vitro as a mechanism by which the cells are directed to the cell death pathway (YAMAMOTO et al. 1999; MANSON et al. 2000). The molecular aspects of COX-2 and its inhibition in apoptosis induction are currently a subject of intensive investigation.

Immunomodulation. Cancer development and growth has long been recognized to be under immunological surveillance, with immunosuppression being conducive to both. Because most PGs and in particular PGE_2, a major PG type produced by tumor cells, are potent immunosuppressants, they may reduce or abolish the ability of the immune surveillance to restrict carcinogenesis, tumor growth, as well as tumor spread. PGE_2 affects various facets of immune reactions including blocking the antitumor activity of lymphocytes, natural killer cells, and macrophages (LEUNG and MIHICH 1980; BRUNDA et al. 1980), mediating immune suppression by T-suppressor cells (FULTON and LEVY 1980), inhibiting production of cytotoxic lymphokines (KAMBAYASHI et al. 1995), and stimulating production of immunosuppressive lymphokines (HUANG et al. 1998). Recently, HUANG et al. (1998) showed that PGE_2 produced by COX-2-expressing NSCLC cell lines may play an immunoregulatory role by inducing IL-10 production. In response to IL-1b stimulation, NSCLC cells increased PGE_2 production up to 50-fold. IL-1b also induced COX-2 mRNA expression and protein production. This IL-1b-induced PGE_2 production was reversed by the pharmacological or antisense oligonucleotide-induced inhibition of COX-2 activity or expression. These investigators further found that PGE_2 stimulated IL-10 production by lymphocytes and macrophages while it inhibited IL-12 production by macrophages. In contrast, by reducing PG production, NSAIDs and COX-2 inhibitors minimize or abolish the immunosuppressive effects of PGs and restore antitumor immunological rejection mechanisms, which can contribute to their antitumor action. Specific inhibition of COX-2 was reported to reduce the growth of Lewis lung carcinoma in vivo by altering the balance in IL-10 and IL-12 synthesis, which led to marked lymphocytic infiltration of the tumor (STOLINA et al. 2000).

Angiogenesis. Angiogenesis, the formation of capillaries from established blood vessels, is an essential requirement for progressive tumor growth beyond small clumps of tumor cells. These capillaries are formed in response to angiogenic substances secreted by tumor cells, as well by normal tissue infiltrates in tumors, such as fibroblasts and macrophages. COX-2 plays an important role in synthesis of angiogenic factors. PGs have long been known to possess angiogenic properties (FORM and AUERBACH 1983; ZICHE et al. 1982). More recent observations showed that there is also a link between COX-2 and VEGF. Cells negative for COX-2 exhibit decreased expression of VEGF (WILLIAMS et al. 2000), and furthermore, COX-2-generated PGs can enhance bFGF-induced angiogenesis through induction of VEGF (MAJIMA et al. 2000). Other factors can also be involved such as stimulation of VEGF production by IL-6 which was in turn induced by PGs (RAK et al. 1996). Thus, PGs can stimulate angiogenesis directly or indirectly through VEGF production.

Both standard NSAIDs and selective COX-2 inhibitors inhibit angiogenesis. The first report on this originated from our group (MILAS et al. 1990), and more recently we observed that the selective COX-2 inhibitor SC-236 was also potent inhibitor of tumor angiogenesis (MILAS et al. 1999; Fig 18.3). This reduction in newly formed vessels by either indomethacin or SC-236 was associated with tumor growth retardation. KOKI et al. (1999) and MASFERRER et al. (2000) showed that the selective COX-2 inhibitor SC-236 and celecoxib profoundly inhibit corneal neovascularization induced in rats and mice by bFGF. In contrast, administration of a selective COX-1 inhibitor, or a regioisomer of celecoxib that does not inhibit COX-2 had no inhibitory effect on bFGF-induced neoangiogenesis. Additional information on COX-2-induced angiogenesis as well as on the inhibition of angiogenesis by COX-2 inhibitors was recently reviewed by GATELY (2000).

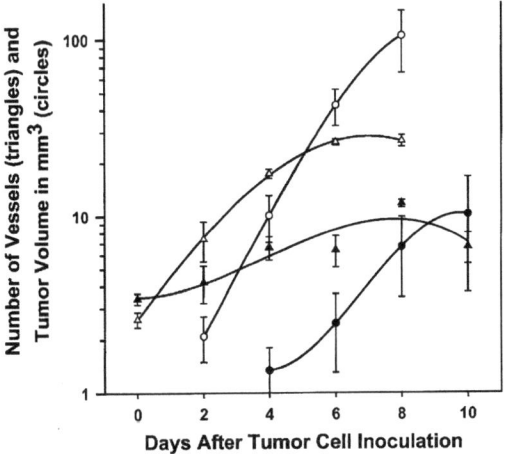

Fig. 18.3. Effect of SC-236 on tumor angiogenesis. The number of newly formed blood vessels was recorded after intradermal injection of 10^6 NFSa cells in mice treated with vehicle (*open triangles*) or SC-236 (*closed triangles*) given at a dose of 6 mg/kg in the drinking water for 9 consecutive days starting 1 day after tumor cell inoculation. Inhibition of tumor angiogenesis was associated with delay in tumor growth (*closed circles*). Vertical bars are SE of the mean values. (From MILAS et al. 1999, with permission)

18.4
Interactions with Ionizing Radiation

18.4.1
Radioprotective Effects of PGs

PGs regulate various protective homeostatic functions guarding cells and tissues from different types of injury, and already in the 1980s it was recognized that they act as radioprotective agents as well (reviewed in HANSON 1998; MILAS and HANSON 1995). The first report of radioprotection came from HANSON and THOMAS (1983) who showed that exogenous administration of PGE_2 prior to the irradiation of mice increased the survival of intestinal epithelial cells. Subsequent studies showed that PGs or their stable analogs radioprotected a variety of other normal cells, including hematopoietic stem cells (HANSON and AINSWORTH 1985), dermal cells (GENG et al. 1992) and spermatogonia (VAN BUUL et al. 1997, 1999). In vitro, PGs were shown to protect both normal and cancer cell lines from radiation injury (HANSON 1998; VAN BUUL et al. 1997, 1999; ZAFFARONI et al. 1993). PGs widely vary in their radioprotective ability; however, the PG analog misoprostol was among the most potent examined when given within a few hours before radiation (HANSON 1998).

Current evidence suggests that radioprotection requires ligand-receptor binding, since in vitro protection could not be achieved in cells that lacked PG receptors or when the receptors were blocked (HANSON et al. 1995). Repair of DNA damage is one of a number of mechanisms controlling radioprotection, as suggested by data showing decreased radioprotection under DNA-repair deficient conditions (VAN BUUL et al. 1997, 1999). Another possible mechanism is reduced cellular sensitivity susceptible to radiation-induced apoptosis (HOUCHEN et al. 2000). Additionally, PGs can radioprotect tissues by stimulating the regeneration of cells surviving radiation exposure (HOUCHEN et al. 2000). Thus, it is clear that multiple mechanisms influence the ability of PGs to protect cells and tissues from radiation damage. These mechanisms of radioprotection provide targets for modulating tumor response to radiotherapy, as discussed in the following sections.

18.4.2
Effect of COX-2 Inhibitors on Tumor Radioresponse

As discussed in Sec. 18.3.1, "Tumorigenesis," 18.3.2, "Established Tumors," and 18.3.3., "Metastasis," there exists a link between tumor expression of COX-2 or excessive production of PGs by tumors and aggressive tumor behavior, which may result in adverse patient prognosis. The poor survival rate observed in those patients could be due to either more aggressive tumor growth or to increased tumor resistance to treatment, such as chemotherapy or radiotherapy. Thus, inhibition of COX-2 activity or PG production has the potential to improve tumor response to cytotoxic therapy.

Printing and Binding: Stürtz AG, Würzburg

enhanced tumor response to irradiation. Radiation enhancement factors for the NFSa tumor were 3.64 for tumor growth delay and 1.77 for the tumor cure endpoint (MILAS et al. 1999). The two other tumors, FSa and U251, also responded dramatically to the combined SC-236 plus radiation treatment (KISHI et al. 2000; PETERSEN et al. 2000). For comparison, Table 18.2 shows the radiation enhancement factors after treatment with indomethacin (NSAID) or SC-236 (COX-2 inhibitor). For example, radioresponse assayed by tumor growth delay was enhanced by a factor of 1.4 by indomethacin but by factors greater than 2.0 by SC-236 for all three tumors: sarcomas NFSa and FSa, and U251 human glioma. The findings clearly show that SC-236 was a more potent enhancer of tumor radioresponse.

KISHI et al. (2000) established proof for the hypothesis that preferential enhancement of tumor vs normal tissue radioresponse (therapeutic gain) could be achieved by specific inhibition of the COX-2 enzyme. Treating the FSa tumor with SC-236 and radiation as described above, tumor growth delay was enhanced by a factor of 2.14 and tumor cure by a factor of 1.87. The study demonstrated no biologically significant increase in normal tissue radioresponse: intestinal epithelium assayed by acute crypt clonogen survival and skin assayed by late contracture of the irradiated leg. Thus, this study was the first investigation to unequivocally establish that therapeutic gain could be achieved with selective inhibition of COX-2 in combination with radiotherapy.

These studies using SC-236 have now been augmented by demonstrating that other selective COX-2 inhibitors such as celecoxib (DAVIS et al. 2002) and NS-398 (PYO et al. 2001) also enhance the effect of radiation both in vitro and in vivo. DAVIS et al. (2002) used celecoxib at 100 mg/kg twice daily by gavage to treat the FSa mouse sarcoma in combination with radiation. Treatment with celecoxib started when the leg tumors were 6 mm in diameter and continued for 20 consecutive days. Irradiation (30-Gy single dose) was given when the tumors grew to 8 mm in diameter. Celecoxib treatment enhanced the tumor radioresponse by a factor of 1.9, an enhancement factor similar to that obtained for SC-236. PYO et al. (2001) obtained a radioenhancement factor of 2.5 for tumor growth delay of the H-460 human lung cancer cell line grown as in vivo xenografts and treated with the selective COX-2 inhibitor NS-398.

Using a variety of murine tumors, FURUTA et al. (1988a) showed that the anti-tumor effect of the NSAID indomethacin critically depended on the tumor's ability to produce PGs: only tumors that produced PGs responded to indomethacin treatment. This observation has recently been confirmed and extended to the action of a specific COX-2 inhibitor. PYO et al. (2001) tested the radioenhancing ability of NS-398 on two human tumors, one of which expressed COX-2 constitutively (NCI-H460 lung cancer) and one that lacked COX-2 expression (HCT-116 colon carcinoma). The radiation response was enhanced, by a factor of 2.5, only for the NCI-H460 tumor that expressed COX-2. This effect was attributed to enhancement of radiation-induced apoptosis. The tumor lacking expression, HCT-116, was not significantly affected by treatment with NS-398. These findings imply that enhancement of tumor radioresponse by COX-2 inhibition will occur only in tumors positive for COX-2 enzyme expression. They further suggest that it may be possible to predict individual tumor treatment response by assaying the tumor either for COX-2 expression or PG profile prior to initiation of radiotherapy.

Table 18.2. Enhancement factors of tumor radioresponse: indomethacin vs SC-236

Drug	Tumor	Growth delay EF	TCD50 EF	References
INDO	NFSa	1.4	1.26	FURUTA et al. (1988b)
Sc-236	NFSa	3.64	1.77	MILAS et al. (1999)
	FSa	2.14	1.87	KISHI et al. (2000)
	U251	2.13		PETERSEN et al. (2000)

EF, enhancement factors; INDO, indomethacin

18.4.3
Effect of COX-2 Inhibitors on Normal Tissue Radioresponse

Any potential radioenhancing agent must increase tumor response more than the response of dose-limiting normal tissues in order to improve therapeutic gain. Limited information regarding this balance between tumor and normal tissue responses is currently available for specific COX-2 inhibitors. As described in Sec. 18.4.2, "Effect of COX-2 Inhibitors on Tumor Radioresponse," KISHI et al. (2000) showed clear therapeutic advantage of treating with SC-236 when comparing tumor radioresponse (EF for FSa tumor cure, 1.87) to that of normal tissue (EF for jejunal crypt survival, 1.03 and EF, 1.0 for leg contraction 120 days after radiation). Clearly, radioenhancement was much greater for tumor than for either acutely responding (jejunum) or late-responding (leg contracture) normal tissue radiation reactions.

Given that treatment with a standard NSAID, indomethacin, has been shown to be radioprotective for some normal tissues such as the hematopoietic system and lung (MILAS et al. 1992; Nishiguchi et al. 1990), we subsequently hypothesized that treatment of select normal tissues with COX-2 inhibitors would also be radioprotective (MILAS 2001). This would particularly affect tissues where inflammation is a significant factor in the pathogenesis of radiation injury. To test this, mice were treated with SC-236 beginning 3 days before local thoracic single-dose irradiation and continued for 10 consecutive days, as was done for the tumor experiments described in Sec. 18.4.2, "Effect of COX-2 Inhibitors on Tumor Radioresponse". Treatment endpoint was the occurrence of lethal pneumonitis 60–180 days after radiation exposure. There was no significant difference between the radiation dose causing 50% fatal pneumonitis in mice treated with radiation only and that in mice treated with SC-236 and radiation (unpublished). Therefore, these preliminary results do not support the hypothesis of radioprotection by inhibition of COX-2 in a normal tissue, but they do support the general concept of enhanced therapeutic gain when radiotherapy is combined with specific COX-2 inhibition.

18.4.4
Clinical Trials Related to Radiotherapy

Rapidly growing preclinical investigations showing the involvement of COX-2 and its products in tumor response to radiation have stimulated clinical research. Currently, two aspects related to radiotherapy are being addressed, one concerning whether the assessment of COX-2 in tumors can be predictive of tumor response to radiotherapy, and the other on whether treatment with selective COX-2 inhibitors can improve treatment outcome of radiotherapy. The former aspect was recently addressed by GAFFNEY et al. (2001) in the case of cervix carcinoma. Tumors from 24 patients were analyzed for COX-2 positivity using immunohistochemistry, and the positivity correlated with patient survival at the median follow-up of 75 months. The results showed that patients with less than 10% of tumor cells staining for COX-2 had significantly better overall survival and disease-free survival compared to patients with 10% or more tumor cells positive for COX-2. Several trials have recently been initiated to address the issue of the therapeutic efficacy of selective COX-2 inhibitors when combined with radiotherapy. Results of these investigations are as yet unavailable.

18.4.5
Mechanisms of Increased Tumor Radioresponse

A paucity of studies limits our understanding of mechanisms by which COX-2 inhibitors enhance tumor response to radiation. However, currently available information suggests that there are multiple modes of action, some of which render tumor cells more sensitive to radiation damage while others affect other determinants of tumor radioresistance. The effect can be inflicted directly on tumor cells or indirectly through modulating tumor cell microenvironment.

Increased Cellular Radiosensitivity. In vitro studies showed that COX-2 inhibitors increase cell radiosensitivity, as demonstrated by clonogenic cell survival (PETERSEN et al. 2000; PYO et al. 2001). A number of mechanisms may be involved and three have been investigated: inhibition of repair from sublethal radiation damage, increased susceptibility to radiation-induced apoptosis, and cell cycle redistribution. Repair from sublethal radiation damage as a mechanism was initially suggested by the lack of shoulder on the radiation survival curve for cells treated with COX-2 inhibitors (PETERSEN et al. 2000; Fig 18.5). The mechanism was subsequently confirmed by demonstrating the inability of treated cells to recover from

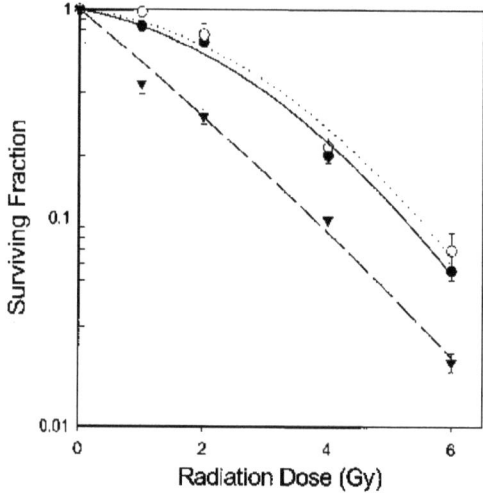

Fig. 18.5. Effect of SC-236 on in vitro radiosensitivity of U251 human glioma cells. Cultures were treated with radiation (●) only or with SC-236 (50 µM) for 1 (○) or 2 (▼) days before irradiation. After irradiation, attached cells were removed and plated, and colony-forming efficiency was determined 10 days later. Survival curves were constructed after normalizing for the cytotoxicity induced by SC-236 alone. Vertical bars are SE of the mean values. (From PETERSEN et al. 2000, with permission)

radiation damage within the time interval between two radiation fractions delivered 4 h apart (Raju et al. 2002). Another possible mechanism whereby COX-2 inhibitors increase sensitivity of tumor cells to radiation-induced apoptosis does not have firm experimental support. Though these inhibitors induced apoptosis on their own, the remaining surviving cells showed no quantitative difference in apoptotic death when exposed to radiation compared to cells not treated with the inhibitors (Petersen et al. 2000; Raju et al. 2002). Finally, investigations related to cell cycle effects as a mechanism for increased cell radiosensitivity by COX-2 inhibitors provided conflicting findings. While some studies showed no cell cycle redistribution, Petersen et al. (2000), Davis et al. (2002), and Raju et al. (2002) showed that SC-236 arrested cells in the radiosensitive G2/M phases of the cell cycle. At the molecular level, the G2/M arrest was associated with down-regulation in the expression of cyclin-A, cyclin-B, as well as cyclin-dependent kinase-1 (cdk-1, also known as cdc-2). In this study, Raju et al. (2002) used murine NFSa sarcoma cells. However, under similar experimental conditions, SC-236 had no effect on cell cycle redistribution of human U251 glioma cell line (Petersen et al. 2000), suggesting that the ability of this agent to induce G2/M arrest may at least partly depend on tumor cell type. In vitro, the induced increase in cellular sensitivity to radiation by COX-2 inhibitors was observed in cells that expressed COX-2 but not in those that were negative for this enzyme (Pyo et al. 2001). Thus, it seems that the presence of COX-2 makes tumor cells more proficient in repairing radiation-induced damage, and that inhibition of this proficiency through inhibition of COX-2 renders cells more sensitive to radiation.

Inhibition of Angiogenesis. As discussed in Sec. 18.3.4, "Mechanisms of COX-2 and Its Inhibitors in Tumorigenesis, Tumor Growth and Metastasis", the ability of COX-2 inhibitors to suppress angiogenesis is one of the mechanisms by which these agents inhibit the growth of tumors and establishment of metastases. SC-236 and celecoxib are highly effective in enhancing tumor response to radiation and both exhibit potent antiangiogenic activity (Milas et al. 1999; Kishi et al. 2000; Masferrer et al. 2000). SC-236 was shown to reduce formation of new blood vessels at the injection site of murine sarcoma cells (Milas et al. 1999; Kishi et al. 2000) and celecoxib inhibited FGF-induced corneal neovascularization in rats (Masferrer et al. 2000). More recently, Dicker et al. (2001) demonstrated that another selective COX-2 inhibitor, rofecoxib, inhibited in vitro proliferation and capillary tube formation of HUVEC endothelial cells. This effect was more pronounced when rofecoxib was combined with radiation, implicating the interaction between the two agents. Poor tumor vascularity is instrumental in the development of tumor hypoxia and consequent emergence of radioresistant hypoxic cells, which are 2.5–3 times more radioresistant than well-oxygenated cells. It has traditionally been thought that the use of agents that inhibit angiogenesis would further increase tumor hypoxia and thus impair tumor response to radiation. Recently, however, increasing evidence shows that the combination of antiangiogenic agents with radiation acts in the opposite direction, i.e., enhances tumor response to radiation (Teicher et al. 1995; Gorski et al. 1998, 1999). Several mechanisms could account for this. Antiangiogenic agents inhibit pro-angiogenic factors produced by tumors, including VEGF, FGF and, in the case of selective COX-2 inhibitors, PGs. VEGF increases blood vessel permeability that could elevate fluid accumulation and pressure in the extracapillary space, and consequently impair blood flow and oxygen supply to tumor cells. Therefore, administration of antiangiogenic agents could prevent these effects of VEGF, and there is a report that treatment with antiangiogenic agents does enhance tumor oxygenation (Teicher et al. 1995). Increased tumor oxygenation could also be the result of tumor cell loss by apoptosis induced by antiangiogenic agents, including COX-2 inhibitors. This mechanism of improved tumor oxygenation has been well documented to occur after tumor treatment with chemotherapeutic agents (Milas et al. 1995; Mason et al. 1999). It should be noted that the effect of selective COX-2 inhibitors on tumor oxygenation has not yet been investigated. Another potential mechanism for improvement of tumor radioresponse by antiangiogenic agents is that these agents may cause vascular collapse in tumors and massive necrosis of tumor cells, as is the case for combretastatin (Li et al. 1998) and C225 antiepidermal growth factor receptor antibody (Milas et al. 2000). Furthermore, since angiogenic substances, such as VEGF (Gorski et al. 1999) and FGF (Haimovitz-Friedman et al. 1991), exhibit radioprotective properties, their inhibition may result in enhanced tumor response to radiotherapy. Abolition of radioprotective effects of PGs is discussed in the following section.

Abolition of PG-rendered Radioprotection. Treatment with selective COX-2 inhibitors reduces PG levels in cultured cells (Raju et al. 2002) and in tumors in vivo (Kishi et al. 2000), and this reduction was associated with enhanced cell and tumor radioresponse. Because PGs are potent radioprotective agents, as described in Sec. 18.4.1, "Radioprotective Effects of PGs", it is logical to attribute, at least partly, the observed radioenhancement to the removal of radioprotective PGs. It was recently observed that radiation increased the expression of COX-2 protein (Steinauer et al. 2000; Davis et al. 2002) and synthesis of PGE_2 in tumor cells (Davis et al. 2002; Raju et al. 2002), suggesting that this represents a cellular survival response to the radiation stress. Addition of SC-236 or celecoxib not only abolished the radiation-induced increase in PGE_2 but it reduced the level of PGE_2 further, to the level in tumor cells treated by the inhibitors only (Davis et al. 2002; Raju et al. 2002). Thus, reduction in PG levels would leave cells without radiation protection by these molecules, leading to increased radiation damage. This conclusion is supported by reports showing that the addition of PGs or their analogs radioprotected a number of cell types (Hanson and Thomas 1983; Riehl et al. 2000; van Buul et al. 1997; Zaffaroni et al. 1993).

Other Potential Mechanisms. As discussed in Sec. 18.3.4, "Mechanisms of COX-2 and Its Inhibitors in Tumorigenesis, Tumor Growth and Metastasis", PGs and especially PGE_2 suppress the immune system by affecting various facets of immunological reaction, which may then facilitate tumor growth and adversely impact the efficacy of tumor radiotherapy (Milas et al. 1990). NSAIDs and selective COX-2 inhibitors were shown to restore immunoreactivity (Milas et al. 1990; Stolina et al. 2000). Also, we previously reported that the indomethacin-induced enhancement of tumor radioresponse was partly mediated by immunological mechanisms (Milas et al. 1990). Thus, it is likely that selective COX-2 inhibitors involve the immune system as a mechanism of their efficacy when combined with radiotherapy or other cytotoxic treatments. However, no studies are available so far that have tested this mechanism. COX-2 inhibitors may modulate various microenvironmental factors present within the tumor that are conducive to tumor cell proliferation. For example, COX-2 inhibitors may interfere with EGFR-mediated signaling pathways (Torrance et al. 2000) and hence inhibit tumor cell growth and enhance tumor response to radiation. With regard to the latter, the blockade of EGFR with C225 anti-EGFR antibody (Milas et al. 2000) or treatment with tyrosine kinase inhibitors that block EGFR signaling pathways (Harari and Huang 2001) were shown to dramatically enhance tumor response to radiotherapy.

18.5
Conclusions

Recent advances in molecular biology have identified a number of molecular determinants and signaling pathways, which function abnormally in tumor cells, and thus play a significant role in the biology of cancer and tumor resistance to therapy. COX-2 is one of these determinants that has recently attracted considerable preclinical and clinical research interest. This enzyme is responsible for the production of prostanoids in tumors, and increasing evidence suggests that its presence in tumors is associated with more aggressive tumor behavior, resistance of tumors to standard treatment modalities and poor patient prognosis. These biological effects are caused mainly by prostanoids, although COX-2 can involve mechanisms unrelated to prostanoids.

Because it stimulates tumor progression and increases tumor resistance to treatments, COX-2 represents a potential target for cancer therapy. Agents that selectively inhibit COX-2 are becoming available at a rapid rate. Already, significant preclinical evidence shows that selective inhibitors of COX-2 are effective in preventing carcinogenesis, slowing the growth of established tumors and inhibiting metastatic spread. These antitumor actions of COX-2 are exerted through multiple mechanisms, including inhibition of tumor cell proliferation, induction of apoptosis, inhibition of neoangiogenesis, and stimulation of the antitumor immune response.

Selective COX-2 inhibitors have also been investigated for their ability to improve tumor response to other cancer treatment modalities, including radiotherapy. A number of preclinical studies, using both animal tumors and human tumor xenografts, demonstrated that these inhibitors can increase tumor response to radiation, with enhancement factors commonly above 2 and as high as 3.6. These enhancement factors are higher than those achieved by common NSAIDs. Moreover, selective COX-2 inhibitors did not appreciably enhance normal tissue response to radiation, indicating that they can provide significant therapeutic gain when combined with radiotherapy.

Mechanisms by which COX-2 inhibitors enhance tumor response to radiation are unclear but they seem to be multiple. Some evidence is already available to show that the inhibitors can prevent cellular repair of radiation damage and increase tumor radioresponse through inhibiting tumor neoangiogenesis. These effects are associated with reduction in PG production, and it is likely that removal of PGs is a major underlying mechanism. However, other mechanisms are possible, including inhibition of the radioprotective cytokines such as FGF and stimulation of antitumor immune rejection responses.

The preclinical findings on COX-2 and its inhibitors have had a rapid impact on clinical research in radiation oncology, where mainly two aspects of COX-2 are being investigated. One aspect is whether COX-2 overexpression is associated with poorer response to radiation treatment and the other is whether administration of selective COX-2 inhibitors improves radiotherapy. Although there are a number of ongoing clinical studies, the findings of these studies are still unknown. Research regarding the effect of COX-2 inhibition on tumor response to radiation or other cytotoxic agents is rapidly evolving. Based on the available preclinical evidence, targeting COX-2 has a significant potential to improve treatment efficacy of radiotherapy and other commonly used cancer therapies.

References

Ahiwa H, Yatabe Y, Hida T et al (1999) Prognostic significance of elevated cyclooxygenase 2 expression in primary, resected lung adenocarcinomas. Clin Cancer Res 5:1001–1005

Bakhle YS (2001) COX-2 and cancer: a new approach to an old problem. Br J Pharmacol 134:1137–1150

Bennett A, Berstock DA, Raja B et al (1979) Survival time after surgery is inversely related to the amounts of prostaglandins extracted from human breast cancers (proceedings). Br J Pharmacol 66:451P

Brunda MJ, Herberman RB, Holden HT (1980) Inhibition of murine natural killer cell activity by prostaglandins. J Immunol 124:2682–2687

Chan G, Boyle JO, Yang EK et al (1999) Cyclooxygenase-2 expression is up-regulated in squamous cell carcinoma of the head and neck. Cancer Res 59:991–994

Chan TA, Morin PJ, Vogelstein B et al (1998) Mechanisms underlying nonsteroidal antiinflammatory drug-mediated apoptosis. Proc Natl Acad Sci U S A 95:681–686

Dannhardt G, Kiefer W (2001) Cyclooxygenase inhibitors – current status and future prospects. Eur J Med Chem 36:109–126

Davis T, Hunter N, Trifan OC, Milas L, Masferrer JL (2002) COX-2 inhibitors as radiosensitizing agents for cancer therapy. Am J Oncol (in press)

Dempke W, Rie C, Grothey A et al (2001) Cyclooxygenase-2: a novel target for cancer chemotherapy? J Cancer Res Clin Oncol 127:411–417

Dicker AP, Williams TL, Grant DS (2001) Targeting angiogenic processes by combination rofecoxib and ionizing radiation. Am J Clin Oncol 24:438–442

Dohadwala M, Luo J, Zhu L et al (2001) Non-small cell lung cancer cyclooxygenase-2-dependent invasion is mediated by CD44. J Biol Chem 276:20809–20812

Eberhart CE, Coffey RJ, Radhika A et al (1994) Up-regulation of cyclooxygenase 2 gene expression in human colorectal adenomas and adenocarcinomas. Gastroenterology 107:1183–1188

Eling TE, Curtis JF (1992) Xenobiotic metabolism by prostaglandin H synthase. Pharmacol Ther 53:261–263

Form DM, Auerbach R (1983) PGE2 and angiogenesis. Proc Soc Exp Biol Med 172:214–218

Forman BM, Tontonoz P, Chen J et al (1995) 15-Deoxy-delta 12, 14-prostaglandin J2 is a ligand for the adipocyte determination factor PPAR gamma. Cell 83:803–812

Forman BM, Chen J, Evans RM (1997) Hypolipidemic drugs, polyunsaturated fatty acids, and eicosanoids are ligands for peroxisome proliferator-activated receptors alpha and delta. Proc Natl Acad Sci U S A 94:4312–4317

Fosslien E (2000) Biochemistry of cyclooxygenase (COX)-2 inhibitors and molecular pathology of COX-2 in neoplasia. Crit Rev Clin Lab Sci 37:431–502

Fu JY, Masferrer JL, Seibert K et al (1990) The induction and suppression of prostaglandin H2 synthase (cyclooxygenase) in human monocytes. J Biol Chem 265:16737–16740

Fulton AM (1987) Interactions of natural effector cells and prostaglandins in the control of metastasis. J Natl Cancer Inst 78:735–741

Fulton AM, Levy JG (1980) The possible role of prostaglandins in mediating immune suppression by nonspecific T suppressor cells. Cell Immunol 52:29–37

Furuta Y, Hall ER, Sanduja S et al (1988a) Prostaglandin production by murine tumors as a predictor for therapeutic response to indomethacin. Cancer Res 48:3002–3007

Furuta Y, Hunter N, Barkley T Jr et al (1988b) Increase in radioresponse of murine tumors by treatment with indomethacin. Cancer Res 48:3008–3013

Gaffney DK, Holden J, Davis M et al (2001) Elevated cyclooxygenase-2 expression correlates with diminished survival in carcinoma of the cervix treated with radiotherapy. Int J Radiat Oncol Biol Phys 49:1213–1217

Garavito RM (1996) The cyclooxygenase-2 structure: new drugs for an old target? Nat Struct Biol 3:897–901

Gately S (2000) The contributions of cyclooxygenase-2 to tumor angiogenesis. Cancer Metastasis Rev 19:19–27

Geng L, Hanson WR, Malkinson FD (1992) Topical or systemic 16, 16 dm prostaglandin E2 or WR-2721 (WR-1065) protects mice from alopecia after fractionated irradiation. Int J Radiat Biol 61:533–537

Gilman AG (1987) G proteins: transducers of receptor-generated signals. Annu Rev Biochem 56:615–649

Gorski DH, Beckett MA, Jaskowiak NT et al (1999) Blockage of the vascular endothelial growth factor stress response increases the antitumor effects of ionizing radiation. Cancer Res 59:3374–3378

Gorski DH, Mauceri HJ, Salloum RM et al (1998) Potentiation of the antitumor effect of ionizing radiation by brief concomitant exposures to angiostatin. Cancer Res 58:5686–5689

Haimovitz-Friedman A, Vlodavsky I, Chaudhuri A et al (1991) Autocrine effects of fibroblast growth factor in repair of radiation damage in endothelial cells. Cancer Res 51:2552–2558

Hansen-Petrik MB, McEntee MF, Jull B et al (2002) Prostaglandin E(2) protects intestinal tumors from nonsteroidal anti-inflammatory drug-induced regression in Apc(Min/+) mice. Cancer Res 62:403–408

Hanson W (1998) Eicosanoid-induced radioprotection and chemoprotection: laboratory studies and clinical applications. In: Bump E, Malaker K (ed) Radioprotectors: chemical, biological and clinical perspectives. CRC Press, Boca Raton, pp 197–221

Hanson W, Geng L, Malkinson FD (1995) Prostaglandin-induced protection from radiation or doxorubicin is tissue specific and dependent upon receptor expression (abstract). Proceedings of the 10th International congress of radiation research, Wurzburg, Germany

Hanson WR, Ainsworth EJ (1985) 16,16-Dimethyl prostaglandin E2 induces radioprotection in murine intestinal and hematopoietic stem cells. Radiat Res 103:196–203

Hanson WR, Thomas C (1983) 16, 16-dimethyl prostaglandin E2 increases survival of murine intestinal stem cells when given before photon radiation. Radiat Res 96:393–398

Harari PM, Huang SM (2001) Radiation response modification following molecular inhibition of epidermal growth factor receptor signaling. Semin Radiat Oncol 11:281–289

Hawkey CJ (1999) COX-2 inhibitors. Lancet 353:307–314

Hida T, Yatabe Y, Achiwa H et al (1998) Increased expression of cyclooxygenase 2 occurs frequently in human lung cancers, specifically in adenocarcinomas. Cancer Res 58:3761–3764

Houchen CW, Stenson WF, Cohn SM (2000) Disruption of cyclooxygenase-1 gene results in an impaired response to radiation injury. Am J Physiol Gastrointest Liver Physiol 279:G858–G865

Huang M, Stolina M, Sharma S et al (1998) Non-small cell lung cancer cyclooxygenase-2-dependent regulation of cytokine balance in lymphocytes and macrophages: up-regulation of interleukin 10 and down-regulation of interleukin 12 production. Cancer Res 58:1208–1216

Jacoby RF, Seibert K, Cole CE et al (2000) The cyclooxygenase-2 inhibitor celecoxib is a potent preventive and therapeutic agent in the min mouse model of adenomatous polyposis. Cancer Res 60:5040–5044

Janne PA, Mayer RJ (2000) Chemoprevention of colorectal cancer. N Engl J Med 342:1960–1968

Kakiuchi Y, Tsuji S, Tsujii M et al (2002) Cyclooxygenase-2 activity altered the cell-surface carbohydrate antigens on colon cancer cells and enhanced liver metastasis. Cancer Res 62:1567–1572

Kambayashi T, Alexander HR, Fong M et al (1995) Potential involvement of IL-10 in suppressing tumor-associated macrophages. Colon-26-derived prostaglandin E2 inhibits TNF-alpha release via a mechanism involving IL-10. J Immunol 154:3383–3390

Kargman SL, O'Neill GP, Vickers PJ et al (1995) Expression of prostaglandin G/H synthase-1 and -2 protein in human colon cancer. Cancer Res 55:2556–2559

Kawamori T, Rao CV, Seibert K et al (1998) Chemopreventive activity of celecoxib, a specific cyclooxygenase-2 inhibitor, against colon carcinogenesis. Cancer Res 58:409–412

Khuri FR, Wu H, Lee JJ et al (2001) Cyclooxygenase-2 overexpression is a marker of poor prognosis in stage I non-small cell lung cancer. Clin Cancer Res 7:861–867

Kishi K, Petersen S, Petersen C et al (2000) Preferential enhancement of tumor radioresponse by a cyclooxygenase-2 inhibitor. Cancer Res 60:1326–1331

Kliewer SA, Forman BM, Blumberg B et al (1994) Differential expression and activation of a family of murine peroxisome proliferator-activated receptors. Proc Natl Acad Sci U S A 91:7355–7359

Koki A, Leahy KM, Masferrer JL (1999) Potential utility of COX-2 inhibitors in chemoprevention and chemotherapy. Exp Opin Invest Drugs 8:1623–1638

Kozaki K, Koshikawa K, Tatematsu Y et al (2001) Multi-faceted analyses of a highly metastatic human lung cancer cell line NCI-H460-LNM35 suggest mimicry of inflammatory cells in metastasis. Oncogene 20:4228–4234

Kujubu DA, Fletcher BS, Varnum BC et al (1991) TIS10, a phorbol ester tumor promoter-inducible mRNA from Swiss 3T3 cells, encodes a novel prostaglandin synthase/cyclooxygenase homologue. J Biol Chem 266:12866–12872

Lemberger T, Desvergne B, Wahli W (1996) Peroxisome proliferator-activated receptors: a nuclear receptor signaling pathway in lipid physiology. Annu Rev Cell Dev Biol 12:335–363

Leung KH, Mihich E (1980) Prostaglandin modulation of development of cell-mediated immunity in culture. Nature 288:597–600

Li L, Rojiani A, Siemann DW (1998) Targeting the tumor vasculature with combretastatin A-4 disodium phosphate: effects on radiation therapy. Int J Radiat Oncol Biol Phys 42:899–903

Li M, Wu X, Xu XC (2001) Induction of apoptosis by cyclo-oxygenase-2 inhibitor NS398 through a cytochrome C-dependent pathway in esophageal cancer cells. Int J Cancer 93:218–223

Lim H, Gupta RA, Ma WG et al (1999) Cyclo-oxygenase-2-derived prostacyclin mediates embryo implantation in the mouse via PPARdelta. Genes Dev 13:1561–1574

Majima M, Hayashi I, Muramatsu M et al (2000) Cyclo-oxygenase-2 enhances basic fibroblast growth factor-induced angiogenesis through induction of vascular endothelial growth factor in rat sponge implants. Br J Pharmacol 130:641–649

Manson MM, Holloway KA, Howells LM et al (2000) Modulation of signal-transduction pathways by chemopreventive agents. Biochem Soc Trans 28:7–12

Marnett LJ (1994) Generation of mutagens during arachidonic acid metabolism. Cancer Metastasis Rev 13:303–308

Marnett LJ (2000) Cyclooxygenase mechanisms. Curr Opin Chem Biol 4:545–552

Marnett LJ, DuBois RN (2002) COX-2: a target for colon cancer prevention. Annu Rev Pharmacol Toxicol 42:55–80

Masferrer JL, Leahy KM, Koki AT et al (2000) Antiangiogenic and antitumor activities of cyclooxygenase-2 inhibitors. Cancer Res 60:1306–1311

Mason KA, Milas L, Hunter NR et al (1999) Maximizing therapeutic gain with gemcitabine and fractionated radiation. Int J Radiat Oncol Biol Phys 44:1125–1135

Milas L (2001) Cyclooxygenase-2 (COX-2) enzyme inhibitors as potential enhancers of tumor radioresponse. Semin Radiat Oncol 11:290–299

Milas L, Hanson WR (1995) Eicosanoids and radiation. Eur J Cancer 31A:1580–1585

Milas L, Furuta Y, Hunter N et al (1990) Dependence of indomethacin-induced potentiation of murine tumor radioresponse on tumor host immunocompetence. Cancer Res 50:4473–4477

Milas L, Nishiguchi I, Hunter N et al (1992) Radiation protection against early and late effects of ionizing irradiation by the prostaglandin inhibitor indomethacin. Adv Space Res 12:265–271

Milas L, Hunter NR, Mason KA et al (1995) Role of reoxygenation in induction of enhancement of tumor radioresponse by paclitaxel. Cancer Res 55:3564–3568

Milas L, Kishi K, Hunter N et al (1999) Enhancement of tumor response to g-radiation by an inhibitor of cyclooxygenase-2 enzyme. J Natl Cancer Inst 91:1501–1504

Milas L, Mason K, Hunter N et al (2000) In vivo enhancement of tumor radioresponse by C225 antiepidermal growth factor receptor antibody. Clin Cancer Res 6:701–708

Murata H, Kawano S, Tsuji S et al (1999) Cyclooxygenase-2 overexpression enhances lymphatic invasion and metastasis in human gastric carcinoma. Am J Gastroenterol 94:451–455

Niki T, Kohno T, Iba S et al (2002) Frequent co-localization of Cox-2 and laminin-5 gamma2 chain at the invasive front of early-stage lung adenocarcinomas. Am J Pathol 160:1129–1141

Nishiguchi I, Furuta Y, Hunter N et al (1990) Radioprotection of hematopoietic tissues in mice by indomethacin. Radiat Res 122:188–192

O'Banion MK (1999) Cyclooxygenase-2: molecular biology, pharmacology, and neurobiology. Crit Rev Neurobiol 13:45–82

Oshima M, Dinchuk JE, Kargman SL et al (1996) Suppression of intestinal polyposis in Apc delta716 knockout mice by inhibition of cyclooxygenase 2 (COX-2). Cell 87:803–809

Petersen C, Petersen S, Milas L, Lang FF, Tofilon P (2000) Human glioma cell radiosensitization by a selective COX-2 inhibitor. Clin Cancer Res 6:2513–2520

Prescott SM, White RL (1996) Self-promotion? Intimate connections between APC and prostaglandin H synthase-2. Cell 87:783–786

Pyo H, Choy H, Amorino GP et al (2001) A selective cyclooxygenase-2 inhibitor, NS-398, enhances the effect of radiation in vitro and in vivo preferentially on the cells that express cyclooxygenase-2. Clin Cancer Res 7:2998–3005

Raju U NE, Yang P, Newman RA, Ang KK, Milas L (2002) In vitro enhancement of tumor cell radiosensitivity by a selective inhibitor of cyclooxygenase-2 enzyme: mechanistic considerations. Int J Radiat Oncol Biol Phys (in press)

Rak J, Filmus J, Kerbel RS (1996) Reciprocal paracrine interactions between tumour cells and endothelial cells: the 'angiogenesis progression' hypothesis. Eur J Cancer 32A:2438–2450

Riehl T, Cohn S, Tessner T et al (2000) Lipopolysaccharide is radioprotective in the mouse intestine through a prostaglandin-mediated mechanism. Gastroenterology 118:1106–1116

Rigas B, Goldman IS, Levine L (1993) Altered eicosanoid levels in human colon cancer. J Lab Clin Med 122:518–523

Sano H, Kawahito Y, Wilder RL et al (1995) Expression of cyclooxygenase-1 and -2 in human colorectal cancer. Cancer Res 55:3785–3789

Sheehan KM, Sheahan K, O'Donoghue DP et al (1999) The relationship between cyclooxygenase-2 expression and colorectal cancer. JAMA 282:1254–1257

Smith ML, Hawcroft G, Hull MA (2000) The effect of non-steroidal anti-inflammatory drugs on human colorectal cancer cells: evidence of different mechanisms of action. Eur J Cancer 36:664–674

Smith WL (1989) The eicosanoids and their biochemical mechanisms of action. Biochem J 259:315–324

Steinauer KK, Gibbs I, Ning S et al (2000) Radiation induces upregulation of cyclooxygenase-2 (COX-2) protein in PC-3 cells. Int J Radiat Oncol Biol Phys 48:325–328

Steinbach G, Lynch PM, Phillips RK et al (2000) The effect of celecoxib, a cyclooxygenase-2 inhibitor, in familial adenomatous polyposis. N Engl J Med 342:1946–1952

Stolina M, Sharma S, Lin Y et al (2000) Specific inhibition of cyclooxygenase 2 restores antitumor reactivity by altering the balance of IL-10 and IL-12 synthesis. J Immunol 164:361–370

Taketo MM (1998a) Cyclooxygenase-2 inhibitors in tumorigenesis, part I. J Natl Cancer Inst 90:1529–1536

Taketo MM (1998b) Cyclooxygenase-2 inhibitors in tumorigenesis, part II. J Natl Cancer Inst 90:1609–1620

Tang D, Honn KV (1994) Eicosanoids and tumor cell metastasis. In: Harris J, Braun DP, Anderson KM (ed) Prostaglandin inhibitors in tumor immunology and immunotherapy. CRC Press, Boca Raton, pp 1073–1108

Teicher BA, Holden SA, Dupuis NP et al (1995) Potentiation of cytotoxic therapies by TNP-470 and minocycline in mice bearing EMT-6 mammary carcinoma. Breast Cancer Res Treat 36:227–236

Teicher BA, Bump EA, Palayoor ST, Northey D, Coleman CN (1996) Signal transduction inhibitors as modifiers of radiation therapy in human prostate carcinoma xenografts. Radiat Oncol Invest 1996:221–230

Thun MJ, Henley SJ, Patrono C (2002) Nonsteroidal anti-inflammatory drugs as anticancer agents: mechanistic, pharmacologic, and clinical issues. J Natl Cancer Inst 94:252–266

Torrance CJ, Jackson PE, Montgomery E et al (2000) Combinatorial chemoprevention of intestinal neoplasia. Nat Med 6:1024–1028

Tsubouchi Y, Mukai S, Kawahito Y et al (2000) Meloxicam inhibits the growth of non-small cell lung cancer. Anticancer Res 20:2867–2872

Tsujii M, DuBois RN (1995) Alterations in cellular adhesion and apoptosis in epithelial cells overexpressing prostaglandin endoperoxide synthase 2. Cell 83:493–501

Tucker ON, Dannenberg AJ, Yang EK et al (1999) Cyclooxygenase-2 expression is up-regulated in human pancreatic cancer. Cancer Res 59:987–990

Van Buul PP, van Duyn-Goedhart A, de Rooij DG et al (1997) Differential radioprotective effects of misoprostol in DNA repair-proficient and -deficient or radiosensitive cell systems. Int J Radiat Biol 71:259–264

Van Buul PP, van Duyn-Goedhart A, Sankaranarayanan K (1999) In vivo and in vitro radioprotective effects of the prostaglandin E1 analogue misoprostol in DNA repair-proficient and -deficient rodent cell systems. Radiat Res 152:398–403

Vane JR (1971) Inhibition of prostaglandin synthesis as a mechanism of action for aspirin-like drugs. Nat New Biol 231:232–235

Watson AJ (1998) Chemopreventive effects of NSAIDs against colorectal cancer: regulation of apoptosis and mitosis by COX-1 and COX-2. Histol Histopathol 13:591–597

Wiese FW, Thompson PA, Kadlubar FF (2001) Carcinogen substrate specificity of human COX-1 and COX-2. Carcinogenesis 22:5–10

Williams CS, DuBois RN (1996) Prostaglandin endoperoxide synthase: why two isoforms? Am J Physiol 270:G393–G400

Williams CS, Tsujii M, Reese J et al (2000) Host cyclooxygenase-2 modulates carcinoma growth. J Clin Invest 105:1589–1594

Wilson KT, Fu S, Ramanujam KS et al (1998) Increased expression of inducible nitric oxide synthase and cyclooxygenase-2 in Barrett's esophagus and associated adenocarcinomas. Cancer Res 58:2929–2934

Wolff H, Saukkonen K, Anttila S et al (1998) Expression of cyclooxygenase-2 in human lung carcinoma. Cancer Res 58:4997–5001

Xie WL, Chipman JG, Robertson DL et al (1991) Expression of a mitogen-responsive gene encoding prostaglandin synthase is regulated by mRNA splicing. Proc Natl Acad Sci U S A 88:2692–2696

Yamamoto Y, Yin MJ, Lin KM et al (1999) Sulindac inhibits activation of the NF-kappaB pathway. J Biol Chem 274:27307–27314

Zaffaroni N, Villa R, Orlandi L et al (1993) Differential effect of 9 beta-chloro-16,16-dimethyl prostaglandin E2 (nocloprost) on the radiation response of human normal fibroblasts and colon adenocarcinoma cells. Radiat Res 135:88–92

Zhang Z, DuBois RN (2000) Par-4, a proapoptotic gene, is regulated by NSAIDs in human colon carcinoma cells. Gastroenterology 118:1012–1017

Ziche M, Jones J, Gullino PM (1982) Role of prostaglandin E1 and copper in angiogenesis. J Natl Cancer Inst 69:475–482

Zimmermann KC, Sarbia M, Weber AA et al (1999) Cyclooxygenase-2 expression in human esophageal carcinoma. Cancer Res 59:198–204

19 Ras Signaling and Its Inhibition with Farnesyltransferase Inhibitors: Effects on Radiation Resistance and the Tumor Microenvironment

E. J. Bernhard, A. K. Gupta, S. M. Hahn, R. J. Muschel, W. G. McKenna

CONTENTS

19.1 Ras and Radiation Resistance 259
19.2 RAS Inhibition and Radiation Resistance 259
19.3 RAS Inhibition with Prenyltransferase Inhibitors 260
19.4 Prenyltransferase Inhibitors and Tumor Growth 260
19.5 Prenyltransferase Inhibitors and Radiosensitization 261
19.6 Ras Pathways Mediating Radiation Resistance 264
19.7 The Effects of FTI Treatment on Radiosensitivity in Vivo 264
19.8 Results from a Clinical Study Combining FTI and Radiation Therapy 266
19.9 Influence of FTI Treatment on the Tumor Microenvironment 267
19.10 FTI Effects on Tumor Metastasis and Collagenolytic Enzyme Production 269
19.11 Conclusions 270
References 271

RAS activation has many effects on the growth and behavior of tumors. This results from its central role in the propagation of growth and survival signals from cell surface receptors. Ras signals to a number of different pathways so that the effects of RAS activation take various forms. In addition to enhancing radiation resistance, the effects of deregulated RAS signaling include promoting tumor growth both through increased cell proliferation and increased tumor cell survival. RAS activation can also contribute to the tumor microenvironment by influencing growth factor production and enzymes involved in tumor metastasis. These factors together make RAS signaling an attractive target for therapeutic intervention.

E. J. Bernhard, PhD; A. K. Gupta, PhD; S. M. Hahn, PhD
W. G. McKenna, MD
Department of Radiation Oncology, University of Pennsylvania School of Medicine, Philadelphia, PA 19104-6072, USA
R. J. Muschel, MD, PhD
Department of Pathology and Laboratory Medicine, University of Pennsylvania School of Medicine, Philadelphia, PA 19104-6072, USA

19.1 Ras and Radiation Resistance

RAS activation can increase radiation resistance in many transformed cells. Oncogenic *ras* was originally shown to increase radiation resistance in rodent cells transformed by N-*ras* (Fitzgerald et al. 1985). Transfection with mutant H-*ras* was subsequently shown to increase radiation survival of both rodent and human cells (Fitzgerald et al. 1990; Ling and Endlich 1989; McKenna et al. 1990a; Miller et al. 1993; Ong et al. 1993; Pirollo et al. 1993; Sklar 1988; Suzuki et al. 1992). Oncogenic H-*ras* also cooperates with other oncogenes including c- and v-*myc*, Adenovirus E1A, and SV40 T-antigen to impart radiation resistance (Ling and Endlich 1989; McKenna et al. 1990b; Su and Little 1993). In addition, human tumor cells overexpressing the H-*ras* proto-oncogene demonstrate increased radioresistance (Samid et al. 1991). In a series of studies carried out by our group, transfection of primary rat embryo fibroblast cells (REF) with oncogenic H-*ras* was shown to impart radiation resistance (Fig. 19.1a; McKenna et al. 1990a,b). Radiation resistance in H-*ras*-transformed REF cells was associated with prolonged G2/M delay after irradiation (McKenna et al. 1991) and reduced apoptosis (McKenna et al. 1996). We subsequently showed that in human tumor cells, expression of oncogenic N-*ras* or K-*ras* increased radiation resistance since radiation survival was diminished after loss of the activated *ras* allele (Fig. 19.1b, c; Bernhard et al. 2000). Radioresistance is not, however, a general effect of oncogene expression and is not promoted by all oncogenes in all cell types (Fitzgerald et al. 1990; Pirollo et al. 1993; Santucci et al. 1992).

19.2 RAS Inhibition and Radiation Resistance

Inhibiting RAS activity using various approaches has provided further evidence for its role in radiation

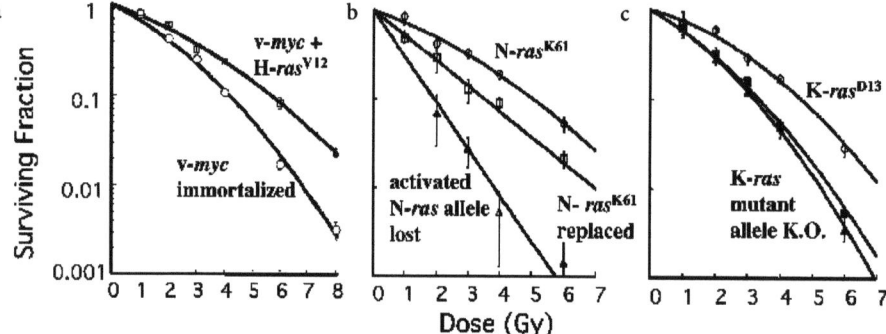

Fig. 19.1a–c. Clonogenic survival of tumor cells is reduced after loss of activated *ras*. Cells in log phase growth were plated and irradiated for clonogenic survival at the doses indicated. After 14–21 days plates were stained and scored for colony formation. a Survival of REF cells transformed with H-*ras*^{V12} and v-*myc* (□) is compared to survival of REF cells immortalized with v-*myc* alone (○). b Survival of HT1080 cells expressing both activated and wild-type endogenous N-*ras* alleles (○) is compared to that of HT1080 expressing only the wild type endogenous N-*ras* allele (△), or expressing the wild type endogenous N-*ras* allele and an activated N-*ras* reintroduced by transfection (□). c Survival of DLD-1 cells expressing both activated and wild type endogenous K-*ras* alleles (○) is compared to the survival of two clones of DLD-1 cells expressing only wild type K-*ras* (▲, ■). Error bars indicate standard deviation from a minimum of three replicates per point. Adapted from (BERNHARD et al. 2000) with permission

resistance. Ras inhibition has been achieved in various cells with antisense oligonucleotides (CUNNINGHAM et al. 2001; DAAKA and WICKSTROM 1990; GRAY et al. 1993; KASHANI-SABET et al. 1994; NAKANO et al. 2001; SORRENTINO et al. 2001) and anti-*ras* ribozymes (TSUCHIDA et al. 2000). PIROLLO et al. (1997) used the anti-sense technique to inhibit RAS or RAF expression in HER-2 overexpressing cells (SK-OV-3) and in cells with mutant H-RAS (T24). In SK-OV-3 cells, signaling through both RAS and RAF is activated by HER-2 while in T24 cells activation results from mutation of the H-*ras* gene. Inhibiting expression of either HER-2 or H-*ras* by antisense resulted in radiosensitization of both cell lines, but did not alter the radiosensitivity of MCF10A cells in which signaling by these oncogenes is not activated. TOFILON et al. (RUSSELL et al. 1999) inhibited RAS activity using an anti-RAS single-chain antibody fragment that recognizes all four RAS isoforms. Using an adenoviral vector for expression of this antibody, they were able to demonstrate reduced radiation resistance in four human tumor cell lines without sensitization of normal fibroblasts. Subsequently, this group showed that radiosensitization using this antibody fragment was specific for tumor lines demonstrating activated RAS signaling (RUSSELL et al. 2002).

19.3
RAS Inhibition with Prenyltransferase Inhibitors

RAS activity is inhibited by disruption of its post-translational processing. H-, K-, and N-RAS are all prenylated by farnesyltransferase under normal conditions. Prenylation is the first step in RAS processing and is required for the function of this protein. A 15-carbon farnesyl group is added to a cysteine residue at the fourth amino acid position from the carboxyl-terminal end of RAS (reviewed in BERNHARD et al. 1999; GELB 1997; GLOMSET and FARNSWORTH 1994). Blocking processing by inhibiting prenylation with inhibitors blocks RAS membrane localization and oncogenic RAS-mediated transformation (reviewed in SEBTI and HAMILTON 1997; WADDICK and UCKUN 1998). In contrast to H-RAS, whose processing is inhibited by blocking the farnesyltransferase enzyme, K- and N-RAS are prenylated by geranylgeranyltransferase-I with a 20-carbon geranylgeranyl- group when farnesylation is blocked (SUN et al. 1998; WHYTE et al. 1997). In order to block both of these enzymes, most studies have used a combination of farnesyltransferase inhibitors (FTI) and geranylgeranyltransferase inhibitors (GGTI) to inhibit K-RAS prenylation (BERNHARD et al. 1998; LERNER et al. 1997; LOBELL et al. 2001).

19.4
Prenyltransferase Inhibitors and Tumor Growth

The effects of prenyltransferase inhibitors on tumor cell growth in vitro and in vivo are now established to be independent of the mutation status of the *ras* oncogenes in these cells (DU et al. 1999; END et al. 2001; KOHL et al. 1994, 1995; LANTRY et al. 2000;

Mangues et al. 1998; Sepp-Lorenzino et al. 1995; Servais et al. 1998; Sun et al. 1995, 1998, 1999). The majority of this work has been done using FTIs. The findings fail to demonstrate a correlation between the presence of H-*ras* mutation and growth inhibition by FTIs (which target H-RAS farnesylation). Some tumors with K-RAS activation (which is resistant to FTIs), or with no *ras* mutations were growth-inhibited by FTIs. This implies either that RAS is not the important target for FTI-mediated growth inhibition, or that RAS signaling is critical to the growth of certain tumors even if RAS is not mutated in these cells. The latter conclusion is supported by the knowledge that RAS can be activated by overexpression or by tyrosine kinase receptor signaling in the absence of mutation. The conclusion that RAS is not the target for FTI-mediated growth inhibition is supported by work from Prendergast et al. These investigators have shown that expression of the small G-protein rho B is needed for FTI-mediated growth inhibition under anchorage-dependent growth conditions (Liu et al. 2000). This may be due to altered rho B function following a shift in prenylation from farnesylation to geranylgeranylation under FTI treatment (Du et al. 1999; Du and Prendergast 1999; Lebowitz et al. 1995, 1997). These investigators have further proposed that geranylgeranylated rho B inhibits Akt, thus promoting apoptosis in epithelial cells (Liu and Prendergast 2000).

In addition to uncertainty about the target of FTI growth inhibition, there remain questions about the mechanism of this inhibition. FTIs have been shown to cause cell cycle arrest in many cell types, but again, there is variability in the data addressing the nature of this arrest. Arrest of cells in G2/M has been shown after FTI treatment of many cultured human tumor cells (Ashar et al. 2001; Hahn et al. 2002; Miquel et al. 1997) and mouse Bcr/Abl-induced leukemia cells (Peters et al. 2001). Accumulation of tetraploid cells was reported in pancreatic ductal cancer cell lines (Song et al. 2000) and M-phase arrest with inhibition of bipolar spindle formation was seen in lung cancer lines (Crespo et al. 2001). In astrocytomas, both G1 and G2/M arrest were observed (Feldkamp et al. 1999). Sepp-Lorenzino (1995) reported induction of p21 and G1 accumulation in p53 +/+ human tumor lines while Barrington et al. (1998) demonstrated little effect of FTI treatment on the cell cycle distribution of MMTV v-H-*ras* mouse salivary and mammary tumors in vivo. This study did detect a small reduction in S-phase and corresponding accumulation in G1 for p53-negative salivary tumors. A consistent finding in these studies was that regardless of the phase in which cells arrested, increased apoptosis was seen in FTI-treated cells. It further appears that the cell cycle blocks induced by FTI and GGTI may differ (Vogt et al. 1996, 1997). Understanding the nature of cell cycle effects of FTIs is important as these effects may guide the clinical development of these agents. A cell cycle block induced by FTIs may antagonize the effect of other cell-cycle-dependent chemotherapy agents such as gemcitabine. On the other hand, cell cycle redistribution may be advantageous for radiotherapy if the cells are blocked in more radiosensitive phases of the cell cycle (G2/M or the G1/S boundary). Alternatively, one would predict that cell cycle blocks due to FTIs would not affect treatment with cell-cycle-independent agents such as cisplatin.

19.5
Prenyltransferase Inhibitors and Radiosensitization

The study of prenyltransferase inhibitors as radiosensitizers differs from the study of their effects on growth inhibition in that radiosensitivity rather than growth inhibition is the end-point measured. These studies are designed to control for the influence of prenyltransferase inhibitors on growth and thus focus on the cytotoxic interaction of radiation with prenyltransferase inhibitors. Inhibiting RAS prenylation was first attempted by Miller et al. using the HMG-CoA reductase inhibitor lovastatin (Miller et al. 1993). Lovastatin inhibits the synthesis of the precursors for farnesyl- and geranylgeranyl isoprenoids required for RAS post-translational processing, but also for the synthesis of many other cellular macromolecules. Lovastatin was shown to inhibit H-RAS prenylation and to radiosensitize human osteosarcoma cells rendered radiation-resistant by transfection with oncogenic H-*ras*. This effect was reversed by addition of mevalonate to the cultures. Radiosensitization was not seen in cells with undetectable expression of H-*ras*. Together these findings supported RAS inhibition as the target for the radiosensitization observed after treatment with lovastatin.

Our studies on radiosensitization have used both FTIs and GGTIs to block RAS prenylation. These inhibitors have greater specificity than lovastatin for blocking RAS processing, but can also block the prenylation of other proteins. Using these inhibitors we assessed radiation survival both in vitro and in vivo.

Our initial studies were done using rat embryo fibroblasts (REF) as a model system. REF cells expressing oncogenic H-*ras* were shown to be radiosensitized by FTI treatment while the radiosensitivity of v-*myc*-immortalized REF and early passage cultures of REF was not affected by FTI treatment (BERNHARD et al. 1996). This study also showed that radiosensitization of *ras*-transformed REF was accompanied by enhanced apoptosis. We next examined the radiosensitization of human tumor lines with mutations in H- and K-*ras*. As shown in Table 19.1, radiosensitization of T24 and HS578T tumor cells with oncogenic mutation of H-*ras* was seen using several different FTIs while no radiosensitization of RT4 or HT29 tumor lines expressing wild type *ras* or GM6096A untransformed fibroblasts was observed.

Our observations on radiosensitization after prenyltransferase inhibition were extended to tumors that did not have *ras* mutations but have activation of RAS by other mechanisms. Overexpression of EGFR causes RAS activity to increase and has also been linked to radiotherapy treatment failure (MIYAGUCHI et al. 1991; ZHU et al. 1996). Inhibition of EGFR signaling has been shown to radiosensitize tumors overexpressing this receptor and is currently under investigation as an antitumor treatment (HARARI and HUANG 2001; LAMMERING et al. 2001; MILAS et al. 2000). Many tumor types that are treated with radiation such as head and neck squamous cell carcinomas (HNSCC) show elevated EGFR expression that could increase RAS signaling (SANTINI et al. 1991; WEICHSELBAUM et al. 1989). Elevated EGFR expression and downstream signaling through RAS have been shown to correlate with treatment resistance (GUPTA et al. 2002). Treatment of two HNSCC cell lines with FTI decreased radiation survival, a finding that implicates RAS signaling in EGFR-mediated radiation resistance. Further studies of radiation resistance in the SQ20B cell line by GUPTA et al. have shown that radiosensitization occurs after inhibition of EGFR with ZD1839 and after inhibition of PI3-kinase with LY294002 (GUPTA et al. 2002). It thus appears that RAS forms part of a pathway leading from the EGFR to PI3-kinase and potentially to Akt. This hypothesis is supported by the findings that sensitization by LY294002 and FTI are equivalent (Fig. 19.2) and that treatment with a combination of these inhibitors is not additive (unpublished). Other groups have reported radiosensitization of tumor cell lines without *ras* mutations as well. Radiosensitization by recombinant adenovirus expressing single-chain anti-RAS antibody was limited to cells

Table 19.1. Surviving fraction of clonogenic cells after 2-Gy irradiation

Cells	Treatment	Inhibition	SF_2 control[a]	SF_2-treated
H-ras mutants				
T24	FTI-277 (5 µM)	Farnesylation	0.86 (.04)	0.50 (.02)
	L744,832 (5 µM)	Farnesylation	0.62 (.04)	0.37 (.02)
HS578T	FTI-277 (5 µM)	Farnesylation	0.79 (.07)	0.63 (.05)
Activated wild type RAS				
SQ20B	L778,123 (1.25 µM)	Farnesylation	0.58 (.05)[b]	0.37 (.01)[b]
	LY294002 (10 µM)	PI3Kinase	0.59 (.06)[b]	0.46 (.03)[b]
	ZD1839 (0.1 µM)	EGFR	0.78 (.04)[b]	0.68 (.02)[b]
	L778 + LY	Farnesylation and PI3 K	0.58 (.05)[b]	0.44 (.08)[b]
Detroit-562	L778,123 (2.5 µM)	Farnesylation	0.80 (.11)[b]	0.63 (.09)b
Wild type ras				
GM6096A	FTI-277 (5 µM)	Farnesylation	0.43 (.03)[b]	0.49 (.04)[b]
	L744,832 (5 µM)	Farnesylation	0.43 (.03)[b]	0.53 (.13)[b]
RT-4	L744,832 (5 µM)	Farnesylation	0.40 (.02)	0.48 (.01)
HT29	FTI-277 (5 µM)	Farnesylation	0.78 (.05)	0.82 (.07)
	L744,832 (5 µM)	Farnesylation	0.72 (.05)	0.68 (.06)

[a]Surviving fraction of clonogenic cells after 2-Gy irradiation (SF2) ± (SE) or (SD)
[b]SF_2 were derived from limiting dilution assays and from standard clonogenic assays at the 2-Gy dose. Both assays compensate for the plating efficiency of unirradiated cells and thus show the effect of FTI on radiosensitivity corrected for any cytotoxic effect of drug alone. Plating of SQ20B appears higher in the ZD1839 experiment due to removal of the drug (and similar manipulation of controls) 24 h after irradiation

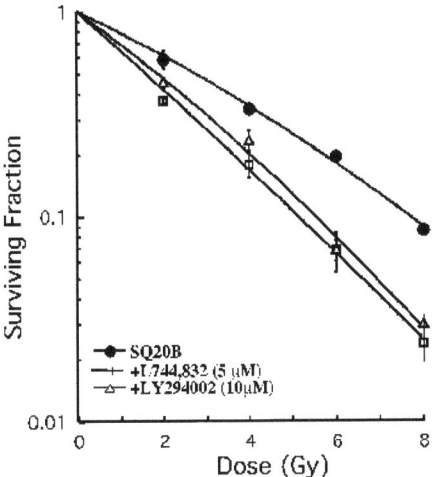

Fig. 19.2. FTI treatment or inhibition of PI3-kinase reduces clonogenic survival of cells with EGFR activation. Clonogenic survival of SQ20B cells was assessed after treatment with 5μM L744,832 or 10μM LY294002 as described in GUPTA et al. (2002). Drug-free medium was added to all cultures 24 h after irradiation. Colonies were stained and counted after 10–14 days. Error bars indicate standard deviation from a minimum of three replicates per point. Adapted with permission from GUPTA et al. (2002)

with high levels of activated (GTP-bound) RAS (RUSSELL et al. 1999, 2002). In addition, bFGF expression in HeLa cells that express wt-*ras* was reported to increase radiation resistance, which was reversed by FTI treatment (COHEN-JONATHAN et al. 1999). These findings indicate that targeting RAS for inactivation is a potential strategy for radiosensitization of tumors that have RAS activation resulting from either mutation or upstream receptor signaling.

Inhibition of K-RAS prenylation also resulted in radiosensitization of human tumors with K-*ras* mutations, but not tumors with wild type ras. In these studies we have combined FTI and GGTI from several sources to inhibit the prenylation of K-RAS in a variety of cell lines in vitro (Fig. 19.3a). Deprenylation with combined FTI + GGTI treatment results in radiosensitization while treatment with either inhibitor alone failed to inhibit K-RAS prenylation and radiosensitize tumors with K-*ras* mutations (Fig. 19.3b; BERNHARD et al. 1998). Using the L778,123 inhibitor with activity for both farnesyl- and geranylgeranyltransferases we have now obtained deprenylation of K-RAS with a single inhibitor (Fig. 19.4) accompanied by radiosensitization that is equivalent to that obtained with combined inhibitor treatment (Fig. 19.5). The L778,123 inhibitor has also been tested in a phase I clinical trial with radiation (see Sec. 19.8, "Results from a Clinical Study Combining FTI and Radiation Therapy").

a   b

Fig. 19.3a, b. Inhibition of K-RAS prenylation and radiosensitization. A Cultures of A549 lung cancer cells (*top panel*) were treated with 5μM FTI-277, 8μM GGTI 298 or 5μM FTI-277+8μM GGTI 298. Cell lysates were harvested at 48 h for analysis. Control cultures were treated with carrier alone. PSN-1 pancreatic cancer cells (*bottom panel*) were treated with the indicated concentrations of FTI-2 and GGTI-2 (Merck & Co. Inc) (LOBELL et al. 2001). Prenylation was assessed by Western blotting with monoclonal antibody specific for K-RAS (Santa Cruz Biotech). *Arrows* indicate unprenylated K-RAS bands. B A549 lung cancer cells were treated for 24 h with 5μM FTI-277 and 8μM GGTI 298 then plated and irradiated to assess clonogenic survival. Carrier-treated cultures were used as controls. Cultures were fed inhibitor-free medium 24 h after irradiation. Plates were stained after 10–14 days allowing unirradiated colonies from treated cultures to reach the same size as control colonies. Error bars indicate standard deviation from a minimum of three replicates per point

Fig. 19.4. Inhibition of RAS prenylation by L778,123. Cultures of A549 lung cancer cells were treated with the indicated concentrations of L778,123 (Merck & Co. Inc). Cell lysates were harvested at 48 h for Western blot analysis with anti-H-RAS (Quality Biotech) and K-RAS (Santa Cruz Biotech) monoclonal antibodies. *Arrows* indicate unprenylated RAS

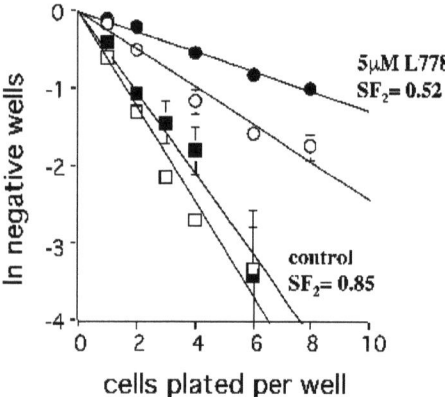

Fig. 19.5. Effect of L778,123 on radiation survival. Cultures of A549 lung cancer cells were treated with 5μM L778,123 (Merck & Co. Inc) for 24 h. Cells were then plated at limiting dilutions in 96 well plates and irradiated with 2 Gy. Cultures were fed inhibitor-free medium 24 h after irradiation. Survival was assessed after 2 weeks by counting wells without colonies using Poisson statistical analysis as described previously (BERNHARD et al. 1998). Control cultures (□), 2-Gy irradiated cultures (■), L778,123-treated cultures (○), 2-Gy irradiated cultures treated with L778,123 (●)

19.6 Ras Pathways Mediating Radiation Resistance

RAS signaling may contribute to intrinsic radioresistance through different downstream pathways in different cells. We have shown that PI3 kinase activation is an important contributor to RAS-mediated radiation resistance. In this study, both pharmacological and genetic approaches were used to inhibit the signaling of selected effectors of RAS signaling, including MEK, p38, PI3-kinase and p70S6-kinase (Fig. 19.6). The results demonstrated that PI3 kinase activity was critical to RAS-mediated radiation resistance in tumor cell lines with activated H- or K-*ras* (GUPTA et al. 2001a). Inhibition of PI3-kinase caused radiosensitization equivalent to that observed after FTI treatment. In addition, expression of active PI3-kinase increased radiation resistance in cells lacking activated RAS, and this increase was reversed by the PI3-kinase inhibitor LY294002 (Fig. 19.7).

In cells with wild type *ras*, however, other signaling pathways downstream of RAS may play a role in radiation resistance. The RAS-to-MAPK pathways are perhaps the most extensively studied and consist of at least three sequential kinase cascades that include the RAS-RAF-MAPK (also known as ERK) pathway, the stress-activated SAPK/JNK pathway, and the p38 pathway. The RAS-to-MAPK pathway has in fact been implicated in radiosensitivity. GOKHALE et al. 1999 transfected a truncated constitutively active *Raf* gene into a human squamous cell carcinoma cell line, leading to increased survival after radiation. The same group has also shown that down-regulation of RAF using *raf* antisense oligonucleotides reduced the radioresistance of human cells, implicating the RAF-MEK-MAPK pathway in radiation sensitivity. DENT's team (CARTEE et al. 2000) have shown that MAP kinase activity contributes to radiation survival in prostate tumor cell lines and monocytic leukemia cells that express wt-*ras* (CARTEE et al. 2000; HAGAN et al. 2000). In our studies on tumor lines with ras mutations, however, inhibition of p38, or MEK, did not reduce radiation survival (GUPTA et al. 2001a,b).

The identification of PI3-kinase as a downstream mediator of RAS and EGFR-induced radioresistance is of considerable interest, because the PI3-kinase pathway may also affect radioresistance independently of RAS activation. This is consistent with our hypothesis that there may be multiple pathways that converge in the induction of radioresistance. The point of convergence could be PI3-kinase (Fig. 19.8). Another prediction from the identification of PI3-kinase as an effector of radiation resistance is that PTEN phosphatase inactivation could affect radiation resistance. Mutations causing PTEN to be functionally inactive are frequently found in many human cancers. The PTEN phosphatase antagonizes PI3-kinase by converting its active product PI(3,4,5)P3 to PI(4,5)P2. Tumor cells with these mutations have increased PI3-kinase signaling. This signaling could be diminished by PI3-kinase inhibition resulting in radiosensitization.

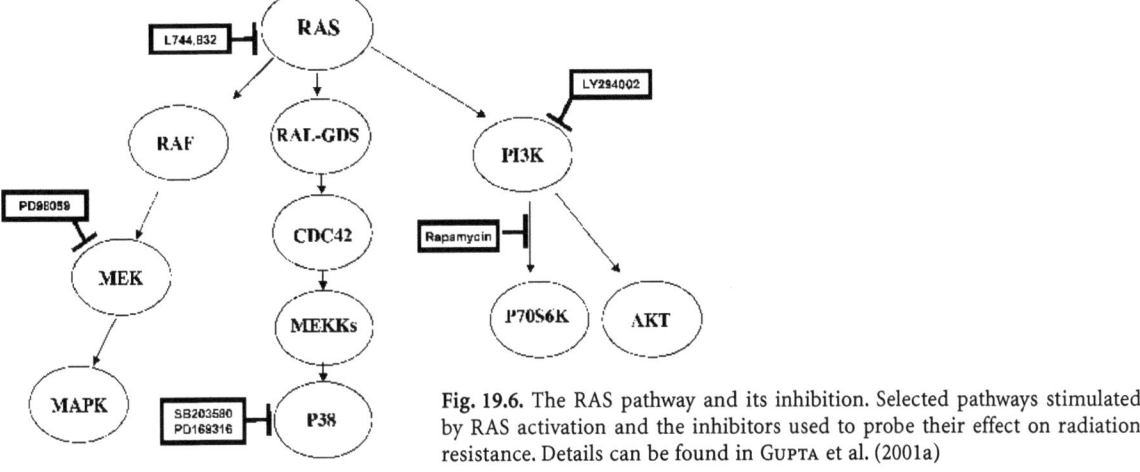

Fig. 19.6. The RAS pathway and its inhibition. Selected pathways stimulated by RAS activation and the inhibitors used to probe their effect on radiation resistance. Details can be found in Gupta et al. (2001a)

Fig. 19.7. PI3-Kinase activation increases radiation survival in cells without activated RAS. The pGRE5/EBV plasmid which has an inducible dexamethasone promoter was used as a vector for a constitutively active p110 unit of PI3-kinase. This plasmid was transiently transfected into MR4 and RT4 cells by electroporation. After 48 h, expression of PI3-kinase was induced by addition of dexamethasone (Sigma, St Louis, MO). Radiation survival experiments were performed and protein samples harvested 24 h after the addition of dexamethasone. LY294002 (10μM) was used to inhibit PI3-kinase at the time of irradiation. Adapted with permission from Gupta et al. (2001a), which contains a detailed description of this experiment

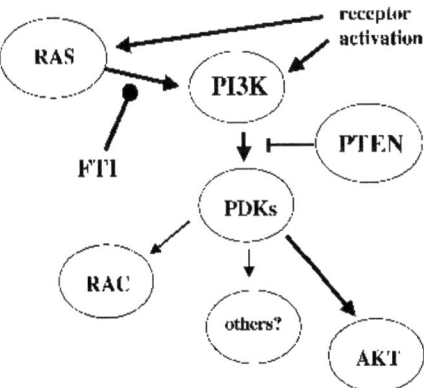

Fig. 19.8. Modulation of PI3-Kinase pathway activity and PI3-Kinase pathway effectors. Potential activation mechanisms, selected signaling pathways and inhibitors of PI3-kinase signaling are shown

19.7
The Effects of FTI Treatment on Radiosensitivity in Vivo

In contrast to the effects of RAS signaling on intrinsic radioresistance measured in vitro, in tumors the environment of the tumor cells can have a large effect on their survival after radiation exposure. We have shown that tumor cell radiosensitization by FTI treatment is achieved in a nude mouse xenograft model (COHEN-JONATHAN et al. 2000). In these studies, radiosensitization was again specific for the human tumor xenografts expressing mutated *ras*. In accordance with the specificity of radiosensitization observed in vitro, no increase in the radiosensitivity of normal tissues was observed in these animal studies, indicating that FTI treatment could potentially increase the therapeutic index of radiation. Our published studies were done using early-generation FTIs. Since that time we have investigated two later-generation FTIs that have been tested in clinical trials. Both R115,777 (END et al. 1998, 2001; KARP et al. 2001; PUNT et al. 2001; ZUJEWSKI et al. 2000) and L778,123 (BRITTEN et al. 1999; HAHN et al. 2002) showed significant radiosensitization of T24 tumor xenografts as measured by evaluating tumor clonogen survival after in vivo treatment with FTI and radiation (Fig. 19.9).

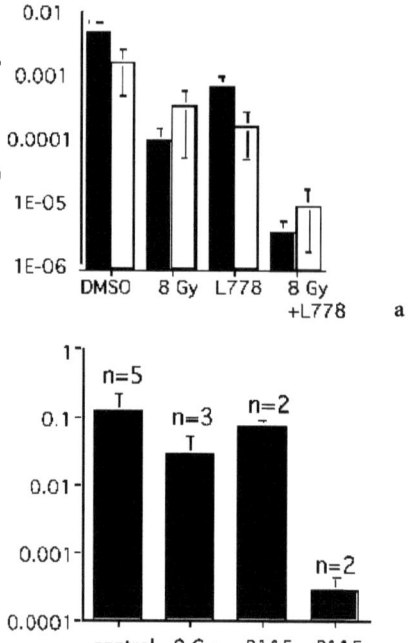

Fig. 19.9a, b. T24 tumor clonogens surviving irradiation and L778,123 or R115777 farnesyltransferase inhibitor treatment in vivo. T24 tumor-bearing animals were treated with (a) L778,123 (Merck & Co. Inc) or with (b) R115,777 (Janssen Pharmaceuticals) prior to irradiation. In (a) each bar represents a single tumor. In (b) each bar represents replicate tumors. After irradiation, mice were killed and the tumors dissociated and plated for clonogenic survival determination. Plating efficiency of tumor cell clonogens was assessed after 10–14 days. Increased plating in (b) is attributed to improved tumor dissociation technique and did not alter the effects of FTI on radiation survival. In b, each bar represents the mean from replicate tumors

19.8
Results from a Clinical Study Combining FTI and Radiation Therapy

The preclinical data demonstrating FTI radiosensitization in human tumor cells in vitro and in vivo led to the initiation of a Phase I clinical trial of the FTI L-778,123 in combination with radiotherapy for selected locally advanced malignancies. L-778,123 is a peptidomimetic inhibitor of farnesyltransferase that was found to be safely tolerated as a 7-day continuous infusion (BRITTEN et al. 2001). The primary objective of the FTI and radiotherapy study was to establish the maximally tolerated dose (MTD) and dose-limiting toxicities (DLTs) of the combination. Patients with locally advanced, unresectable non-small cell lung cancer (NSCLC), head and neck cancer (HNC), and pancreatic cancer were enrolled on this trial. The presence of a *ras* mutation was not required for study entry. The results of this study in NSCLC and HNC patients have recently been reported (HAHN et al. 2002).

Patients on this trial were treated with standard radiotherapy over 7 weeks. L-778,123 was administered as a continuous infusion of 280 mg/M^2/day for 7 days during weeks 1, 2, 4, and 5 of radiation (dose level 1) and as a continuous infusion of 560 mg/M^2/day during weeks 1, 2, 4, 5, and 7 of radiation (dose level 2). Nine patients with NSCLC and HNC were enrolled, six patients on dose level 1 and three patients on dose level 2. No dose-limiting toxicities (DLTs) were observed on the first dose level. One DLT, grade IV neutropenia, was observed on dose level 2. No episodes of dose-limiting mucositis, esophagitis, or pneumonitis were observed. Four patients with NSCLC had evaluable disease and three patients had a complete response to treatment. The remaining NSCLC patient had a partial response. Two HNC patients who completed treatment had complete responses. The remaining HNC patient was taken off study shortly after completion of therapy.

A cell line, AdrM, was established from an adrenal metastasis obtained from one of the NSCLC patients enrolled on this study. Radiosensitization of this cell line, which did not contain an activating *ras* mutation, was observed with L-778,123. Furthermore, treatment of AdrM cells with L-778,123 resulted in an accumulation of cells in G2/M (HAHN et al. 2002).

L-778,123 and radiation was well tolerated with no DLTs at the first dose level studied in this trial. Interestingly, no increase in mucosal toxicities was observed in these patients. This is especially important to emphasize because one of the major toxicities of combined modality therapy with conventional chemotherapy agents and radiation in NSCLC and HNC patients is mucositis and esophagitis (DILLMAN 1996; HAHN et al. 2002; LANGER et al. 1996). It is difficult to draw firm conclusions regarding the responses observed in this study. Nonetheless, it is encouraging that local responses have been observed.

19.9 Influence of FTI Treatment on the Tumor Microenvironment

The maintenance of an adequate blood supply to a growing solid tumor requires the formation of new blood vessels and capillaries through tumor angiogenesis. Angiogenesis is promoted by several growth factors produced by tumor cells, including basic fibroblast growth factor (bFGF) and vascular endothelial growth factor/vascular permeability factors (VEGF/VPF or VEGF) (RAK et al. 1995). VEGF/VPFs that act as endothelial cell-specific mitogens are expressed by a variety of solid tumors, including brain tumors as well as breast, kidney, colon, ovarian, bladder carcinomas, and melanomas (reviewed in DVORAK et al. 1995; KOLCH et al. 1995; SENGER et al. 1993). VEGF/VPF was first isolated as a cytokine from lectin-stimulated lymphocytes that increased the permeability of guinea pig capillaries (SOBEL et al. 1977). Thus, in addition to its mitogenic properties, VEGF/VPF causes increased vascular permeability and influences both angiogenesis and tumor interstitial pressure.

RAS activation has been implicated in the up-regulation of VEGF/VPF expression in a number of studies (reviewed in KERBEL et al. 1998). H-RAS activation has been associated with increased VEGF/VPF expression in murine 3T3 cells, keratinocytes and endothelial cells, including immortalized rat intestinal epithelial (RIE) cells (FELESZKO et al. 1999; LARCHER et al. 1996; RAK et al. 1995). Stimulation of VEGF expression by growth factors involves a pathway that includes RAS, MAP kinase and SP1 (MILANINI-MONGIAT et al. 2002). In contrast, VEGF induction by HIF-1 under hypoxia has been shown to result from RAS signaling through the PI3 kinase pathway (BLANCHER et al. 2001; MAZURE et al. 1997). K-RAS has been shown to up-regulate VEGF in experimental models and in human tumors (KONISHI et al. 2000; RAK et al. 1995). The effects of normal RAS signaling on VEGF/VPF expression was also observed in astrocytoma cells.

We initially postulated that FTIs would act as antiangiogenic agents since FTIs inhibit RAS function and RAS signaling promotes VEGF/VPF expression. This was initially proposed by Kerbel and his colleagues (RAK et al. 1995). Evidence supporting this hypothesis was also obtained in several studies. Cells transfected to express the dominant inhibitory mutant H-*ras*^{N17} demonstrated a reduction in VEGF/VPF secretion under both normoxic and hypoxic conditions. Similar reductions in VEGF/VPF secretion were obtained when these cells were treated by the farnesyltransferase inhibitor L-744,832 (FELDKAMP et al. 1999). Lovastatin treatment of murine 3T3-ras cells resulted in decreased VEGF production and reduced vascularization at the site of tumor cell injection (FELESZKO et al. 1999). FTI treatment was also associated with a two-fold decrease in VEGF/VPF expression in H-*ras*-transfected HaCaT cells (CHARVAT et al. 1999). If FTI treatment completely blocked angiogenesis, then it would be predicted to cause decreased tumor perfusion and increase the level of hypoxia. Increased hypoxia is induced by some antiangiogenic agents (DING et al. 2001). But increased hypoxia would reduce, not enhance radiation-killing of tumor cells.

For this reason we examined the oxygenation of tumors after FTI treatment. Hypoxia was detected using the pentafluorinated 2-nitroimidazole EF5 (KOCH et al. 1995; LORD et al. 1993). EF5 forms covalent adducts with cellular proteins under hypoxic conditions in viable cells (AYENE et al. 1995; BRITTEN et al. 1996; EVANS et al. 1995; FENTON et al. 1999; GREENLEE et al. 2000; LORD et al. 1993; WALEH et al. 1995). These adducts are detected with a monoclonal antibody that is highly specific for EF5 (KOCH et al. 1995). This method of determining tumor oxygenation is independent of cell or tissue type, has been found to detect biologically relevant increases in hypoxia, and has been repeatedly validated (EVANS et al. 1995; KAVANAGH et al. 1999; LEE et al. 1996).

Contrary to our prediction that FTI treatment would induce hypoxia, the levels of hypoxia were diminished in tumors with oncogenic *ras* after FTI treatment, raising the possibility that FTI inhibition of RAS is not exclusively antiangiogenic. We showed that treatment of tumor-bearing mice with the FTI L744,832 caused a decrease in the incidence and degree of tumor hypoxia in T24 human bladder tumor xenografts and in 141-1 prostate tumor grafts. No change in the hypoxia of HT29 colon or RT4 bladder xenografts that express wild type RAS was detected (COHEN-JONATHAN et al. 2001) (Fig. 19.10). The improved oxygenation was evident as early as 3 days after the initiation of FTI treatment and lasted through 2 weeks, which was the latest time examined. Further studies with L778,123 have confirmed that FTI treatment can reduce hypoxia in tumors with H-*ras* mutations. These studies also confirmed the timing of this effect, and demonstrated that the enhanced oxygenation by FTIs is not compound-specific (Fig. 19.11). Experiments to determine the mechanisms responsible for this change in tumor oxygenation are currently in progress.

These results raise the possibility that there is more than one mechanism of FTI-mediated radiosensitization occurring in vivo. Radiation oncologists and radiobiologists have long been interested in tumor oxygenation because hypoxic cells may limit radiation treatment outcome. It is well established that hypoxic cells survive irradiation to a significantly greater extent than cells in an oxygenated environment. The magnitude of the difference in survival is dose-dependent, but in general hypoxic cells require a two- to threefold higher dose to effect the same cell killing in vitro as that obtained in normoxic cells (PALCIC and SKARSGARD 1984). In addition, hypoxia induces apoptosis in tumors and may lead to more aggressive tumors by selecting for cells that are deficient in apoptosis induction (GRAEBER et al. 1996; MAZURE et al. 1997).

From clinical studies it is known that human tumors containing hypoxic cells are more prone to recurrence following radiation therapy. GATENBY et al. (1988) demonstrated that the short-term clinical response of irradiated, well-oxygenated cervical node metastases from head and neck tumors was superior to that of poorly oxygenated lymph nodes. Similarly, Overgaard's group showed that pO2 values less than 2.5 mmHg were significantly predictive of locoregional failure using three methods of data analysis ($P=.01-P=.018$) (NORDSMARK et al. 1996). BRIZEL et al. (1997) demonstrated a marked decrease in disease-free survival for patients with head and neck cancer and median pO_2 less than 10 mmHg. The average tumor median pO_2 for relapsing patients was 4.1 mmHg and 17.1 mmHg in nonrelapsing patients.

Other studies have also demonstrated that hypoxia negatively affects the outcome of radiotherapy in patients with carcinoma of the cervix. In two studies, HOCKEL et al. (1993, 1996) showed that patients with hypoxic cervix carcinoma tumors treated with radiotherapy with or without chemotherapy, or with radiotherapy or surgery had significantly worse disease-free and overall survival probabilities compared to patients with nonhypoxic tumors. ROFSTAD et al. (2000) found that radiotherapy treatment failure in advanced cervical carcinoma was primarily associated with increased tumor hypoxia. FYLES et al. also found that hypoxic tumors were predictive of lower disease-free survival (FYLES et al. 1998). However, this group has now reported that hypoxia is predictive only in node-negative cervical cancer and may be related to metastatic probability (FYLES et al. 2002).

Studies have also shown that tumor reoxygenation can occur following irradiation (reviewed in KALLMAN 1988) Interestingly, irradiation lowers tumor interstitial pressure (ZNATI et al. 1996), which could contribute to better oxygenation. However, the net effect of radiation alone on tumor hypoxia and perfu-

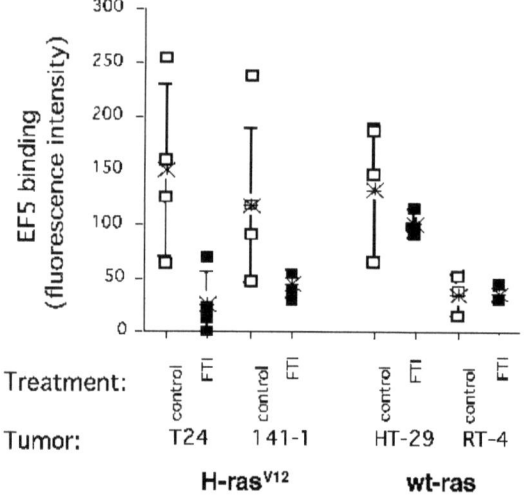

Fig. 19.10. Tumor oxygenation is increased (EF5 binding is decreased) in tumors expressing oncogenic H-*ras*. Mean EF5 staining intensity was quantitated in tumor regions staining with intensities 20 fluorescence channels above background. The mean fluorescence intensities of the positively staining regions in individual tumors are shown. Tumor-bearing mice were treated with L-744,832 40 mg/kg per day for 3–7 days (■) and control tumors treated with carrier alone (□). The mean of values obtained in each group are indicated (∗). Mann-Whitney analysis demonstrated statistical significance for the difference between FTI-treated and control T24 tumors ($n=4$ each group; $\alpha(D)$ value of 0.05) and for the difference in FTI-treated and control 141-1 tumors ($n=5$ each group; a (D) of 0.025). From COHEN-JONATHAN et al. (2001) with permission

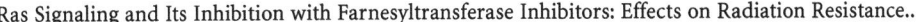

Fig. 19.11a–d. Hypoxia in T24 tumor xenografts after FTI treatment. T24 tumor-bearing animals were implanted with Alzet microosmotic pumps containing carrier (**a**) or 40 mg/kg/day L778,123 (**b, c, d**). Animals received continuous infusion of drug or carrier for 1 day (**a** and **b**), for 4 days (**c**) or 2 weeks (**d**). Tumor sizes at sacrifice were: (**a**) 411mm³, (**b**) 353mm³, (**c**) 533mm³, (**d**) 506mm³. The exposure time for EF5 fluorescence image capture was 0.41 s in **a** and **b**, 4.0 s in **c, d** so the hypoxia in **a** and **b** relative to **c** and **d** is 10× greater than shown. Details of the experimental method can be found in Cohen-Jonathan et al. (2001)

sion of tumor vessels, even at the relatively high doses of 10 Gy, appears to be transient (Fenton et al. 1998).

Taken as a whole, the studies outlined above indicate that continuously enhanced oxygenation of tumors prior to and during a course of irradiation could promote the effectiveness of radiation in tumor cell killing. Our studies with FTIs provide evidence that these inhibitors may be effective in promoting tumor oxygenation. Furthermore, since normal tissues are not hypoxic, enhanced oxygenation resulting from FTI treatment could preferentially sensitize tumor, and not normal tissues.

19.10 FTI Effects on Tumor Metastasis and Collagenolytic Enzyme Production

In addition to its influence on intrinsic radiosensitivity and on tumor hypoxia, RAS signaling also promotes expression of collagenolytic enzymes implicated in metastasis. Expression of one of these enzymes, the 92-kDa gelatinase (MMP-9) has been strongly associated with the metastatic phenotype in a number of rodent and human cells (reviewed in Himelstein et al. 1994; John and Tuszynski 2001). We therefore examined the effect of RAS inhibition with FTI on the expression of MMP-9 in a model where MMP-9 expression has been shown to affect metastasis (Bernhard et al. 1990, 1994, 1995). Treatment of metastatic REF cells transformed with oncogenic H-ras with the FTI L744,832 resulted in a dose-dependent and marked decrease in MMP-9 expression (Fig. 19.12). Expression of other collagenases was also reduced but to a lesser extent. The reduction in collagenolytic enzyme expression was accompanied by reduced metastatic potential when FTI-treated cells were injected IV and lung metastases enumerated. The number of metastatic nodules in treated mice was reduced fivefold relative to controls (Fig. 19.13a). Survival of mice injected with the

Fig. 19.12. Inhibition of gelatinase expression in v-myc + H-ras-transformed REF cells. Serum-free supernatants of 2.10.10 REF cell cultures were harvested after 24 h in medium containing the indicated concentrations of L744,832. Gelatinase activity was assayed after nondenaturing gel electrophoresis and zymography, as described in BERNHARD et al. (1990). Gelatinase activity appears as bands of clearing due to gelatin substrate cleavage. The migration of the 92-kDA and 72-kDa gelatinases is indicated

treated cells was also prolonged, though they eventually succumbed to the few metastases that did occur when these reached a large enough size to compromise their breathing (Fig. 19.13b). The reduction in tumor growth rate after FTI treatment (Fig. 19.13c) was not sufficient to account for either the reduced number of metastases, but may have contributed to the prolonged survival. Similar results were obtained when untreated cells were injected into FTI-treated mice and in a 141-1 H-ras-transformed murine prostate tumor model (SEHGAL et al. 1998; THOMPSON et al. 1993, 1995) (not shown). We had previously shown that oncogenic H-ras expression promoted metastasis (BERNHARD et al. 1990; MUSCHEL et al. 1985) and that inhibiting gelatinase expression could reduce metastatic potential (BERNHARD et al. 1994, 1995; SEHGAL et al. 1998) The results presented here demonstrate that inhibition of H-RAS by FTIs can significantly reduce metastatic potential in these cells coincident with a substantial reduction in gelatinase expression.

19.11
Conclusions

RAS activation has many effects that contribute to tumor aggressiveness and resistance to therapy. Molecular targeting of RAS using prenyltransferase inhibition has shown that blocking RAS can reverse many of these effects. Clinical studies have shown that these agents are well tolerated, including their use as adjuvants to radiotherapy. However, despite the defined molecular target for which FTIs were developed, it is apparent that the mechanisms of their activity are not fully understood. Further study of the mechanism of FTI action may better define the conditions under which these inhibitors will be most

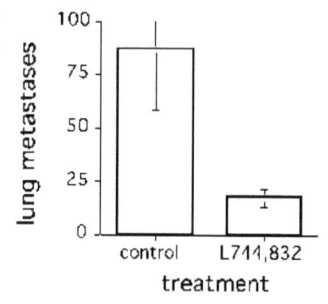

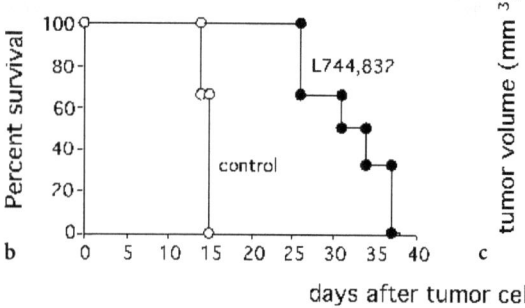
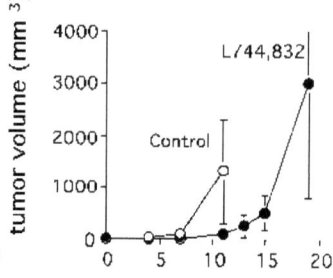

Fig. 19.13a–c. Inhibition of metastasis by FTI treatment. 2.10.10 cells were pretreated in vitro for 24 h with 5μM L744,832 or carrier, then injected into the tail vein (a and b, 4.5×10^4 cells, n=6 per group) or flank (c, 5×10^5 cells, n=4 per group) of nude mice. Animals were followed until they showed signs of labored breathing or discomfort, at which time they were killed. Metastases were counted in lungs (a) after inflation under a dissecting microscope. Events in b were scored at the time of death

days after tumor cell injection

effective. These studies may also uncover unknown targets that are important for the activity of FTIs and potentially define new strategies for molecular therapeutic intervention.

Acknowledgements. This work was supported by NIH grants CA73820 and CA75138 and Department of Defense award DAMD17-98-1-8546. Additional support was provided by a sponsored research agreement with Merck & Co., Inc. and from the Department of Radiation Oncology at the University of Pennsylvania.

References

Ashar HR, James L, Gray K et al (2001) The farnesyl transferase inhibitor SCH 66336 induces a G(2)®M or G(1) pause in sensitive human tumor cell lines. Exp Cell Res 262:17–27

Ayene IS, Koch CJ, Krisch RE (1995) Modification of radiation-induced strand breaks by glutathione: comparison of single- and double-strand breaks in SV40 DNA. Radiat Res 144:1–8

Barrington RE, Subler MA, Rands E et al (1998) A farnesyltransferase inhibitor induces tumor regression in transgenic mice harboring multiple oncogenic mutations by mediating alterations in both cell cycle control and apoptosis. Mol Cell Biol 18:85–92

Bernhard EJ, Muschel RJ, Hughes EN (1990) Mr 92,000 gelatinase release correlates with the metastatic phenotype in transformed rat embryo cells. Cancer Res 50:3872–3877

Bernhard EJ, Gruber SB, Muschel RJ (1994) Direct evidence linking expression of matrix metalloproteinase 9 (92-kDa gelatinase/collagenase) to the metastatic phenotype in transformed rat embryo cells. Proc Natl Acad Sci U S A 91: 4293–4297

Bernhard EJ, Hagner B, Wong C et al (1995) The effect of E1A transfection on MMP-9 expression and metastatic potential. Int J Cancer 60:718–724

Bernhard EJ, Kao G, Cox AD et al (1996) The farnesyltransferase inhibitor FTI-277 radiosensitizes H-ras-transformed rat embryo fibroblasts. Cancer Res 56:1727–1730

Bernhard EJ, McKenna WG, Hamilton AD et al (1998) Inhibiting Ras prenylation increases the radiosensitivity of human tumor cell lines with activating mutations of ras oncogenes. Cancer Res 58:1754–1761

Bernhard EJ, McKenna WG, Muschel RJ (1999) Radiosensitivity and the cell cycle. Cancer J Sci Am 5:194–204

Bernhard EJ, Stanbridge EJ, Gupta S et al (2000) Direct evidence for the contribution of activated N-ras and K-ras oncogenes to increased intrinsic radiation resistance in human tumor cell lines. Cancer Res 60:6597–6600

Blancher C, Moore JW, Robertson N et al (2001) Effects of ras and von Hippel-Lindau (VHL) gene mutations on hypoxia-inducible factor (HIF)-1alpha, HIF-2alpha, and vascular endothelial growth factor expression and their regulation by the phosphatidylinositol 3'-kinase/Akt signaling pathway. Cancer Res 61:7349–7355

Britten C, Rowinsky E, Yao S-L et al (1999) The farnesyl protein transferase (FPTase) inhibitor L-778,123 in patients with solid cancer (abstract). Proc Am Soc Clin Oncol 18:155a

Britten RA, Evans AJ, Allalunis-Turner MJ et al (1996) Effect of cisplatin on the clinically relevant radiosensitivity of human cervical carcinoma cell lines. Int J Radiat Oncol Biol Phys 34:367–374

Britten CD, Rowinsky EK, Soignet S et al (2001) A phase I and pharmacological study of the farnesyl protein transferase inhibitor L-778,123 in patients with solid malignancies. Clin Cancer Res 7:3894–3903

Brizel DM, Sibley GS, Prosnitz LR et al (1997) Tumor hypoxia adversely affects the prognosis of carcinoma of the head and neck. Int J Radiat Oncol Biol Phys 38:285–289

Cartee L, Vrana JA, Wang Z et al (2000) Inhibition of the mitogen activated protein kinase pathway potentiates radiation-induced cell killing via cell cycle arrest at the G2/M transition and independently of increased signaling by the JNK/c-Jun pathway. Int J Oncol 16:413–422

Charvat S, Duchesne M, Parvaz P et al (1999) The up-regulation of vascular endothelial growth factor in mutated Ha-ras HaCaT cell lines is reduced by a farnesyl transferase inhibitor. Anticancer Res 19:557–561

Cohen-Jonathan E, Toulas C, Ader I et al (1999) The farnesyltransferase inhibitor FTI-277 suppresses the 24-kDa FGF2-induced radioresistance in HeLa cells expressing wild-type RAS. Radiat Res 152:404–411

Cohen-Jonathan E, Muschel RJ, Gillies McKenna W et al (2000) Farnesyltransferase inhibitors potentiate the antitumor effect of radiation on a human tumor xenograft expressing activated HRAS. Radiat Res 154:125–132

Cohen-Jonathan E, Evans SM, Koch CJ et al (2001) The farnesyltransferase inhibitor L744,832 reduces hypoxia in tumors expressing activated H-ras. Cancer Res 61:2289–2293

Crespo NC, Ohkanda J, Yen TJ et al (2001) The farnesyltransferase inhibitor, FTI-2153, blocks bipolar spindle formation and chromosome alignment and causes prometaphase accumulation during mitosis of human lung cancer cells. J Biol Chem 276:16161–16167

Cunningham CC, Holmlund JT, Geary RS et al (2001) A phase I trial of H-ras antisense oligonucleotide ISIS 2503 administered as a continuous intravenous infusion in patients with advanced carcinoma. Cancer 92:1265–1271

Daaka Y, Wickstrom E (1990) Target dependence of antisense oligodeoxynucleotide inhibition of c-Ha-ras p21 expression and focus formation in T24-transformed NIH3T3 cells. Oncogene Res 5:267–275

Dillman RO (1996) Concurrent chemoradiation in unresectable stage III non-small cell lung cancer: too much pain for no gain. Cancer J Sci Am 2:76

Ding I, Sun JZ, Fenton B et al (2001) Intratumoral administration of endostatin plasmid inhibits vascular growth and perfusion in MCa-4 murine mammary carcinomas. Cancer Res 61:526–531

Du W, Prendergast GC (1999) Geranylgeranylated RhoB mediates suppression of human tumor cell growth by farnesyltransferase inhibitors. Cancer Res 59:5492–5496

Du W, Lebowitz PF, Prendergast GC (1999) Cell growth inhibition by farnesyltransferase inhibitors is mediated by gain of geranylgeranylated RhoB. Mol Cell Biol 19:1831–1840

Dvorak HF, Brown LF, Detmar M et al (1995) Vascular permeability factor/vascular endothelial growth factor, microvascular hyperpermeability, and angiogenesis. Am J Pathol 146: 1029–1039

End D, Skrzat S, Devine A (1998) R115777, a novel imidazole farnesyl protein transferase inhibitor (FTI): biochemical and cellular effects in H-ras and K-ras dominant systems. Proc Am Assoc Cancer Res 39:270

End DW, Smets G, Todd AV et al (2001) Characterization of the antitumor effects of the selective farnesyl protein transferase inhibitor R115777 in vivo and in vitro. Cancer Res 61: 131–137

Evans SM, Joiner B, Jenkins WT et al (1995) Identification of hypoxia in cells and tissues of epigastric 9L rat glioma using EF5 [2-(2-nitro-1H-imidazol-1-yl)-N-(2,2,3,3,3-pentafluoropropyl) acetamide]. Br J Cancer 72:875–882

Feldkamp MM, Lau N, Guha A (1999) Growth inhibition of astrocytoma cells by farnesyl transferase inhibitors is mediated by a combination of anti-proliferative, pro-apoptotic and anti-angiogenic effects. Oncogene 18:7514–7526

Feleszko W, Balkowiec EZ, Sieberth E et al (1999) Lovastatin and tumor necrosis factor-alpha exhibit potentiated antitumor effects against Ha-ras-transformed murine tumor via inhibition of tumor-induced angiogenesis. Int J Cancer 81:560–567

Fenton BM, Paoni SF, Koch CJ et al (1998) Effect of local irradiation on tumor oxygenation, perfused vessel density, and development of hypoxia. Adv Exp Med Biol 454:619–628

Fenton BM, Paoni SF, Lee J et al (1999) Quantification of tumour vasculature and hypoxia by immunohistochemical staining and HbO2 saturation measurements. Br J Cancer 79:464–471

FitzGerald TJ, Daugherty C, Kase K et al (1985) Activated human N-ras oncogene enhances x-irradiation repair of mammalian cells in vitro less effectively at low dose rate. Implications for increased therapeutic ratio of low dose rate irradiation. Am J Clin Oncol 8:517–522

FitzGerald TJ, Henault S, Sakakeeny M et al (1990) Expression of transfected recombinant oncogenes increases radiation resistance of clonal hematopoietic and fibroblast cell lines selectively at clinical low dose rate. Radiat Res 122:44–52

Fyles AW, Milosevic M, Wong R et al (1998) Oxygenation predicts radiation response and survival in patients with cervix cancer. Radiother Oncol 48:149–156

Fyles AW, Milosevic M, Hedley D et al (2002) Tumor hypoxia has independent predictor impact only in patients with node-negative cervix cancer. J Clin Oncol 20:680–687

Gatenby RA, Kessler HB, Rosenblum JS et al (1988) Oxygen distribution in squamous cell carcinoma metastases and its relationship to outcome of radiation therapy. Int J Radiat Oncol Biol Phys 14:831–838

Gelb MH (1997) Protein prenylation, et cetera: signal transduction in two dimensions (comment). Science 275:1750–1751

Glomset JA, Farnsworth CC (1994) Role of protein modification reactions in programming interactions between ras-related GTPases and cell membranes. Annu Rev Cell Biol 10:181–205

Gokhale PC, McRae D, Monia BP, Bagg A, Rahman A, Dritschilo A, Kasid U (1999) Antisense raf oligodeoxyribonucleotide is a radiosensitizer in vivo. Antisense Nucleic Acid Drug Dev 9:191–202

Graeber TG, Osmanian C, Jacks T et al (1996) Hypoxia-mediated selection of cells with diminished apoptotic potential in solid tumours (see comments). Nature 379:88–91

Gray GD, Hernandez OM, Hebel D et al (1993) Antisense DNA inhibition of tumor growth induced by c-Ha-ras oncogene in nude mice. Cancer Res 53:577–580

Greenlee RT, Murray T, Bolden S et al (2000) Cancer statistics 2000. CA Cancer J Clin, 50:7–33

Gupta AK, Bakanauskas VJ, Cerniglia GJ et al (2001a) The Ras radiation resistance pathway. Cancer Res 61:4278–4282

Gupta AK, Bakanauskas VJ, McKenna WG et al (2001b) Ras regulation of radioresistance in cell culture. Methods Enzymol 333:284–290

Gupta AK, McKenna WG, Weber CN et al (2002) Local recurrence in head and neck cancer: relationship to radiation resistance and signal transduction. Clin Cancer Res 8: 885–892

Hagan M, Wang L, Hanley JR et al (2000) Ionizing radiation-induced mitogen-activated protein (MAP) kinase activation in DU145 prostate carcinoma cells: MAP kinase inhibition enhances radiation-induced cell killing and G2/M-phase arrest. Radiat Res 153:371–383

Hahn SM, Bernhard EJ, Regine W et al (2002) A phase I trial of the farnesyltransferase inhibitor L-778,123 and radiotherapy for locally advanced lung and head and neck cancer. Clin Cancer Res 8:1065–1072

Harari PM, Huang SM (2001) Head and neck cancer as a clinical model for molecular targeting of therapy: combining EGFR blockade with radiation. Int J Radiat Oncol Biol Phys 49:427–433

Himelstein BP, Canete-Soler R, Bernhard EJ et al (1994) Metalloproteinases in tumor progression: the contribution of MMP-9. Invasion Metastasis 14:246–258

Hockel M, Knoop C, Schlenger K et al (1993) Intratumoral pO2 predicts survival in advanced cancer of the uterine cervix. Radiother Oncol 26:45–50

Hockel M, Schlenger K, Aral B et al (1996) Association between tumor hypoxia and malignant progression in advanced cancer of the uterine cervix. Cancer Res 56:4509–4515

John A, Tuszynski G (2001) The role of matrix metalloproteinases in tumor angiogenesis and tumor metastasis. Pathol Oncol Res 7:14–23

Kallman RF (1988) Reoxygenation and repopulation in irradiated tumors. Front Radiat Ther Oncol 22:30–49

Karp JE, Lancet JE, Kaufmann SH et al (2001) Clinical and biologic activity of the farnesyltransferase inhibitor R115777 in adults with refractory and relapsed acute leukemias: a phase 1 clinical-laboratory correlative trial. Blood 97:3361–3369

Kashani-Sabet M, Funato T, Florenes VA et al (1994) Suppression of the neoplastic phenotype in vivo by an anti-ras ribozyme. Cancer Res 54:900–902

Kavanagh MC, Tsang V, Chow S et al (1999) A comparison in individual murine tumors of techniques for measuring oxygen levels. Int J Radiat Oncol Biol Phys 44:1137–1146

Kerbel RS, Viloria-Petit A, Okada F et al (1998) Establishing a link between oncogenes and tumor angiogenesis. Mol Med 4:286–295

Koch C, Evans S, Lord E (1995) Oxygen dependence of cellular uptake of EF5 [2-(2-nitro-1H-imidazol-1-yl)-N-(2,2,3,3,3-pentaluoropropyl)acetamide]: analysis of drug adducts by fluorescent antibodies versus bound radioactivity. Br J Cancer 72:869–874

Kohl N, Wilson F, Mosser S et al (1994) Protein farnesyl transferase inhibitors block the growth of ras-dependent tumors in nude mice. Proc Natl Acad Sci U S A 91:9141–9251

Kohl N, Omer C, Conner M et al (1995) Inhibition of farnesyltransferase induces regression of mammary and salivary carcinomas in ras transgenic mice. Nat Med 1:792–797

Kolch W, Martiny-Baron G, Kieser A et al (1995) Regulation of the expression of the VEGF/VPS and its receptors: role in tumor angiogenesis. Breast Cancer Res Treat 36:139–155

Konishi T, Huang CL, Adachi M et al (2000) The K-ras gene regulates vascular endothelial growth factor gene expression in non-small cell lung cancers. Int J Oncol 16:501–511

Lammering G, Valerie K, Lin PS et al (2001) Radiosensitization of malignant glioma cells through overexpression of dominant-negative epidermal growth factor receptor. Clin Cancer Res 7:682–690

Langer CJ, Curran WJ, Keller SM et al (1996) Long-term survival results for patients with locally advanced, initially unresectable non-small cell lung cancer treated with aggressive concurrent chemoradiation. Cancer J Sci Am 2:99

Lantry LE, Zhang Z, Yao R et al (2000) Effect of farnesyltransferase inhibitor FTI-276 on established lung adenomas from A/J mice induced by 4-(methylnitrosamino)-1-(3-pyridyl)-1-butanone. Carcinogenesis 21:113–116

Larcher F, Robles AI, Duran H et al (1996) Up-regulation of vascular endothelial growth factor/vascular permeability factor in mouse skin carcinogenesis correlates with malignant progression state and activated H-ras expression levels. Cancer Res 56:5391–5396

Lebowitz PF, Davide JP, Prendergast GC (1995) Evidence that farnesyltransferase inhibitors suppress Ras transformation by interfering with Rho activity. Mol Cell Biol 15:6613–6622

Lebowitz PF, Casey PJ, Prendergast GC et al (1997) Farnesyltransferase inhibitors alter the prenylation and growth-stimulating function of RhoB. J Biol Chem 272:15591–15594

Lee J, Siemann DW, Koch CJ et al (1996) Direct relationship between radiobiological hypoxia in tumors and monoclonal antibody detection of EF5 cellular adducts. Int J Cancer 67:372–378

Lerner EC, Zhang TT, Knowles DB et al (1997) Inhibition of the prenylation of K-Ras, but not H- or N-Ras, is highly resistant to CAAX peptidomimetics and requires both a farnesyltransferase and a geranylgeranyltransferase I inhibitor in human tumor cell lines. Oncogene 15:1283–1288

Ling CC, Endlich B (1989). Radioresistance induced by oncogenic transformation. Radiat Res 120:267–279

Liu A, Prendergast GC (2000) Geranylgeranylated RhoB is sufficient to mediate tissue-specific suppression of Akt kinase activity by farnesyltransferase inhibitors. FEBS Lett 481: 205–208

Liu A, Du W, Liu JP et al (2000) RhoB alteration is necessary for apoptotic and antineoplastic responses to farnesyltransferase inhibitors. Mol Cell Biol 20:6105–6113

Lobell RB, Omer CA, Abrams MT et al (2001) Evaluation of farnesyl:protein transferase and geranylgeranyl:protein transferase inhibitor combinations in preclinical models. Cancer Res 61:8758–8768

Lord EM, Harwell L, Koch CJ (1993) Detection of hypoxic cells by monoclonal antibody recognizing 2-nitroimidazole adducts. Cancer Res 53:5721–5726

Mangues R, Corral T, Kohl NE et al (1998) Antitumor effect of a farnesyl protein transferase inhibitor in mammary and lymphoid tumors overexpressing N-ras in transgenic mice. Cancer Res 58:1253–1259

Mazure NM, Chen EY, Laderoute KR et al (1997) Induction of vascular endothelial growth factor by hypoxia is modulated by a phosphatidylinositol 3-kinase/Akt signaling pathway in Ha-ras-transformed cells through a hypoxia inducible factor-1 transcriptional element. Blood 90:3322–3331

McKenna WG, Weiss MC, Bakanauskas VJ et al (1990a) The role of the H-ras oncogene in radiation resistance and metastasis. Int J Radiat Oncol Biol Phys 18:849–859

McKenna WG, Weiss MC, Endlich B et al (1990b) Synergistic effect of the v-myc oncogene with H-ras on radioresistance. Cancer Res 50:97–102

McKenna WG, Iliakis G, Weiss MC et al (1991) Increased G2 delay in radiation-resistant cells obtained by transformation of primary rat embryo cells with the oncogenes H-ras and v-myc. Radiat Res 125:283–287

McKenna WG, Bernhard EJ, Markiewicz DA et al (1996) Regulation of radiation-induced apoptosis in oncogene-transfected fibroblasts: influence of H-ras on the G2 delay. Oncogene 12:237–245

Milanini-Mongiat J, Pouyssegur J, Pages G (2002) Identification of two Sp1 phosphorylation sites for p42/p44 mitogen-activated protein kinases. Their implication in vascular endothelial growth factor gene transcription. J Biol Chem 277:20631–20639

Milas L, Mason K, Hunter N et al (2000) In vivo enhancement of tumor radioresponse by C225 antiepidermal growth factor receptor antibody. Clin Cancer Res 6:701–708

Miller AC, Kariko K, Myers CE et al (1993) Increased radioresistance of EJras-transformed human osteosarcoma cells and its modulation by lovastatin, an inhibitor of p21ras isoprenylation. Int J Cancer 53:302–307

Miquel K, Pradines A, Sun J et al (1997) GGTI-298 induces G0-G1 block and apoptosis whereas FTI-277 causes G2-M enrichment in A549 cells. Cancer Res 57:1846–1850

Miyaguchi M, Olofsson J, Hellquist HB (1991) Expression of epidermal growth factor receptor in glottic carcinoma and its relation to recurrence after radiotherapy. Clin Otolaryngol 16:466–469

Muschel R, Williams J, Lowy D et al (1985) Harvey ras induction of metastatic potential depends upon oncogene activation and the type of recipient cell. Am J Pathol 121:1–8

Nakano M, Aoki K, Matsumoto N et al (2001) Suppression of colorectal cancer growth using an adenovirus vector expressing an antisense K-ras RNA. Mol Ther 3:491–499

Nordsmark M, Overgaard M, Overgaard J (1996) Pretreatment oxygenation predicts radiation response in advanced squamous cell carcinoma of the head and neck. Radiother Oncol 41:31 39

Ong A, Li WX, Ling CC (1993) Low-dose-rate irradiation of rat embryo cells containing the Ha-ras oncogene. Radiat Res 134:251–255

Palcic B, Skarsgard LD (1984) Reduced oxygen enhancement ratio at low doses of ionizing radiation. Radiat Res 100: 328–339

Peters DG, Hoover RR, Gerlach MJ et al (2001) Activity of the farnesyl protein transferase inhibitor SCH66336 against BCR/ABL-induced murine leukemia and primary cells from patients with chronic myeloid leukemia. Blood 97: 1404–1412

Pirollo KF, Tong YA, Villegas Z et al (1993) Oncogene- transformed NIH 3T3 cells display radiation resistance levels indicative of a signal transduction pathway leading to the radiation-resistant phenotype. Radiat Res 135:234–243

Pirollo KF, Hao Z, Rait A et al (1997) Evidence supporting a signal transduction pathway leading to the radiation-resistant phenotype in human tumor cells. Biochem Biophys Res Commun 230:196–201

Punt CJ, van Maanen L, Bol CJ et al (2001) Phase I and pharmacokinetic study of the orally administered farnesyl transferase inhibitor R115777 in patients with advanced solid tumors. Anticancer Drugs 12:193–197

Rak J, Mitsuhashi Y, Bayko L et al (1995) Mutant ras oncogenes upregulate VEGF/VPF expression: implications for induction and inhibition of tumor angiogenesis. Cancer Res 55: 4575–4580

Rofstad EK, Sundfor K, Lyng H et al (2000) Hypoxia-induced treatment failure in advanced squamous cell carcinoma of the uterine cervix is primarily due to hypoxia-induced radiation resistance rather than hypoxia-induced metastasis. Br J Cancer 83:354–359

Russell JS, Lang FF, Huet T et al (1999) Radiosensitization of human tumor cell lines induced by the adenovirus-mediated expression of an anti-Ras single-chain antibody fragment. Cancer Res 59:5239–5244

Russell JS, Raju U, Gumin GJ et al (2002) Inhibition of radiation-induced nuclear factor-kappaB activation by an anti-Ras single-chain antibody fragment: lack of involvement in radiosensitization. Cancer Res 62:2318–2326

Samid D, Miller AC, Rimoldi D et al (1991) Increased radiation resistance in transformed and nontransformed cells with elevated ras proto-oncogene expression. Radiat Res 126: 244–250

Santini J, Formento JL, Francoual M et al (1991) Characterization, quantification, and potential clinical value of the epidermal growth factor receptor in head and neck squamous cell carcinomas. Head Neck 13:132–139

Santucci MA, Anklesaria P, Anderson SM et al (1992) The v-src oncogene may not be responsible for the increased radioresistance of hematopoietic progenitor cells expressing v-src. Radiat Res 129:297–303

Sebti S, Hamilton A (1997) Inhibition of ras prenylation: a novel approach to cancer chemotherapy. Pharmacol Ther 74:103–114

Sehgal G, Hua J, Bernhard EJ et al (1998) Requirement for matrix metalloproteinase-9 (gelatinase B) expression in metastasis by murine prostate carcinoma. Am J Pathol 152:591–596

Senger DR, Van de Water L, Brown LF et al (1993) Vascular permeability factor (VPF, VEGF) in tumor biology. Cancer Metastasis Rev 12:303–324

Sepp-Lorenzino L, Ma Z, Rands E et al (1995) A peptidomimetic inhibitor of Farnesyl:protein transferase blocks the anchorage-dependent and -independent growth of human tumor cell lines. Cancer Res 55:5302–5309

Servais P, Gulbis B, Fokan D et al (1998) Effects of the farnesyltransferase inhibitor UCF-1C/manumycin on growth and p21-ras post-translational processing in NIH3T3 cells. Int J Cancer 76:601–608

Sklar MD (1988) The ras oncogenes increase the intrinsic resistance of NIH 3T3 cells to ionizing radiation. Science 239:645–647

Sobel AT, Branellec AI, Blanc CJ et al (1977) Physicochemical characterization of a vascular permeability factor produced by con A-stimulated human lymphocytes. J Immunol 119: 1230–1234

Song SY, Meszoely IM, Coffey RJ et al (2000) K-Ras-independent effects of the farnesyl transferase inhibitor L-744,832 on cyclin B1/Cdc2 kinase activity, G2/M cell cycle progression and apoptosis in human pancreatic ductal adenocarcinoma cells. Neoplasia 2:261–272

Sorrentino R, Porcellini A, Spalletti-Cernia D et al (2001) Inhibition of MAPK activity, cell proliferation, and anchorage-independent growth by N-Ras antisense in an N-ras-transformed human cell line. Antisense Nucleic Acid Drug Dev 11:349–358

Su LN, Little JB (1993) Prolonged cell cycle delay in radioresistant human cell lines transfected with activated ras oncogene and/or simian virus 40 T-antigen. Radiat Res 133:73–79

Sun J, Qian Y, Hamilton A et al (1995) Ras CAAX peptidomimetic FTI 276 selectively blocks tumor growth in nude mice of a human lung carcinoma with k-ras mutation and p53 deletion. Cancer Res 55:4243–4247

Sun J, Qian Y, Hamilton AD et al (1998) Both farnesyltransferase and geranylgeranyltransferase I inhibitors are required for inhibition of oncogenic K-ras prenylation but each alone is sufficient to suppress human tumor growth in nude mouse xenografts. Oncogene 16:1467–1473

Sun J, Blaskovich MA, Knowles D et al (1999) Antitumor efficacy of a novel class of non-thiol-containing peptidomimetic inhibitors of farnesyltransferase and geranylgeranyltransferase I: combination therapy with the cytotoxic agents cisplatin, Taxol, and gemcitabine. Cancer Res 59: 4919–4926

Suzuki K, Watanabe M, Miyoshi J (1992) Differences in effects of oncogenes on resistance of gamma rays, ultraviolet light, and heat shock. Radiat Res 129:157–162

Thompson TC, Truong LD, Timme TL et al (1993) Transgenic models for the study of prostate cancer. Cancer 71: S1165–S1171

Thompson TC, Park SH, Timme TL et al (1995) Loss of p53 function leads to metastasis in ras+myc-initiated mouse prostate cancer. Oncogene 10:869–879

Tsuchida T, Kijima H, Hori S et al (2000) Adenovirus-mediated anti-K-ras ribozyme induces apoptosis and growth suppression of human pancreatic carcinoma. Cancer Gene Ther 7: 373–383

Vogt A, Qian Y, McGuire TF et al (1996) Protein geranylgeranylation, not farnesylation, is required for the G1 to S phase transition in mouse fibroblasts. Oncogene 13:1991–1999

Vogt A, Sun J, Qian Y et al (1997) The geranylgeranyltransferase-I inhibitor GGTI-298 arrests human tumor cells in G0/G1 and induces p21(WAF1/CIP1/SDI1) in a p53-independent manner. J Biol Chem 272:27224–27229

Waddick KG, Uckun FM (1998) Innovative treatment programs against cancer. I. Ras oncoprotein as a molecular target. Biochem Pharmacol 56:1411–1426

Waleh NS, Brody MD, Knapp MA et al (1995) Mapping of the vascular endothelial growth factor-producing hypoxic cells in multicellular tumor spheroids using a hypoxia-specific marker. Cancer Res 55:6222–6226

Weichselbaum RR, Dunphy EJ, Beckett MA et al (1989) Epidermal growth factor receptor gene amplification and expression in head and neck cancer cell lines. Head Neck 11:437–442

Whyte DB, Kirschmeier P, Hockenberry TN et al (1997) K- and N-Ras are geranylgeranylated in cells treated with farnesyl protein transferase inhibitors. J Biol Chem 272: 14459–14464

Zhu A, Shaeffer J, Leslie S et al (1996) Epidermal growth factor receptor: an independent predictor of survival in astrocytic tumors given definitive irradiation. Int J Radiat Oncol Biol Phys 34:809–815

Znati CA, Rosenstein M, Boucher Y et al (1996) Effect of radiation on interstitial fluid pressure and oxygenation in a human tumor xenograft. Cancer Res 56:964–968

Zujewski J, Horak ID, Bol CJ et al (2000) Phase I and pharmacokinetic study of farnesyl protein transferase inhibitor R115777 in advanced cancer. J Clin Oncol 18:927–941

Subject Index

Acetylsalicylic Acid   62, 244
Acidic Fibroblast Growth Factor (aFGF)   61
Acidosis   180
Adhesion Molecules   32-33
AKT   19, 79, 165, 172
Alveolar Membranes   29
Amifostine   162
– and intestine   59
– and central nervous system   80
– and lung   43-44
Anaplastic Astrocytoma   140
Anemia   90
– in solid tumors   90
– pathophysiology   90-91
– prognostic impact   91
Angiogenesis   131, 140, 179, 248, 267
Angiostatin   179
Angiotensin-converting enzyme (ACE)   31
– ACE inhibitors   42
Antigen Presenting Cell (APC)   207
Ataxia Teleangiectasia-mutated (ATM) protein kinase   19, 164, 168
Apoptosis   15, 50, 55, 74, 89, 132, 162, 195, 227-232
Arachidonic Acid   32, 60, 242
ASMase   168
Astrocyte   74

B
BAD   18
Basic Fibroblast Growth Factor (bFGF)   19, 32, 39, 45, 61, 78, 104, 148, 183
BAX   17, 133
BCL-2   18, 132, 163, 232
Bestatin   149
BID   232
Blood Transfusion   92-97
Bone Marrow   104-105
Bowel see Intestine
Brain see Central Nervous System
Breast Cancer
– and lung irradiation   37
BRCA1   166

C
Capsaicin   58
Caspases   17-18, 163, 230-232
Capillary   16, 31, 77
Carbonic Anhydrase IX   131
CD40   45
CD95 (s. Fas)   163, 228
Celecoxib   245, 247, 251

Cell Cycle Arrest   166
Cell Death
– modes of   162-164
Central Nervous System (CNS)   73-87
– tumors   139-146
Ceramide   17, 168, 231
Cervical Cancer   126
– and COX-2   132, 252
– and VEGF   130
– and HER-2/neu   130
Cetuximab (C225)   129, 167, 197-201
Chelerythrine   170
Ciliary Neurotrophic Factor (CNTF)   79
c-Jun Kinase (JNK)   168
Clopidogrel   64
Collagen   20, 29, 53
Colon Cancer   152
Connexin43   10
Corticosteroids
– and fibrosis   24
– and central nervous system   80
– and lung   44
Cyclin D1   192
Cyclin-dependent Kinases (CDK)   22, 166
– inhibition   23
– inhibitors   32
Cyclooxygenase (COX)   131, 150, 241-254
– and intestine   60
– inhibition   243-255
Cytochrome C   18, 163, 232
Cytokines   205-218

D
Death Ligands   227-232
Death Receptor   17, 227-232
Demyelination   74
Dendritic Cell   108, 207
Difluoromethylornithine   81
DNA-dependent Protein Kinase (DNA PK)   19, 199

E
Effective Doubling Time   3
Endometrial Cancer   128
Endostatin   179
Endothelial Cell   15, 29, 55, 74, 163, 180
Endothelial Cell Adhesion Factor-1 (ECAM-1)   16
Endothelin   77
Ependymoma   141
Epidermal Growth Factor Receptor (EGFR, Erb-B1)   9, 126, 140, 147, 150, 167, 189-196
– and radioresponse   192-196

– inhibition 9, 129, 133, 197
Epidermis 4
ErbB-2 (HER2/neu) 126, 130-131, 147, 150
Erythropoietin 89-101
Esophageal Cancer 151-152
Extracellular Matrix 131
Ezrin 127

F

Farnesyltransferase 260
– inhibitors 260-271
Fas (CD95) 228
– associated death domain (FADD) 18, 229
– ligand 163, 212, 228
Fibroblast 20, 29, 53
Fibroblast Progenitor Cell 15
Fibrocyte 20
Fibrosis 15, 20, 52
– antifibrotic strategies 24
Functional Imaging 158

G

Gastric Cancer 152
Gemcitabine 161
Gene Therapy
– and IL-2 212
– and IL-12 215
– and SOD 59
– and GM-CSF 108
– and p53 169
– and TNF 234
Glial Growth Factor 78
Glioblastoma multiforme 139
Glutamine 62
Glutathione 80
Granulocyte 104
Granulocyte Colony-stimulating Factor (G-CSF) 32, 103-107
Granulocyte Macrophage Colony-stimulating Factor (GM-CSF) 33, 103-108

H

Head and Neck Cancer
– and COX-2 246
– and EGFR 150, 193
– and farnesyltransferase inhibitor 266
– expression of growth factors 150
– overall treatment time 4
– treatment of mucositis 107, 118
Heat Shock Proteins 207
Hemoglobin 92-93, 98
Heparin 57
Heparinase 16
HER2/neu (s. ErbB-2) 126, 130-131, 147, 150
Hirudin 64
Human Papilloma Virus (HPV) 126
Hypoxia 89-94, 131, 161, 180, 184, 267-269
Hypoxia-inducible factor 89, 130-131

I

Immune System 205-208, 248
– cellular 206
– humoral 206
– – and radiation effects 211-212

Indomethacin 44, 250
Insulin-like Growth Factor-1 (IGF-1) 32, 61, 75, 83, 140, 148
Integrins 33
Intensity Modulated Radiotherapy (IMRT) 157-158
Intercellular Adhesion Molecule-1 (ICAM-1) 33, 45, 75
Interferons
– and fibrosis 24
– alpha 149, 209-210, 215-217
– beta 150, 209-210, 215-217
– gamma 32-33, 149, 210, 217-218
Interleukins
– IL-1 21, 33, 39, 55, 60, 74, 209, 212
– IL-2 209, 212-213
– IL-3 209, 212
– IL-4 32, 55, 209, 213
– IL-5 209
– IL-6 33, 39, 209, 212
– IL-7 60
– IL-8 32-33
– IL-10 209
– IL-11 45, 60, 109
– IL-12 209, 214, 215
– IL-15 61, 209
– IL-18 209
Intestine 49-72
Intracoronary Brachytherapy 108
Iressa (ZD-1839) 197
Iron Substitution 98
Ischemia 16, 78

K

Keratinocyte 8, 23, 113
Keratinocyte Growth Factor (KGF) 10, 61, 113-122

L

Latency-associated Peptide (LAP) 24
Lentinan 151
Ligand-binding Assay (LBA) 127
Lovastatin 261, 267
Lung
– – Cancer 37, 147
– – adenocarcinoma 148
– – small cell carcinoma 38, 148
– – squamous cell carcinoma 147
– – and COX-2 246
– – and farnesyltransferase inhibitor 266
– – and VEGF antibody 181
– Diffusion capacity of carbon monoxide 40
– Fibrosis 24, 29, 37
– – and Tamoxifen 24, 40
– Perfusion 41
– Toxicity 37-46
– – and Paclitaxel 40
Lymphocyte 32, 206

M

Macrophages 29, 74
– macrophage colony-stimulating factor 108
– macrophage inflammatory protein-1alpha (MIP-1α) 33, 62
Major Histocompatibility Complex (MHC) 206-208
Malignant Glioma 139
Mannose 6-phosphate/insulin-like growth factor-2 receptor (M6P/IGF-2R) 39

Subject Index

Mast Cells 56
Matrix Metalloproteinase 57, 107, 269-270
MDM2 164
Megakaryocyte Growth and Development Factor 109
Meningeoma 142
Microenvironment of Tumors 131, 158
Microglia 74
Misoprostol 60, 249
Mitogen-activated Protein Kinase (MAPK/ERK) 17, 79
Monocyte Chemotactic Protein-1 (MCP-1) 33, 54, 62
Mucositis 4, 107, 114
Myelopathy 73
Myelosuppression 103

N

N-acetyl-L-cysteine (NAC) 80
Natural Killer (NK) Cells 54, 60, 206, 229
Nerve
– sensory 57
– growth factor 75
Neuregulins 126
Neuron 74
Neutropenia 103
Nimorazole 161
Normal Tissue Complications 15
– acute reactions 15, 37, 50, 73
– late reactions 15, 37, 50, 73
– normal tissue complication probability (NTCP) in lung 39
Nuclear Factor (NF)-kappaB 63, 75, 248

O

Octreotide 63
OK-432 153
Oligodendrocyte 74
Oligodendroglioma 141
Oral Mucosa 4, 107, 114
Ovarian Cancer 127-129

P

P15 22, 32
P16 32
P21 17, 22, 32, 166, 196
P27 22, 32, 194
P38 264
P53 17, 19, 127, 164, 169
Paclitaxel 161
Pancreatic Cancer 152, 246
Penicillamine 42
Pentoxifylline
– and fibrosis 24
– and intestine 60
– and lung toxicity 43
Phosphatidyl-inositol-3'-kinase (PI3K) 19, 79, 165, 172, 264
– inhibition of 172, 265
Pifithrin 162
Pituitary Adenoma 142
Plasminogen-activating factor 31
Plasminogen activator inhibitor type 1 (PAI-1) 141
Platelet-activating factor (PAF) 55
Platelet-derived Growth Factor (PDGF) 20, 32, 78, 82, 140, 148, 150, 179
Pneumocytes 29
Pneumonitis 24, 29, 37-46, 252

Predictive Assay 65
Prenyltransferase inhibitors 260-264
Prostacyclin 55
Prostaglandins 242-243
– E1 60
– E2 33, 60, 77, 131, 150, 242-243
– D2 242-243
– F2 242-243
– G2 242
– I2 31, 77, 242-243
Prostanoids 242-243
Protease-activated Receptors (PAR) 55
Protein C 55
Protein Kinase B *see* AKT
Protein Kinase C (PKC) 17, 168-169
– inhibitors of 170
PTEN 264

R

RAC1 17
Radiosensitivity 158-160
Radiosensitization 160
RAF1 17, 264
RANTES 33, 62
Rapamycin 172, 265
RAS 164, 172, 259-271
Reactive Oxygen Species (ROS) 22, 32-33, 52
Receptor Tyrosine Kinases 166
Reoxygenation 6
Repopulation 3, 196
– accelerated 3
Rituximab 106

S

Schwannoma 142
Serotonin 77
Signal Transduction Proteins 15
Sizofiran 151
Smad Proteins 22
Smooth Muscle Cells 53-55, 77
Sphingomyelinase 17, 168
Spinal Cord *see* Central Nervous System
Squamous Cell Carcinoma 4
Stem Cell 3, 15, 30, 74, 104, 119-120
Stem Cell Factor (SCF) 61
Steroids *see* Corticosteroids
Stress-activated Protein Kinase (SAPK/JNK) 79
Substance P 58
Sucralfate 63, 107
Sulfasalazine 62
Sulindac 248
Superoxid Dismutase (SOD) 24, 33, 45, 59, 81
Suramin 184
Surfactant Factor 30, 108
Surfactant Protein D 39

T

Tamoxifen 24
Tarceva (OSI774) 197
Taxanes 161
Teleangiectasia 16, 73
Therapeutic Index 159
Thoracic Radiation Therapy 37-46

Thrombin 55
Thrombocytopenia 108
Thrombomodulin 16, 55
Thrombopoietin 108-109
Thrombosis 73
Thromboxanes 242-243
Thyroid Cancer 150
Tirapazamine 161
Tissue Plasminogen Activator 57
Tissue Remodelling 15
TRAIL 163, 228, 234-238
Transforming Growth Factor (TGF) 20, 31, 39, 54, 140, 147, 150
Transforming Growth Factor Receptor (TGFR) 22
Tirilazad 60
Tumor Cell Vaccines 218
Tumor Necrosis Factor (TNF) 18, 21, 32, 43, 54-55, 74, 227
– and radiation 232-234
Tumor Necrosis Factor Receptor (TNFR) 18, 163, 228-232
– TNFaR-associated death domain (TRADD) 18, 228
Tyrosine Kinases (s. Receptor Tyrosine Kinases) 166

U
Urokinase Plasminogen Activator 57

V
Vaccines (s. Tumor Cell Vaccines) 218
Vascular Endothelial Growth Factor (VEGF) 32, 61, 77, 130, 140, 148, 150, 179-185, 248, 267
– receptor inhibition 168, 180
Vascular System 15, 50, 77
Vitamin E 60
Von Willebrand Factor 16, 55
Vulvar Cancer 128

List of Contributors

NICOLAUS ANDRATSCHKE, MD
Department of Radiation Oncology
Klinikum rechts der Isar
Technical University Munich
Ismaninger Strasse 22
81675 München
Germany

K. KIAN ANG, MD, PhD
Department of Radiation Oncology
The University of Texas M. D.
Anderson Cancer Center
1515 Holcombe Blvd.
P.O. Box 66
Houston, TX 77030-4009
USA

MICHAEL BAUMANN, MD, PhD
Department of Radiation Oncology
University Hospital Carl Gustav Carus
Experimental Center
Medical Faculty Carl Gustav Carus
Technical University Dresden
Fetscherstrasse 74, PF 58
01307 Dresden
Germany

ERIC J. BERNHARD, PhD
Department of Radiation Oncology
Division of Oncology Research
University of Pennsylvania School of Medicine
Room 185 John Morgan Building
3620 Hamilton Walk
Philadelphia, PA 19104-6072
USA

STEPHAN BODIS, MD
Laboratory for Molecular Radiobiology
Department of Radiation Oncology
University Hospital Zurich
Raemistrasse 100
8091 Zurich
Switzerland

JAMES M. BONNER, MD
Merle M. Saltr Professor and Chairman
Department of Radiation Oncology
University of Alabama at Birmingham
1530 3rd Ave. S
Birmingham, AL 35294-1150
USA

JAMES W. DENHAM, MD
Department of Radiation Oncology
Newcastle Mater Misericordiae Hospital
Newcastle University
NSW 2310, Newcastle
Australia

JENNIFER F. DE LOS SANTOS, MD
Department of Radiation Oncology
University of Alabama at Birmingham
1530 3rd Ave. S
Birmingham, AL 35294-1150
USA

WOLFGANG DÖRR, DVM, PhD
Professor, Medical Faculty Carl Gustav Carus
Technical University Dresden
Fetscherstrasse 74, PF 58
01307 Dresden
Germany

JUERGEN DUNST, MD
Professor, Department of Radiotherapy
Martin-Luther-University Halle-Wittenberg
Dryanderstrasse 4
06097 Halle
Germany

Z. FAN, MD
Department of Experimental Therapeutics
The University of Texas M. D.
Anderson Cancer Center
1515 Holcombe Blvd., P.O. Box 66
Houston, TX 77030-4009
USA

ANTHONY W. FYLES, MD
Gynecologic Cancer Program Head
Department of Radiation Oncology
Princess Margaret Hospital
610 University Avenue
Toronto, Ontario M5G 2M9
Canada

SHANNON GODDARD, MD
Research Assistant, Department of Radiation Oncology
Princess Margaret Hospital
610 University Avenue
Toronto, Ontario M5G 2M9
Canada

ANJALI K. GUPTA, PhD
Department of Radiation Oncology
Division of Oncology Research
University of Pennsylvania School of Medicine
3620 Hamilton Walk
Philadelphia, PA 19104-6072
USA

STEPHEN M. HAHN, PhD
Department of Radiation Oncology
University of Pennsylvania School of Medicine
John Morgan Building
3620 Hamilton Walk
Philadelphia, PA 19104-6072
USA

MARTIN HAUER-JENSEN, MD, PhD, FACS
Arkansas Cancer Research Center
4301 West Markham, Slot 725
Little Rock, AR 72205
USA

THOMAS HERRMANN, MD
Medical Faculty Carl Gustav Carus
Technical University Dresden
Fetscherstrasse 74, PF 58
01307 Dresden
Germany

CARSTEN HERSKIND, PhD
Department of Experimental Clinical Oncology
Aarhus University Hospital
Norrebrogade 44, Building 5
8000 Aarhus C
Denmark

AMIR HUSAIN, MD
Department of Experimental Radiation Oncology
The University of Texas M. D.
Anderson Cancer Center
1515 Holcombe Blvd.
P.O. Box 66
Houston, TX 77030
USA

BRANISLAV JEREMIC, MD
Department of Radiation Oncology
Klinikum rechts der Isar
Technical University Munich
Ismaninger Strasse 22
81675 München
Germany

CHUAN-YUAN LI, PhD
Department of Radiation Oncology
Medical Center
Duke University
201B MSRB, Box 3455
Durham, NC 27710
USA

ZHONGXING LIAO, MD
Department of Radiation Oncology
The University of Texas M. D.
Anderson Cancer Center
1515 Holcombe Blvd.
P.O. Box 66
Houston, TX 77030
USA

THOMAS LICHT, MD
Department of Hematology and Medical Oncology
Klinikum rechts der Isar
Technical University Munich
Ismaninger Strasse 22
81675 München
Germany

FRANK LOHR, MD
Sektion Strahlentherapie
Institut für Klinische Radiologie
Universitätsklinikum Mannheim
Theodor-Kutzer Ufer 1-3
68167 Mannheim
Germany

JENS LOHR, MD
Department of Pathology
San Francisco School of Medicine
University of California
Parnassus Avenue
San Francisco, CA 94143
USA

KATHY A. MASON
Department of Experimental Radiation Oncology
The University of Texas M. D.
Anderson Cancer Center
1515 Holcombe Blvd.
P.O. Box 66
Houston, TX 77030-4009
USA

W. GILLIES MCKENNA, PhD
Department of Pathology and Laboratory Medicine
University of Pennsylvania School of Medicine
3620 Hamilton Walk
Philadelphia, PA 19104-6072
USA

RAYMOND E. MEYN, PhD
Kathryn O'Connor Research Professor
Anderson Cancer Center
The University of Texas M. D.
Box 66
1515 Holcombe Blvd.
Houston, TX 77030
USA

LUKA MILAS, MD, PhD
Department of Experimental Radiation Oncology
The University of Texas M. D.
Anderson Cancer Center
1515 Holcombe Blvd.
P.O. Box 66
Houston, TX 77030-4009
USA

List of Contributors

MIRA MILAS, MD
Department of General Surgery
The Cleveland Clinic Fondation
Cleveland, OH 44195
USA

ANUPAMA MUNSHI, MD
Instructor, The University of Texas M. D.
Anderson Cancer Center
Box 66
1515 Holcombe Blvd.
Houston, TX 77030
USA

Ruth J. Muschel, MD, PhD
Department of Pathology and
Laboratory Medicine
University of Pennsylvania
School of Medicine
Philadelphia, PA 19104-6072
USA

CARSTEN NIEDER, MD
Department of Radiation Oncology
Klinikum rechts der Isar
Technical University Munich
Ismaninger Strasse 22
81675 München
Germany

MARTIN PRUSCHY, PhD
Laboratory for Molecular Radiobiology
Department of Radiation Oncology
University Hospital Zurich
Raemistrasse 100
8091 Zurich
Switzerland

UMA RAJU, PhD
Department of Experimental Radiation Oncology
The University of Texas M. D.
Anderson Cancer Center
1515 Holcombe Blvd.
P.O. Box 66
Houston, TX 77030
USA

OLIVER RIESTERER, MD
Laboratory for Molecular Radiobiology
Department of Radiation Oncology
University Hospital Zurich
Raemistrasse 100
8091 Zurich
Switzerland

HANS-PETER RODEMANN, PhD
Professor, Department of Radiation Oncology
Section of Radiobiology and Molecular
Environmental Research
Eberhard-Karls University Tubingen
Röntgenweg 11
72076 Tübingen
Germany

JÜRGEN SCHLEGEL, MD
Department of Pathology
Klinikum rechts der Isar
Technical University Munich
Ismaninger Strasse 22
81675 München
Germany

GEORG STÜBEN, MD
Klinik für Strahlentherapie und
Radiologische Onkologie der
Universität Essen
Hufelandstrasse 55
45122 Essen
Germany

MARTIN STUSCHKE, MD
Professor, Klinik für Strahlentherapie und
Radiologische Onkologie der
Universität Essen
Hufelandstrasse 55
45122 Essen
Germany

KLAUS-RÜDIGER TROTT, MD
Professor, St. Bartholomew's Medical College QMW
Charterhouse Square
London, EC1M 6BQ
UK

JUNRU WANG, MD, PhD
Department of Surgery
University of Arkansas for Medical Sciences
Little Rock, AR 72205
USA

FREDERIK WENZ, MD
Sektion Strahlentherapie
Institut für Klinische Radiologie
Universitätsklinikum Mannheim
Theodor-Kutzer Ufer 1-3
68167 Mannheim
Germany

FRANK B. ZIMMERMANN, MD
Department of Radiation Oncology
Klinikum rechts der Isar
Technical University Munich
Ismaninger Strasse 22
81675 München
Germany

DANIEL ZIPS, MD
Department of Radiation Oncology
University Hospital Carl Gustav Dresden
Fetscherstrasse 74
01307 Dresden
Germany

MEDICAL RADIOLOGY Diagnostic Imaging and Radiation Oncology
Titles in the series already published

RADIATION ONCOLOGY

Lung Cancer
Edited by C.W. Scarantino

Innovations in Radiation Oncology
Edited by H. R. Withers and L. J. Peters

Radiation Therapy of Head and Neck Cancer
Edited by G. E. Laramore

Gastrointestinal Cancer – Radiation Therapy
Edited by R.R. Dobelbower, Jr.

Radiation Exposure and Occupational Risks
Edited by E. Scherer, C. Streffer, and K.-R. Trott

Radiation Therapy of Benign Diseases
A Clinical Guide
S.E. Order and S. S. Donaldson

Interventional Radiation Therapy Techniques – Brachytherapy
Edited by R. Sauer

Radiopathology of Organs and Tissues
Edited by E. Scherer, C. Streffer, and K.-R. Trott

Concomitant Continuous Infusion Chemotherapy and Radiation
Edited by M. Rotman and C. J. Rosenthal

Intraoperative Radiotherapy – Clinical Experiences and Results
Edited by F. A. Calvo, M. Santos, and L.W. Brady

Radiotherapy of Intraocular and Orbital Tumors
Edited by W. E. Alberti and R. H. Sagerman

Interstitial and Intracavitary Thermoradiotherapy
Edited by M. H. Seegenschmiedt and R. Sauer

Non-Disseminated Breast Cancer
Controversial Issues in Management
Edited by G. H. Fletcher and S.H. Levitt

Current Topics in Clinical Radiobiology of Tumors
Edited by H.-P. Beck-Bornholdt

Practical Approaches to Cancer Invasion and Metastases
A Compendium of Radiation Oncologists' Responses to 40 Histories
Edited by A. R. Kagan with the Assistance of R. J. Steckel

Radiation Therapy in Pediatric Oncology
Edited by J. R. Cassady

Radiation Therapy Physics
Edited by A. R. Smith

Late Sequelae in Oncology
Edited by J. Dunst and R. Sauer

Mediastinal Tumors. Update 1995
Edited by D. E. Wood and C. R. Thomas, Jr.

Thermoradiotherapy and Thermochemotherapy
Volume 1:
Biology, Physiology, and Physics
Volume 2:
Clinical Applications
Edited by M.H. Seegenschmiedt, P. Fessenden, and C.C. Vernon

Carcinoma of the Prostate
Innovations in Management
Edited by Z. Petrovich, L. Baert, and L.W. Brady

Radiation Oncology of Gynecological Cancers
Edited by H.W. Vahrson

Carcinoma of the Bladder
Innovations in Management
Edited by Z. Petrovich, L. Baert, and L.W. Brady

Blood Perfusion and Microenvironment of Human Tumors
Implications for Clinical Radiooncology
Edited by M. Molls and P. Vaupel

Radiation Therapy of Benign Diseases
A Clinical Guide
2nd Revised Edition
S. E. Order and S. S. Donaldson

Carcinoma of the Kidney and Testis, and Rare Urologic Malignancies
Innovations in Management
Edited by Z. Petrovich, L. Baert, and L.W. Brady

Progress and Perspectives in the Treatment of Lung Cancer
Edited by P. Van Houtte, J. Klastersky, and P. Rocmans

Combined Modality Therapy of Central Nervous System Tumors
Edited by Z. Petrovich, L. W. Brady, M. L. Apuzzo, and M. Bamberg

Age-Related Macular Degeneration
Current Treatment Concepts
Edited by W. A. Alberti, G. Richard, and R. H. Sagerman

Radiotherapy of Intraocular and Orbital Tumors
2nd Revised Edition
Edited by R. H. Sagerman, and W. E. Alberti

Clinical Target Volumes in Conformal and Intensity Modulated Radiation Therapy
A Clinical Guide to Cancer Treatment
Edited by V. Grégoire, P. Scalliet, and K. K. Ang

Biological Modification of Radiation Response
Edited by C. Nieder, L. Milas, and K. K. Ang

Palliative Radiation Oncology
R. G. Parker, N. A. Janjan, and M. T. Selch

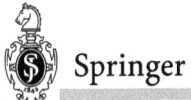 Springer

MEDICAL RADIOLOGY Diagnostic Imaging and Radiation Oncology
Titles in the series already published

Diagnostic Imaging

Innovations in Diagnostic Imaging
Edited by J. H. Anderson

Radiology of the Upper Urinary Tract
Edited by E. K. Lang

The Thymus - Diagnostic Imaging, Functions, and Pathologic Anatomy
Edited by E. Walter, E. Willich, and W. R. Webb

Interventional Neuroradiology
Edited by A. Valavanis

Radiology of the Pancreas
Edited by A. L. Baert, co-edited by G. Delorme

Radiology of the Lower Urinary Tract
Edited by E. K. Lang

Magnetic Resonance Angiography
Edited by I. P. Arlart, G. M. Bongartz, and G. Marchal

Contrast-Enhanced MRI of the Breast
S. Heywang-Köbrunner and R. Beck

Spiral CT of the Chest
Edited by M. Rémy-Jardin and J. Rémy

Radiological Diagnosis of Breast Diseases
Edited by M. Friedrich and E.A. Sickles

Radiology of the Trauma
Edited by M. Heller and A. Fink

Biliary Tract Radiology
Edited by P. Rossi

Radiological Imaging of Sports Injuries
Edited by C. Masciocchi

Modern Imaging of the Alimentary Tube
Edited by A. R. Margulis

Diagnosis and Therapy of Spinal Tumors
Edited by P. R. Algra, J. Valk, and J. J. Heimans

Interventional Magnetic Resonance Imaging
Edited by J. F. Debatin and G. Adam

Abdominal and Pelvic MRI
Edited by A. Heuck and M. Reiser

Orthopedic Imaging
Techniques and Applications
Edited by A. M. Davies and H. Pettersson

Radiology of the Female Pelvic Organs
Edited by E. K.Lang

Magnetic Resonance of the Heart and Great Vessels
Clinical Applications
Edited by J. Bogaert, A. J. Duerinckx, and F. E. Rademakers

Modern Head and Neck Imaging
Edited by S. K. Mukherji and J. A. Castelijns

Radiological Imaging of Endocrine Diseases
Edited by J. N. Bruneton
in collaboration with B. Padovani and M.-Y. Mourou

Trends in Contrast Media
Edited by H. S. Thomsen, R. N. Muller, and R. F. Mattrey

Functional MRI
Edited by C. T. W. Moonen and P. A. Bandettini

Radiology of the Pancreas
2nd Revised Edition
Edited by A. L. Baert
Co-edited by G. Delorme and L. Van Hoe

Emergency Pediatric Radiology
Edited by H. Carty

Spiral CT of the Abdomen
Edited by F. Terrier, M. Grossholz, and C. D. Becker

Liver Malignancies
Diagnostic and Interventional Radiology
Edited by C. Bartolozzi and R. Lencioni

Medical Imaging of the Spleen
Edited by A. M. De Schepper and F. Vanhoenacker

Radiology of Peripheral Vascular Diseases
Edited by E. Zeitler

Diagnostic Nuclear Medicine
Edited by C. Schiepers

Radiology of Blunt Trauma of the Chest
P. Schnyder and M. Wintermark

Portal Hypertension
Diagnostic Imaging-Guided Therapy
Edited by P. Rossi
Co-edited by P. Ricci and L. Broglia

Recent Advances in Diagnostic Neuroradiology
Edited by Ph. Demaerel

Virtual Endoscopy and Related 3D Techniques
Edited by P. Rogalla,
J. Terwissscha Van Scheltinga, and B. Hamm

Multislice CT
Edited by M. F. Reiser, M. Takahashi, M. Modic, and R. Bruening

Pediatric Uroradiology
Edited by R. Fotter

Transfontanellar Doppler Imaging in Neonates
A. Couture and C. Veyrac

Radiology of AIDS
A Practical Approach
Edited by J.W.A.J. Reeders and P.C. Goodman

CT of the Peritoneum
Armando Rossi and Giorgio Rossi

Magnetic Resonance Angiography
2nd Revised Edition
Edited by I. P. Arlart, G. M. Bongratz, and G. Marchal

Pediatric Chest Imaging
Edited by Javier Lucaya and Janet L. Strife

Applications of Sonography in Head and Neck Pathology
Edited by J. N. Bruneton in collaboration with C. Raffaelli and O. Dassonville

Imaging of the Larynx
Edited by R. Hermans

3D Image Processing
Techniques and Clinical Applications
Edited by D. Caramella and C. Bartolozzi

Imaging of Orbital and Visual Pathway Pathology
Edited by W. S. Müller-Forell

Pediatric ENT Radiology
Edited by S. J. King and A. E. Boothroyd

Radiological Imaging of the Small Intestine
Edited by N. C. Gourtsoyiannis

Imaging of the Knee
Techniques and Applications
Edited by A. M. Davies and V. N. Cassar-Pullicino

Perinatal Imaging
From Ultrasound to MR Imaging
Edited by Fred E. Avni

Radiological Imaging of the Neonatal Chest
Edited by V. Donoghue

Diagnostic and Interventional Radiology in Liver Transplantation
Edited by E. Bücheler, V. Nicolas, C. E. Broelsch, X. Rogiers, and G. Krupski

Radiology of Osteoporosis
Edited by S. Grampp

Imaging and Intervention in Abdominal Trauma
Edited by R. F. Dondelinger

Imaging of the Foot and Ankle
Techniques and Applications
Edited by A. M. Davies, R. W. Whitehouse, and J. P. R. Jenkins

Interventional Radiology in Cancer
Edited by A. Adam, R. F. Dondelinger, and P. R. Mueller

Imaging of the Pancreas
Cystic and Rare Tumors
Edited by C. Procacci and A. J. Megibow

Intracranial Vascular Malformations and Aneurysms
From Diagnostic Work-Up to Endovascular Therapy
Edited by M. Forsting

Imaging Pelvic Floor Disorders
Edited by C. I. Bartram and J. O. L. DeLancey
Associate Editors: S. Halligan, F. M. Kelvin, and J. Stoker

High Resolution Sonography of the Peripheral Nervous System
Edited by S. Peer and G. Bodner

Radiology Imaging of the Ureter
Edited by F. Joffre, Ph. Otal, and M. Soulie

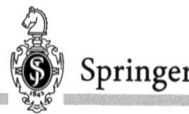

Printing and Binding: Stürtz AG, Würzburg

If you have any concerns about our products,
you can contact us on
ProductSafety@springernature.com

In case Publisher is established outside the EU,
the EU authorized representative is:
**Springer Nature Customer Service Center GmbH
Europaplatz 3, 69115 Heidelberg, Germany**

Printed by Libri Plureos GmbH
in Hamburg, Germany